Reducing Suicide

A NATIONAL IMPERATIVE

SK Goldsmith, TC Pellmar, AM Kleinman, WE Bunney, editors

Committee on Pathophysiology and Prevention of
Adolescent and Adult Suicide
Board on Neuroscience and Behavioral Health
INSTITUTE OF MEDICINE
OF THE NATIONAL ACADEMIES

THE NATIONAL ACADEMIES PRESS
Washington, D.C.
www.nap.edu

THE NATIONAL ACADEMIES PRESS • 500 Fifth Street, N.W. • Washington, DC 20001

NOTICE: The project that is the subject of this report was approved by the Governing Board of the National Research Council, whose members are drawn from the councils of the National Academy of Sciences, the National Academy of Engineering, and the Institute of Medicine. The members of the committee responsible for the report were chosen for their special competences and with regard for appropriate balance.

Support for this project was provided by the Centers for Disease Control and Prevention, the National Institute of Mental Health, the National Institute on Drug Abuse, the National Institute on Alcohol Abuse and Alcoholism, the Substance Abuse and Mental Health Services Administration, and the Veterans Administration. The views presented in this report are those of the Institute of Medicine Committee on Pathophysiology and Prevention of Adolescent and Adult Suicide and are not necessarily those of the funding agencies.

Library of Congress Cataloging-in-Publication Data

Reducing suicide : a national imperative / S.K. Goldsmith ... [et al.], editors ; Committee on Pathophysiology & Prevention of Adolescent & Adult Suicide, Board on Neuroscience and Behavioral Health, Institute of Medicine.
    p. ; cm.
Includes bibliographical references and index.
  ISBN 0-309-08321-4 (pbk.)
  1. Suicide—United States. 2. Suicide—United States—Prevention. 3. Suicidal behavior—Treatment—United States. 4. Suicidal behavior—Risk factors—United States.
  [DNLM: 1. Suicide—prevention & control—United States. 2. Psychotherapy—United States. 3. Risk Factors—United States. 4. Social Support—United States. 5. Suicide—psychology—United States.
] I. Goldsmith, Sara K. II. Institute of Medicine (U.S.). Committee on Pathophysiology & Prevention of Adolescent & Adult Suicide.
  HV6548.U5 R43 2002
  362.28'7'0973—dc21

                              2002012032

Additional copies of this report are available for sale from the National Academies Press, 500 Fifth Street, N.W., Box 285, Washington, DC 20055. Call (800) 624-6242 or (202) 334-3313 (in the Washington metropolitan area); Internet, http://www.nap.edu.

For more information about the Institute of Medicine, visit the IOM home page at **www.iom.edu.**

Printed in the United States of America.

The serpent has been a symbol of long life, healing, and knowledge among almost all cultures and religions since the beginning of recorded history. The serpent adopted as a logotype by the Institute of Medicine is a relief carving from ancient Greece, now held by the Staatliche Museen in Berlin.

*"Knowing is not enough; we must apply.
Willing is not enough; we must do."*
—Goethe

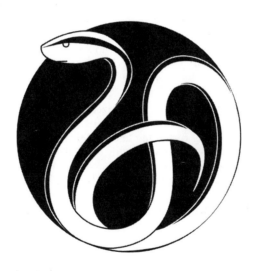

INSTITUTE OF MEDICINE

Shaping the Future for Health

THE NATIONAL ACADEMIES
Advisers to the Nation on Science, Engineering, and Medicine

The **National Academy of Sciences** is a private, nonprofit, self-perpetuating society of distinguished scholars engaged in scientific and engineering research, dedicated to the furtherance of science and technology and to their use for the general welfare. Upon the authority of the charter granted to it by the Congress in 1863, the Academy has a mandate that requires it to advise the federal government on scientific and technical matters. Dr. Bruce M. Alberts is president of the National Academy of Sciences.

The **National Academy of Engineering** was established in 1964, under the charter of the National Academy of Sciences, as a parallel organization of outstanding engineers. It is autonomous in its administration and in the selection of its members, sharing with the National Academy of Sciences the responsibility for advising the federal government. The National Academy of Engineering also sponsors engineering programs aimed at meeting national needs, encourages education and research, and recognizes the superior achievements of engineers. Dr. Wm. A. Wulf is president of the National Academy of Engineering.

The **Institute of Medicine** was established in 1970 by the National Academy of Sciences to secure the services of eminent members of appropriate professions in the examination of policy matters pertaining to the health of the public. The Institute acts under the responsibility given to the National Academy of Sciences by its congressional charter to be an adviser to the federal government and, upon its own initiative, to identify issues of medical care, research, and education. Dr. Harvey V. Fineberg is president of the Institute of Medicine.

The **National Research Council** was organized by the National Academy of Sciences in 1916 to associate the broad community of science and technology with the Academy's purposes of furthering knowledge and advising the federal government. Functioning in accordance with general policies determined by the Academy, the Council has become the principal operating agency of both the National Academy of Sciences and the National Academy of Engineering in providing services to the government, the public, and the scientific and engineering communities. The Council is administered jointly by both Academies and the Institute of Medicine. Dr. Bruce M. Alberts and Dr. Wm. A. Wulf are chair and vice chair, respectively, of the National Research Council.

www.national-academies.org

Reviewers

This report has been reviewed in draft form by individuals chosen for their diverse perspectives and technical expertise, in accordance with procedures approved by the NRC's Report Review Committee. The purpose of this independent review is to provide candid and critical comments that will assist the institution in making its published report as sound as possible and to ensure that the report meets institutional standards for objectivity, evidence, and responsiveness to the study charge. The review comments and draft manuscript remain confidential to protect the integrity of the deliberative process. We wish to thank the following individuals for their review of this report:

Daniel Blazer, Duke University Medical Center
Gregory Fricchione, The Carter Center
Douglas G. Jacobs, Harvard Medical School
David Lester, Richard Stockton College
Marsha M. Linehan, University of Washington
Anthony J. Marsella, University of Hawaii
David O. Meltzer, The University of Chicago, Pritzker School of Medicine
Charles O'Brien, University of Pennsylvania
Lee N. Robins, Washington University School of Medicine
David Satcher, Morehouse School of Medicine
Richard D. Todd, Washington University School of Medicine

Although the reviewers listed above have provided many constructive comments and suggestions, they were not asked to endorse the conclusions or recommendations nor did they see the final draft of the report before its release. The review of this report was overseen by **Joseph Coyle**, Harvard Medical School and **Henry W. Riecken**, University of Pennsylvania. Appointed by the National Research Council and Institute of Medicine, they were responsible for making certain that an independent examination of this report was carried out in accordance with institutional procedures and that all review comments were carefully considered. Responsibility for the final content of this report rests entirely with the authoring committee and the institution.

Preface

When Kevin Carter, a celebrated South African photo-journalist who was in his 30's and only months before had won the highly prestigious Pulitzer Prize, killed himself several years ago, it was at first assumed that his suicide was linked to the consequences in trauma, moral desolation, and guilt that he experienced in filming some of Africa's great human tragedies: wars and famines. Indeed his suicide note indicates as much. Soon afterward it was learned that he had been abusing drugs and suffered from bipolar disorder. Later still, it surfaced that he had experienced a wrenching divorce and was deeply upset about the separation from his young daughter. As this case shows, suicide can be a complex process. If ever a condition begged for an integrated understanding that takes into account biological, clinical, subjective, and social factors, this is it.

It is for this reason that global data on suicide loom large and usefully balance findings from the United States that are the primary focus of this report. For example, although American psychiatrists have found that 90 percent of suicides in our country appear to be associated with a mental illness, data from China suggest that probably less than half of suicides there have such a correlation. In China, unlike most countries, more women than men kill themselves. Eastern European societies experience suicide rates 4 to 6 times higher than in the United States. Whereas in Hungary there has long been a very high rate of suicide, in other countries formerly part of the Soviet Union, the elevated rates correlate with a period of deep and disruptive social change. Suicide may have a basis in depression or substance abuse, but it simultaneously may relate to social factors like community breakdown, loss of key social relations, economic depression, or political violence. Indeed, it may be that emotional states like hopelessness and impulsiveness link these different levels of human experience. It is important not to lose this sense of complexity if we are to fashion intervention programs that can prevent suicide.

This report reflects different perspectives and levels of analysis. It embodies tensions between medical and social analyses of suicide that date back at least 100 years. Given the uncertain status of the science, it is not always possible or even useful to try to resolve these distinctive points of view. But we have tried to place all the relevant materials before the reader; even where the tensions can not be resolved by efforts at integration of analytic approaches, we have tried to present the uncertainties and contradictions. That way we feel we have done justice to the science *and* to the resonantly human characteristics of this crucial subject. Indeed, it is inconceivable that policy and programs will be up to the challenge unless they engage the different sides of suicide.

Suicide is a medical issue; but it is also an economic, social relational, moral, and as September 11's tragic global spectacle of suicide terrorist attack made clear, a political issue as well. Suicide prevention, in turn, holds medical, social, psychological, economic, moral and political significance. Our Committee of medical and social scientists grappled as best it could with this complex reality and has written a report that suggests that this is precisely what policy makers need to do to advance the science and improve health and social responses.

I wish to acknowledge the crucial role played by the Committee's staff in assembling this report from the Committee's diverse perspectives.

Arthur Kleinman, M.D.

***

Suicide represents a major national and international public health problem with about 30,000 deaths in the United States and 1,000,000 deaths in the world each year and every year. The estimated cost to this nation in lost income alone is 11.8 billion dollars per year. There has been in the past and is currently a dramatic mismatch in terms of the federal dollars devoted to the understanding and prevention of suicide contrasted with other diseases of less public health impact. Research tools and opportunities currently exist to attack the problem of suicide. Recent successful programs for the prevention of suicide demand further testing. This report recommends a comprehensive approach to suicide and the development of a network of research laboratories for the study of suicide. There is every reason to expect that a national consensus to declare war on suicide and to fund research and prevention at a level commensurate with the severity of the problem will be successful and will lead to highly significant discoveries as have the wars on cancer, Alzheimer's disease, and AIDS.

Suicide is the eleventh leading cause of death for all ages in the United States and the third leading cause of death among adolescents. A great deal of local and national funding and effort has been devoted to the problem of homicide in contrast to suicide. However, suicides in this country outnumber homicides by a third. During the period of the Vietnam War, four times the number of Americans died by suicide than died in combat. Two hundred thousand more people died of suicide than died of AIDS in the past 20 years. These mortality figures do not capture the intense suffering of the suicidal patient. One patient stated the night before she committed suicide: "The pain is all consuming, overwhelming. The pain has become excruciating, constant and endless."

A great deal has been learned about the risk factors contributing to suicide, biological changes that are associated with suicide, links between childhood trauma and suicide, and the impact of social and cultural influences, medical and psychosocial interventions. But a fundamental understanding of the suicide process remains unknown, and national prevention efforts have not been successful. The establishment of 60 centers throughout the United States to fight a war on cancer, and 28 Alzheimer disease centers, to fight a war on Alzheimer's disease, provide highly successful models for the committee recommendation to develop a network of eight population-based research laboratories for war on suicide and investigation of the suicidal process.

In 2000, the National Institute of Mental Health, the National Institute of Drug Abuse, the Veterans Administration, the National Institute on Alcohol Abuse and Alcoholism, Substance Abuse and Mental Health Services Administration and the Centers for Disease Control and Prevention asked the Institute of Medicine to assess the science base of suicide etiology, evaluate the current status of primary and secondary prevention including risk and protective factors, develop strategies for studying suicide and comment on gaps in knowledge, research opportunities and strategies for prevention. The Institute of Medicine formed a Committee on the Pathophysiology and Prevention of Adolescent and Adult Suicide.

In conducting this study, the 13-member committee met six times during 2001. The Committee was informed by two hosted workshops, *Suicide Prevention* and *Risk Factors for Suicide*, the deliberations of which have been subsequently published. The meeting agendas are in Appendix C of this report. At these workshops the committee was informed by a number of presentations by experts in the field. These included: Aaron T. Beck, C. Hendricks Brown, Gregory Brown, William Byerley, Katherine

Comtois, David Goldston, Madelyn Gould, David Hemenway, John Kalafat, Ronald Maris, Eve Mościcki, Ghanshayam Pandey, Robert Post, Herbert C. Schulberg, Edwin Shneidman, and Martin Teicher. Additional experts in the field of suicide made presentations to the Committee: Paul Appelbaum, Alan Berman, Robert Gebbia, Scott Kim, Bernice Pescosolido, and Leonardo Tondo. Several representatives from government agencies provided their perspectives: Steven M. Berkowitz, Alexander Crosby, Robert DeMartino, David Litts, Jacques Normand, Jane Pearson, and Deidra Roach. Still others prepared background papers or provided analyses and data: Robert Anderson, Lois Fingerhut, David Jobes, Thomas Joiner, Jeremy Pettit, Ramani Pilla, Morton Silverman, and Shirley Zimmerman. The names and affiliations of these expert consultants are listed in Appendix B. Subsequently, individual committee members prepared draft chapters. Analysis and data collection, development, and writing of the final study report required an extensive staff effort. The Study Director, Sara K. Goldsmith, organized our discussions and prepared drafts of important components of the report. She was assisted by Sandra P. Au, Research Associate, Daria K. Boeninger, Research Assistant, Allison M. Panzer, Senior Project Assistant, and Miriam Davis, Consultant. The Director of the Board of Neuroscience and Behavioral Health, Terry C. Pellmar, prepared the initial project proposal and provided outstanding oversight of the entire effort and participated in writing and organizing the final draft. We thank each of the individuals and organizations for their assistance and advice over the course of this effort to analyze and attack the crisis of suicide in this nation.

William E. Bunney, M.D.

Contents

Executive Summary

Every year approximately 30,000 people die by suicide in the United States, and one million worldwide. Approximately 650,000 people yearly receive emergency treatment after attempting suicide in the United States. It is the third leading cause of death among American youths and the eleventh for Americans of all ages. Over the last 100 years suicides have out-numbered homicides by at least 3 to 2. Almost 4 times as many Americans died by suicide than in the Vietnam War during the same time period. The rates of suicide are exceptionally high among certain populations: white males over 75 years of age, Native Americans, and certain professions (e.g., health professions, police). The rates among youth are rising.

For decades, the federal government of the United States has been concerned about high suicide rates. Thirty years after the first national effort was established at the National Institute of Mental Health in 1969, the Surgeon General of the United States issued a "Call to Action to Prevent Suicide." Soon after, a National Strategy for Suicide Prevention (2001) presented a comprehensive assessment of future goals and objectives to combat suicide. Several federal agencies (the National Institute of Mental Health, the National Institute of Drug Abuse, the Veterans Administration, the Centers for Disease Control and Prevention, Substance Abuse and Mental Health Services Administration, and the National Institute on Alcohol Abuse and Alcoholism) joined together to ask the Institute of Medicine to convene the Committee on Pathophysiology and Prevention of Adolescent and Adult Suicide to examine the state of the science base, gaps in our knowledge, strategies for prevention, and research designs for the study of suicide.

RISK AND PROTECTIVE FACTORS

Biological, psychological, social, and cultural factors all have a significant impact on the risk of suicide. The report reviews many of these risk factors individually, but the Committee emphasizes the need for an integrated understanding of their influence.

Over 90 percent of suicides in the United States are associated with mental illness and/or alcohol and substance abuse. Yet it is important to remember that as many as 10 percent of people who complete suicide do not have any known psychiatric diagnosis. This percentage appears higher still in non-Western societies such as China. It is also important to remember that over 95% of those with mental disorders do not complete suicide. The relationship between suicide and mental illness is a conundrum. Suicidality, although clearly overlapping the symptomatology of the associated disorders, does not appear to respond to treatment in exactly the same way. Depressive symptoms can be reduced by medicines without reduction in suicidality. And psychotherapy can reduce suicide without significant changes in affective symptoms.

Over 30 years of research confirms the relationship between hopelessness and suicide across diagnoses. Hopelessness can persist even when other symptoms of an associated disorder, such as depression, have abated. Impulsivity, especially among youth, is increasingly linked to suicidal behavior. Resiliency and coping skills, on the other hand, can reduce the risk of suicide. Research suggests that coping skills can be taught.

Biological changes are associated with completed and attempted suicide. Abnormal functioning of the hypothalamic-pituitary-adrenal (HPA) axis, a major component of adaptation to stress, has been shown to be promising for the prediction of *future* suicides, but not consistently for suicide attempts. Serotonergic function is reduced and noradrenergic function is altered in the central nervous systems of both suicide attempters and completers. Several lines of evidence, including adoption, twin, and family studies, point to a link between genetic inheritance and risk of suicide. Having a first-degree relative who completed suicide increases an individual's risk of suicide 6-fold. The genetic liability may be linked to the heritability of mental illness and/or impulsive aggression. Since the heritability of liability to suicidal behavior appears to be on the order of 30–50%, interactions with social and cultural influences must also be significant.

Childhood trauma has emerged as a strong risk factor for suicidal behavior in adolescents *and* adults. The official rate of child victimization in 1999 was about 12 per 1000 and but the rates are even higher in surveys of children and parents. Independent of psychopathology and other known risk factors, child sexual abuse has been reported in 9–20 percent of suicide attempts in adults.

Social support is a protective factor. Those who enjoy close relationships cope better with various stresses, including bereavement, job loss, and illness, and enjoy better psychological and physical health. Divorced, separated and widowed persons are more likely to die by suicide. Being a parent, particularly for mothers, appears to decrease the risk of suicide. Discord within the family is correlated with increased suicide, while parental and family connectedness has a protective effect, especially among youth. Participation in religious activities is a protective factor for suicide, perhaps in part because of the social support it affords, but belief structures and spiritualism may also be important factors. Furthermore, epidemiological analyses reveal that occupation, employment status, and socioeconomic status affect the risk of suicide. These factors are not specific to the United States or even to the Western world, but global.

At both the individual and collective levels, the suicide rate has long been understood to correlate with cultural, social, political, and economic forces. Political coercion or violence can increase suicide. For example, in the former Soviet Union, areas experiencing sociopolitical oppression (the Baltic States) and forced social change (Russia) had higher suicide rates compared to other regions. Twenty years of civil war in Sri Lanka are associated with increased suicide rates, as well. Vast social changes associated with modernization and globalization are thought to break down traditional values and practices and result in increased suicide. Since the fall of the Soviet Union and its Eastern European satellite states much of East Europe has reported worsening health statistics, including adult mortality, alcohol and drug abuse, and some of the highest suicide rates in the world today. Here suicide is correlated with societal breakdown, severe economic dislocation, major cultural change and new political systems. Suicide carries a social and moral meaning in all societies. A society's perception of suicide, or its stigma, can influence its rate, preventing suicide in those societies and social groups where it is frowned upon but increasing suicide where it is a culturally acceptable option in certain situations.

Despite the extensive knowledge that research has provided regarding these risk and protective factors, we are still far from being able to integrate these factors so as to understand how they work in concert to evoke suicidal behavior or to prevent it. We do not understand why significant proportions (20–49 percent) of maltreated children do not display suicidal symptoms or why the majority of individuals affected with mental illness do not complete suicide. We also need to understand the large numbers of people who commit suicide in the absence of pathology, how suicide varies with social and cultural forces, and how it relates to individual, group, and contextual experiences.

Without a combination of a population-based approach and studies at the level of the individual patient within higher risk sub-groups, macrosocial trends cannot be related to biomedical measures. Most existing studies are retrospective or cross-sectional, involve few correlates, and do not address prediction of risk. Without specific data from well-defined and characterized populations whose community-level social descriptives are well known, normative behavior and abnormality cannot be estimated.

TREATMENT

Suicidality can be treated. There is evidence that lithium treatment of bipolar disorder significantly reduces suicide rates. In fact, lithium may have specific anti-suicidal effects for people with this disorder since these effects may be *separate* from its antidepressant and antimanic effects. Rates are reduced only while the patients take lithium; after discontinuation of lithium, the rates begin to rise to levels similar to those seen prior to lithium treatment. Despite the encouraging evidence, the protective effects of lithium are not consistent across studies. Other psychiatric medications, including anti-psychotic (especially clozapine) and antidepressants, also show promise for the reduction of suicide. A correlation has been observed between an increase in prescription rates for antidepressants, in particular the serotonin re-uptake inhibitors (SSRIs), and a decline in suicide rates in a number of countries. However, randomized clinical trials with antidepressants have failed to reveal significant differences versus placebo, perhaps due to methodological limitations.

Medications alone are not sufficient for treating mental disorders or suicidality, nor are treatments equally effective across individuals and diagnoses. Psychotherapy provides a necessary therapeutic relationship that reduces the risk of suicide. Cognitive-behavioral approaches that include problem-solving training seem to reduce suicidal ideation and attempts more effectively than treatment as usual or nondirective therapy.

Patients are at much greater risk of suicide in the weeks immediately following discharge from the hospital. Discharged patients who committed suicide were 3.7 times more likely to have had their outpatient care reduced at their last session. On the other hand, patients who continued care either through community services or with pharmacotherapy had lower suicide rates.

Psychological autopsy studies reveal that only 6–14 percent of depressed suicide victims were adequately treated and only 8–17 percent of all suicides were under treatment with prescription psychiatric medications. Yet significant opportunities to deliver adequate care exist since over 50–70 percent of those who complete suicide have contact with health services in the days to months before their death. However, suicide risk is difficult to assess. Individuals making serious suicide attempts may knowingly withhold their intentions. Currently, no psychological test, clinical technique, or biological marker is sufficiently sensitive and specific to accurately assess acute prediction of suicide in an individual.

There are significant barriers to receiving effective mental health treatment. About two-thirds of people with diagnosable mental disorders do not receive treatment. The stigma of mental illness deters people who need treatment from seeking it. The fragmented organization of mental health services and the cost of care are among the most frequently cited barriers to mental health treatment. Economic analyses of patterns of use of mental health services clearly indicate that use is sensitive to price: use falls as costs rise, while use increases with better insurance coverage. Physicians are reticent to talk to their patients about suicide; they often do not ask about intent or ideation, and patients often do not spontaneously report it. The goal of suicide treatment in specialty care is to develop and implement a treatment plan, which includes monitoring of medication efficacy and safety, as well as discharge planning. The details of treatment of suicidality, however, are not spelled out in any clinical guidelines. And many physicians are inadequately prepared to address suicide in their practices.

Primary care has become a critical setting for detection of the two most common risk factors for suicide: depression and alcoholism. According the American Medical Association, a diagnostic interview for depression is comparable in sensitivity and specificity to many radiologic and laboratory tests commonly used in medicine. Yet, currently only about 30–50 percent of adults with diagnosable depression are accurately diagnosed by primary care physicians. Treatment of depression in primary care is associated with reduced rates of completed suicide as shown by an ecological study on the Swedish Island of Gotland. Substance use disorders are especially important in suicide among young adults. Substance abuse and mood disorders frequently co-occur, with 51 percent of suicide attempters having both. In the primary care setting, numerous professional groups recommend routine screening for problem drinking in all patients.

PREVENTION

A number of prevention programs have been explored to reduce the incidence of suicide and suicidal behaviors. At multiple levels (universal, selective, and indicated) interventions attempt to address risk factors and to enhance protective factors. Programs that integrate prevention at multiple levels are likely to be the most effective. The Air Force's prevention program is one example of an integrated program that appears to have effectively reduced suicide rates in the community by removing barriers to treatment; increasing knowledge, attitudes, and competencies within the community; and increasing access to help and support with a consequent decrease in suicide rates. While there are several promising programs that have been implemented, long-term assessments and rigorous evaluation of their effectiveness are unavailable. Furthermore, some programs may work only in certain populations under certain circumstances; it is not yet evident whether these programs can be generalized to other populations or what characteristics of the programs are broadly applicable.

Reducing the availability or the lethality of a method (such as using blister packs for pills or enacting stricter gun control laws) results in a decline in suicide by that method; method substitution does not invariably occur. Education of the media regarding appropriate reporting of suicides can limit imitation effects and thereby reduce suicide rates.

Comprehensive school-based programs have shown some success in reducing suicidality. It is important to distinguish these programs from simple awareness interventions that can be detrimental. Screening programs, gatekeeper training programs, support/skills training groups, and school-based crisis response teams/plans can create a coordinated effort that identifies youth at risk for suicide and provides individual follow-up. If done appropriately, these interventions can provide the skills that allow youth to cope effectively with their life's stresses.

Lack of longitudinal and prospective studies are a critical barrier to understanding and preventing suicide. Many prevention programs do not have the long-term funding that would allow them to assess reduction in the completion of suicide as an endpoint. The low-base rate of suicide, combined with the short duration of assessment and the relatively small populations under study, makes it difficult to acquire sufficient power for such trials. Some intervention analyses have increased their power by using alternate endpoints such as suicide attempts or ideation. Prevention studies sometimes use proximal outcomes like attitude or knowledge. There are statistical approaches used in other disciplines that can facilitate analyses of these low-rate events and would be worthwhile to apply to suicide. Refinements of Poisson regression models can be applied to low-base rate events and expand our understanding of suicide by sorting out the effects of age, race, and sex on clustered suicides (i.e., within counties) and improving our capability for assessment in prevention programs.

ADDITIONAL CHALLENGES IN SUICIDE RESEARCH

Reporting Problems

Because suicide has a low base-rate, studies need large populations to yield significant results. This problem is exacerbated by the poor reporting of suicides. Official suicide statistics capture completed suicides only and are fraught with inaccuracies. The numbers are inaccurate because of classification as death from undetermined causes and because of under-reporting. It is estimated that most if not all of the undetermined cases are actually suicides. The quality of data on suicide attempts is even more tenuous than that of completed suicides.

Part of the reporting problem stems from the marked differences in the training and background of the person who by law certifies a death as a suicide. In the United States, the qualifications range from simply having an interest in the job (e.g., Indiana) to specialized training in forensic pathology (e.g., Oklahoma). Medico-legal officials may be elected, appointed or serve ex-officio (e.g., outside of the larger California counties, elected county sheriffs). Investigations may be centralized within a state (e.g., Rhode Island) or organized by each county (e.g., Utah). Internationally, differences in the organization and functioning of the officials monitoring suicide as a cause of death can produce artifactual differences even between similar countries such as England and Scotland. Most developing societies lack registries and expertly trained officials to record suicide. Further, there are cross-national differences in the underlying logic of classifications systems. In India, for example, the classification scheme focuses on social stresses and not psychopathology. Countries with religious sanctions against suicide tended to report suicide rates that were lower than for countries without sanctions. Furthermore, difference among countries may reflect the capacity of the emergency health care system to respond rather than differences in the intent of the individuals. The high rate of suicide among young Chinese women may result from their ready access to extremely toxic pesticides in the face of limited availability of emergency treatment. Each of these factors affects the nature, extent, and quality of the investigation and the classification of deaths as suicide.

Exclusion from Clinical Trials

Screening out clinical trial participants for suicidality has been the industry standard for trials of psychoactive medicines in an effort to reduce the risk of death. However, excluding those at risk for suicide precludes evaluation of treatments for this population. Suicide is, unfortunately, a medically expectable outcome of many mental illnesses. Death in a cancer clinical trial may be predictable or even inevitable, but trials do not exclude terminally ill patients. One might consider the outcome of suicide as a result of the mental illness, not the research or therapeutic intervention. The practice of excluding these patients from trials limits the opportunity for this population to benefit from such research. Excluding high-risk patients from these trials has been shown to weaken the sensitivity of intervention trials. Thus, suicide raises unique ethical issues. Furthermore, distinctive social and cultural contexts create different concerns for studying suicidal risk. These contexts must be taken into account, especially in global research.

Including participants at risk for suicide in clinical trials can be challenging. Before a person can consent to be part of a clinical trial, they must understand the purpose, the risks, and the possible benefits of the research. It has been argued that a suicidal person might understand the risks of a research protocol but not care about, or even welcome, the risks. Additional safeguards to ensure safety and ethical conduct of research can be provided, such as involving family members or other surrogates and ensuring that risks are not greater than under ordinary, usual, or standard care. In addition to the commonly used guidelines for protection of human subjects, a study design that affords greater protection to the participants can be used. For example, a risk-based allocation design, which assures that all of the sickest patients receive the experimental treatment, may be effective in research with suicidal patients.

NEXT STEPS

To effectively study suicide requires a large population base, better reporting of completed and attempted suicide, careful control and analysis of risk and protective factors, common databases, and banks of biological tissues for analysis. Because of its low base rate, the difficulties in assessment, and the long-term nature of the risk and protective factors, the optimal approach to suicide is to use large populations with cultural and genetic diversity for long-duration, interdisciplinary studies.

Research centers have often been the mechanism used to address similar obstacles. Large research centers have the additional advantage of being able to provide training opportunities and thereby attract new researchers to a difficult field. Furthermore, centers provide the opportunities for tissue banks and registries that are necessary resources to advance the field, and would enable ethnic, economic, and other social comparisons.

Suicide is responsible for about 30,000 deaths each year. Mental illness, the primary risk factor, afflicts over 80 million people in the United States; almost 15 million people have a serious mental illness (i.e., a mental disorder that leads to a functional impairment). For comparison, breast cancer claims the lives of about 40,000 women per year and between 10–15 million people are living with the diagnosis of breast cancer. In 1998 over $400 million was allocated to research into the prevention, treatment, and cure of breast cancer. From estimates of the portfolios of SAMHSA, CDC, and NIMH, the funding for suicide was less than $40 million in 2000. The committee finds that this is disproportionately low, given the magnitude of the problem of suicide. A substantial investment of funds is needed to make meaningful progress.

In recognition of the current funding and research shortage in the area of suicide, the committee provides the following recommendation for establishing population research centers that will integrate the talents of experts from many disciplines and will draw upon a large population base with continuity over a long duration to improve prevention and treatment interventions. In addition, the recommendations aim to improve the monitoring of suicide, to increase the recognition and consequently the treatment of the primary risk factors in primary care, and to expand the efforts in prevention.

Recommendation 1

The National Institute of Mental Health (in collaboration with other agencies) should develop and support a national network of suicide research Population Laboratories devoted to interdisciplinary research on suicide and suicide prevention across the life cycle. The network of Population Laboratories should be administered by NIMH and funded through partnerships among federal agencies and private sources, including foundations. Very large study samples of at least 100,000 are necessary because of the relatively low frequency of suicide in the general public. A number of Population Laboratories (e.g., 5–10) are necessary to capture the data for numerous and complex interacting variables including the profound effects of demographics, region, culture, socioeconomic status, race, and ethnicity. Extending the efforts into the international arena where cultural differences are large may provide new information and can be fostered and guided by such global organizations as the World Health Organization and the World Bank and by the Fogarty International Center at NIH.

◆ **The network should be equipped to perform safe, high-quality, large-sample, multi-site studies on suicide and suicide prevention.**

❖ Each Laboratory would have a population base of approximately 100,000. At a base-rate of 10–12 suicides per 100,000 people, this population base of the network would significantly improve the available data for estimates of suicide incidence, capacity for longitudinal studies, development of brain repositories, access to representative samples for prevention and intervention studies, and studies of genetic risk for suicide. Several such laboratories would provide adequate data to assess the numerous and complex interacting variables including the profound effects of demographics, regions, culture, socioeconomic status, race, and ethnicity. Coordination and collaboration among centers should be encouraged to further enhance the breadth of the database.

❖ The laboratories would cover an ethnically and socially diverse and representative population and would recruit higher risk individuals and subgroups in communities within the population laboratories for longitudinal and more detailed studies.

❖ Treatment and prevention studies would be carried out in

high-risk patients recruited from within the population laboratories.

❖ With these defined populations, the centers would conduct prospective studies—integrating biological, psychosocial, ethnographic, and ethical dimensions—that would be of great importance in advancing science and meeting public health needs. These studies would include such research initiatives as identified in the committee report including:

Evaluating means and effectiveness of promoting greater continuity of care, treatment adherence, and access to emergency services.

The effects of reducing hopelessness on suicide.

The potential of pharmacotherapies to reduce suicidal behavior.

The types and aspects of psychotherapy that are effective in reducing suicide.

The influence of HPA axis function on suicidality. Brain mapping studies on biological predictors of suicidal behavior.

The relationship between genetic markers and suicidal behavior and between suicide and aggression/impulsivity.

Prospective studies of populations at high risk for the onset of suicidal behavior.

Risk and protective effects of hospitalization, the relationships between length of stay and outcomes, and the factors post-hospital that account for the increased risk for suicide.

Outcomes of prophylactic/short-term versus maintenance/long-term treatment for suicidality.

Interactions of genetics and psychosocial, socio-political, and socioeconomic context.

Ethnographic research and other qualitative methods to obtain greater detail about the setting, conditions, process, and outcome of suicide.

◆ **Funding should be provided for the necessary infrastructure for these centers.** This should include support for dedicated full-time staff at NIH to provide long-term (at least 10 years) continuity and consistency in these efforts. Furthermore, funding for centers should include support for the following:

❖ Population cores to coordinate the social science, ethnographic data and to maintain registries of deaths by suicide and suicide attempts.

❖ Pathology cores to maintain the repositories for tissue samples from suicide victims.

❖ Statistical cores to manage the databases on risk and protective factors including genetic markers and cultural contexts.

❖ Clinical cores to recruit patients and to ensure their safe and ethical treatment.

❖ Research efforts that encompass both program projects and individual projects. Centers should encourage collaborations across the centers and facilitate the sharing of data maintained by the cores.

◆ In an effort to recruit excellent scientists to research in suicide, **supported sites should develop training programs** to provide local and distance mentoring, to attract new investigators from a wide variety of disciplines into the field, **and to form research and research training partnerships with developed and developing countries.**

Recommendation 2

National monitoring of suicide and suicidality should be improved. Steps toward improvement should include the following:

◆ **Funding agencies (including NIMH, NIA, NICHD, NIDA, NIAAA, CDC, SAMHSA, and DVA) should encourage that measures of suicidality (e.g., attempts) be included in all large and/or long-term studies of health behaviors, mental health interventions, and genetic studies of mental disorder.** Funding agencies should issue program announcements for supplements to ongoing longitudinal studies to include the collection and analysis of these additional measures.

◆ **Suicidal patients should be included in clinical trials when appropriate safeguards are in place.**

◆ **A national suicide attempt surveillance system should be de-**

veloped and coordinated through the CDC. It might be developed as part of a broader injury reporting database. Modeled after Oregon's program for the reporting of adolescent suicide attempts and the HIV/AIDS registry, pilot programs should be developed, tested, and implemented as soon as feasible. State participation should be encouraged by requiring reporting as a prerequisite for receiving funding for related programs.

◆ **Federal funding should be provided to support a surveillance system such as the National Violent Death Reporting System that includes data on mortality from suicide.** The system should have sufficient funding to support a national effort. CDC would be the most appropriate agency to coordinate this database given their experience with HIV/AIDS surveillance. Efforts to create such registries in other countries should be encouraged and, where feasible, assisted.

Recommendation 3

Because primary care providers are often the first and only medical contact of suicidal patients, tools for recognition and screening of patients should be developed and disseminated. Furthermore, since over half of suicides occur in populations receiving treatment for mental disorders, it is critical to enhance the capacity of mental health professionals to recognize and address both chronic and acute suicide risk factors.

◆ **NIMH and other funding agencies should provide funds to clinical researchers to develop and evaluate screening tools that assess risk factors for suicide** such as substance use, history of abuse and/or trauma, involvement with the criminal justice system, mental illness, psychological and personality traits such as impulsivity and hopelessness, abnormal neurobiology or genetic markers, employment problems, bereavement and other relationship stresses, etc. Funding agencies should issue program announcements to encourage efforts in this area.

◆ **Physicians should refer patients with multiple risk factors to consultation with a mental health professional.** This should be standard in the same way finding high blood cholesterol levels dictates further medical and behavioral interventions. This will only be effective if the issue of parity is addressed and insurance benefits are expanded adequately to cover mental health care.

◆ **Professional medical organizations should provide training to health care providers for assessment of suicide risk and provide them with existing tools.** Mental health professional associations should encourage (or require, when appropriate) their memberships to increase their skills in suicide risk detection and intervention. National, state, county, and city public health organizations should build on their existing infrastructure to facilitate suicide screening especially in high-risk populations.

◆ **Medical and nursing schools should incorporate the study of suicidal behavior into their curricula or expand existing education.**

◆ **NIMH and Agency for Health Care Research and Quality (AHRQ) should work with physician associations including American College of Physicians, American College of Family Physicians, American Academy of Pediatrics, American Society of Internal Medicine to implement these recommendations.** In addition, through their health services research funds they should support efforts to improve approaches to identifying and treating those at risk.

Recommendation 4

Programs for suicide prevention should be developed, tested, expanded, and implemented through funding from appropriate agencies including NIMH, DVA, CDC, and SAMHSA.

◆ **Partnerships should be formed among federal, state, and local agencies to implement effective suicide prevention programs.** Collaboration should be sought with professional organizations (including the American Psychiatric Association and the American Psychological Association) and non-profit organizations dedicated to the prevention of suicide (such as the American Foundation for the Prevention of Suicide or the American Association of Suicidology). NIMH and SAMHSA should work with the Department of

Education and the Administration on Aging to encourage national programs for youth and elderly populations.

◆ **Programs that have shown success within select populations should be expanded.** For example, the Air Force program should be adopted by hierarchical organizations that employ groups with increased suicide rates, including police and rescue workers. Gatekeeper training programs and screening programs for youth and elderly should be implemented more broadly within work and educational settings to identify and intervene with those at suicide-risk. There should be a systemic identification of high suicide risk groups for targeted intervention.

◆ **Pilot programs for coping and resiliency training as part of the curriculum for school-aged children should be implemented, evaluated, and scaled up when feasible.** Given the involvement of cumulative life-stressors in suicide and the existing efficacy data on these programs, it is expected that this intervention will reduce suicidality as well as other unwanted outcomes.

◆ **Restriction of access or reduced lethality of common means of suicide should be legislated** (e.g., gun safety, barriers on bridges, altering the content of cooking gas, packaging of commonly used pills, and poison control).

◆ **Long-term public education campaigns and media training should be evaluated** for their effectiveness both to change the public's knowledge and attitudes and to reduce suicide and suicidal behaviors.

My life felt so cluttered and obstructed that I could hardly breathe. I inhabited a closed, concentrated world, airless and without exits . . . I had entered the closed world of suicide, and my life was being lived for me by forces I couldn't control.

—ALFRED ALVAREZ
   The Savage God: A Study of Suicide

1

Introduction

Every year there are approximately 30,000 suicides in the United States (NCIPC, 2000), and one million worldwide (WHO, 1999). Approximately 650,000 people per year in the United States are seen in emergency rooms after attempting suicide (PHS, 2001). It is the third leading cause of death among American youths and among the top 12 for Americans of all ages. For the past hundred years, the number of reported suicides has been higher than the number of homicides, by approximately three to two. The rates of suicide among some populations are exceptionally high, for example, white males over 75 years of age and Native American Indians. Unfortunately, the rate of suicide has held relatively steady in the United States for the past 50 years (Bureau of the Census, 1976; Hoyert et al., 2001; Minino and Smith, 2001; NCHS, 2001; NCIPC, 2000).

To put this in perspective: between 1964 and 1973 (between the Gulf of Tonkin Resolution and the Paris Peace Accords) approximately 58,000 U.S. servicemen and women lost their lives in the Vietnam War (Center for Electronic Records, 1998). During this same period, approximately 220,000 citizens died by suicide (Bureau of the Census, 1976; NCHS, 2001). From 1979 to 1999, 448,060 people in the United States died from AIDS and HIV-related diseases; over this same 20 years, 626,226 people died by suicide (Figure 1-1). The suicide crisis continues unabated.

PERSONAL SUFFERING

Suicide is ultimately a private act. It is difficult to put into words the suffering and agonized state of mind of those who kill themselves. But

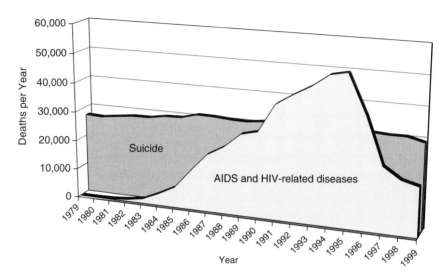

FIGURE 1-1 Deaths from Suicide and AIDS and HIV-related Diseases. Based on data from the CDC (2001), NCHS (2001), and NCIPC (2000).

personal accounts of those who have completed or attempted suicide provide a glimpse of the psychological pain that culminates in a desperate act. A minority of those who kill themselves actually write suicide notes, and these only infrequently try to communicate the complex reasons for the act. Still, some consistent psychological themes emerge. Clearest of these is the presence of an unendurable heartache, captured in the simple phrase, "I can't stand the pain any longer," a phrase often seen in suicide notes or heard by clinicians after an attempt. One woman expressed it this way in her suicide note:

> I wish I could explain it so someone could understand it. I'm afraid it's something I can't put into words.
>
> There's just this heavy, overwhelming despair—dreading everything. Dreading life. Empty inside, to the point of numbness. It's like there's something already dead inside. My whole being has been pulling back into that void for months.
>
> Everyone has been so good to me—has tried so hard. I truly wish that I could be different, for the sake of my family. Hurting my family is the worst of it, and that guilt has been wrestling with the part of me that wanted only to disappear.
>
> But there's some core-level spark of life that just isn't there. Despite what's been said about my having "gotten better" lately—the voice in

my head that's driving me crazy is louder than ever. It's way beyond being reached by anyone or anything it seems. I can't bear it any more. I think there's something psychologically—twisted—reversed that has taken over, that I can't fight any more. I wish that I could disappear without hurting anyone. I'm sorry. (Jamison, 1999: 81-82)

One young journalist, only 20 years old at the time of her suicide, described in her journals the pain, abject hopelessness, and numbing exhaustion brought about by her depression. "I am," she wrote, "growing more and more tired, more and more desperate . . . The fog keeps rolling in . . ." The night before she died she wrote, "the pain has become excruciating, constant and endless." The next morning she drowned herself (unpublished journals of Dawn Renee Befano, quoted in Jamison, 1999: 94-97).

Ten years after the family tragedy that nearly destroyed his life, Les Franklin is haunted by memories. "It's the gray eyes," he says, describing a vision that comes to him at night as he struggles to find sleep. They are the eyes of his late son Shaka, a 16-year-old high school football star who fatally shot himself in the family's Denver home one day in 1990. "It's seeing him lying on the table in the hospital with plastic gloves on his hands and a sheet up over him, a bullet hole through his head," says Franklin, 61. "I see his mother laying her head on his chest and just sobbing, sobbing her heart out." . . .

[Years later] Franklin has suffered a second tragedy . . . . Franklin and his second wife . . . found the decomposing body of his only other child, Jamon, 31, who had killed himself, possibly a week earlier by inhaling carbon monoxide fumes . . . . Jamon Franklin, who was living at home at the time of his death, had apparently never recovered from his brother's suicide, which was followed just five months later by the death of the boys' mother . . . from cancer . . . .

Since [then], Franklin's mood has swung between guilt and anger, self-doubt and despair. "I'm just trying to hang on," he says . . . (Rogers and Bane, 2000: 166).

THE FEDERAL RESPONSE

For decades, the federal government of the United States has been concerned about the high suicide rates. In 1966, the Center for Studies of Suicide Prevention (later the Suicide Research Unit) was established at the National Institute of Mental Health. The Centers for Disease Control and Prevention's efforts in violence prevention in the mid-1980s high-lighted the high rates of suicide among youth and led to a task force on youth suicide. Suicide became a central issue worldwide in the mid-1990s. At this time, several private foundations and public-private partnerships became active in the United States. A seminal conference was held in Reno, Nevada in 1998 that summarized recommendations for action. In 1999, the Surgeon General of the United States issued a "Call to Action to Prevent Suicide" (PHS, 1999), and soon after presented a comprehensive assessment of future goals and objectives to combat suicide (PHS, 2001). The federal commitment to reducing suicide rate is further illustrated by the goals of *Healthy People 2010* to reduce the overall suicide rate to 6 per 100,000 by the year 2010 and to reduce adolescent suicide attempts by one percent each year (US DHHS, 2000).

STATEMENT OF TASK

Despite its long history and the deep suffering it causes, despite the increased understanding that has come with research over the past de-cades, suicide continues to claim tens of thousands of lives each year. While the National Strategy presents 11 goals and multiple objectives, specific actions still need to be designed. In 2000, several federal agencies (the National Institute of Mental Health, the National Institute of Drug Abuse, the Veterans Administration, the Centers for Disease Control and Prevention, Substance Abuse and Mental Health Services Administra-tion, and the National Institute on Alcohol Abuse and Alcoholism) joined together to fund an Institute of Medicine study in an effort to explore new directions for the field. In the autumn of 2000, the Committee on Patho-physiology and Prevention of Adolescent and Adult Suicide was formed to examine the state of the science base, gaps in our knowledge, strategies for prevention, and research designs for the study of suicide. A committee was constituted with a broad range of expertise, including neuroscience, genetics, epidemiology, sociology, anthropology, psychology, psychiatry, and community interventions. While some members of the committee were experts in suicidology, the committee also included many who were not suicidologists but whose relevant expertise could contribute to a fresh view of the subject. The committee was asked to address the following tasks:

• An assessment of the science base of suicide etiology, including cognitive, affective, behavioral, sociological, epidemiological, genetic, epi-genetic, and neurobiological components. This will include an examination of the vulnerability of specific populations (e.g., American Indians) and age groups (e.g., adolescents and aged).

• An evaluation of the current status of primary and secondary prevention including risk, protective factors, and issues of contagion. Access to methods of suicide and the availability of emergency interventions will be considered. The committee will consider strategies for prevention of suicide, including an examination of the efficacy of national and international intervention and prevention efforts.

• Strategies for studying suicide. This effort will consider the ethics of incorporating suicidal patients into drug trials, the current classifications of suicide and suicidal behavior, behavioral measures to evaluate suicide risk and outcomes, and statistical methods.

• Conclusions concerning gaps in knowledge, research opportunities, and strategies for prevention of suicide.

The committee decided that it would focus on suicide and suicide attempts that were self-inflicted with an intent to die. Although important subjects in their own right, three types of self-destructive behavior were beyond the scope of this report. They are:

• Self-destructive behaviors with high immediate or long-term physical risk and that may be motivated by a wish to die (Poussaint and Alexander, 2000)
• Assisted suicide
• Suicides in the face of terminal illness and/or suffering.

It should also be noted that this study is not intended as an all-inclusive review of the field. For such a review, we refer readers to a number of recent excellent books (e.g., Hawton and van Heeringen, 2000; Jacobs, 1999; Lester, 2001; Wasserman, 2001). Rather, this report aims to identify the next steps necessary to significantly reduce suicide, and within this task, discuss the most relevant information.

SUICIDE THROUGH HISTORY

Suicide is not a new phenomenon. Strikingly, accounts of suicide across the last millennium catalog the same factors associated with suicide as those revealed by modern scientific study in western cultures: serious mental illness, alcohol and substance abuse, co-morbidity, childhood abuse, loss of a loved one, fear of humiliation, and economic dislocation and insecurity. In Box 1.1, accounts of suicides in Europe across several centuries are presented.

BOX 1.1
Suicide in Western History

1293. Adam Le Yep, a freeholder in Worcestershire, was reclassified a serf because of his extreme poverty. Rejecting the social demotion, he drowned himself in the Severn.

1302. Raoul de Nesles rushed headlong into the melee during the Battle of the Golden Spurs at Courtrai, preferring certain death to the humiliation of defeat.

1394. After several days of illness, Jean Masstoier decided to drown himself in the river. Saved in time but still suffering from "melancholy of the head," he threw himself down a well.

1418. When his wife fell ill, Pierre le Vachier, a retired butcher from Sarcelles who had been ruined by the civil war and had lost two of his children, not only was left destitute but also felt totally abandoned. He "went to hang himself from a tree, where he died and strangled himself."

1426. Jeannette Mayard, a shoemaker's wife and a good Catholic but given to drink and jealousy, hanged herself.

1447. A woman known to be insane got up in the middle of the night. "Her husband asked her where she was going and she answered that she wanted to go relieve herself. Thus the said woman went about the house stark naked, then threw herself into a well a good thirteen arm-widths deep."

1728. Joseph Castille, a peasant, hanged himself from an apple tree near Domagné. Alcohol had clearly affected his mental faculties. Witnesses were unanimous: "He drank continually"; "he was perturbed." He had hallucinations, danced about in nothing but his chemise, talked to the birds, washed himself at the holy water font, and had become morbidly jealous. . . .

1769. A young girl of fifteen, François Royer, drowned herself at Fougères. She had for some time been abused by her mother, who sent her out to beg, gave her hardly enough to eat, threw her out into the street in the middle of the night calling her a whore, and beat her with a stick. . . .

1787. Yves Barguil, a known drunkard thirty years of age who had already attempted to kill himself on several occasions, hanged himself near Quimperlé. He had long declared his intention and was considered mad, as his mother had been. Alcohol aggravated his condition; his wife had hidden all the ropes and locked up the barn.

SOURCE: Minois, 1999: 8-9, 278-280. © 1999. Reprinted by permission of the Johns Hopkins University Press.

Most but not all current societies and religious traditions ban suicide. Some traditions sanction suicide under certain conditions, such as acts perceived in some Islamic sects as martyrdom in war against an enemy (Dale, 1988), and suicide deaths of widowed women in Hinduism (Inamdar et al., 1983). In Japan, for example, homicide–suicide may be a culturally acceptable response to disgrace and dishonor, or untenable circumstances (Iga, 1996; Sakuta, 1995). In traditional Chinese society, suicide was seen as an available option for coping with humiliation and also as a means for upright officials to criticize immoral and corrupt times. Examples are given in Box 1.2 below.

In western, Judeo-Christian culture, prohibition of suicide came after much-heated debate by the Church leaders during the first three centuries of the Common Era. These leaders were concerned by what they observed as unacceptably high suicide rates, which they related to increasing acts of martyrdom, following the example of Christ (Minois, 1999). This early struggle by governing leadership on how to reduce suicide rates culminated with St. Augustine's clear proscription in his *City of God*:

> This we declare and affirm and emphatically accept as true: No man may inflict death upon himself at will merely to escape from temporal difficulties—for this is but to plunge into those which are everlasting; no man may do so even on account of another's sins, fearing they may lead to a sin of one's own—for we are not sullied by others' sins; no man may do so on account of past sins—for to expiate them by penance we need life all the more; no one may end his own life out of a desire to attain a better life which he hopes for after death, because a better life after death is not for those who perish by their own hand (St. Augustine, ca. 426 CE/1950).

The prohibition in canon law was reinforced by changes in law of the Roman Empire during the same period. Plagues, famine, and war continually took their toll on the population, and both the Catholic Church and the Roman Empire needed to sustain their population. The Romans outlawed all manners of reducing the population including contraception, abortion, infanticide, and suicide by the end of the fourth century, and instituted forfeiture of worldly goods of suicides by the government. This contrasted with the earlier social acceptance of suicide.

These perspectives continued to pervade the thinking about suicide in early modern England and colonial United States. In 967 King Edgar decreed that the goods of a person who completed suicide were to be forfeit—based on the earlier canon laws. Henry de Bracton, a mid-thirteenth-century jurist, stated that suicide was a crime: "Just as a man commit felony by slaying another, so he may do so by slaying himself, the

BOX 1.2
Suicide in Eastern History

295 B.C. The Chinese poet, Qu Yuan (332–295 B.C.) drowned himself as a protest against official persecution. His act has traditionally symbolized the loss of legitimacy of an unjust social order through an act of moral courage (Kleinman, 1995).

1944. [Prior to his kamikaze mission] ". . . Second Lieutenant Shigeyuki Suzuki wrote: 'People say that our feeling is of resignation, but that does not know at all how we feel, and think of us as a fish about to be cooked . . . Young blood does flow in us . . . There are persons we love, we think of, and many unforgettable memories. However, with those, we cannot win the war'" (Sasaki, 1996: 186).

1976. Lao She, a famous Chinese writer, drowned himself in the Lake of Peace in Beijing during the Cultural Revolution (1966–1976) because he could not bear the great social suffering (Ji et al., 2001).

1996. "After an accident and cover-up at a nuclear-power plant, a manager in charge of an in-house investigation faced the press. Hours later, he went up to the roof of a Tokyo hotel and jumped off. 'I feel grave responsibility for my poorly considered actions,' he wrote." (Lev, 1998).

1998. With his arrest on corruption charges imminent, a member of the Japanese parliament Shokei Arai hanged himself with the belt from a bathrobe in a hotel room in Tokyo. A Japanese sword and several notes were found in the room (Lev, 1998).

2001. Volodymr Oleksandrenko, chief of city construction in the Crimean capital city Simferopol, poured a flammable liquid over himself in an attempt at self-immolation during a session of the municipal council. He told council members he was being persecuted by bureaucrats in Kiev, and made the apparent suicide attempt as a protest against these corrupt officials (Tulubiev, 2001).

2001. New Delhi. Jangarh Singh Shyam, India's most prominent tribal artist, completed suicide in Japan by hanging himself from the ceiling of his room. Shyam was at the Mithila Museum in Niigata as an artist in residence and reportedly felt depressed after being denied permission to return home (Sinha, 2001).

felony is said to be done to himself." In seventeenth-century colonial America, suicides were brought to trial where they were considered criminal (even if there was evidence of mental illness). This history provides the backdrop for our modern perspectives on suicide. It continues to negatively impact accurate identification of patients at risk and the reporting of suicides and suicide attempts.

SUICIDE AS AN INTERDISCIPLINARY EFFORT

The approaches and findings of sociology, psychology, medicine, and public health are all critical components of our current understanding of suicide. To understand the current status of the field, the development of thought within each discipline is worth exploring.

Two schools of thought provided the foundation for present-day sociological study of suicide: the work of Emile Durkheim, the pre-eminent French sociologist in suicidology who lived at the turn of the twentieth century; and the "Chicago School" of sociology founded in the 1920s at the University of Chicago. Durkheim (1897/1951) purported that suicide was an index of societal well-being and that suicide could be divided into four categories based on individual motivation and the balance of individual and society. These categories are:

- egoistic, focus on individual functioning and lack of social integration;
- altruistic, insufficient independence and over-identification with a group or cults;
- anomic, abrupt disruptions of normative restraint as in wartime or after the stock market crash;
- fatalistic, excessive constraints such as in incarcerated populations.

Durkheim contrasted higher suicide in Northern European Protestant societies with lower suicide in Southern European Catholic societies, which he attributed to religion. This line of cross-cultural comparison continues in contemporary anthropological research. The "Chicago School" of sociology, led by William I. Thomas, was responsible for the establishment of statistical analysis as the foundation for scientific objectivity. Although a contribution to the field in terms of population-based risk, the statistical approach was limited in its ability to provide predictions at an individual level, as evidenced by the work of Cavan (1965).

In contrast, psychological approaches to suicide address changes at the individual level. The basic tenet of all psychological and psychoanalytic theories is that personal psychological conflict, related to individual history, is responsible for suicide (Freud, 1957b), and that prevention and intervention occurs through resolving these conflicts and learning more adaptive coping strategies for dealing with stressors and conflicts (Freud, 1957a). Three types of psychological study inform the current understanding of suicide: psychoanalysis, developmental psychology, and cognitive-behavioral psychology. Psychoanalysis stems from Freud and focuses on the links between suicide and mourning a loss due to death or other separation. Developmental psychological efforts of Bowlby (1953; 1970; 1978) led to the formulation of attachment theory.[1] This approach served as the basis for neurobiological research in attachment that revealed disruptions in the hypothalamic-pituitary-adrenal stress-response system, and changes in the serotonin system associated with suicide (see Chapter 4). Cognitive-behavioral psychology, developed by Aaron T. Beck (1987), suggests that an individual's distress can be reduced by teaching them how to change their behavioral and thought habits. The measurement scales that evolved from this approach (e.g., the Beck Hopelessness Scale) are widely used in clinical settings to assess suicidality.

A third school of thought, starting with Emil Kraepelin in the nineteenth century, is a medical approach with the premise that there are physical causes for mental illnesses. Current research on suicide reveals alterations in neurotransmitters and other biological markers specific in those who have completed or attempted suicide.

The old boundaries of scientific disciplines have faded, and many new interdisciplinary fields in behavior (e.g., medical anthropology, psychoneuroimmunology, the behavioral neurosciences) are blossoming. Cross-disciplinary fields burgeoning over the last 20 years have now demonstrated that psychological and social changes can also lead to alterations of the physiological systems. Almost all states of health and disease result from interactions between individual and environmental factors (IOM, 2001). Suicide is a clear example of the interaction of multiple factors including individual biological and psychological factors, life-stressors, and cultural and social factors. Suicide is a consequence of complex interactions among biological, psychological, cultural, and sociological factors. Mental disorders and substance abuse, childhood and adult trauma, social isolation, economic hardship, relationship loss, and indi-

---

[1]Attachment theory "deals with the affectional bonds between individuals, their origins in childhood and adolescent relationships, the distress caused by involuntary severance of such bonds or by their faulty development, and the treatment of these disturbances" (Bowlby, 1978).

vidual psychological traits such as hopelessness and impulsiveness all increase the risk. The presence of multiple risk factors further increases the risk. Yet, simply identifying the risk factors is not adequate for the development of effective interventions.

The Surgeon General's 1999 Call to Action (PHS, 1999) and subsequent reports on mental illness in the United States (US DHHS, 1999; US DHHS, 2001) raised public awareness of the complexity of the issue and the need for multifaceted approaches.

DEFINITIONS

The lack of universally accepted definitions for suicide and suicidal behaviors hampers progress. Comparisons across studies that are critical for a low-base rate behavior such as suicide are critical but difficult with the use of variable terminology. The Committee consensus was that universally accepted definitions of suicide, suicide attempts, suicidal ideation, and suicidal communications are needed to facilitate efforts in the field. Early classifications of suicidal behavior were typologies with implied causal relationships, but were not evidence-based. These efforts incorporate useful clinical and sociological observations, but do not serve the need for a classification system. For the purpose of this study, the Committee chose a classification system that does not speak to causal hypotheses. Rather, it selected the system initiated at the National Institute of Mental Health Center for the Studies of Suicidal Prevention meeting in 1972–1973 that has been refined through subsequent research (O'Carroll et al., 1996). These definitions, listed below, best described how the committee chose to think about the terms used throughout the report. This choice allowed them to move forward with their task but is not meant as a recommendation for the field. The terms are defined here to provide guidance to the reader in understanding what is meant in the report when this terminology is used.

Suicide: Fatal self-inflicted destructive act with explicit or inferred intent to die. Multiaxial description includes: Method, Location, Intent, Diagnoses, and Demographics.

Suicide attempt: A non-fatal, self-inflicted destructive act with explicit or inferred intent to die. (Note: important aspects include the frequency and recency of attempt(s), and the person's perception of the likelihood of death from the method used, or intended for use, medical lethality and/or damage resulting from method used, diagnoses, and demographics.)

Suicidal ideation: Thoughts of harming or killing oneself. (Frequency, intensity, and duration of these thoughts are all posited as important to determining the severity of ideation.)

Suicidal communications: Direct or indirect expressions of suicidal ideation or of intent to harm or kill self, expressed verbally or through writing, artwork, or other means. The more concrete and explicit the plan is and the more lethal the intended method, the greater the seriousness of suicidal communications. Suicidal threats are a special case of suicidal communications, used with the intent to change the behavior of other people.

High-risk groups: Those that are known to have a higher than average suicide rate.

Suicidality: All suicide-related behaviors and thoughts including completing or attempting suicide, suicidal ideation or communications.

ORGANIZATION OF THE REPORT

The report explores what is known about the epidemiology, risk factors, and interventions for suicide and suicide attempts. Overarching recommendations are presented at the end of the report, but each chapter provides some new directions that might help us advance our battle against suicide.

Chapter 2 reviews the epidemiology and explores the magnitude of the problem.

Chapter 3 describes the psychiatric and psychologic factors contributing to risk of suicide.

Chapter 4 explores the biological changes that are associated with suicide.

Chapter 5 reviews the links between childhood trauma and suicide.

Chapter 6 examines the impact of societal and cultural influences.

Chapter 7 explores the medical and psychosocial interventions for suicide.

Chapter 8 looks at programs for suicide prevention.

Chapter 9 explores the barriers to treatment.

Chapter 10 looks at the barriers in research.

Chapter 11 presents the overarching recommendations of the committee for new directions.

Through the evaluation of the currently available scientific information on suicide, this study aimed to identify the best approaches to reducing suicide now, as well as the best paths for the future: what must be done if we as a nation are committed to reducing suicide significantly.

REFERENCES

Beck AT. 1987. Cognitive models of depression. *Journal of Cognitive Psychotherapy*, 1(1): 5-37.

Bowlby J. 1953. Critical phases in the development of social responses in man and other animals. *New Biology*, 14: 25-32.

Bowlby J. 1970. Disruption of affectional bonds and its effects on behavior. *Journal of Contemporary Psychotherapy*, 2(2): 75-86.

Bowlby J. 1978. Attachment theory and its therapeutic implications. *Adolescent Psychiatry*, 6: 5-33.

Bureau of the Census. 1976. *Historical Statistics of the United States: Colonial Times to 1970, Part 1*. Washington, DC: U.S. Department of Commerce.

Cavan RS. 1965. *Suicide*. New York: Russell & Russell. The University of Chicago Sociological Series.

CDC (Centers for Disease Control and Prevention). 2001. *CDC Wonder: Scientific Data*. [Online]. Available: http://wonde.cdc.gov/wonder/sci_data.asp [accessed October 15, 2001].

Center for Electronic Records. 1998. *Statistical Information About Casualities of the Vietnam Conflict*. Reference Report #18. College Park, MD: National Archives and Records Administration. [Online]. Available: http://www.nara.gov/nara/electronic/vnstat.html [accessed December 2001].

Dale SF. 1988. Religious suicide in Islamic Asia: Anticolonial terrorism in India, Indonesia, and the Philippines. *Journal of Conflict Resolution*, 32(1): 37-59.

Durkheim E. 1897/1951. Translated by JA Spaulding and G Simpson. *Suicide: A Study in Sociology*. New York: Free Press.

Freud S. 1957a. Freud's psychoanalytic procedure. 1904. Reprint. Strachey J, Editor and Translator. *Standard Edition of the Complete Psychological Works of Sigmund Freud*. Vol. 7, No. 249-256. London: The Hogarth Press.

Freud S. 1957b. Mourning and melancholia. 1917. Reprint. Strachey J, Editor and Translator. *Standard Edition of the Complete Psychological Works of Sigmund Freud*. Vol. 14. (pp. 239-258). London: The Hogarth Press.

Hawton K, van Heeringen K, Editors. 2000. *The International Handbook of Suicide and Attempted Suicide*. Chichester, UK: John Wiley and Sons.

Hoyert DL, Arias E, Smith BL, Murphy SL, Kochanek KD. 2001. Deaths: Final data for 1999. *National Vital Statistics Reports*, 49(8): 1-113.

Iga M. 1996. Cultural aspects of suicide: The case of Japanese oyako shinju (parent-child suicide). *Archives of Suicide Research*, 2: 87-102.

Inamdar SC, Oberfield RA, Darrell EB. 1983. A suicide by self-immolation: Psychosocial perspectives. *International Journal of Social Psychiatry*, 29(2): 130-133.

IOM (Institute of Medicine). 2001. *Health and Behavior: The Interplay of Biological, Behavioral, and Societal Influences*. Washington, DC: National Academy Press.

Jacobs DG, Editor. 1999. *The Harvard Medical School Guide to Suicide Assessment and Intervention*. San Francisco: Jossey-Bass Publishers.

Jamison KR. 1999. *Night Falls Fast: Understanding Suicide*. New York: Alfred A Knopf.

Ji J, Kleinman A, Becker AE. 2001. Suicide in contemporary China: A review of China's distinctive suicide demographics in their sociocultural context. *Harvard Review of Psychiatry*, 9(1): 1-12.

Kleinman A. 1995. *Writing at the Margin: Discourse Between Anthropology and Medicine*. Berkeley, CA: University of California Press.

Lester D, Editor. 2001. *Suicide Prevention: Resources for the Millennium*. Philadelphia: Brunner-Routledge. Neimeyer RA, Editor. Series in Death, Dying, and Bereavement.

Lev MA. 1998, February 27. Suicide imbedded in Japan's culture. *Seattle Times.* [Online]. Available: http://seattletimes.nwsource.com/news/nation-world/html98/ altjpan_022798 [accessed January 4, 2002].

Minino AM, Smith BL. 2001. Deaths: Preliminary data for 2000. *National Vital Statistics Reports,* 49(12): 1-40.

Minois G. 1999. Translated by LG Cochrane. *History of Suicide: Voluntary Death in Western Culture.* Baltimore: Johns Hopkins University Press.

NCHS (National Center for Health Statistics). 2001. *Data From the National Vital Statistics System.* Hyattsville, MD: Centers for Disease Control and Prevention. [Online]. Available: http://www.cdc.gov/nchs/nvss.htm [accessed September 2001].

NCIPC (National Center for Injury Prevention and Control). 2000. *Web-Based Injury Statistics Query and Reporting System.* [Online]. Available: http://www.cdc.gov/ncipc/ wisqars/ [accessed December 13, 2001].

O'Carroll PW, Berman AL, Maris RW, Moscicki EK, Tanney BL, Silverman MM. 1996. Beyond the Tower of Babel: A nomenclature for suicidology. *Suicide and Life-Threatening Behavior,* 26(3): 237-252.

PHS (Public Health Service). 1999. *The Surgeon General's Call to Action to Prevent Suicide.* Rockville, MD: U.S. Department of Health and Human Services.

PHS (Public Health Service). 2001. *National Strategy for Suicide Prevention: Goals and Objectives for Action.* Rockville, MD: U.S. Department of Health and Human Services.

Poussaint AF, Alexander A. 2000. *Lay My Burden Down: Unraveling Suicide and the Mental Health Crisis Among African-Americans.* Boston: Beacon Press.

Rogers P, Bane V. 2000, December 4. The cruelest blow. *People.* p. 165-173.

Sakuta T. 1995. A study of murder followed by suicide. *Medicine and Law,* 14(1-2): 141-153.

Sasaki M. 1996. Who became kamikaze pilots, and how did they feel towards their suicide mission? *The Concord Review,* 7: 175-209.

Sinha G. 2001, July 7. Indian artist commits suicide in Japan. *The Hindu.* [Online]. Available: http://www.hinduonnet.com/thehindu/2001/07/07/stories/02070003.htm [accessed January 4, 2002].

St. Augustine. ca. 426 CE/1950. Translated by GG Walsh and DB Zema. *The City of God: Books I-VII.* New York: Fathers of the Church.

Tulubiev Y. 2001, February 16. News from Ukraine. *Ukrinform.* [Online]. Available: http:// www.ukremb.com/ news/Ukrinform/2001/february/160201UI1.htm [accessed January 4, 2002].

US DHHS (U.S. Department of Health and Human Services). 1999. *Mental Health: A Report of the Surgeon General.* Rockville, MD: U.S. Department of Health and Human Services, Substance Abuse and Mental Health Services Administration, Center for Mental Health Services, National Institutes of Health, National Institute of Mental Health.

US DHHS (U.S. Department of Health and Human Services). 2000. *Healthy People 2010.* Washington, DC: U.S. Department of Health and Human Services.

US DHHS (U.S. Department of Health and Human Services). 2001. *Mental Health: Culture, Race and Ethnicity—A Supplement to Mental Health: A Report of the Surgeon General.* Rockville, MD: U.S. Department of Health and Human Services, Substance Abuse and Mental Health Services Administration, Center for Mental Health Services, National Institutes of Health, National Institute of Mental Health.

Wasserman D, Editor. 2001. *Suicide: An Unnecessary Death.* London: Martin Dunitz.

WHO (World Health Organization), Department of Mental Health. 1999. *Mental and Behavioural Disorders: Figures and Facts About Suicide.* Geneva.

After great pain, a formal feeling comes—
The Nerves sit ceremonious, like Tombs—
The stiff Heart questions was it He, that bore,
And Yesterday, or Centuries before?

The Feet, mechanical, go round—
Of Ground, or Air, or Ought—
A wooden way
Regardless grown,
A quartz contentment, like a stone—

This is the Hour of Lead—
Remembered, if outlived,
As Freezing persons, recollect the Snow—
First—Chill—then Stupor—then the letting go—

—EMILY DICKINSON

2

Magnitude of the Problem

Suicide is a global problem, a leading cause of death in the world claiming about 30,000 lives in the United States each year, almost 1 million annually world-wide. In the United States, the suicide rate was 10.7 per 100,000 in 1999. It greatly exceeded the rate of homicide (6.2 per 100,000) in 1999, as it has for the last 100 years (Figure 2-1) (Bureau of Justice Statistics, 2001; Bureau of the Census, 1976; Hoyert et al., 2001; Minino and Smith, 2001; NCHS, 2001; NCIPC, 2000). Suicide is the third leading cause of death in youth 15–24 years old. White males over 85 have the highest rate of suicide, about 65 per 100,000. Suicide rates are also elevated in some ethnic groups. For example, suicide is about 1.5 times more prevalent than average among Native Americans. While whites continue to have higher suicide rates than blacks, the gap seems to be narrowing in young males.

Suicides in males outnumber those in females in almost all nations, including the United States. While males are more likely to complete suicide, females are more likely to attempt suicide. Nationally and internationally there is geographic heterogeneity, suggesting that social and cultural differences have a significant impact on suicide rates (see also Chapter 6). In the United States in 1998, firearms accounted for the majority of suicides both in general (57.0%) and among youth 15–24 (61%) (NCIPC, 2000). Suffocation (18.7%; 25%), poisoning (16.6%, 7%), and falls (2.0% both) follow in usage. This differs in other nations; for example, self-poisoning, especially with insecticides, is the most common method in both Pakistan (Khan and Reza, 2000) and rural China (Yip, 2001).

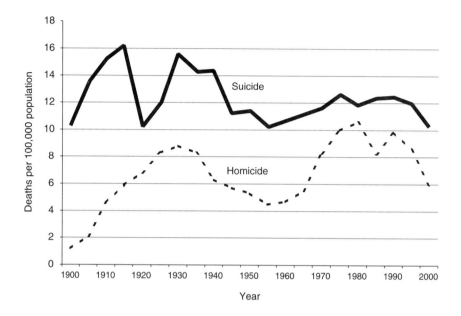

FIGURE 2-1 Rates of Suicide and Homicide in the United States: 1900–2000. Based on data from the Bureau of Justice Statistics (2001), Bureau of the Census (1976), Hoyert et al. (2001), Minino and Smith (2001), and NCHS (2001). Inconsistencies in reporting before 1933 may account for some of the early fluctuations in rates.

This chapter reviews the characteristics of some of the populations at risk, describes the geographical differences, and briefly explores the limitations of the epidemiological data. The chapter closes with an analysis of the economic cost to society that suicide presents.

GEOGRAPHIC TRENDS

Suicide rates are generally higher in northern European nations than in southern European nations (see Table 2-1). For example, Hungary's suicide rate was over 33 per 100,000 as of 1999 (WHO, 2001a). In comparison, Greece has had low suicide rates, only 3.8 per 100,000 as of 1998 (WHO, 2001a). Suicide rates have been high in recent years in many, but not all, of the former Soviet states. For example, suicide rates are over 35 per 100,000 in the Russian Federation and Lithuania, but are less than 5 per 100,000 in Armenia, Azerbaijan, and Georgia (WHO, 2001a).

TABLE 2-1 National Suicide Rates per 100,000 for Selected Countries. Most Recent Data from the World Health Organization (WHO, 2001a)

Country	Total	Male	Female	Year
Armenia	1.8	2.7	0.9	1999
Austria	19.2	28.7	10.3	1999
Azerbaijan	0.7	1.1	0.2	1999
Belarus	34.0	61.1	10.0	1999
Brazil	4.1	6.6	1.8	1995
Canada	12.3	19.6	5.1	1997
China	14.1	13.4	14.8	1998
Rural Areas	23.3	21.9	24.8	1998
Urban Areas	6.8	6.8	6.8	1998
Finland	23.8	38.3	10.1	1998
Georgia	4.3	6.6	2.1	1992
Greece	3.8	6.1	1.7	1998
Hungary	33.1	53.1	14.8	1999
India	10.7	12.2	9.1	1998
Italy	8.2	12.7	3.9	1997
Japan	18.8	26.0	11.9	1997
Kuwait	2.2	2.7	1.6	1999
Lithuania	41.9	73.8	13.6	1999
Mexico	3.1	5.4	1.0	1995
Norway	12.1	17.8	6.6	1997
Philippines	2.1	2.5	1.7	1993
Poland	14.3	24.1	4.6	1996
Republic of Korea	13.0	17.8	8.0	1997
Russian Federation	35.5	62.6	11.6	1998
Singapore	11.7	13.9	9.5	1998
Sri Lanka	31.0	44.6	16.8	1991[a]
Sweden	14.2	20.0	8.5	1996
Tajikistan	3.5	5.1	1.8	1995
Thailand	4.0	5.6	2.4	1994
Ukraine	29.1	51.2	10.0	1999
United Kingdom of Great Britain & Northern Ireland	7.4	11.7	3.3	1998
United States	10.7	17.6	4.1	1999

[a]The more recent total suicide rate for 1996 was 21.6, but rates by sex were not available.

Overall, suicide rates are lower in other Asian nations compared to China, including Singapore (11.7 per 100,000), Japan (18.8 per 100,000), and Thailand, which reports a very low rate of 4.0 per 100,000 (Table 2-1, WHO, 2001a). The suicide rate for China has decreased dramatically in recent years, dropping from 23 per 100,000 in 1999 to 17 per 100,000 in 2000 (WHO, 2001b).

Studies from across the world find higher rates of suicide in rural versus urban areas (Plotnikov, 2001; Yip, 2001; Yip et al., 2000). In China, for example, the rate is two to five times greater in rural regions (Ji et al., 2001; Jianlin, 2000; Phillips et al., 1999; Yip, 2001). Higher rates in rural regions have also been documented for young males in Australia (Wilkinson and Gunnell, 2000) and in the Ukraine (Kryzhanovskaya and Pilyagina, 1999). Even among adolescents in Greece, where the suicide rate is relatively low, urban areas report significantly lower rates than rural areas (Beratis, 1991). In China (Yip et al., 2000), unlike Australia for example (Morrell et al., 1999), the usual pattern of more suicides among men than women is reversed in rural areas due to the very high female suicide rate, especially among young women (Ji et al., 2001; Yip, 2001; Yip et al., 2000).

Like the United States (see below), suicide rates are higher in rural areas in China. In 1998, women in rural China completed suicide at a rate of over 30 per 100,000 for ages 25–34 and 45–64, with increasing rates at older ages (WHO, 2001a). The male rate surpasses that for women starting at age 55, with over 129 per 100,000 dying by suicide over the age of 75 in rural China (WHO, 2001a). In comparison, the overall rate for females and males in urban China is 6.8 per 100,000 in 1998, with the highest rate for males over 75 at about 32 per 100,000 (WHO, 2001a).

Suicide rates vary greatly across the United States, with higher rates generally in the western states. New Jersey is the lowest with 6.4/100,000 in 1998. Nevada and Alaska are the highest with rates in excess of 21/ 100,000 (Murphy, 2000). Mapping the rates by county (see Appendix A and Figure 2-2) illustrates that those counties with the highest rates are predominantly in the western states with lowest population density. Counties with the lowest rates (7.5 suicides per 100,000) appear to be clustered in the central United States. Finally, counties classified with intermediate rates are largely in the eastern portion of the United States. Population density has been suggested as a factor in these differences (Saunderson and Langford, 1996). Examining the suicide rates by urbanization in the United States reveals that the rates are higher in less populated area compared to densely populated cities (Figure 2-3). For the most part this difference is a reflection of the decrease in firearm suicides with urbanization (Figure 2-4). This relationship of suicide by firearms and population density is even more dramatic when suicide among elderly persons is explored. Among the elderly, suicide by firearms decreases dramatically with increased urbanization (Figure 2-5), but non-firearm suicides are more common in urban areas. When controlling for education, employment status, and divorce rate, Birckmayer and Hemenway (2001) also found that living in urban areas was associated with increases in U.S. suicide rates for non-firearm suicides among adults.

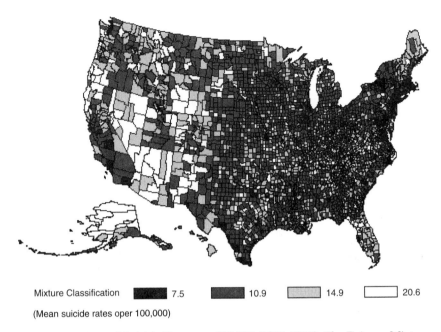

FIGURE 2-2 Annual Suicide Rates per 100,000 (1996–1998). The Poisson Mixture Model applied to county-level data.

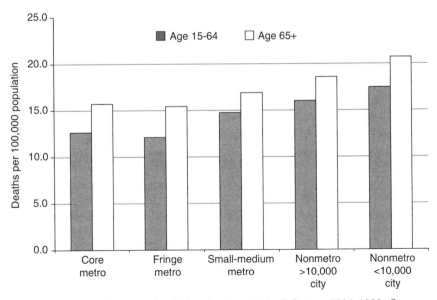

FIGURE 2-3 Suicide Rates by Urbanization: United States, 1996–1998. Source: NCHS (2001). Provided by LA Fingerhut.

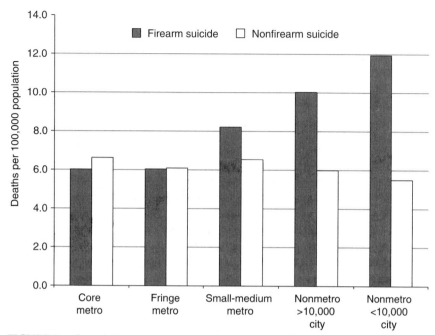

FIGURE 2-4 Suicide Rates by Urbanization and Use of Firearms Among Persons 15–64 Years: United States, 1996–1998. Source: NCHS (2001). Provided by LA Fingerhut.

Limited access to mental health services and to emergency care have been implicated in the increased rates seen in some rural areas. Rural residents suffer higher overall mortality rates from accidents and injuries of all intents because of isolation from care facilities (IOM, 1999). Mental health services are poor in many rural areas (e.g., Howland, 1995) and travel distance to mental health treatment impedes use by rural residents (Fortney et al., 1999, see also Chapter 9).

The reported suicide rates are confounded by the effects of race, sex, and age. A statistical analysis described in Appendix A illustrates an approach to adjust rates for these variables. That analysis reveals that even after accounting for these important demographic variables, considerable spatial variability remains. Again, the highest adjusted rates are typically found in the less densely populated areas of the western United States. The analysis also reveals that there are spatial anomolies; in the western United States and Alaska, where suicide rates are typically high, there are a few counties that have calculated estimates that are consistent with the national average. Similarly, in the central United States, where

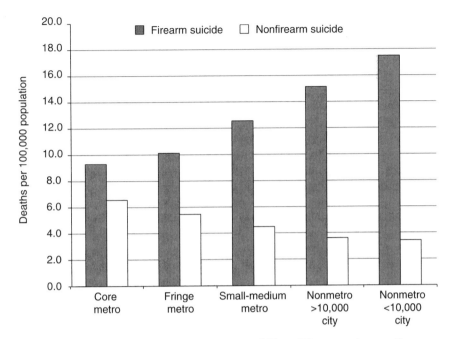

FIGURE 2-5 Suicide Rates by Urbanization and Use of Firearms Among Persons 65 Years and Older: United States, 1996–1998. Source: NCHS (2001). Provided by LA Fingerhut.

there is a high concentration of counties with the lowest suicide rates, there are a few counties that exhibit the highest suicide rates. What are the protective factors that have produced these spatial anomalies? Are these spatial anomalies simply due to reporting bias or some other unmeasured characteristic that has produced the outliers? Examining these spatial anomalies in greater detail is certainly a fruitful area for further research.

POPULATIONS AT RISK

Gender Differences

In western nations such as Greece, Mexico, and the United States, male suicides outnumber female suicides 3- to 5-fold (WHO, 2001a). The gender gap is narrower in Asian nations, where the difference tends to be less than 2-fold. China is singular in this regard, with *more* female than male suicides, although this gap has narrowed in recent years (WHO, 2001a). Risk factors for suicide differ significantly by gender. Although women are twice as likely as men to experience episodes of major depression in the United States, they are 25 percent less likely than men to complete suicide (Murphy, 1998). There are several factors that may explain this. Men who are depressed have a higher prevalence of comorbid alcohol and substance abuse than women. Also, men's depression in later life is more likely to go unrecognized and untreated than women's depression (Rihmer et al., 1995). Murphy (1998) suggests that men may regard a need for help as a weakness and consequently avoid help seeking; while women may place a higher value on interdependence and consider how their actions will affect others to a greater degree than do men.

A comparison of male and female suicide victims provides additional clues as to the gender differences for completed suicide (Brent et al., 1999). First, females are more likely to engage in suicidal behavior using potentially reversible methods, such as overdose. Second, females are less likely to use alcohol during a suicide completion. Third, alcohol intoxication in the context of a suicide increases the likelihood of use of a gun for completion of suicide in males, but not females.

Youth

Although suicide rates for all age groups have been relatively stable since the 1950s, the reported rate among adolescents has increased markedly. Between 1970 and 1990, the rates for youth aged 15 through 19 nearly doubled; the rate tripled since the mid 1950s. Since 1990, the overall suicide rate for this age group has stabilized at approximately 11 deaths per 100,000. One national school-based study of youth found high one-year prevalence rates for suicide attempts (7.7 percent), ideation (20.5 percent), and making a plan (15.7 percent) (Kann et al., 1998). The increase in the suicide rate is thought to be attributable to an increase in alcohol and substance abuse and increased availability of firearms over this period of time (Brent et al., 1987). Being unemployed or out of school was associated with completed suicide in a large case-control study completed in New York (Gould et al., 1996; Shaffer et al., 1996). In other countries that experienced a dramatic increase in suicide in the past 10 years, such as New Zealand and in the province of Quebec, social change, including diminishing opportunities for employment, is thought to be a primary factor (Beautrais, 2000).

Suicide victims under the age of 30 are more likely to have problems with substance abuse, impulsive aggressive personality disorders, and precipitants such as interpersonal and legal problems (Rich et al., 1986b) than those over 30. Co-occurrences of mental illness, substance abuse, conduct disorder, or all three are significant risk factors for suicide, but especially in adolescent males (Brent et al., 1999; Shaffer et al., 1996). In general, suicidal behavior is a more impulsive act in younger people. Younger people are less likely to complete a suicide than older people. Even within the adolescent age range, younger adolescents who complete suicide show lower suicidal intent than older ones (Brent et al., 1999; Groholt et al., 1998). Furthermore, youth are more likely to be influenced by media presentations of suicide and to die in cluster suicides[1] (although even so, only about 5% of youth suicides occur in clusters; Gould and Shaffer, 1986; Gould et al., 1990; Phillips and Carstensen, 1986).

Guns are the most common mechanism of suicide among youths. In a case-control study of suicide, the availability of guns in the home conveyed the largest risk in adolescents and young adults (Kellermann et al., 1992). A comparison of the suicide rates in Seattle and Vancouver (see also Chapter 8) showed that when gun control was absent (in the United States) youth (15–24) suicide was significantly greater, with 10-fold more suicide by firearms (Sloan et al., 1990).

Moreover, guns in the home, particularly loaded guns, pose up to a 30-fold increased risk for suicide, especially among individuals *without* major mental disorder (Brent et al., 1993; Kellermann et al., 1992). The rate of psychopathology among younger adolescent suicide victims is much lower than among older adolescents, so that the availability of guns becomes the paramount risk factor for younger, impulsive individuals (Brent et al., 1999; Shaffer et al., 1996).

Elderly

In almost all industrialized countries, men 75 years of age and older have the highest suicide rate among all age groups (Pearson et al., 1997). Of the countries that provide suicide data, Hungary has the highest suicide rates for both elderly men and women: in 1991–1992, the suicide rate for men 75 years and older was as high as 177.5/100,000 (Sartorius, 1996). The lowest rates for both elderly men and women were in Northern Ireland and England/Wales, with rates for men of 20/100,000 and 18/100,000, respectively (Schweizer et al., 1988).

In 1990 the United States had a suicide rate of 24.9/100,000 for men aged 75–84. In 1998 the rate had risen to 42.0/100,000. Although older individuals comprise approximately 10% of the U.S. population, they account for 20% of the completed suicides (Hoyert et al., 2001; Hoyert et al., 1999). Men account for about four out of five completed suicides among those older than 65. This is partly explained by the fact that men are more

---

[1]The term cluster suicides refers to higher-than-expected numbers of suicides occurring in a small geographic area within a limited time period.

likely to use more lethal methods. Seventy-six percent of men and 33% of women who completed suicide used firearms, while 3% of men and 33% of women who completed suicide used overdose on medications in the United States (NCHS, 1992).

Risk factors that predispose to suicide differ across the life span. Widowhood (Smith et al., 1988), serious medical illness, and social isolation (Draper, 1994) are more likely to be salient vulnerability factors among older as opposed to younger adults. Whereas affective illness is a vulnerability factor across all age groups (Asgard, 1990; Rich et al., 1986b), the limited findings for dual diagnosis tend to be weak or negative in later life but consistently positive among young people (Asgard, 1990; Barraclough et al., 1974; Rich et al., 1986b). It is important to note that risk factors often co-occur, such as social isolation and depression, or social isolation and drug abuse, or depression and drug abuse. Considerations specific to suicide in the elderly include: (1) the greater likelihood that the elderly will die in or following a suicide attempt; (2) the greater prevalence of indirect self-destructive behaviors such as poor-adherence to treatment regimens in the elderly; and (3) co-morbid conditions that increase suicide risk, including bereavement, depression, and terminal illness.

There is greater likelihood of death in or following a suicide attempt in the elderly. While in younger age groups suicide attempts are more often impulsive and communicative acts, in later life most attempts can be considered "failed suicides." Older individuals make fewer suicide attempts per completed suicide. The highest suicide attempt to completion rate is in younger women (200:1), compared with 4:1 in the elderly. Suicide attempts in the elderly are more likely to lead to completed suicide than in any other age group: 6% of individuals aged 55 and older died by suicide within a year of a suicide attempt compared to 2% of younger attempters (Gardner et al., 1964). The reasons for this low attempt to completion ratio are complex. The elderly are more medically fragile and frequently live alone, which increases the probability of a fatal outcome. Suicides in older people are often with high intent, long-planned and frequently involve highly lethal methods. The elderly are often less rescuable because of these aspects of their suicidal behavior. Furthermore, suicide methods selected by the elderly are less likely to be affected by short-term modeling effects, such as suicide epidemics. Although most people who kill themselves give direct or indirect warnings, older people are less likely to directly communicate their intent to die. As the elderly are often preoccupied with death and dying, their environment is more likely to miss the indirect warning that they give, such as "nothing is in front of me anymore." However, contrary to common belief, lack of hope and depression are not part of normal aging, not even in the terminally ill elderly.

Indirect self-destructive behavior in the elderly are particularly notable. In addition to overt suicide attempts, there are subtle behaviors especially in the elderly, with conscious or unconscious intent to die, such as refusal to eat or drink, noncompliance with treatment, or extreme self-neglect. Farberow (1980) used the term "sub-intentional suicide" to refer to indirect self-destructive behaviors which often lead to premature death, and are common in certain settings such as nursing homes (where more immediate means to complete suicide are limited), and among people whose religion forbids suicide. Osgood et al. (1991) found that the rate of completed suicide among elderly nursing home residents was 15.8/100,000 as compared to 19.2/100,000 for elderly living in the community. By contrast they estimated the rate of indirect self-destructive behavior leading to death to be 79.9/100,000 among nursing home residents, and the rate of such behavior not resulting in death to be 227/100,000. Kastenbaum and Mishara (1971) found that 44% of men and 22% of women who were hospitalized for chronic medical illnesses exhibited indirect self-destructive behavior during a 1-week period.

Bereavement is an important risk factor in the elderly. The effect of spousal loss on suicidality appears to be the most pronounced in elderly men. In the United States, the highest suicide rate is among bereaved elderly white men: 84/100,000 (NCHS, 1992). Rates of suicidal ideation are also elevated in elderly with complicated or traumatic grief, which differs from bereavement-related depression and includes PTSD-like symptoms (Szanto et al., 1997).

Although chronic physical illness has been associated with an increased suicide risk in depressed patients (Duggan et al., 1991), depression and not physical illness differentiated elderly suicide completers from non-completers (Conwell et al., 2000). A 1-year follow-up study of psychiatric register cases observed that depressed patients aged 55 years or older had more than twice the rate of suicide (475/100,000) than younger depressed patients (207/100,000) (Gardner et al., 1964). In the 60–90 year old age group, the rates of suicide attempts associated with untreated mood disorders increase with each subsequent decade (Bostwick and Pankratz, 2000). Psychological autopsy studies have found depression to be the most common psychiatric diagnosis in elderly suicide victims, while alcoholism is the most common diagnosis in younger adults (Conwell and Brent, 1996; Dorpat and Ripley, 1960). Conwell and Brent (1996) reported that 76 percent of elderly suicide victims had diagnosable psychopathology, including 54 percent with major depression and 11 percent with minor depression.

Seventy percent or more of elderly suicide victims were seen by their primary care physician within one month from their death (Barraclough et al., 1971; Conwell, 1994; Miller, 1976). Terminal illness needs to be considered when assessing risk factors, particularly in the elderly, although only 2–4 percent of terminally ill elderly complete suicide. Suicidal ideation is rare without depression even in the terminally ill. Untreated or under-treated pain, anticipatory anxiety regarding the progression of medical illness, fear of dependence, and fear of burdening the family are the major contributing factors in the suicidality of elderly with medical illness. Adequate management of chronic pain decreases the request to die among cancer patients (Foley, 1991). When pain and depression are adequately treated, most previously suicidal elderly express a wish to live (Hendin, 1999). In one study, two-thirds of the patients who requested euthanasia changed their minds during a 2-week follow-up period (Hendin, 1999).

Race and Ethnicity

Suicide, like many health outcomes, varies widely across different racial and ethnic groups in the United States (IOM, 2002). Over the last twenty years, when considering all age groups and both sexes, whites and Native Americans have the highest suicide rates, varying from approximately 11 to 14 per 100,000 (NCIPC, 2000). Asian-Pacific Islanders and African-Americans and Hispanics[2] have rates at approximately half—averaging 6.14 to 6.53 per 100,000 across this same time-span (NCIPC, 2000). These differences are even more complex when examined by gender (Figure 2-6), as well as age group. Mining the reasons underlying such differences may hold important information for reducing suicide (Chapter 6). Below we discuss the differences in suicide rates for African Americans and Native Americans in greater detail.

African-Americans

The rate of suicide among African Americans has historically been lower than that of whites, but in young black males the gap has been gradually closing (see Table 2-2; Griffith and Bell, 1989). In fact, the rate of increase in young black males has been a cause for concern. From 1980 to 1995, the suicide rates for black youth ages 10–19 increased from 2.1 to 4.5 per 100,000—an increase of 114 percent. For comparison over the same time, the rates in white males of the same ages increased from 5.4 to 6.4 per 100,000. The suicide rate increased the most for blacks ages 10–14 years (233 percent; CDC, 1998). The convergence of black and white rates was more dramatic with different age groups. For example in 1986 in

---

[2]Data for Hispanic individuals has only been collected since 1990 (NCIPC, 2000).

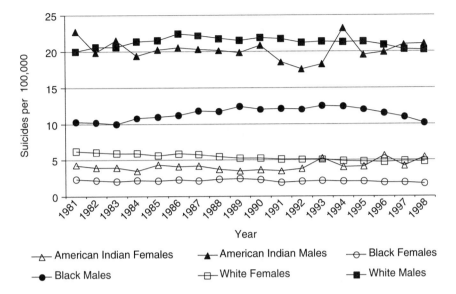

FIGURE 2-6 Suicides Rates by Race and Gender: United States, 1981–1998. Source: NCIPC (2000).

black men 25–34 the rate (20/100,000) was nearly the same as in the same aged white male (26/100,000) (Griffith and Bell, 1989; Hollinger et al., 1994). In 1993 for ages 25–34 the suicide rates for white men was 25.6/100,000 and for black men was 24.0/100,000.

The suicide rates for black women are remarkably low. The suicide rates among black women have held steady at about 2/100,000 for the past two decades (Griffith and Bell, 1989). The difference between black and white women is diminished when suicide attempts, rather than completed suicides are considered. The suicide rate among elderly black men is also strikingly low, in dramatic contrast to elderly white men. For men over 65, the rates are currently approximately 12/100,000 in African Americans compared to 37/100,000 in white men (NCIPC, 2000).

The rising rates among African American males has been noted with considerable concern. As early as 1938, Prudhome (1938) predicted that as Blacks acculturated into White middle class society, their suicide rates would go up. In support of this hypothesis, Clark (1965) noted that the suicide rates in Harlem were half those of New York City rates, but there were three middle class black communities in Harlem where the suicide rates were equal to the city as a whole. Others have suggested that young black men, like elderly white men, feel that society has no place for them (Bell, 1986; Bell and Clark, 1998; Robins et al., 1977).

TABLE 2-2   Suicide Rate per 100,000 for
Young (15–24) Black and White Males

Year	Black	White
1989	16.63	22.48
1990	15.13	23.19
1991	16.43	23.08
1992	17.92	22.68
1993	20.00	23.07
1994	20.53	23.94
1995	17.94	23.34
1996	16.72	20.99
1997	16.00	19.64
1998	14.98	19.28

The statistical analysis using detailed county-level data (as described in Chapter 10 and Appendix A) can be applied to the question of the rise in rate of suicides in young black males. Comparing suicide rates in young white and black males, ages 15–24, from 1989–1998 reveals that the overall suicide rates have been decreasing over the past ten years and that, in 1989, the suicide rate in white males was significantly larger than the suicide rate in black males. However, the rate of young black suicides was increasing relative to young white males over the past 10 years. The increase in young black suicides was largest in 1993 and 1994, but has decreased somewhat since then.

The low rates of suicide among African Americans, especially women, has also been subject to some debate. Spirituality is one of the leading hypotheses regarding the low rates of suicide among black women. This may extend some protection to black males. While almost half the whites believed that suicide is sometimes justified, only one-fifth of blacks did (Robins et al., 1977). Furthermore, fewer whites believe in an after-life. One might also propose that similar to young white males, young black males may have more secular attitudes toward suicide and an after-life, but these attitudes change with age as black men mature. Another suggestion put forward (Comer, 1973) is that black women's connections to community institutions such as the black church would protect black women from suicide. In fact, two-thirds of the African-American respondents to a National Mental Health Association (NMHA) survey on attitudes and beliefs about depression reported that they believed prayer and faith alone will successfully treat depression "almost all of the time" or "some of the time" (NMHA, 2000).

Since mental illness is a risk factor for suicide (see Chapter 3), the high prevalence of mental disorders among African-Americans compared with

Whites must be considered. In the Epidemiologic Catchment Area study (ECA) of the 1980s, African Americans had higher levels of any lifetime or current disorder than whites (Robins and Regier, 1991). This was true both over the respondent's lifetime (Robins and Regier, 1991) and over the past month (Regier et al., 1993). When the ECA study and the more recent National Comorbidity Survey (NCS) (Kessler et al., 1994) took into account differences in age, gender, marital status, and socioeconomic status, the black–white difference was eliminated.

The impact of these findings on suicide is difficult to discern, especially in light of the findings of the NMHA (2000) survey on attitudes and beliefs about depression in the African-American community. This survey revealed that the majority think depression is a "personal weakness" and only a third (compared to 69% of the general population) recognize depression as a "health problem" for which they would be willing to take prescribed medication. For further discussion of these issues, see Chapter 6, and the sections in Chapter 7 on faith-based interventions, and Chapter 9 on barriers to treatment.

Native Americans[3] and Alaska Natives

The rate of suicide among Indians and Alaska Natives of the United States is about 1.7 times the rate of the nation as a whole (Indian Health Service, 1999). Between 1975 and 1977 the rates peaked at 22.5/100,000 and decreased to a low of 16.0 in 1984 through 1986. Since then it increased to its current rate of 19.3 per 100,000 in 1995 (Indian Health Service, 1999). In contrast, over the past 40 years, rates of violence have generally declined for American Indians (Hisnanick, 1994). Suicide takes a significant toll.

As illustrated in Figure 2-6, suicide deaths for American Indian males are substantially higher overall than for other ethnic groups. They also show a different pattern across the life-span. For ages 5 through 14 the suicide rate is three times higher for Indian males than the general population, ages 15 through 34 years it is 2.5 times higher, and for ages 35 through 44 years it is 1.5 times higher (Indian Health Service, 1999). The male rate peaks at 67 per 100,000 in ages 25–34, and is somewhat lower for the next youngest age group (15–24) at 54 per 100,000. However, by age 45 Indian males complete suicide at a rate that is approximately the same as

---

[3]The term American Indian is used throughout this manuscript to denote those residents of the United States and Canada who belong to ethnic groups indigenous to North America (prior to 1492). This is the general term preferred by many Natives in the United States, when it is not possible to denote specific tribal affiliation.

males in the general population. Over the age of 55 the rate declines dramatically to half that of general population males. For Indian and Alaska Native males, the risk is highest in the young years but tapers off substantially in the older years, the very years when white males most commonly complete suicide.

Young Indian females (5–34) have rates of suicide that are 2.2 to 3.6 times higher than females in the general population. For example, for ages 15–24 the rate is 11/100,000. However, by 35 through 44 years, the rate is 1.5 times the general population, and 45 years to 75 years is approximately the same as or slightly less than the general female population. At 55–75, the rate is 5/100,000. American Indian women 75 years of age and older do not complete suicide with any measurable frequency. Therefore, while Indian and Alaska Native females have substantially lower rates than Indian and Alaska Native males, their rates are higher than other women in the country until age 44, and then they are approximately the same until age 75, when suicides no longer occur (Indian Health Service, 1999).

The decrease in Indian suicide during the early 1980s has been attributed to the changing denominators in the United States, stemming from better enumeration of Indians in Census data and an increased tendency for self-identification as Indian or Native. But the more stable and easily-monitored data from the State of New Mexico, where neither of these phenomena have occurred over the same time period, has also shown a definite and similar reduction in incidence of suicide among Indians. Among the three major Indian cultural groups (the Navajo, Pueblo, and Apache) in the late 1980s, a substantial drop occurred and a leveling of rates was evident in the 1990s (New Mexico Vital Records and Health Statistics, 2000; VanWinkle and May, 1993). In fact, the aggregate rates for the nineteen Pueblo Indian tribes have continued to drop throughout the 1990s (VanWinkle and Williams, 2001).

Among American Indian and Alaska Native suicide, gunshot wounds, hanging, and other violent means predominate (Wallace et al., 1996). American Indians also have high rates of other violent deaths including motor vehicle crashes (Guerin, 1991; Guerin, 1998; Jarvis and Boldt, 1982; Katz and May, 1979; May, 1989), a small percentage of which are believed to be covert suicides (Hackenberg and Gallagher, 1972; May, 1987; Stull, 1972; Stull, 1973; Stull, 1977; Wills, 1969). In studies of Alaska Natives, firearms have been the predominant method of suicide at 75 to 85 percent (Forbes and Van Der Hyde, 1988; Hlady and Middaugh, 1988; Kost-Grant, 1983), as in studies of the American Plains, and 55 percent in the American Southwest during the same period (Shuck et al., 1980; VanWinkle and May, 1986; VanWinkle and May, 1993). In Canada the same pattern prevails where firearms account for 55 to 82 percent (Butler,

1965; Garro, 1988; Jarvis and Boldt, 1982; Spaulding, 1985–1986). Hanging is the second most common cause of suicidal death among Indians and Alaska Natives in most studies in most areas of the continent (Kraus, 1974; Wallace et al., 1996; Wissow, 2000). The range is great, with hanging accounting for an unusually low 7 percent in one study to a more usual 26–40 percent in others (Butler, 1965; Garro, 1988; Spaulding, 1985–1986; VanWinkle and May, 1993). In a state like New Mexico, suicide by fire-arms and hanging combined account for over 90 percent of all American Indian suicides (VanWinkle and May, 1993).

Social and familial disruption, cultural conflict, and social disorgani-zation are often cited as major influences on American Indian suicide rates. Suicide rates among American Indians vary with the degree of social and cultural change and acculturation pressure (Garro, 1988; Levy, 1965; VanWinkle and May, 1986; 1993). The high suicide rates among youth in Indian families and communities have been attributed to acute acculturation stress (Levy, 1965; May and Dizmang, 1974; Spaulding, 1985–1986; Travis, 1984; VanWinkle and May, 1986; 1993), cultural con-flict (Kahn, 1982; Kettl and Bixler, 1991; Opler, 1969; Patterson, 1969) and social disorganization (EchoHawk, 1997; Expert Working Group, 1994; Joe, 2001; Resnik and Dizmang, 1971). While American Indian and Alaska Native adolescents face the same turmoil as mainstream youth, they are also challenged by self-identity and actualization in their minority status and complex choices as to whether to adhere to mainstream or tradi-tional, native culture (Bechtold, 1994; Howard-Pitney et al., 1992; Sack et al., 1994; U.S. Congress, 1990). The stress of these dilemmas can increase the risk of alcohol or drug abuse, depression or other psychopathology, and parasuicidal and suicidal behavior (Beauvais, 1998; Elliot et al., 1990; Kettl and Bixler, 1993; Manson et al., 1989; May, 1982; Norton et al., 1995; Prince, 1988; Sack et al., 1994).

Immigrants and Refugees

Between 1980 and 1991 the United States immigrant population tripled; almost 20 million immigrants resided in the United States in 1990. Suicide in immigrants is a public health concern because this population is subject to many sociocultural risk factors. Immigration also provides opportunities to study the impact of culture and environment on preva-lence of mental illness and suicide. In general, suicide rates tend to reflect that of the country of origin, with convergence toward that of the host country over time (Singh and Siahpush, 2001).

A careful review of the data on immigrants reveals some interesting patterns, which may differ across nations. Higher suicide rates have been reported for immigrants to some countries. For example, Finnish immigrants in Sweden had a higher rate of suicide (similar to that in Finland) than native-born Swedes and other immigrants. Social isolation and low social class acted as confounding factors, although they do not completely account for the increased rates (Ferrada-Noli et al., 1995). A comparison of suicide rates in high- and low-income areas of Stockholm county revealed the highest suicide rates in the low-income areas, regardless of ethnicity, though low-income immigrants still completed suicide at higher rates (Ferrada-Noli and Asberg, 1997). In contrast, immigrants to the United State have lower or comparable rates to native-born individuals. In their review of death certificates from 1970 to 1992 in California for 15–34 year olds, Sorenson and Shen (1996) found that although foreign-born individuals had significantly higher rates of homicide deaths, they had fewer suicides. This study did not control for demographic variables, however. Singh and Siapush (2001) reviewed national death certificate data investigating all-cause and cause-specific mortality of foreign-born versus native-born in the United States, controlling for the demographic factors sex, race/ethnicity, age, income, and education. They found that foreign-born males had 52 percent *lower* suicide rate than U.S.-born males when demographic variables were controlled. On the other hand, demographically adjusted suicide rates for foreign-born females did not significantly differ from that of native-born U.S. females. While some studies in Britain and Australia found a similar concordance of foreign- versus native-born suicide rates in women (e.g., Morrell et al., 1999), others have found increased suicides and suicide attempts in female immigrants compared to their male counterparts or to native-born females (Merrill and Owens, 1988; Patel and Gaw, 1996).

Research on immigration and suicide has initiated contextual psychological studies on the stresses of immigration as related to suicidality. These studies all involved immigrants to the United States unless otherwise noted. Hovey and King (1997) for example, expanded previous models of acculturation (i.e., Williams and Berry, 1991) to include the development of depression and suicidality. Aspects of acculturative stress include disrupted social support and family support networks, low education and income, lack of knowledge of the language and culture of the new country, motives for immigrating, spiritual beliefs, tolerance of the host country toward immigrants, and positive or negative views of the acculturative process itself. Studies of various Hispanic and Asian immigrant groups demonstrate that lack of English skills predicts distress, depression, and suicidal ideation among immigrants, sometimes over and above the effects of pre-arrival trauma (Hinton et al., 1997; Hovey, 2000a; Hovey, 2000b). Spiritual beliefs, social support, and marital status, protective factors and processes (see Chapter 6), appear to buffer the effects of acculturation stress on suicidality both in the United States (Hovey, 1999) and in Israel (Hinton et al., 1997; Hovey, 2000b; Ponizovsky et al., 1997). Disagreement with the decision to migrate and expectations for the future have predicted depression and sucidial ideation in samples of Hispanic immigrants (Hovey, 2000a; 2000b).

Guarnaccia and Lopez (1998) note that since children do not wield the power to decide whether to migrate, those children with refugee experiences and those whose families evidence significant migratory stress likely represent a particularly vulnerable group. In corroboration, Tousignant and colleagues (1999) note that familial variables such as father's long-term *un*employment after migration correlates with youth psychopathology. Two recent reports from the National Academies (NRC 1998; 1999) provide in-depth analyses of the physical and mental health of immigrant children in the United States.

Refugee status among immigrants is often associated with trauma. Recent Southeast Asian and Central American immigrants represent refugee populations with high prevalence of trauma exposure who have increasingly immigrated to the U.S. (Holman et al., 2000; Hovey, 2000a; O'Hare and Van Tran, 1998). While various studies show Mexican-born and overall numbers of Asian-born immigrants attempt and complete suicide less frequently than their American-born peers (Shiang et al., 1997; Sorenson and Golding, 1988; Sorenson and Shen, 1996), studies have not differentiated between suicide rates of Central American versus other Hispanic or Southeast Asian versus other Asian immigrants. Some studies document higher rates of Posttraumatic Stress Disorder (PTSD), depression, and anxiety in these sub-groups (Hinton et al., 1997; Hovey, 2000a). Given the relationship between such disorders and suicide (see Chapter 3), studying suicidality in these populations is likely pertinent.

Incarcerated Populations

Suicide rates for jail inmates are 9 times greater than that of the general population (Hayes, 1989) and 15 times higher for men alone. For example, in county jail rates are 107 per 100,000. Most suicide victims in jails of all types and sizes (e.g., rural and urban county jails, city jails, and police department lock-ups) are young white males arrested for non-violent offenses and intoxicated upon arrest (Hayes, 1998). Suicide was usually by hanging within 24 hours of incarceration (Hayes, 1989). Patterns in prisons were similar but considerably lower than in jails, about 1.5 times higher than in the general population (Anno, 1985; Anno, 1991).

The reasons for the higher rate of suicide in jails and prisons are unclear. However, mental illness, a strong risk factor for suicide (see Chapter 3), is prevalent in correctional facilities.

Studies in jails and prisons estimate that between 6 and 15 percent of the population have serious and persistent mental illnesses (Bland et al., 1990; Brooke et al., 1996; Jemelka et al., 1989; Manderscheid and Sonnenschein, 1999; Morrissey et al., 1993; National Commission on Correctional Health Care, 2000; Steadman et al., 1987; Taylor and Gunn, 1984; Veysey and Bichler-Robertson, 1999). In jails, prevalence rates of mental illness are two to three times higher than those in the general population (Teplin, 1990). In prison, with the longer terms, nearly 10 percent of state prison inmates received some form of mental health counseling or psychotherapy from a physician, nurse, psychologist, or social worker (Morrissey et al., 1993). State and federal prisons have a minimum of 13 percent who will require psychiatric care for an acute episode of serious mental illness at some time during their incarceration (National Commission on Correctional Health Care, 2000).

In addition, more than 30 percent of male mentally ill inmates and 78 percent of females reported prior physical or sexual abuse (Ditton, 1999), another risk factor for suicide (see Chapter 5). Mentally ill in correctional facilities are more likely than other offenders to have a higher prevalence of homelessness, unemployment, alcohol and drug abuse, and physical and sexual abuse before their current incarceration (US DHHS, 2001). These risk factors are likely to contribute to the prevalence of suicide among those incarcerated.

Occupations at Risk

Several professions (e.g. police, doctors, dentists) have been noted as having suicide rates that are higher than the population averages. These assessments, however, are confounded by demographic variables including age, sex, socioeconomic class and marital status, all of which affect suicide rates independently from occupation (Stack, 2001). For example, suicide rates for elementary school teachers are 44 percent lower than the general population, but this difference is not significant when controlling for gender (Stack, 2001).

Models of occupation's influence on suicidality propose stressors and access to lethal means as the causal variables. Stressors includes level of prestige and dependency on a client base (e.g., Labovitz and Hagedorn, 1971). Holding infrequent roles, such as female chemists and soldiers, or other rare roles, appears to increase suicide rates, as well (Bedeian, 1982; Seiden and Gleiser, 1990; Stack, 1995). Studies regarding the effect of availability of lethal means such as firearms or lethal drugs on suicide rates for certain occupations have found inconsistent results, though the evidence is stronger for medical professions (see Stack, 2001 review).

Higher rates of suicide are more frequent in occupations of lower prestige, class, and salary (Boxer et al., 1995). When demographic factors of race, gender, age, and, particularly, marital status are controlled, this relationship between manual labor occupations and suicide does not remain significant (Charlton, 1995; Stack, 2001). In fact, Stack's (2001) recent study found that clerks are 15 percent and farm workers 30 percent *less* likely to complete suicide after controlling for demographic variables.

A population-based study from Denmark examining the income-suicide relationship suggests that for higher income/occupational level, hospital admission for serious mental illness may be associated with greater suicide risk (Agerbo et al., 2001). These investigators speculate that those in prestigious occupations may face greater stigma, and may have greater illness severity before hospital admittance due to delaying treatment. A smaller study in the United States found similar results with high education level (Martin et al., 1985). A large, prospective Finnish study found fewer violent suicides and greater admissions for psychoses among those in higher occupational levels (Koskinen et al., in press).

Health professions carry increased suicide risk independently from demographic factors. Adjusted odds ratios for suicide have been calculated as 5.4 for dentists, 2.3 for physicians, and 1.6 for nurses (Stack, 2001). The reasons for high suicide risk within medical professions remain unclear; these occupations are largely client-dependent and afford easy access to lethal methods. Mathematicians and scientists, artists, and social workers also appear to experience occupation-related increased suicide risk (Stack, 2001).

The police force has often been cited as at higher risk for suicide, but closer examination reveals inconsistent results. A few controlled studies (e.g., Schmidtke et al., 1999) show moderately increased suicide rates for police that vary according to region and across time (Hem et al., 2001). Violanti and colleagues (1998) conducted a cohort mortality survey from 1950 to 1990 and found higher than expected mortality rates among male officers for all-cause mortality, including suicide. When compared to other working-age men, as opposed to the general population, however, police appear to have only a slightly increased suicide risk (Burnett et al., 1992; Hem et al., 2001; Stack and Kelly, 1994).

Sexual Orientation

Fewer than 5 percent of adults in the United States identify themselves as homosexual or bisexual (Michaels, 1996). This population faces societal stigma, discrimination, and violence victimization, among other stressors (Faulkner and Cranston, 1998; Herek, 1996; Hershberger and

D'Augelli, 1995). Awareness of their exposure to stressful events has spawned a growing research literature on whether they face an increased risk of suicidality.

Young homosexual or bisexual males are at greater risk than heterosexuals for suicide *attempts*, but findings are less clear regarding suicide *completion* (McDaniel et al., 2001). According to two population-based studies in San Diego (Rich et al., 1986a) and New York City (Shaffer et al., 1995), rates of suicide completion do not appear to be higher for gay men and lesbians than for heterosexuals. These two studies were the first psychological autopsy studies to assess retrospectively the sexual orientation of those who completed suicide. Such assessment can be inaccurate because individuals may conceal their sexual orientation and because baseline prevalence for homosexuality in the relevant comparison population is difficult to obtain. A recent review of these studies determined that firm conclusions were unwarranted (McDaniel et al., 2001).

For suicide attempts, several recent population- and school-based studies provide strong support for a relationship between sexual orientation and suicidal behavior in males. Population-based studies of homosexual or bisexual males (ages 18 to 40 or so) found them to be 5–14 times more likely than heterosexual males to have reported a suicide attempt (Bagley and Tremblay, 1997; Cochran and Mays, 2000). Similarly, five studies of high school students in several states found elevated rates of suicide attempts among males engaging in same-sex behavior compared to their heterosexual peers (DuRant et al., 1998; Faulkner and Cranston, 1998; Garofalo et al., 1998; Garofalo et al., 1999; Remafedi et al., 1998), with relative risk calculated at 2- to 5-fold. Strikingly, most of the school-based studies among gay or bisexual adolescents found about 30 percent had attempted suicide. In young adult and middle-aged homosexuals, the prevalence is lower but still significantly elevated compared to controls (Cochran and Mays, 2000; Herrell et al., 1999).

Most studies on suicidality in homosexuals document the elevation of risk in young males (McDaniel et al., 2001), not young females. This contrasts with the general population, in which female teenagers and young adults attempt suicide more frequently than do males. The reasons for this reversal are not well understood (McDaniel et al., 2001). However, a recent nationally representative study (Russell and Joyner, 2001) of adolescents found increased risk for suicide ideation and attempts for *both* males and females when factors such as depression, hopelessness, and substance use were controlled. The authors speculate this difference may have arisen because the study measured self-reported same-sex romantic attraction/relationships, not self-identification as gay or lesbian.

Several studies explored the reasons behind the elevated risk of suicidality in homosexual or bisexual men. A longitudinal study of children from New Zealand (birth to age 21) found that gay, lesbian, and bisexual youth had higher risk not only of suicidal behavior, but also of depression, anxiety, substance abuse. The increased risk was greatest (a 6-fold increase) for suicide behavior and having multiple mental disorders (Fergusson et al., 1999). Harrell et al. (1999) used a co-twin control method to assess suicidality in relation to sexual orientation. They found that middle-aged male twins reporting same-gender sexual orientation were at higher risk for several lifetime measures of suicidality. The strong association could not be explained by abuse of alcohol and other substances, by depressive symptoms, or by unmeasured genetic and familial factors. The contribution of unique risk factors such as disclosure of sexual orientation to friends and family (McDaniel et al., 2001) remains to be fully assessed.

LIMITATIONS OF DATA

Official suicide rates capture completed suicides only. They have been used to chart trends in suicide, monitor the impact of change in legislation, treatment policies, and social change, and to compare suicides across regions, both within and across countries. In addition, suicide rates have offered a way to assess risk and protective factors for geographical areas (counties, states, and countries). However, official suicide statistics are fraught with inaccuracies. Undetermined cases and open verdicts and under-reporting limit their strength. The methodological weaknesses and promising approaches to resolve them are discussed more fully in Chapter 10. In brief, there are four primary sources of variability in suicide statistics (Jobes et al., 1987; O'Carroll, 1989). First, there are regional differences in the definition of suicide and in how ambiguous cases are classified. Legally a classification of suicide requires that it be beyond a reasonable doubt (O'Donnell and Farmer, 1995). Second, there are regional differences in the training and background of the coroner or medical examiner. Third, there are differences in terms of the extent to which cases are investigated. Fourth, there are sources of variability that have to do with the quality of data management involved in preparing official statistics. In fact, in many developing countries, suicide statistics are imputed, rather than based on actual death registries (Kleinman, 2001). This is discussed further in Chapter 6.

COST TO SOCIETY

The emotional cost of suicide is severe, and for family and friends of suicide victims, the personal loss is paramount. There is an additional economic cost that society incurs with these untimely deaths. The economic[4] cost of suicide encompasses four factors. (1) Medical expenses of emergency intervention and non-emergency treatment for suicidality. These medical costs are not borne by the health care industry alone, but by all of society through higher health care costs that are ultimately passed on to workers and taxpayers. (2) The lost and/or reduced productivity of people suffering from suicidality. (3) The lost productivity of the loved ones' grieving a suicide. (4) Lost wages of those completing suicide, with the greatest absolute numbers of suicides occurring before retirement. Even if the analysis is restricted to the estimate of lost wages of suicide victims, the financial impact of suicide is enormous. By doing this analysis, the Committee found that for suicide in 1998 alone, **the value of lost productivity was calculated to be $11.8 billion** (in 1998 dollars). The basis of this analysis is described below.

Lost productivity was defined as the discounted present value of expected future age-, sex- and race-specific earnings. The average annual earnings by age, race/origin, and sex were estimated from the March 1998 supplement to the Current Population Survey (Bureau of Labor Statistics, 1998). The Current Population Survey (CPS) is a monthly survey of about 50,000 households conducted by the Bureau of the Census for the Bureau of Labor Statistics. The March supplement CPS contains detailed information on income and work experience in the United States. In constructing our estimates of average annual earnings, we did not weight observations by their probability of being sampled for the CPS. This should not have much impact on the representativeness of our estimates, except in cases where there were a very small number of observations in a stratum (e.g., the average annual earnings of female Asian/Pacific Islanders, 85 years old and over was based on seven observations in this stratum). Even in such cases, the lack of sample weighting in estimating earnings is not likely to have a meaningful influence on the overall estimate of lost productivity due to suicide. Average annual earnings were estimated for the mid-point age of each of seven age intervals: 15–24 years old, 25–34, 35–44, 45–54, 55–64, 65–74, 75–84, and 85 and over. In addition, it should be noted that this estimate using the cross-sectional perspective probably underestimates the real economic loss from suicide for two reasons. First, real wages are likely to rise over time. Second the non-market productivity of older persons (for example in caring for a disabled spouse) has also not been included in this analysis of the cost of suicide.

We used five mutually exclusive categories of race/ethnicity: white non-Hispanic, black-non-Hispanic, American Indian/Aleutian/Eskimo

---

[4]It is noted that a common estimate of the monetary value of lost life is how much people are willing to pay to extend their lives. Such an analysis was not undertaken here, in part because the intent to die in suicide complicates the assumption in such an analysis.

non-Hispanic, Asian/Pacific Islander non-Hispanic, and Hispanic of any race. Next, we estimated the present value of future earnings by discounting and summing the stream of expected annual earnings. Race- and sex-adjusted life expectancy at the mid-point of each age interval was taken from the 1998 U.S. Life Tables (Anderson, 2001). This method of estimating future earnings is based on a cross-sectional perspective, rather than a longitudinal birth cohort perspective. For example, the 1998 earnings of a 60 year old black man are used to estimate the annual earnings of a 50 year old black man 10 years later. Future earnings were discounted at an annual rate of 3 percent to yield their present values. This is based on the real value of the short-term United States T-bill, in an effort to approximate the risk-free time-value of money.

To estimate the total lost earnings due to suicide, we multiplied the number of suicides in each age/sex/race group (data from the National Center of Disease Control's WISQARS™, Web-based Injury Statistics Query and Reporting System) in 1998 by age-, sex-, race-specific estimated future earnings and summed across groups. As described above, the cost of lost earnings from suicide in just the one year (1998) was calculated to be $11.8 billion.

A similar analysis was done for suicides in New Brunswick, Canada, during 1996 (Clayton and Barcelo, 1999). The direct costs (health care services, autopsies, funerals, and police investigations) for the 94 reported suicides came to $535,158. Indirect costs, which include the lost productivity, came to $79,353,354 for a mean total cost per suicide death in 1996 of $849,878. For 30,000 deaths each year, this totals about 25 billion dollars.

Although the issue can be raised that any premature death (e.g., from smoking) can save society money (Viscusi, 1995), the Committee decided not to even broach this argument, considering it contrary to the goals of public health and morally unacceptable.

FINDINGS

• Suicide rates vary widely across demographic groups. African Americans have had significantly lower rates historically than whites despite higher incidence of major risk factors. The rates of completed suicide are particularly low among African American women. In contrast, the suicide rates among Native Americans have been and continue to be extremely high. Older white males have the highest rate in the United States. Males have higher rates across the globe except in rural China where women complete suicide at a higher rate.

• The suicide rate in the United States has remained relatively unchanged for the last 50 years. The rate for youth in the United States, however, has been increasing. While the rates in African American adolescents has increased through the 1990s, the rates appear to have leveled off.

• The differences in suicide rates among ethnic groups in the United States, among immigrant populations, and among countries throughout the world point to the influence of social and cultural factors. Risk factors vary in their importance for different groups. Youth suicide is more highly associated with impulsiveness than for other age groups. On the other hand, older persons are at greater risk for completing suicide because of the seriousness of the intent and social isolation.

> Studies of the differences in the risk of suicide among populations can enhance our understanding of the impact of risk and protective factors. This is best accomplished by collection of specific data from well defined and characterized populations whose community level social descriptions are well known, which would allow the integration of population-based approaches with studies of individual characteristics.

• Suicide rates vary across geographic region. Rates are lower in more densely populated areas around the world. When rates within the United States are analyzed county by county, striking variations in some adjacent counties are revealed. This approach bridges traditional sociological and anthropological studies that use ecological data and case-controlled approaches that examine individual risk factors for suicide.

> Future studies could identify social factors that differ between two communities that are adjacent, or otherwise similar, but have dramatically different suicide rates. This approach could provide more precise assessments of the roles of social factors in suicide including public health issues such as access to and the quality of health care.

• Costs to Society: The annual cost of lost productivity due to suicide deaths was calculated to be $11.8 billion (in 1998 dollars). This does not include medical care costs, or costs incurred by loss of productivity of either those suffering from suicidality or the close family and friends of a suicide victim.

REFERENCES

Agerbo E, Mortensen PB, Eriksson T, Qin P, Westergaard-Nielsen N. 2001. Risk of suicide in relation to income level in people admitted to hospital with mental illness: Nested case-control study. *British Medical Journal*, 322(7282): 334-335.

Anderson RN. 2001. United States Life Tables, 1998. *National Vital Statistics Report*, 48(18): 1-40.

Anno BJ. 1985. Patterns of suicide in the Texas Department of Corrections, 1980-1985. *Journal of Prison and Jail Health*, 2: 82-93.

Anno BJ. 1991. *Prison Health Care: Guidelines for the Management of an Adequate Delivery System*. Washington, DC: U.S. Department of Justice, Department of Corrections.

Asgard U. 1990. A psychiatric study of suicide among urban Swedish women. *Acta Psychiatrica Scandinavica*, 82(2): 115-124.

Bagley C, Tremblay P. 1997. Suicide behaviors in homosexual and bisexual males. *Crisis*, 18(1): 24-34.

Barraclough B, Bunch J, Nelson B, Sainsbury P. 1974. A hundred cases of suicide: Clinical aspects. *British Journal of Psychiatry*, 125: 355-373.

Barraclough BM, Nelson B, Bunch J, Sainsbury P. 1971. Suicide and barbiturate prescribing. *Journal of the Royal College of General Practitioners*, 21(112): 645-653.

Beautrais AL. 2000. Risk factors for suicide and attempted suicide among young people. *Australian and New Zealand Journal of Psychiatry*, 34(3): 420-436.

Beauvais F. 1998. American Indians and alcohol. *Alcohol Health and Research World*, 22(4): 253-259.

Bechtold DW. 1994. Indian adolescent suicide: Clinical and developmental considerations. *American Indian and Alaska Native Mental Health Research Monograph Series*, 4: 71-80.

Bedeian AG. 1982. Suicide and occupation: A review. *Journal of Vocational Behavior*, 21(2): 206-223.

Bell CC. 1986. Impaired black health professionals: Vulnerabilities and treatment approaches. *Journal of the National Medical Association*, 78(10): 925-930.

Bell CC, Clark DC. 1998. Adolescent suicide. *Pediatric Clinics of North America*, 45(2): 365-380.

Beratis S. 1991. Suicide among adolescents in Greece. *British Journal of Psychiatry*, 159: 515-519.

Birckmayer J, Hemenway D. 2001. Suicide and firearm prevalence: Are youth disproportionately affected? *Suicide and Life-Threatening Behavior*, 31(3): 303-310.

Bland RC, Newman SC, Dyck RJ, Orn H. 1990. Prevalence of psychiatric disorders and suicide attempts in a prison population. *Canadian Journal of Psychiatry*, 35(5): 407-413.

Bostwick JM, Pankratz VS. 2000. Affective disorders and suicide risk: A reexamination. *American Journal of Psychiatry*, 157(12): 1925-1932.

Boxer PA, Burnett C, Swanson N. 1995. Suicide and occupation: A review of the literature. *Journal of Occupational and Environmental Medicine*, 37(4): 442-452.

Brent DA, Baugher M, Bridge J, Chen T, Chiappetta L. 1999. Age- and sex-related risk factors for adolescent suicide. *Journal of the American Academy of Child and Adolescent Psychiatry*, 38(12): 1497-1505.

Brent DA, Perper JA, Allman CJ. 1987. Alcohol, firearms, and suicide among youth: Temporal trends in Allegheny County, Pennsylvania, 1960 to 1983. *Journal of the American Medical Association*, 257(24): 3369-3372.

Brent DA, Perper JA, Moritz G, Baugher M, Schweers J, Roth C. 1993. Firearms and adolescent suicide. A community case-control study. *American Journal of Diseases of Children*, 147(10): 1066-1071.

Brooke D, Taylor C, Gunn J, Maden A. 1996. Point prevalence of mental disorder in unconvicted male prisoners in England and Wales. *British Medical Journal*, 313(7071): 1524-1527.

Bureau of Justice Statistics, U.S. Department of Justice. 2001. *Homicide Victimization, 1950–1999*. [Online]. Available: http://www.ojp.usdoj.gov/bjs/ [accessed October 12, 2001].

Bureau of Labor Statistics, U.S. Department of Labor and Bureau of the Census, U.S. Department of Commerce. 1998. *Current Population Survey, Annual Demographic Supplement*.

Bureau of the Census. 1976. *Historical Statistics of the United States: Colonial Times to 1970, Part 1.* Washington, DC: U.S. Department of Commerce.

Burnett C, Boxer P, Swanson N. 1992. *Suicide and Occupation: Is There a Relationship?* Cincinnati, OH: National Institute for Occupational Safety and Health.

Butler GC. 1965. Incidence of suicide among ethnic groups of the Northwest Territories and Yukon Territory. *Medical Services Journal of Canada*, 21(4): 252-256.

CDC (Centers for Disease Control and Prevention). 1998. Suicide among black youths— United States, 1980–1995. *Morbidity and Mortality Weekly Report*, 47(10): 193-196.

Charlton J. 1995. Trends and patterns in suicide in England and Wales. *International Journal of Epidemiology*, 24 (Suppl 1): S45-S52.

Clark K. 1965. *Dark Ghetto.* New York: Harper and Row.

Clayton D, Barcelo A. 1999. The cost of suicide mortality in New Brunswick, 1996. *Chronic Diseases in Canada*, 20: 89-95.

Cochran SD, Mays VM. 2000. Lifetime prevalence of suicide symptoms and affective disorders among men reporting same-sex sexual partners: Results from NHANES III. *American Journal of Public Health*, 90(4): 573-578.

Comer JP. 1973. Black suicide: A hidden crisis. *Urban Health*, 2: 41-44.

Conwell Y. 1994. Suicide in elderly patients. In: Schneider LS, Reynolds CFIII, Lebowitz BD, Friedhoff AJ, Editors. *Diagnosis and Treatment of Depression in Late Life: Results of the NIH Consensus Development Conference.* (pp. 397-418). Washington, DC: American Psychiatric Press.

Conwell Y, Brent D. 1996. Suicide and aging I: Patterns of psychiatric diagnosis. In: Pearson JL, Conwell Y, Editors. *Suicide and Aging: International Perspectives.* (pp. 15-30). New York: Springer Publishing.

Conwell Y, Lyness JM, Duberstein P, Cox C, Seidlitz L, DiGiorgio A, Caine ED. 2000. Completed suicide among older patients in primary care practices: A controlled study. *Journal of the American Geriatrics Society*, 48: 23-29.

Ditton PM. 1999. *Mental Health and Treatment of Inmates and Probationers.* NCJ 174463. Washington, DC: U.S. Department of Justice, Office of Justice Programs, Bureau of Justice Statistics.

Dorpat TL, Ripley HS. 1960. A study of suicide in the Seattle area. *Comprehensive Psychiatry*, 1: 349-359.

Draper B. 1994. Suicidal behaviors in the elderly. *International Journal of Geriatric Psychiatry*, 8: 655-661.

Duggan CF, Sham P, Lee AS, Murray RM. 1991. Can future suicidal behaviour in depressed patients be predicted? *Journal of Affective Disorders*, 22(3): 111-118.

DuRant RH, Krowchuk DP, Sinal SH. 1998. Victimization, use of violence, and drug use at school among male adolescents who engage in same-sex sexual behavior. *Journal of Pediatrics*, 133(1): 113-118.

EchoHawk M. 1997. Suicide: The scourge of Native American people. *Suicide and Life-Threatening Behavior*, 27(1): 60-67.

Elliot CA, Kral MJ, Wilson KG. 1990. Suicidal concerns among native youth. In: Lester D, Editor. *Suicide '90: Proceedings of the 23rd Annual Meeting of the American Association of Suicidology.* (pp. 283-285). Denver, Colorado: American Association of Suicidology.

Expert Working Group. 1994. *Suicide in Canada: Update of the Report of the Task Force on Suicide in Canada.* Ottawa: Minister of National Health and Welfare.

Farberow NL. 1980. Indirect self-destructive behavior: Classification and characteristics. In: Farberow NL, Editor. *The Many Faces of Suicide: Indirect Self-Destructive Behavior.* (pp. 15-27). New York: McGraw-Hill.

Faulkner AH, Cranston K. 1998. Correlates of same-sex sexual behavior in a random sample of Massachusetts high school students. *American Journal of Public Health*, 88(2): 262-266.

Fergusson DM, Horwood LJ, Beautrais AL. 1999. Is sexual orientation related to mental health problems and suicidality in young people? *Archives of General Psychiatry*, 56(10): 876-880.

Ferrada-Noli M, Asberg M. 1997. Psychiatric health, ethnicity and socioeconomic factors among suicides in Stockholm. *Psychological Reports*, 81(1): 323-332.

Ferrada-Noli M, Asberg M, Ormstad K, Nordstrom P. 1995. Definite and undetermined forensic diagnoses of suicide among immigrants in Sweden. *Acta Psychiatrica Scandinavica*, 91(2): 130-135.

Foley KM. 1991. The relationship of pain and symptom management to patient requests for physician-assisted suicide. *Journal of Pain and Symptom Management*, 6(5): 289-297.

Forbes N, Van Der Hyde V. 1988. Suicide in Alaska from 1978 to 1985: Updated data from state files. *American Indian and Alaska Native Mental Health Research*, 1(3): 36-55.

Fortney J, Rost K, Zhang M, Warren J. 1999. The impact of geographic accessibility on the intensity and quality of depression treatment. *Medical Care*, 37(9): 884-893.

Gardner EA, Bahn AK, Mack M. 1964. Suicide and psychiatric care in the aging. *Archives of General Psychiatry*, 10(6): 547-553.

Garofalo R, Wolf RC, Kessel S, Palfrey SJ, DuRant RH. 1998. The association between health risk behaviors and sexual orientation among a school-based sample of adolescents. *Pediatrics*, 101(5): 895-902.

Garofalo R, Wolf RC, Wissow LS, Woods ER, Goodman E. 1999. Sexual orientation and risk of suicide attempts among a representative sample of youth. *Archives of Pediatrics and Adolescent Medicine*, 153(5): 487-493.

Garro LC. 1988. Suicides by status Indians in Manitoba. *Arctic Medical Research*, 47 (Suppl 1): 590-592.

Gould MS, Fisher P, Parides M, Flory M, Shaffer D. 1996. Psychosocial risk factors of child and adolescent completed suicide. *Archives of General Psychiatry*, 53(12): 1155-1162.

Gould MS, Shaffer D. 1986. The impact of suicide in television movies. Evidence of imitation. *New England Journal of Medicine*, 315(11): 690-694.

Gould MS, Wallenstein S, Kleinman M. 1990. Time-space clustering of teenage suicide. *American Journal of Epidemiology*, 131(1): 71-78.

Griffith EEH, Bell CC. 1989. Recent trends in suicide and homicide among blacks. *Journal of the American Medical Association*, 262(16): 2265-2269.

Groholt B, Ekeberg O, Wichstrom L, Haldorsen T. 1998. Suicide among children and younger and older adolescents in Norway: A comparative study. *Journal of the American Academy of Child and Adolescent Psychiatry*, 37(5): 473-481.

Guarnaccia PJ, Lopez S. 1998. The mental health and adjustment of immigrant and refugee children. *Child and Adolescent Psychiatric Clinics of North America*, 7(3): 537-553, viii-ix.

Guerin PE. 1991. *Alcohol-Related Traffic Fatalities in New Mexico*. Masters Thesis, Department of Sociology, University of New Mexico.

Guerin PE. 1998. *Motor Vehicle Crashes in New Mexico: Developing Risk Profiles Utilizing Race/ Ethnicity and Alcohol Involvement*. Doctoral Dissertation, University of New Mexico.

Hackenberg RA, Gallagher MM. 1972. The costs of cultural change: Accident injury and modernization among the Papago Indians. *Human Organization*, 31(2): 211-226.

Hayes LM. 1989. National study of jail suicides: Seven years later. *Psychiatric Quarterly*, 60(1): 7-29.

Hayes LM. 1998. Suicide prevention in correctional facilities: An overview. In: Puisis M, Editor. *Clinical Practice in Correctional Medicine*. (pp. 245-256). St. Louis, MO: Mosby.

Hem E, Berg AM, Ekeberg AO. 2001. Suicide in police—a critical review. *Suicide and Life-Threatening Behavior*, 31(2): 224-233.

Hendin H. 1999. Suicide, assisted suicide, and euthanasia. In: Jacobs DG, Editor. *The Harvard Medical School Guide to Suicide Assessment and Intervention*. (pp. 540-560). San Fransisco: Jossey-Bass Publishers.

Herek GM. 1996. Heterosexism and homophobia. In: Cabaj RP, Stein TS, Editors. *Textbook of Homosexuality and Mental Health.* (pp. 101-113). Washington, D.C.: American Psychiatric Press.

Herrell R, Goldberg J, True WR, Ramakrishan V, Lyons M, Eisen S, Tsuang MT. 1999. Sexual orientation and suicidality: A co-twin control study in adult men. *Archives of General Psychiatry*, 56: 867-874.

Hershberger SL, D'Augelli AR. 1995. The impact of victimization on the mental health and suicidality of lesbian, gay and bisexual youths. *Developmental Psychology*, 31: 65-74.

Hinton WL, Tiet Q, Tran CG, Chesney M. 1997. Predictors of depression among refugees from Vietnam: A longitudinal study of new arrivals. *Journal of Nervous and Mental Disease*, 185(1): 39-45.

Hisnanick JJ. 1994. Comparative analysis of violent deaths in American Indians and Alaska Natives. *Social Biology*, 41(1-2): 96-109.

Hlady WG, Middaugh JP. 1988. Suicides in Alaska: Firearms and alcohol. *American Journal of Public Health*, 78(2): 179-180.

Hollinger PC, Offer D, Barter JT, Bell. C.C. 1994. *Suicide and Homicide Among Adolescents.* New York: The Guilford Press.

Holman EA, Silver RC, Waitzkin H. 2000. Traumatic life events in primary care patients: A study in an ethnically diverse sample. *Archives of Family Medicine*, 9(9): 802-810.

Hovey JD. 1999. Religion and suicidal ideation in a sample of Latin American immigrants. *Psychological Reports*, 85(1): 171-177.

Hovey JD. 2000a. Acculturative stress, depression, and suicidal ideation among Central American immigrants. *Suicide and Life-Threatening Behavior*, 30(2): 125-139.

Hovey JD. 2000b. Acculturative stress, depression, and suicidal ideation in Mexican immigrants. *Cultural Diversity and Ethnic Minority Psychology*, 6(2): 134-151.

Hovey JD, King CA. 1997. Suicidality among acculturating Mexican Americans: Current knowledge and directions for research. *Suicide and Life-Threatening Behavior*, 27(1): 92-103.

Howard-Pitney B, LaFromboise TD, Basil M, September B, Johnson M. 1992. Psychological and social indicators of suicide ideation and suicide attempts in Zuni adolescents. *Journal of Consulting and Clinical Psychology*, 60(3): 473-476.

Howland RH. 1995. The treatment of persons with dual diagnoses in a rural community. *Psychiatric Quarterly*, 66(1): 33-49.

Hoyert DL, Arias E, Smith BL, Murphy SL, Kochanek KD. 2001. Deaths: Final data for 1999. *National Vital Statistics Reports*, 49(8): 1-113.

Hoyert DL, Kochanek KD, Murphy SL. 1999. Deaths: Final data for 1997. *National Vital Statistics Reports*, 47(19): 1-104.

Indian Health Service. 1999. *Trends in Indian Health, 1998-1999.* Rockville, MD: U.S. Department of Health and Human Services.

IOM (Institute of Medicine). 1999. Bonnie RJ, Fulco CE, Liverman CT, Editors. *Reducing the Burden of Injury: Advancing Prevention and Treatment.* Washington, DC: National Academy Press.

IOM (Institute of Medicine). 2002. B.D. Smedley, A.Y. Stith, A.R. Nelson, Editors. *Unequal Treatment: Confronting Racial and Ethnic Disparities in Healthcare.* Washington, DC: National Academy Press.

Jarvis GK, Boldt M. 1982. Death styles among Canada's Indians. *Social Science and Medicine*, 16(14): 1345-1352.

Jemelka R, Trupin E, Chiles JA. 1989. The mentally ill in prisons: A review. *Hospital and Community Psychiatry*, 40(5): 481-491.

Ji J, Kleinman A, Becker AE. 2001. Suicide in contemporary China: A review of China's distinctive suicide demographics in their sociocultural context. *Harvard Review of Psychiatry*, 9(1): 1-12.

Jianlin J. 2000. Suicide rates and mental health services in modern China. *Crisis*, 21(3): 118-121.

Jobes DA, Berman AL, Josselson AR. 1987. Improving the validity and reliability of medical–legal certifications of suicide. *Suicide and Life-Threatening Behavior*, 17(4): 310-325.

Joe JR. 2001. Out of harmony: Health problems and young Native American men. *Journal of American College Health*, 49(5): 237-242.

Kahn MW. 1982. Cultural clash and psychopathology in three Aboriginal cultures. *Academic Psychology Bulletin*, 4(3): 553-561.

Kann L, Kinchen SA, Williams BI, Ross JG, Lowry R, Hill CV, Grunbaum JA, Blumson PS, Collins JL, Kolbe LJ. 1998. Youth Risk Behavior Surveillance—United States, 1997. State and Local YRBSS Coordinators. *Journal of School Health*, 68(9): 355-369.

Kastenbaum R, Mishara BL. 1971. Premature death and self-injurious behavior in old age. *Geriatrics*, 26(7): 71-81.

Katz PA, May PA. 1979. *Motor Vehicle Accidents on the Navajo Reservation: 1973–1975*. Window Rock, AZ: The Navajo Health Authority.

Kellermann AL, Rivara FP, Somes G, Reay DT, Francisco J, Banton JG, Prodzinski J, Fligner C, Hackman BB. 1992. Suicide in the home in relation to gun ownership. *New England Journal of Medicine*, 327(7): 467-472.

Kessler RC, McGonagle KA, Zhao S, Nelson CB, Hughes M, Eshleman S, Wittchen HU, Kendler KS. 1994. Lifetime and 12-month prevalence of DSM-III-R psychiatric disorders in the United States. Results from the National Comorbidity Survey. *Archives of General Psychiatry*, 51(1): 8-19.

Kettl P, Bixler EO. 1993. Alcohol and suicide in Alaska Natives. *American Indian and Alaska Native Mental Health Research*, 5(2): 34-45.

Kettl PA, Bixler EO. 1991. Suicide in Alaska Natives, 1979-1984. *Psychiatry: Interpersonal and Biological Processes*, 54(1): 55-63.

Khan MM, Reza H. 2000. The pattern of suicide in Pakistan. *Crisis*, 21(1): 31-35.

Kleinman A. 2001. Cross-cultural psychiatry: A psychiatric perspective on global change. *Harvard Review of Psychiatry*, 9(1): 46-47.

Koskinen O, Pukkila K, Hakko H, Tiihonen J, Väisänen E, Säkioja Teal. in press. Is occupation relevant for suicide. *Journal of Affective Disorders*.

Kost-Grant BL. 1983. Self-inflicted gunshot wounds among Alaska Natives. *Public Health Reports*, 98(1): 72-78.

Kraus R. 1974. Suicidal behavior in Alaska natives. *Alaska Medicine*, 16(1): 2-6.

Kryzhanovskaya L, Pilyagina G. 1999. Suicidal behavior in the Ukraine, 1988–1998. *Crisis*, 20(4): 184-190.

Labovitz S, Hagedorn R. 1971. An analysis of suicide rates among occupational categories. *Sociological Inquiry*, 41: 67-72.

Levy JE. 1965. Navaho suicide. *Human Organization*, 24(4): 308-318.

Manderscheid RW, Sonnenschein MA, Editors. 1999. *Mental Health, United States, 1998*. Rockville, MD: U.S. Department of Health and Human Services.

Manson SM, Beals J, Dick RW, Duclos C. 1989. Risk factors for suicide among Indian adolescents at a boarding school. *Public Health Reports*, 104(6): 609-614.

Martin RL, Cloninger CR, Guze SB, Clayton PJ. 1985. Mortality in a follow-up of 500 psychiatric outpatients. II. Cause-specific mortality. *Archives of General Psychiatry*, 42: 58-66.

May PA. 1982. Substance abuse and American Indians: Prevalence and susceptibility. *International Journal of the Addictions*, 17(7): 1185-1209.

May PA. 1987. Suicide and self-destruction among American Indian youths. *American Indian and Alaska Native Mental Health Research*, 1(1): 52-69.

May PA. 1989. Motor vehicle crashes and alcohol among American Indians and Alaska Natives. In: *The Surgeon General's Workshop on Drunk Driving: Background Papers*. (pp. 207-223). Washington, DC: U.S. Department of Health and Human Services.

May PA, Dizmang LH. 1974. Suicide and the American Indian. *Psychiatric Annals*, 4(11): 22-28.

McDaniel JS, Purcell D, D'Augelli AR. 2001. The relationship between sexual orientation and risk for suicide: Research findings and future directions for research and prevention. *Suicide and Life-Threatening Behavior*, 31 (Suppl): 84-105.

Merrill J, Owens J. 1988. Self-poisoning among four immigrant groups. *Acta Psychiatrica Scandinavica*, 77(1): 77-80.

Michaels S. 1996. The prevalence of homosexuality in the United States. In: Cabaj RP, Stein TS, Editors. *Textbook of Homosexuality and Mental Health*. (pp. 43-63). Washington, D.C.: American Psychiatric Press.

Miller M. 1976. Geriatric suicide: The Arizona Study. *Gerontologist*, 18: 488-495.

Minino AM, Smith BL. 2001. Deaths: Preliminary data for 2000. *National Vital Statistics Reports*, 49(12): 1-40.

Morrell S, Taylor R, Slaytor E, Ford P. 1999. Urban and rural suicide differentials in migrants and the Australian-born, New South Wales, Australia 1985–1994. *Social Science and Medicine*, 49(1): 81-91.

Morrissey JP, Swanson JW, Goldstrom I, Rudolph L, Manderscheid RW. 1993. Overview of mental health services provided by state adult correctional facilities: United States, 1988. *Mental Health Statistical Note*, 207: 1-13.

Murphy GE. 1998. Why women are less likely than men to commit suicide. *Comprehensive Psychiatry*, 39(4): 165-175.

Murphy SL. 2000. Deaths: Final data for 1998. *National Vital Statistics Reports*, 48(11): 1-105.

National Commission on Correctional Health Care. 2000. *The Health Status of Soon-to-Be-Released Inmates*. Chicago, IL: National Commission on Correctional Health Care.

National Mental Health Association. 2000. *Depression and African-Americans Fact Sheet*. Alexandria, VA: National Mental Health Association.

NCHS (National Center for Health Statistics). 2001. *Data From the National Vital Statistics System*. Hyattsville, MD: Centers for Disease Control and Prevention. [Online]. Available: http://www.cdc.gov/nchs/nvss.htm [accessed September 2001].

NCHS (National Center for Health Statistics). 1992. Advance report of final mortality statistics, report No. 40. *NCHS Monthly Vital Statistics Report*.

NCIPC (National Center for Injury Prevention and Control). 2000. *Web-Based Injury Statistics Query and Reporting System*. [Online]. Available: http://www.cdc.gov/ncipc/wisqars/ [accessed December 13, 2001].

New Mexico Vital Records and Health Statistics. 2000. *1998 New Mexico Selected Health Statistics: Annual Report*.

Norton GR, Rockman GE, Malan J, Cox BJ, Hewitt PL. 1995. Panic attacks, chemical abuse, and suicidal ideation: A comparison of native and non-native Canadians. *Alcoholism Treatment Quarterly*, 12(3): 33-41.

NRC (National Research Council). 1998. Hernandez DJ, Charney E, Editors. *From Generation to Generation: The Health and Well-Being of Children in Immigrant Families*. Washington, DC: National Academy Press.

NRC (National Research Council). 1999. Hernandez DJ, Editor. *Children of Immigrants: Health, Adjustment, and Public Assistance*. Washington, DC: National Academy Press.

O'Carroll PW. 1989. A consideration of the validity and reliability of suicide mortality data. *Suicide and Life-Threatening Behavior*, 19(1): 1-16.

O'Donnell I, Farmer R. 1995. The limitations of official suicide statistics. *British Journal of Psychiatry*, 166(4): 458-461.

O'Hare T, Van Tran T. 1998. Substance abuse among Southeast Asians in the U.S.: Implications for practice and research. *Social Work in Health Care*, 26(3): 69-80.

Opler MK. 1969. International and cultural conflicts affecting mental health. Violence, suicide and withdrawal. *American Journal of Psychotherapy*, 23(4): 608-620.

Osgood NJ, Brant BA, Lipman A. Suicide Among the Elderly in Long-Term Care Facilities. 1991. New York: Greenwood Press.

Patel SP, Gaw AC. 1996. Suicide among immigrants from the Indian subcontinent: A review. *Psychiatric Services*, 47(5): 517-521.

Patterson HL. 1969. Suicide among the youth on the Quinault Indian Reservation. In *U.S. Senate Committee on Labor and Public Welfare, Part 5, Subcommittee on Indian Education*. (pp. 2016-2021). Washington, DC: U.S. Government Printing Office.

Pearson JL, Conwell Y, Lindesay J, Takahashi Y, Caine ED. 1997. Elderly suicide: A multinational view. *Aging and Mental Health*, 1(2): 107-111.

Phillips DP, Carstensen LL. 1986. Clustering of teenage suicides after television news stories about suicide. *New England Journal of Medicine*, 315(11): 685-689.

Phillips MR, Liu H, Zhang Y. 1999. Suicide and social change in China. *Culture, Medicine and Psychiatry*, 23: 25-50.

Plotnikov N. 2001. Suicide in Russia. *Russian Social Science Review*, 42(3): 41-43.

Ponizovsky A, Safro S, Ginath Y, Ritsner M. 1997. Suicide ideation among recent immigrants: An epidemiological study. *Israel Journal of Psychiatry and Related Sciences*, 34(2): 139-148.

Prince C. 1988. Recognition of predisposing factors which affect the high suicide rate of Canadian Indians. *Arctic Medical Research*, 47 (Suppl 1): 588-589.

Prudhome C. 1938. The problem of suicide in the American negro. *Psychoanalytic Review*, 25: 187-204; 372-391.

Regier DA, Farmer ME, Rae DS, Myers JK, Kramer M, Robins LN, George LK, Karno M, Locke BZ. 1993. One-month prevalence of mental disorders in the United States and sociodemographic characteristics: The Epidemiologic Catchment Area study. *Acta Psychiatrica Scandinavica*, 88(1): 35-47.

Remafedi G, French S, Story M, Resnick MD, Blum R. 1998. The relationship between suicide risk and sexual orientation: Results of a population-based study. *American Journal of Public Health*, 88(1): 57-60.

Resnik HLP, Dizmang LH. 1971. Observations on suicidal behavior among American Indians. *American Journal of Psychiatry*, 127(7): 882-887.

Rich CL, Fowler RC, Young D, Blenkush M. 1986a. San Diego suicide study: Comparison of gay to straight males. *Suicide and Life-Threatening Behavior*, 16(4): 448-457.

Rich CL, Young D, Fowler RC. 1986b. San Diego suicide study. I. Young vs old subjects. *Archives of General Psychiatry*, 43(6): 577-582.

Rihmer Z, Rutz W, Pihlgren. 1995. Depression and suicide on Gotland: An intensive study of all suicides before and after a depression—training programme for general practitioners. *Journal of Affective Disorders*, 35: 147-152.

Robins L, Regier DA. 1991. *Psychiatric Disorders in America: The Epidemiologic Catchment Area Study*. New York: The Free Press.

Robins LN, West PA, Murphy GE. 1977. The high rate of suicide in older White men: A study testing ten hypotheses. *Social Psychiatry*, 12(1): 1-20.

Russell ST, Joyner K. 2001. Adolescent sexual orientation and suicide risk: Evidence from a national study. *American Journal of Public Health*, 91(8): 1276-1281.

Sack WH, Beiser M, Baker-Brown G, Redshirt R. 1994. Depressive and suicidal symptoms in Indian school children: Findings from the Flower of Two Soils. *American Indian and Alaska Native Mental Health Research Monograph Series*, 4: 81-94; discussion 94-6.

Sartorius N. 1996. Recent changes in suicide rates in selected eastern European and other European countries. In: Pearson JL, Conwell Y, Editors. *Suicide and Aging: International Perspectives*. (pp. 169-176). New York: Springer Publishing.

Saunderson TR, Langford IH. 1996. A study of the geographical distribution of suicide rates in England and Wales 1989-92 using empirical bayes estimates. *Social Science and Medicine*, 43(4): 489-502.

Schmidtke A, Fricke S, Lester D. 1999. Suicide among German federal and state police officers. *Psychological Reports*, 84(1): 157-166.

Schweizer E, Dever A, Clary C. 1988. Suicide upon recovery from depression. A clinical note. *Journal of Nervous and Mental Disease*, 176(10): 633-636.

Seiden RH, Gleiser M. 1990. Sex differences in suicide among chemists. *Omega—Journal of Death and Dying*, 21(3): 177-189.

Shaffer D, Fisher P, Hicks RH, Parides M, Gould M. 1995. Sexual orientation in adolescents who commit suicide. *Suicide and Life-Threatening Behavior*, 25 (Suppl): 64-71.

Shaffer D, Gould MS, Fisher P, Trautman P, Moreau D, Kleinman M, Flory M. 1996. Psychiatric diagnosis in child and adolescent suicide. *Archives of General Psychiatry*, 53: 339-348.

Shiang J, Blinn R, Bongar B, Stephens B, Allison D, Schatzberg A. 1997. Suicide in San Francisco, CA: A comparison of Caucasian and Asian groups, 1987–1994. *Suicide and Life-Threatening Behavior*, 27(1): 80-91.

Shuck LW, Orgel MG, Vogel AV. 1980. Self-inflicted gunshot wounds to the face: A review of 18 cases. *Journal of Trauma*, 20(5): 370-377.

Singh GK, Siahpush M. 2001. All-cause and cause-specific mortality of immigrants and native born in the United States. *American Journal of Public Health*, 91(3): 392-399.

Sloan JH, Rivara FP, Reay DT, Ferris JAJ, Path MRC, Kellermann AL. 1990. Firearms regulations and rates of suicide: A comparison of two metropolitan areas. *New England Journal of Medicine*, 322(6): 369-373.

Smith JC, Mercy JA, Conn JM. 1988. Marital status and the risk of suicide. *American Journal of Public Health*, 78(1): 78-80.

Sorenson SB, Golding JM. 1988. Prevalence of suicide attempts in a Mexican-American population: Prevention implications of immigration and cultural issues. *Suicide and Life-Threatening Behavior*, 18(4): 322-333.

Sorenson SB, Shen H. 1996. Youth suicide trends in California: An examination of immigrant and ethnic group risk. *Suicide and Life-Threatening Behavior*, 26(2): 143-154.

Spaulding JM. 1985–1986. Recent suicide rates among ten Ojibwa Indian bands in northwestern Ontario. *Omega—Journal of Death and Dying*, 16(4): 347-354.

Stack S. 1995. Gender and suicide among laborers. *Archives of Suicide Research*, 1(1): 19-26.

Stack S. 2001. Occupation and suicide. *Social Science Quarterly*, 82(2): 384-396.

Stack S, Kelly T. 1994. Police suicide: An analysis. *American Journal of Police*, 13(4): 73-90.

Steadman HJ, Fabisiak S, Dvoskin J, Holohean EJ Jr. 1987. A survey of mental disability among state prison inmates. *Hospital and Community Psychiatry*, 38(10): 1086-1090.

Stull DD. 1972. Victims of modernization: Accident rates and Papago Indian adjustment. *Human Organization*, 31(2): 227-240.

Stull DD. 1973. *Modernization and Symptoms of Stress: Attitudes, Accidents and Alcohol Use Among Urban Papago Indians*. Doctoral Dissertation, University of Colorado.

Stull DD. 1977. New data on accident victims rates among Papago Indians: The urban case. *Human Organization*, 36(4): 395-398.

Szanto K, Prigerson H, Houck P, Ehrenpreis L, Reynolds CF 3rd. 1997. Suicidal ideation in elderly bereaved: The role of complicated grief. *Suicide and Life-Threatening Behavior*, 27(2): 194-207.

Taylor PJ, Gunn J. 1984. Violence and psychosis. I. Risk of violence among psychotic men. *British Medical Journal (Clinical Research Edition)*, 288(6435): 1945-1949.

Teplin LA. 1990. The prevalence of severe mental disorder among male urban jail detainees: Comparison with the Epidemiologic Catchment Area Program. *American Journal of Public Health*, 80(6): 663-669.

Tousignant M, Habimana E, Biron C, Malo C, Sidoli-LeBlanc E, Bendris N. 1999. The Quebec Adolescent Refugee Project: Psychopathology and family variables in a sample from 35 nations. *Journal of the American Academy of Child and Adolescent Psychiatry*, 38(11): 1426-1432.

Travis RM. 1984. Suicide and economic development among the Inupiat Eskimo. *White Cloud Journal*, 3(3): 14-21.

U.S. Congress, Office of Technology Assessment. 1990. *Indian Adolescent Mental Health OTA-H-446*. Washington, DC: U.S. Government Printing Office.

US DHHS (U.S. Department of Health and Human Services). 2001. *Mental Health: Culture, Race and Ethnicity—A Supplement to Mental Health: A Report of the Surgeon General*. Rockville, MD: U.S. Department of Health and Human Services, Substance Abuse and Mental Health Services Administration, Center for Mental Health Services, National Institutes of Health, National Institute of Mental Health.

VanWinkle NW, May PA. 1986. Native American suicide in New Mexico, 1957-1979: A comparative study. *Human Organization*, 45(4): 296-309.

VanWinkle NW, May PA. 1993. An update on American Indian suicide in New Mexico, 1980-1987. *Human Organization*, 52(3): 304-315.

VanWinkle NW, Williams M. 2001. *Evaluation of the National Model Adolescent Suicide Prevention Project: A Comparison of Suicide Rates Among New Mexico American Indian Tribes, 1980-1998*. Tulsa, Oklahoma: Oklahoma State University, College of Osteopathic Medicine.

Veysey BM, Bichler-Robertson G. 1999. *Prevalence Estimates for Psychiatric Disorders in Correctional Settings*. Chicago, IL: National Commission on Correctional Health Care.

Violanti JM, Vena JE, Petralia S. 1998. Mortality of a police cohort: 1950-1990. *American Journal of Industrial Medicine*, 33(4): 366-373.

Viscusi WK. 1995. Cigarette taxation and the social consequences of smoking. In: National Bureau of Economic Research. *Tax Policy and the Economy*. Vol. 9. (pp. 51-101). Cambridge, MA: MIT Press.

Wallace LJ, Calhoun AD, Powell KE, O'Neil J, James SP. 1996. *Homicide and Suicide Among Native Americans, 1979-1992*. Atlanta, Georgia: National Center for Injury Prevention and Control Violence Surveillance Summary Series, No.2.

WHO (World Health Organization). 2001a. *Mental Health and Brain Disorders. Suicide Rates (Per 100,000)*. Geneva: World Health Organization. [Online]. Available: http://www.who.int/mental_health/Topic_Suicide/ Suicide_rates.html [accessed January 7, 2002].

WHO (World Health Organization). 2001b. *The World Health Report, 2001. Mental Health: New Understanding, New Hope*. Geneva: World Health Organization.

Wilkinson D, Gunnell D. 2000. Youth suicide trends in Australian metropolitan and non-metropolitan areas, 1988-1997. *Australian and New Zealand Journal of Psychiatry*, 34(5): 822-828.

Williams CL, Berry JW. 1991. Primary prevention of acculturative stress among refugees. Application of psychological theory and practice. *American Psychologist*, 46(6): 632-641.

Wills JE. 1969. Psychological problems of the Sioux Indians resulting in the accident phenomenon. *Pine Ridge Research Bulletin*, 8: 49-63.

Wissow LS. 2000. Suicide among American Indians and Alaska Natives. In: Rhoades ER, Editor. *American Indian Health*. (pp. 260-280). Baltimore, MD: The Johns Hopkins University Press.

Yip PS. 2001. An epidemiological profile of suicides in Beijing, China. *Suicide and Life-Threatening Behavior*, 31(1): 62-70.

Yip PS, Callana C, Yuen HP. 2000. Urban/rural and gender differentials in suicide rates: East and west. *Journal of Affective Disorders*, 57(1-3): 99-106.

Psychosis can create a particularly terrible kind of pain that leads to suicidal behavior. Robert Bayley, who suffered for years from schizophrenia, recounted his struggles with extremely frightening hallucinations:

The reality for myself is almost constant pain and torment. The voices and visions, which are so commonly experienced, intrude and so disturb my everyday life. The voices are predominantly destructive, either rambling in alien tongues or screaming orders to carry out violent acts. They also persecute me by way of unwavering commentary and ridicule to deceive, derange, and force me into a world of crippling paranoia. Their commands are abrasive and all-encompassing and have resulted in periods of suicidal behavior and self-mutilation. I have run in front of speeding cars and severed arteries while feeling this compulsion to destroy my own life. As their tenacity gains momentum, there is often no element of choice, which leaves me feeling both tortured and drained.

—ROBERT BAYLEY
"First person account: Schizophrenia"

3

Psychiatric and Psychological Factors

In the United States, over 90 percent of suicides are associated with mental illness including alcohol and/or substance use disorders (Conwell et al., 1996; Harris and Barraclough, 1997; Robins et al., 1959). Recent estimates indicate 28–30 percent of the U.S. population has a mental or addictive disorder, or approximately 80 million people in the year 2000 (Kessler et al., 1994; Regier et al., 1993a). With 30,000 suicides each year, however, over 95 percent of these affected individuals do not complete suicide. Determining who among those with mental disorders will attempt suicide is paramount for individual intervention and prevention.

It is important to note that mental illness and substance abuse are *not always* the greatest risk factors for suicide. For instance, in a cross-cultural study, Bhatia and colleagues (1987) found that humiliation, shame, economic hardship, examination failure, and family disputes were the greatest risk factors for suicide in India, compared to the United States where mental illnesses and/or alcoholism, personal loss, and increased age were associated with the greatest risk. Psychopathology is less important as a risk factor for suicide in China as well. Despite the 30 percent overall higher suicide rate in China compared to the United States, the prevailing evidence is that there is a significantly *lower* prevalence of mental illnesses and substance use disorders in China (Shen et al., 1992). Since China and India are the world's most populous countries, accounting for approximately 40 percent of the global population, it is important to keep in mind that suicide evidence in the United States and other Western countries may not be globally representative.

This chapter explores the associations of mental illness and substance abuse that are risk factors for suicide in the United States and Europe. The first section of this chapter discusses suicide risk associated with mental and/or addictive disorders and what is known about who among those with these disorders is at greatest risk. Suicides in adolescents appear to be associated with a somewhat different set of variables, as discussed in a separate section. Next, the chapter explores psychological variables, including protective factors: those associated with *reduced* risk for suicide. Certain psychological factors distinguish and predict those who complete or attempt suicide. These include habits of thinking, problem solving, and expectations about the future, termed cognitive style or factors. These factors are modifiable through counseling and training, and their modification holds promise in reducing suicide. Finally, the chapter turns to temperament. Temperament has a significant genetic component (Goldsmith and Lemery, 2000) that interacts with environmental adversities to increase vulnerability to a number of unwanted outcomes, including suicide.

PSYCHIATRIC/SUBSTANCE USE
DISORDERS AND SUICIDE RISK

Almost all psychiatric disorders, including alcohol and substance disorders, are associated with an increased risk of suicide. Depressive disorders are found in 30–90 percent of those who complete suicide, including the approximately 5 percent with bipolar disorder (Lönnqvist, 2000). Approximately another 5 percent are associated with schizophrenia (De Hert and Peuskens, 2000), 30 percent with a personality disorder (Davis et al., 1999; Henriksson et al., 1993; Isometsa et al., 1996), and 25 percent with alcohol abuse disorders (Murphy, 2000). Anxiety disorders including post-traumatic stress disorder (PTSD) are associated with approximately 20 percent of suicides (Allgulander, 2000). As many as 10 percent of those who complete suicide do not have a known psychiatric diagnosis. Around 20–25 percent of individuals who die by suicide are intoxicated with alcohol at death (see section on Alcohol Use below). Many individuals have multiple diagnoses concurrently, and comorbidity may in and of itself increase risk (Kessler et al., 1999), although there are little data on this issue, in part due to the hierarchical nature of the current psychiatric diagnostic system, in which mood and psychotic disorders are more heavily considered.

Diagnoses associated with suicide attempts present a similar profile. Though there may be distinctions between sub-types of attempters and completers, they appear to be generally overlapping populations; current data do not allow resolution of this issue. This differentiation is further complicated by the difficulties in defining suicide attempts as distinct from self-mutilation and/or other self-destructive behaviors including risk-taking behaviors (Poussaint and Alexander, 2000). Data from the National Comorbidity Survey (NCS) reveal that serious suicide attempters closely resemble suicide completers (Molnar et al., 2001). For men, substance abuse disorders were associated with a 6.2 times greater risk of serious suicide attempts, and mood disorders were associated with a 13.5 times greater risk. Women with substance abuse disorders had a 4.4 times greater risk of a serious suicide attempt, a 4.8 times risk with anxiety disorders (excluding PTSD), and an 11.8 time greater risk with a mood disorder. Overall, this study found that between 74 and 80 percent of the population attributable risk (PAR[1]) for serious suicide attempts was accounted for by psychiatric illness.

Psychiatric disorders are diagnosed through interviews, including current and past behaviors, moods, and thoughts. The psychological autopsy technique is used to make post-humous diagnoses when there is no medical history of mental illness available (see Chapter 10). Diagnostic criteria used in the United States are those in the *Diagnostic and Statistical Manual* developed through a task force overseen by the American Psychiatric Association. The version used at this writing is the DSM-IV (APA, 1994). The DSM-IV provides five axes to describe the individual's functioning. The mental and substance use disorders are coded on Axis I or Axis II. The Axis I disorders most frequently associated with suicide (also referred to as the major or serious mental disorders) include schizophrenia, bipolar disorder, depressive disorders, and alcohol and substance use disorders. The Axis II disorders are the personality disorders. Borderline personality and antisocial personality disorders are those most frequently associated with suicide.

Mood Disorders

Suicides in many nations including the United States are most commonly associated with a diagnosis of a mood disorder in adults (Lönnqvist, 2000) and adolescents (Goldman and Beardslee, 1999). Best estimates of lifetime risk of suicide for those with mood disorders is approximately 4 percent (see Chapter 10 for discussion of risk calculations). Estimated rates vary greatly depending on the severity of the illness (Goodwin and Jamison, 1990). These disorders are very common in the United States, with approximately 18.8 million American adults (Narrow, unpublished, cited by NIMH), or about 9.5 percent of those 18 and older

---

[1]Population-attributable risk expresses the proportion of an outcome that could be eliminated if the risk factor were removed.

(Regier et al., 1993b), afflicted in a given year. Also called affective disorders, they include three diagnoses: (1) major depressive disorder, (2) dysthymic disorder, and (3) bipolar disorder. Each year, almost two times as many women (12.0 percent) as men (6.6 percent) suffer from a depressive disorder. These percentages correspond to 12.4 million women and 6.4 million men in the United States (Narrow, unpublished, cited by NIMH). For those born in recent decades, depressive disorders may be appearing earlier in life compared to prior cohorts (Klerman and Weissman, 1989). In addition, depressive disorders often co-occur with other mental and bodily disorders, including schizophrenia and anxiety, personality, and substance use disorders (Regier et al., 1998), as well as cardiac disease (e.g., Appels, 1997; Lesperance and Frasure-Smith, 2000).

Major Depressive Disorder and Dysthmia

Major depression, which is often episodic, recurrent, or even chronic, is diagnosed upon the occurrence of a major depressive episode. A major depressive episode includes at least five of a list of nine criteria symptoms persisting for a minimum of 2 weeks including: depressed or irritable mood, diminished interest in usual activities and pleasures, changes in eating and sleeping, and suicidal thoughts. A major depressive episode and borderline personality disorder are the only diagnostic entities in the DSM-IV system that include suicidality as a symptom. Dysthymic disorder is diagnosed when an individual is depressed and sad more days than not for at least 2 years, but does not have symptoms that meet criteria for a major depressive disorder.

Death from many causes is increased in major depression. For example, Zheng and colleagues (1997), using data from the U.S. National Health Interview Survey in 1989, found a 3.1 adjusted hazard rate ratio for white males for all-cause mortality in major depression during a 2.5-year follow-up study, and a 1.7 rate for white females. In Harris and Barraclough's meta-analysis of suicide in mental illness (1998), they found that deaths in those with major depressive disorder from natural causes were 1.3 times more frequent than expected, whereas suicide deaths were 21 times the population rate, and deaths by other violent causes 2.3 times expected. The lifetime risk of suicide in those with major depression is difficult to ascertain for a number of reasons. Most studies examining lifetime mortality from suicide follow patients after release from the hospital and compare their rate of suicide compared to either other patients or the population at large. Rates reported from such estimates may be artificially higher since they often follow the most severely affected patients (those hospitalized) for only a few years after hospitalization, which is also the time of highest risk (Lönnqvist, 2000). In addition, a commonly used calculation for suicide mortality, as Bostwick and Pankratz (2000) evaluated, appears to have artificially increased estimates of lifetime suicide mortality rate as discussed in Appendix A. Taking all of this into account, the best estimates are that approximately 4 percent of those with depressive disorders will die by suicide.

More than half of those with depressive disorders have thoughts of suicide. The severity of their thoughts, plans, and attempts increase with increasing severity of the disorder. The suicidality often remits along with the other symptoms of depression (e.g., Harrington et al., 1998; Joiner et al., 2001b, see Chapter 7). A study of over 35,000 insured people receiving treatment for depression showed greater rates of suicide by those receiving more intensive treatments, considered an indication of the severity of the depression. The highest suicide rate was among those receiving inpatient treatment and lowest among those receiving outpatient treatment with medication. No suicides were observed in those being treated on an outpatient basis without medication (Simon and Von Korff, 1998). Other studies suggest a disconnect between the response of depressive symptoms and suicidal behavior (Brent et al., 1997; Lerner and Clum, 1990).

Other depressive symptoms predictive of suicidality are hopelessness (Beck et al., 1975; Beck, 1986) as well as feelings of guilt, loss of interest in usual activities, and low self-esteem (Van Gastel et al., 1997). Mann and colleagues (1999) showed that the objective severity of current depression or psychosis did *not* distinguish the 184 patients of 347 consecutive psychiatric admissions who had attempted suicide compared to those who never attempted. Rather, higher scores of *subjective* depression and higher scores of suicidal ideation, as well as fewer "reasons for living" as measured by the Reasons for Living Inventory (Linehan et al., 1983) distinguished those who had attempted suicide (Mann et al., 1999). Hopelessness, as discussed in the psychological factors section below, is a better predictor of suicide than the objective measures of depressed affect, not only in depressive disorders (Beck et al., 1993) but in physical illnesses as well (Chochinov et al., 1998).

Bipolar Disorder

Bipolar disorder affects approximately 1.2 percent of the U.S. population age 18 and older (Weissman et al., 1988). Twenty-five to 50 percent of those with bipolar disorder will attempt suicide at least once (Goodwin and Jamison, 1990). Suicides by those with bipolar disorder account for only 1–5 percent of all suicides as found in a number of countries including Finland, New Zealand, the United States, and Northern Ireland (Conwell et al., 1996; Foster et al., 1997; Isometsa et al., 1994; Joyce et al., 1994). A review of 14 studies by Harris and Barraclough (1997) from seven countries, for a total population of 3700 people with bipolar disorder, found a rate of suicide 15-fold higher than would be expected in the general population. The risk of death from suicide in bipolar disorder is greater than the mortality rate for some types of heart disease (Goodwin and Jamison, 1990).

Bipolar disorder (also called manic depressive disorder), is a biological disorder with significant genetic heritability (Alda, 1997; Blackwood et al., 2001). Bipolar disorder includes depressive and manic episodes (APA, 1994). Depressive episodes are described in the section above on depressive disorders and include long-lasting sad, apathetic or irritable mood, altered thinking, activity, and bodily functions. Manic episodes include periods of abnormally and persistently elevated, expansive, or irritable mood; inflated self-esteem; decreased need for sleep; extreme talkativeness; distractibility; high levels of activity; and increased pleasure-seeking and risk-taking behaviors. Symptoms of psychosis including delusions and hallucinations can also occur in bipolar disorder (APA, 1994). Currently, there are two recognized types of bipolar disorder, Type I and Type II. Bipolar II may have an increased risk for suicide and differs from Type I in that the manic periods are less severe and thus are termed hypomania. Bipolar II disorder is frequently misdiagnosed as major depression (Goodwin and Jamison, 1990).

Whereas much is known about variables associated with increased risk for all of those with mood disorders, few studies have examined bipolar disorder separately. Unlike the usual gender difference with more men than women completing suicide, women with bipolar illness complete suicide at a rate almost equal to that of men with bipolar illness (Weeke, 1979). The greatest risk of suicide is early in the course of illness, within the first 5 years of the initial diagnosis (Guze and Robins, 1970; Roy-Byrne et al., 1988; Weeke, 1979). Severity of the disorder is also associated with increased risk for suicide (Hagnell et al., 1981), and those with more severe cases of bipolar disorder will have more frequent hospitalizations. Discharge from the hospital is a period of high risk. Inadequate treatment, whether due to non-adherence, unavailability, or lack of treatment response, is associated with increased suicide risk; inadequate levels of mood stabilizers or antidepressants are found in the majority of those who die by suicide (Isometsa et al., 1994). The time after discharge from the hospital may also carry high risk because the person must rebuild their life while facing a future with a recurrent, life-disrupting disorder. In addition, family and employers may inadvertently increase stress on the individual by having unrealistic expectations of an immediate return to full functioning (Appleby, 2000; Goodwin and Jamison, 1990).

Those with bipolar type II disorder, which includes periods of *hypomania*, but not mania, is associated with increased risk of suicide (Dunner et al., 1976; Stallone et al., 1980). One study found that out of 100 consecutive suicides, 46 percent had bipolar II, 1 percent had bipolar I, and 53 percent had non-bipolar major depression (Rihmer et al., 1990). This particular vulnerability of those with bipolar II may be due to increased mixed states that include depressive and manic symptoms at the same time (see Chapter 7), and can also include severe agitation. There is a significantly increased rate of alcohol and/or substance use disorder in individuals with bipolar disorder (Brady and Sonne, 1995; Goodwin and Jamison, 1990), understood in part as an attempt to "self-medicate." The co-occurrence of these two disorders is associated with increased rates of suicide above that for each single disorder (see section on alcohol and substance use below).

Anxiety Disorders

Anxiety disorders are ubiquitous across the globe and are the most common mental disorders in the United States (Kessler et al., 1994; Regier et al., 1993a; Weissman et al., 1997). The 1-year prevalence for the adult population has been estimated between 16 and 25 percent (Kessler et al., 1994; Regier et al., 1993a; Weissman et al., 1997). Anxiety disorders carry significant comorbidity with mood and substance abuse disorders (Goldberg and Lecrubier, 1996; Magee et al., 1996; Regier et al., 1998) that seem to eclipse the general clinical significance of anxiety disorders.

Although a few psychological autopsy studies of adult suicides have included a focus on comorbid conditions (Conwell and Brent, 1995), it is likely that the specific contribution of anxiety disorders to suicidality has been underestimated. Research from the last decade has started correcting this, however. A recent study using the National Comorbidity Survey data (Molnar et al., 2001) found that for all anxiety disorders *including* PTSD, the population attributable risk for serious suicide attempts is almost 60 percent for females, and 43 percent for males.

Anxiety disorders encompass a group of eight conditions[2] (APA, 1994) that share extreme or pathological anxiety and fear as the principal disturbance of mood, with accompanying disturbances of thinking, behavior, and physiological activity. The longitudinal course of these disorders is characterized by relatively early ages of onset, chronicity, relapsing or recurrent episodes of illness, and periods of disability (Gorman and

---

[2]The eight anxiety disorders in the DSM-IV: panic disorder (with and without a history of agoraphobia), agoraphobia (with and without a history of panic disorder), generalized anxiety disorder, specific phobia, social phobia, obsessive-compulsive disorder, acute stress disorder, and post-traumatic stress disorder.

Coplan, 1996; Keller and Hanks, 1995; Liebowitz, 1993; Marcus et al., 1997). Of the eight anxiety disorders diagnosed via the DSM-IV, the two most frequently associated with suicide in existent studies are panic disorder (Schmidt et al., 2000) and PTSD (Kessler, 2000), discussed in turn below.

Panic Disorder

Weissman and colleagues (1989) provided the first overview of panic disorder in relation to suicide and found an almost 20-fold increased risk for suicide attempts compared to those without any psychiatric disorder. Follow-up studies of completed suicides suggest approximately 20 percent of suicide deaths are due to panic disorder (Schmidt et al., 2000). A large follow-up study in Sweden found a suicide rate for pure panic disorder comparable to major depression and other serious psychiatric illness requiring inpatient care (Allgulander and Lavori, 1991).

The comorbidity of panic disorder with other mental illnesses conveys the greatest suicide risk (Schmidt et al., 2000). In one of the few studies investigating clinical predictors of suicidality in panic disorder, Schmidt and colleagues (2000) confirmed that co-occurring agoraphobia as well as depression significantly increase risk for suicidality, but found that depression likely mediates the relationship between panic disorder and suicidality. This suggests that co-occurring depression in panic disorder may actually be a secondary disorder that develops in response to the panic disorder. This study also found that patients' avoidance of bodily sensations and their anticipatory anxiety significantly predict suicide attempt, offering clues for assessment and intervention regarding suicidality in this population.

Post-Traumatic Stress Disorder

Post-traumatic stress disorder has demonstrated the strongest association with suicidality of any of the anxiety disorders (Kessler, 2000; Molnar et al., 2001). It predicts subsequent first onset of a suicide attempt with an odds ratio of 6, as compared to other anxiety disorders with an odds ratio of 3, and mood disorders at 12.9 times the increased risk (Kessler et al., 1999). Furthermore, PTSD appears to have an equal or greater odds ratio than mood disorders or other anxiety disorders for making a suicide *plan* and for making *impulsive* suicide attempts (Kessler et al., 1999).

Recent analyses of the data from the National Comorbidity Survey have significantly increased knowledge about PTSD within the U.S. population, including finding it far more common (7.8 percent lifetime prevalence) than earlier, less sensitive estimates (Kessler, 2000; Kessler et al., 1995). Using time series analysis, Kessler (2000) found that current PTSD significantly predicts subsequent first onset of all other anxiety disorders, substance use disorders, major depression, and dysthymia for males and females. Furthermore, PTSD predicts the onset of mania in males, with an odds ratio of 15.5. Given the overwhelming presence of co-occurring mental disorders in those with PTSD (Chu, 1999), Kessler (2000) made another significant discovery in demonstrating that only those with active PTSD are at increased risk for comorbidity. With remission of PTSD symptoms, this increased risk for secondary diagnoses disappeared.

Animal and human research on neurobiological changes in the body's stress response system after trauma suggests a physiological mechanism for the development of post-trauma affective disorder and PTSD (Garland et al., 2000; Heim and Nemeroff, 2001; Heim et al., 1997). Post-traumatic stress disorder involves unusual physiological and metabolic patterns of the major stress hormones such as cortisol and norepinephrine. The disorder further alters the serotonergic, dopamine, and opioid systems. Those with the diagnosis also suffer psychophysiological effects of trauma such as hyper-arousal and conditioned startle responses, and evidence abnormalities in the regions of the brain involved in memory and emotion (see van der Kolk, 1996). These same neurobiological pathways are consistently shown to be involved in substance use disorders (below), developmental trauma (Chapter 5), and in suicide (Chapter 4).

Schizophrenic Disorders

Approximately 2.2 million American adults (Narrow, unpublished, cited by NIMH) or about 1.1 percent of the population age 18 and older in a given year (Regier et al., 1993b) have schizophrenia. Schizophrenia affects men and women with equal frequency and has an onset in early adulthood (Robins and Regier, 1991). Symptoms of schizophrenia include delusions, hallucinations, disorganized speech, thought and movements. These are also termed "positive symptoms," in that they are additional behaviors. Others, termed "negative symptoms" are the *absence* of normative behaviors such as flattened emotions or reduced spontaneous behaviors, social interaction, and volition (APA, 1994). Schizoaffective disorder includes periods of illness during which there is either a major depressive episode, a manic or mixed episode, concurrent with the criterion symptoms for schizophrenia. People with this disorder are often diagnosed with schizophrenia upon expression of those symptoms, making calculation of the prevalence as a separate disorder difficult. For the purpose of this report, those with either diagnosis will be referred to as those with schizophrenic disorders.

The schizophrenic disorders are associated with premature death, with approximately a 4–10 percent lifetime risk of suicide (Tsuang et al., 1980). The risk of suicide for those with schizophrenic disorders is approximately 30–40 times that of the general population (Caldwell and Gottesman, 1992; Harris and Barraclough, 1998). Individuals with schizophrenic disorders account for 25–33 percent of suicides occurring in psychiatric hospitals (Proulx et al., 1997; Roy, 1982). Suicide attempts among this population are more likely to be moderately to severely lethal with high levels of intent (Funahashi et al., 2000; Harkavy-Friedman et al., 1999; Radomsky et al., 1999). Approximately 50 percent of those who complete suicide had made prior attempts (Drake et al., 1985; Heila et al., 1997; 1998). This is markedly lower than the 65 percent rate of prior attempts among people who complete suicide with borderline personality disorder, which likely reflects in part the high lethality of suicidal behavior in those with schizophrenia.

Suicide risk may be highest early in the disorder (within the first 5–10 years) (Funahashi et al., 2000; Harkavy-Friedman et al., 1999; Mortensen and Juel, 1993; Nyman and Jonsson, 1986; Saarinen et al., 1999). Those with suicidal behavior have more frequent hospitalizations either directly due to the suicidal behaviors or to the exacerbation of symptoms (Roy et al., 1984). The greatest risk for suicidal behavior is during hospitalization and within the first 6 months post-discharge (Funahashi et al., 2000; Landmark et al., 1987; Peuskens et al., 1997; Qin et al., 2000; Rossau and Mortensen, 1997). For those in outpatient treatment, the majority of the suicide victims have been recently seen by a mental health professional (Heila et al., 1998; Saarinen et al., 1999). Often the suicidality was communicated to the clinician, but it is not always acted on clinically (Breier and Astrachan, 1984; Qin et al., 2000). In schizophrenic disorders as compared to the population at large, gender differences in rates are non-existent for suicide attempts (Bromet et al., 1992; Roy et al., 1984) and reduced for completions (Caldwell and Gottesman, 1990; Drake et al., 1985; Wiersma et al., 1998).

Co-occurrence of schizophrenia with depressive symptoms increases risk of suicide (Amador et al., 1996; Fenton et al., 1997; Roy, 1990). Severity of positive symptoms including command hallucinations (voices repeatedly ordering the individual to do something) also have been related to increased suicide rates (Falloon and Talbot, 1981), while negative symptoms may be related to *lower* suicide rates (Fenton et al., 1997; Hellerstein et al., 1987). Self-awareness of symptoms is related to increased suicide rates (Amador et al., 1996).

Better premorbid functioning (prior to the onset of the illness) is associated with less severe morbidity of the disorders, but possibly with *increased* suicide rates. For example, some researchers find higher suicide rates among those with higher IQ and educational attainment—indications of better premorbid functioning (Dingman and McGlashan, 1986; Drake et al., 1984; Peuskens et al., 1997; Westermeyer et al., 1991). This may be due to the more severely dashed life's hopes and aspirations these individuals experience upon onset of this severe mental disorder. Related to this, those with better premorbid functioning also tend to have fewer negative symptoms (Bailer et al., 1996; Fennig et al., 1995).

Personality Disorders

Approximately 10–15 percent of the population has a personality disorder (Ottoson et al., 1998; Ucok et al., 1998; Weissman, 1993). Personality disorders are enduring patterns of behaviors and inner experiences that both deviate from an individual's cultural norms and significantly impede functioning (APA, 1994). There are 10 types of personality disorders grouped into three clusters. Less is known about etiology and effective treatment for personality disorders than for other psychiatric illnesses. In addition, there is a general tendency to consider Axis II disorders subordinate in their effect on the clinical condition of the individual, possibly leading to the underestimation of the importance of the Axis II disorders for clinical outcomes including suicide. Yet, increasing evidence indicates that personality disorders interfere with treatment for numerous comorbid Axis I mental and substance use disorders (e.g., Green and Curtis, 1988; Jenike et al., 1986; Kroll and Ryan, 1983; Reich, 1988; Turner, 1987), including depression (Pfohl et al., 1984; Pilkonis and Frank, 1988; Poldrugo and Forti, 1988).

Borderline Personality Disorder

Borderline personality disorder (BPD) is the most frequently studied personality disorder in relation to suicide, in part due to the high rate of self-injurious behaviors and suicide attempts. In fact BPD is one of only two diagnoses in the DSM system for which suicidal behavior is listed as a symptom, with depressive episode as the other (APA, 1994). Borderline personality disorder is a serious mental illness characterized by pervasive instability in moods, interpersonal relationships, self-image, and behavior, which seriously interferes with functioning. Originally thought to be at the "borderline" of psychosis, people with BPD suffer from a disorder of emotion regulation. Borderline personality disorder is *more prevalent* than either schizophrenia or bipolar disorder, affecting 2 percent of adults, mostly young women (Swartz et al., 1990). There is a high rate of self-injury without suicide intent, as well as a significant rate of suicide attempts and completed suicide in severe cases (Gardner and Cowdry, 1985;

Soloff et al., 1994b). Patients often need extensive mental health services; studies have shown that individuals with BPD have more extensive histories of psychiatric outpatient, inpatient, psychopharmacologic and psychosocial treament than both patients with major depressive disorder (Bender et al., 2001) and patients with other Axis II disorders (Zanarini et al., 2001). Yet newly developed specialty psychotherapy treatment called Dialectical Behavioral Therapy (DBT) can significantly improve functioning (Koerner and Linehan, 2000, see Chapter 7).

Between 4 and 8 percent of those with a personality disorder complete suicide (Linehan et al., 2000). Borderline personality disorder specifically carries approximately 10 percent lifetime risk of completed suicide (Frances et al., 1986; Stone et al., 1987), within the same range as for schizophrenia and major depressive disorder (Guze and Robins, 1970; Winokur and Tsuang, 1975). Approximately 40–90 percent of those with personality disorders have attempted suicide (Ahrens and Haug, 1996; Bornstein et al., 1988; Corbitt et al., 1996; Garvey and Spoden, 1980; Modestin et al., 1997). A large, psychological autopsy study of completed suicides in Finland found that personality disorder and major depressive disorder were diagnosed in equal percentages (31 percent) among completed suicides, while 59 percent had any mood disorder, and 7 percent had schizophrenia (Henriksson et al., 1993). Since BPD has a higher population prevalence, it may in fact account for more suicides than either schizophrenia or bipolar disorder.

Up to 65 percent of those with BPD have a concurrent major depressive episode (Paris et al., 1989; Soloff et al., 1994a), which increases the risk of suicide. Isometsa et al. (1996) found that 95 percent of suicide victims with cluster B personality disorders had comorbid depressive disorders, substance use disorders, or both. Fyer and colleagues (1988) found that individuals with comorbid BPD and mood or substance use disorders were more likely than other patients to make high lethality suicide attempts. In addition, borderline symptoms that do not reach criteria for a diagnosis of BDP in depressed patients increases the likelihood of a suicide attempt (Corbitt et al., 1996; Friedman et al., 1983; Joffe and Regan, 1989). In contrast, Soloff (1994a) found no increased risk of suicide attempt with comorbid affective or substance use disorders. Often suicidal behaviors in BPD occur in the *absence* of serious depressive symptoms, which some attribute to the impulsivity associated with BPD (Brodsky et al., 1997; Corbitt et al., 1996).

A history of child abuse or neglect in those with BPD increases risk of suicide (Brodsky et al., 1997; Brown and Anderson, 1991; Dubo et al., 1997; van der Kolk et al., 1991). There is a high frequency of abuse histories in those with BPD, and childhood abuse is posited to be a causative factor (Figueroa and Silk, 1997; Gunderson and Sabo, 1993; Paris, 1998).

The effects of childhood trauma on suicide risk are discussed in Chapter 5.

Alcohol Use

As of 1999, 64 percent of all American adults report some use of alcoholic beverages (non-abstention), and this has not changed appreciably since 1939 (The Gallup Organization, 2001). Annual consumption currently averages to the equivalent of approximately 2.2 gallons of pure ethanol per capita (NIAAA, 2001). Approximately 15–18 million Americans have an alcohol abuse disorder (NIAAA, 2001) with 8.2 million Americans dependent on alcohol in a 1999 government survey (SAMHSA, 1999).

Alcohol-related suicides vary by state and jurisdiction, from 28 percent in Ohio to 53 percent in Alaska (Table 3-1), consistent with increased frequency of alcohol associated suicides reported for the western "frontier" states (Hlady and Middaugh, 1988; May, 1995). Alcohol-related suicides are more frequently associated with death by firearms (Brent et al., 1987; Hlady and Middaugh, 1988). However, among some subpopulations of American Indians (May et al., In press), and in other countries such as Australia (Hayward et al., 1992), alcohol-related suicides are no more likely to be associated with firearms than with other methods (e.g., hanging and carbon monoxide poisoning).

As with the psychiatric disorders, the majority of those who consume alcohol and/or meet diagnostic criteria for alcohol abuse disorders do not attempt or complete suicide. Alcohol use, particularly heavy use and alcohol dependence, is highly associated with suicide in three ways:

- Alcohol through its disinhibiting effects is related to suicide attempts and completions
- Individuals with alcohol use disorders are at an increased risk of suicide as compared to the population at large
- At the population level (nationally and internationally) alcohol consumption is correlated with suicide rate

Impulsivity, Relationship Loss, and Hopelessness

Acute alcohol intoxication acts as a disinhibitor in impulsive, angry suicides, often precipitated by loss of a relationship (Mayfield and Montgomery, 1972). On average (see Table 3-1) almost 25 percent of suicide victims are intoxicated (generally 0.10 gm/dl blood alcohol concentration or greater) at the time of death. The highest prevalence of intoxication is generally found among males under the age of 50 in most every popula-

TABLE 3-1 The Nature and Extent of Alcohol-Related Suicide in Selected Studies of Large Populations

Study Population (years)	N of Suicides	% Alcohol-Related	% (Legally) Intoxicated[a]	Avg. BAC	Reference
Cuyahoga County (Cleveland), OH (1959-1974)	(830)	28	20	—	Ford et al., 1979
Alaska (1983-84)	(195)	53	31	—	Hlady & Middaugh, 1988
Alaska Natives		(79)	(54)		
Alaska Whites		(48)	(20)		
Erie County (Buffalo), NY (1972-1984)	(806)	33	20	28% > .05	Welte et al., 1988
North Carolina (1973-1983)	(8,146)	35	26	—	Smith et al., 1989
Western Australia (1986-1988)	(515)	36	20	—	Hayward et al., 1992
Oklahoma (1978-1984)	(3,082)	40	24	—	Goodman et al., 1991
New Mexico (1990-1999)	(3,044)	44	—	—	May et al., in press
NM American Indians (1980-1998)	(439)	(69)	(62)	.136 (all suicides) .197 (alcohol positive only)	

— = 38.4   — = 23.5
sd = 8.2   sd = 4.5
md = 36   md = 22
weighted — = 37.4   weighted — = 24.7

[a]Defined in most studies in the United States as BAC > 0.10 gm/dl of blood and in the Australia and New Mexico studies, as > 0.08 gm/dl, the same as legal intoxication for driving a motor vehicle.
—data not available

tion studied (Ford et al., 1979; Hayward et al., 1992) and in suicides that occur at night and on weekends (Smith et al., 1989; Welte et al., 1988). Alcohol was involved for 15–64 percent of attempters (Roizen, 1982).

Common among alcohol-related suicides are impulsivity and relationship loss, both in adults (Welte et al., 1988) and youth (Brent et al., 1987). Similar patterns of impulsivity have been linked to alcohol-related suicide in particular cultures such as younger adults in Finland (Makela, 1996) and Native Americans (Bechtold, 1988; Ward, 1984). Relationship problems are frequently precipitants in alcohol-related suicides (Miles, 1977; Murphy and Robins, 1967; Rich et al., 1988) especially when there is ready access to a high-lethality means (Hayward et al., 1992; Welte et al., 1988). Suicides associated with chronic conditions such as long-term depression or physical disability are less likely to involve alcohol (Welte et al., 1988).

> . . . Mostly, I'm a social drinker. Like everyone else, I've been drunk in my time but it's not really my style; I value my control too highly. This time, however, I went at the bottle with a pure need, as though parched. I drank before I got out of bed, almost before my eyes were open. I continued steadily throughout the morning until, by lunchtime, I had half a bottle of whiskey inside me and was beginning to feel human . . . The important thing was not to stop. In this way, I got through a bottle of whiskey a day, a good deal of wine and beer. Yet it had little effect. Toward evening, when the child was in bed, I suppose I was a little tipsy, but the drinking was merely part of a more jagged frenzy. . . .
>
> After that, I remember nothing at all until I woke up in the hospital and saw my wife's face swimming vaguely toward me through a yellowish fog. She was crying. But that was three days later, three days of oblivion, a hole in my head. . . . only gradually have I been able to piece together the facts from hints and snippets, recalled reluctantly and with apologies. Nobody wants to remind an attempted suicide of his folly, or be reminded of it (Alvarez, The Savage God: A Study of Suicide, 1971/1990: 294-297).

Interpersonal loss seems to be a major acute precursor of suicide among many with alcohol use disorders (Murphy, 1992; Murphy et al., 1979). Murphy and colleagues (1979) demonstrated that 26–33 percent of alcoholics had experienced a loss of affectional relationships within 6 weeks of suicide and 48–50 percent had similar losses within the previous year. Duberstein et al. (1993) more recently replicated these findings among alcoholics/substance abusing subjects in finding that interpersonal stressors were present within 6 weeks (77 percent) or 1 year (90 percent) of suicides by alcoholics as compared to 22 and 59 percent, respectively, among suicides by persons with mood or anxiety disorders. Hopelessness significantly predicted suicidal ideation more accurately than depression in alcoholics, as well as non-alcoholics (Beck et al., 1982). Alcohol has an effect on depression as well. Large doses of alcohol over time are associated with depressive activity (Mirin and Weiss, 1986; Tamerin and Mendelson, 1969). Some suggest that depression is secondary to the effects of heavy and chronic alcohol consumption, since depression wanes with withdrawal (Flavin et al., 1990; Nakamura et al., 1983). However, drinking can also begin as a reaction to depression.

Alcohol Use Disorders

Estimating the prevalence of suicide among those with alcohol use disorders is difficult because the data come from studies using varying approaches (retro- and prospective, and population studies) as well as highly variable follow-up periods. Harris and Barraclough (1997) found in their meta-analysis of 32 studies that alcohol-dependence and abuse increased suicide risk almost 6-fold. Murphy (1992) estimates that in a year, 25 percent of all suicides (approximately 7600 of 30,400) in the United States are of individuals with alcohol use disorders, and that these individuals have 115 times the risk of suicide compared to a psychiatrically healthy population. Lifetime risk of suicide has been estimated at 3.4 percent for those with severe alcohol abuse disorders requiring hospitalization (Murphy, 1992). Alcohol dependent individuals who complete suicide are most frequently male, white, middle-aged, unmarried, with hospitalization in the past year, and with a history of previous attempts (Roy and Linnoila, 1986). Yet alcohol-dependent females have a 20- to 30-fold greater risk of completing suicide than non-clinical female populations (Harris and Barraclough, 1997; Medhus, 1975).

Severity and time-course of the alcohol use disorder are associated with suicide risk. In a mortality study of 8060 individuals matched for age, sex, race, and cigarette smoking, the effects of alcohol intake were examined on a variety of causes of death over 10 years (Klatsky et al., 1981). Suicide accounted for 3.5 percent of all the deaths, and the heaviest drinkers, those consuming 6+ drinks daily, accounted for almost half of the suicides. Merrill and colleagues (1992) in England found increased alcohol consumption associated with increased rates of suicide attempt for males and females. The risk of suicide is highest in the late stages of chronic alcohol abuse, and is associated with similar high risk events and psychiatric symptoms found among non-alcoholic individuals (Kendall, 1983).

Population Correlation

Over the last century alcohol and suicide rates have co-varied in a number of countries. A precipitous drop in suicide rates in the United States (from 15.3 to 10.2 per 100,000 between 1910 to 1920) occurred during the period of most acute reduction of alcohol consumption (Lester, 1995). Reductions in alcohol consumption secondary to rationing in the 1950s in Sweden, and large increases in price in Denmark in the early part of the twentieth century both coincided with significant reductions in the suicide rates (Wasserman, 1992). In Finland, a significant positive correlation was observed between alcohol consumption and suicide rates for males aged 15–49 from 1950 to 1991, but not for older males (Makela, 1996). A study examining the relationship between alcohol consumption and suicide in Denmark, Finland, Norway, and Sweden for up to 50 years found significant relationships only in Sweden and Norway (Norstrom, 1988). No relationship was observed for Finland (Norstrom, 1988). The single largest reduction in male suicides in the last 30 years occurred during the Perestroika in the USSR during the second half of the 1980s. This reduction was seen in all 15 republics of the USSR, with the greatest decrease, from over 65 per 100,000 to less than 40 per 100,000 occurring in the Russian Republic from 1984 to 1986 (Wasserman et al., 1998). During this time, alcohol consumption was significantly reduced due to a broad, multi-level national campaign to reduce alcoholism and to immeasurably increased hope from the economic and social restructuring under Gorbachev (Wasserman and Varnik, 2001). Population-level observations are difficult to interpret, since it is not known if the variables of interest are correlated within individuals (see also Chapter 6). Possible confounding issues include income, divorce and unemployment (e.g., Makela, 1996).

Substance Use Disorders

In 1999 almost 15 million Americans used illicit drugs and 3.5 million were dependent on these substances (SAMHSA, 1999). Drug dependence has been experienced by 7.5 percent of the population, and drug use without dependency by 4.4 percent of the population (Kessler et al., 1994). Substance abuse prevalence is increasing among younger cohorts (Kessler et al., 1994).

Abuse of illicit substances, like alcohol abuse, is associated with increased risk for suicide and suicide attempts. Treated opiate abusers had a suicide attempt rate 4 times that of the community surveyed, with a lifetime prevalence of 17.3 percent (Murphy et al., 1983). Reported estimates for completed suicide associated with illicit substance abuse (mainly opiate use) range from 7 to 25 percent proportionate mortality[3] (Flavin et al., 1990). Molnar and colleagues (2001) estimated the PAR for serious suicide attempts among substance abusers (including alcohol) to be 30.2 percent for females and 52.9 percent for males. The vast majority of studies focus either on alcohol disorders alone or combine alcohol and other substance abuse disorders in their analyses. Murphy (2000) in a recent review argues that such an approach is warranted because of the common co-morbidities and the similarities among those with alcohol use disorders and those with illicit substance use disorders. On the other hand, others find clinical factors that distinguish those who abuse illicit substances from those who abuse alcohol (Porsteinsson et al., 1997; Vaillant, 1966).

Substance abusers frequently have comorbid Axis I and II disorders. A cross-national investigation found that mood and anxiety disorders are often comorbid in substance-abusing individuals, and that of the Axis II disorders, conduct disorder and antisocial personality disorder are at increased prevalence in this population (Merikangas et al., 1998). Almost 18 percent of individuals with substance use disorders (non-alcohol) have anti-social personality disorder (Kessler et al., 1994), while 10–30 percent of treatment-seeking cocaine abusing and opioid dependent individuals have comorbid depression (Weiss and Hufford, 1999). The relationship of substance abuse disorders and comorbid psychiatric diagnoses to suicidal behavior is complex, since it is often unclear in what order the conditions arose, what causal links exist, and whether other characteristics of psychology, biology or social circumstance may mediate the relationships.

The same suicide risk factors are found in substance abusers as in other populations: family psychopathology (especially maternal depression), hopelessness, comorbid disorders, use of multiple substances, and poorer psychosocial functioning (Flavin et al., 1990). Impulsivity (Block et al., 1988) is associated with increased risk for developing substance use disorders, as are novelty-seeking/impulsive personality traits (see section below) (Fergusson and Lynskey, 1996; Fergusson et al., 2000). In addition to the associated risk factors, individuals who abuse substances often diminish their protective social networks, secondary to their drug-related behaviors (Vaillant and Blumenthal, 1990).

---

[3]Proportionate mortality describes the proportion of deaths in a specified population over a period of time attributable to different causes.

Special Issues for Youth

Youth and Mental Disorders

About 20 percent of children ages 9–17 are estimated to have mental disorders with at least mild functional impairment, 6.2 percent of which have a mood disorder (Shaffer et al., 1996). Longitudinal data from New Zealand (Feehan et al., 1993) found a 21.5 percent prevalence rate of DSM-III disorders at age 15 and a 36 percent prevalence rate at age 18. The most prevalent conditions at age 15 were anxiety (8 percent) and conduct disorders (5 percent). At age 18, they were major depressive episode (17 percent), alcohol dependence (10 percent), and social phobia (11 percent). In the United States, depression is the strongest correlate of suicide for adolescent suicide victims and attempters (Brent et al., 1993; Shaffer, 1988), although some studies find conduct disorder more strongly associated with suicide attempts in adolescents (Borst and Noam, 1989). In four studies, between 40 and 53 percent of the youth suicides were diagnosed with a personality disorder (Brent et al., 1994; Lesage et al., 1994; Rich and Runeson, 1992; Rich et al., 1986). The prevalence of personality disorders in suicide appears to decline with age (Rich et al., 1986), perhaps due to a decreased population prevalence of personality disorders across the lifespan (Ames and Molinari, 1994; Cohen et al., 1994).

The nature and distribution, as well as symptom presentation, of mental disorders are somewhat different in children and youth as compared to adults, although the overall prevalence is comparable. Youth are more likely to exhibit irritability, acting out behaviors, and anger rather than exhibiting sad and depressed affect (APA, 1994). Bipolar disorder in youth often presents with symptoms typically diagnosed as conduct disorder and/or attention deficit disorder (Berenson, 1998; Mohr, 2001). It also may be that bipolar disorder in youth is frequently comorbid with these other disorders, complicating diagnosis and treatment (Berenson, 1998; Mohr, 2001).

Hopelessness, an important risk and predictive factor for adult suicide (see below), is also associated with suicidality in adolescents. Hopelessness predicts repeat suicide attempts and differentiates suicidal from non-suicidal psychiatrically disturbed youths (for reviews, see Brent et al., 1990; Weishaar and Beck, 1990). The severity of depression may be a stronger predictor of suicidality than hopelessness in younger populations (e.g., Asarnow et al., 1987; Cole, 1989; Goldston et al., 2001), which may reflect the time-course of cognitive development (c.f., Nolen-Hoeksema et al., 1992). On the other hand, positive expectations are one of the strongest predictors of resilient people from childhood through adulthood in longitudinal studies (Werner, 1995; Werner and Smith, 2001; Wyman et al., 1993).

Adolescents, Alcohol, and Substance Abuse

The relationship between alcohol and younger suicide victims (i.e., those younger than 35 years of age) is not simple. Brent et al. (1987) found a very strong link between alcohol use prior to suicide and firearm use among youth less than 20 years of age. Teenage suicide victims who use firearms to complete suicide are 4.9 times more likely to have been drinking than those who used other methods.

Substance abuse among youth is another of the most significant risk factors for suicidal behavior (for review, see Brent and Kolko, 1990). The 3-fold rise in adolescent suicide that occurred in the United States throughout the 1960s and 1980s has been attributed to a rise in use of alcohol and illicit drugs. Among the youthful suicides in San Diego, California, the occurrence of drug abuse was reported more frequently in the 1970s and early 1980s; it was the major difference between suicide precursors in younger and older victims (Rich et al., 1986). Multiple substance use or polysubstance abuse (alcohol and other drugs) was common among younger suicide victims in San Diego, although the direction of the relationship of substance abuse to other diagnoses such as depression was not clear (Fowler et al., 1986). Difficulty in pinning down the extant relationship between alcohol, drugs, and suicide has been noted elsewhere (Neeleman and Farrell, 1997).

Family dysfunction and personality traits can contribute to the effects of alcohol and substance abuse on suicide among youth. Frequent illicit substance abuse and intoxication with alcohol can be an important predictor of hopelessness, particularly among lonely youth (Page et al., 1993). A psychological autopsy of 20 adolescents revealed a history of drug or alcohol abuse in 70 percent of those completing suicide compared with 29 percent of controls (Shafii et al., 1985). Other significant risk factors were antisocial behavior, an inhibited personality, and previous suicide attempts or suicide communications. Surveys of youth, parents, and respondents in psychological autopsies of deceased youth in California point to alcohol and substance abuse as important risk factors for suicide. Family dysfunction, individual psychopathology and distress, and interpersonal problems were also cited as contributing factors (Nelson et al., 1988).

King et al. (1993) examined the relationship between alcohol consumption, family dysfunction, and depression to suicidality in adolescent female inpatients. Both alcohol consumption and family dysfunction predicted the severity of clinician documented suicidal ideation and behavior. Self-reported ideation, however, was not predicted by alcohol consumption, but rather by the severity of depression and family dysfunction.

Comorbidity of Psychiatric Disorders

Comorbidity of psychiatric disorders with other psychiatric illnesses including substance use disorders or with somatic disorders increases risk of suicide (Lönnqvist, 2000). Co-occurrence of mental disorders and substance abuse disorders increases the risk of suicide beyond that for each of these disorders singly (Suominen et al., 1996). Methodological practices in psychiatry present obstacles to understanding this increased risk posed by comorbidity. It is common to provide only one "primary" psychiatric diagnosis (e.g., Roy and Draper, 1995). Since this primary diagnosis is often the only one analyzed, important data on co-occurrence of disorders is minimized or lost. Some researchers believe it is the co-occurrence of psychiatric disorders itself that mediates suicide risk (Goldsmith et al., 1990). The importance of comorbidity may be part of the increased risk for suicide that cumulative risk factors confer.

PSYCHOLOGICAL DIMENSIONS OF SUICIDE RISK

Information from a number of fields has converged over the last 30 years on an understanding of how genetic, developmental, environmental, physiological, and psychological factors all effect health through multiple, complex causal pathways (IOM, 2001). A growing body of data shows that the physiological responses to stress are potent contributors to physical illnesses including cardiac diseases and cancer, as well as mental disorders including depression and post-traumatic stress disorder (Heim et al., 1997; Nemeroff, 1996). The physiological response to stress can be modified through psychosocial components (e.g., Koenig et al., 1997), including learning new coping skills and thinking habits (Antoni et al., 2000; Bandura, 1992; Cruess et al., 2000a; 2000b).

These psychosocial and learning interventions significantly improve psychological responses to stressors, as well (e.g., Antoni et al., 2001; Cruess et al., 2000b; Gillham et al., 1995; Jaycox et al., 1994; Wyman et al., 2000). "Resilience" represents positive adaptations in the face of life stress. Resilience has been studied alternately as an individual trait or quality, an outcome, or, more recently, as an interactive process of positive factors and negative factors within and between individuals and their environments (see Glantz and Sloboda, 1999; Kaplan, 1999; Kumpfer, 1999, for reviews). Psychological research on resilient outcomes largely focuses on habits of thinking, problem solving, and expectations about the future that appear to protect individuals from developing psychiatric disorders, and on how to enhance such "cumulative competence and stress protection" (Wyman et al., 2000). The enhancement of resiliency through modification of these factors has developed into a field of study and is used in prevention programs for numerous unwanted outcomes including suicide, both in the United States and in other nations (see Chapter 8). Building resiliency is included in one of the four aims of the Surgeon General's National Strategy for Suicide Prevention (PHS, 2001) and is promoted as a necessary part of national and school-based suicide reduction strategies by the United Nations (1996) and World Health Organization (1999).

The opportunity for enlisting these psychosocial factors to reduce suicide appears potent, but remains largely untested. This section discusses the psychological factors in these stress–response pathways, their relationship to suicide, and what is known about their protective effects against suicide. Chapter 5 provides a developmental context for the role of psychological factors in responses to trauma. These psychological processes form the basis for some of the treatment and prevention strategies described in Chapters 7 and 8.

Psychological Variables

The psychological variables that have been studied in relation to suicide include aspects of thinking, reasoning, and behavior, as listed below.

- Memory and Cognitive Distortions
- Hopelessness and Hope
- Self-Efficacy
- Locus of Control
- Coping Style and Affect Regulation

Memory and Cognitive Distortions

Individuals with mental disorders, especially those with depression, often display cognitive distortions such as rigid or dichotomous thinking, overgeneralization, exaggeration or minimization of events, drawing conclusions based on insufficient/contradictory evidence or selectively attending to relevant information, and falsely attributing causality to themselves (for review, see Weishaar and Beck, 1990). Unlike self-reports of high depression, which predict depression remission after treatment, high levels of cognitive distortion appear difficult to modify and may predict continued depression (Brent et al., 1998). Studies have found greater cognitive distortions among suicidal youths and adults than among nonsuicidal mentally ill or healthy controls (see Brent and Kolko, 1990;

Weishaar and Beck, 1990). In particular, cognitive rigidity (dichotomous thinking) seems to more strongly characterize suicidal than nonsuicidal individuals. Such rigid thinking appears related to the interpersonal and general problem-solving deficits commonly seen in suicidal individuals (see below). Cognitive behavioral and problem-solving therapy specifically target such variables and appear effective in reducing suicidality (see Chapter 7).

Recent reports address the association between suicidality and memory. A neuropsychological study indicated that executive function deficits, and not general memory deficits, differentiate suicidal from nonsuicidal mentally ill and nonmentally ill individuals (Keilp et al., 2001). Several studies have found a pattern of "over-general," or non-specific, autobiographical memory in suicidal vs. nonsuicidal persons that demonstrates high correlations with interpersonal problem-solving deficits (Evans et al., 1992; Pollock et al., 2001; Sidley et al., 1997). Investigators posit that the inability to retrieve specific memories of negative events may serve as a means of emotion regulation (e.g., Startup et al., 2001), but hinders effective problem-solving by restricting information retrieval (Pollock et al., 2001). These findings suggest a benefit of targeting problem-solving treatments for suicidality (Chapter 7) to this memory pattern (Pollock et al., 2001).

Hopelessness and Hope

The relationship between hopelessness and suicidality has been studied for over 25 years (for reviews, see Abramson et al., 2000; Beck et al., 1975; Brent and Kolko, 1990; Weishaar and Beck, 1990). Hopelessness predicted suicide ideation better than depression in a sample of 1306 people with at least one mood disorder and 488 patients without mood disorders (Beck et al., 1993). In longitudinal studies, Beck and colleagues (1990; 1989; 1985) found that elevated scores on the Beck Hopelessness Scale (Beck et al., 1974) predicted 91–94 percent of suicides in both inpatients and outpatients over 5–10 years. Hopelessness appears trait-like, exhibiting stability and chronicity over the course of mental illness and remaining even after remission of major depression (Brent et al., 1998; Minkoff et al., 1973; Rifai et al., 1994). A high level of hopelessness during one psychiatric episode predicts high hopelessness in later episodes (Beck et al., 1985). Evidence suggests that hopelessness represents a distinct phenomenon that can arise separately from mood disorders and occurs across psychiatric diagnoses (Bonner and Rich, 1991; Joiner et al., 2001a; Minkoff et al., 1973). Treatment strategies that focus solely on the mood symptoms may therefore miss a critical, modifiable risk factor for reducing suicide.

Hopelessness appears to arise from multiple sources, including low self-esteem combined with interpersonal losses and the lack of confidence in one's ability to regulate mood or solve personal problems (negative coping efficacy beliefs, e.g., Catanzaro, 2000; Dieserud et al., 2001). Cognitive behavioral therapy (CBT) is designed to reduce clinical symptoms by changing thoughts and behaviors (Weishaar and Beck, 1990). Numerous studies show CBT is effective in reducing depression and hopelessness in various populations including adolescents (Brent et al., 1999; Brent et al., 1998). Reductions in suicidal ideation and attempt have also been reported (see Chapter 7), but there are no published findings on the *specific* effect of reducing hopelessness on rates of suicidality.

Alternatively, positive expectations regarding the future (hope) and positive ways of assigning causality to events (optimistic attributional style) powerfully buffer the effects of life stress on mental, behavioral, and physical health (e.g., Beck et al., 1976; Linehan et al., 1983; Range and Penton, 1994; Scheier and Carver, 1992; Taylor et al., 2000; Werner, 1996; Wyman et al., 1993). Research suggests that optimism enables individuals to procure and engage potent protective factors such as adaptive coping skills and increased self-efficacy (described below), reinterpreting adverse experiences to find meaning and benefit, and seeking and perceiving social support (Antoni et al., 2001; Benight et al., 1999a; Brissette et al., 2002; Scheier et al., 1986). Chapter 6 discusses how religious beliefs and involvement can increase hope. Several research groups have designed cognitive–behavioral interventions that teach optimism, and results suggest that children and adults can learn positive, hopeful thinking patterns that attenuate psychological distress and depression and make subsequent episodes of depression less likely (Antoni et al., 2001; Brissette et al., 2002; Gillham and Reivich, 1999; Gillham et al., 1995; Jaycox et al., 1994). Although studies indicate that hope protects against suicidality (Linehan et al., 1983; Malone et al., 2000; Range and Penton, 1994), no published studies on the effect of optimism training on suicidality are currently available.

Self-Efficacy

Self-efficacy beliefs, the assessment of one's ability to manage or control external and internal threats, exert a primary influence on human emotion, cognition, and behavior (Bandura, 1982; 1991). Positive self-efficacy beliefs represent the opposite of hopelessness and appear to protect individuals from suicidality (Linehan et al., 1983; Malone et al., 2000; Range and Penton, 1994; Strosahl et al., 1992). Coping self-efficacy beliefs affect physiological stress responses involving the catecholamines, opioids, and the hypothalamic-pituitary-adrenal axis (see Chapter 4)

(Bandura, 1982; 1992; Bandura et al., 1988; 1985; Benight et al., 1997), and directly contribute to emotional arousal, psychological distress and well-being, and anxiety (Bandura, 1988; 1991; Benight et al., 1997; 1999a; 1999b; 2001; Catanzaro and Mearns, 1999). Positive self-efficacy beliefs further increase the establishment and use of protective factors such as social support and active coping strategies (e.g., Bandura, 1982; 1988; 1992; Benight et al., 1999a; Green and Rodgers, 2001). Although some studies show coping efficacy beliefs buffering suicidality, very little research exists on modifying suicidality via increasing self-efficacy. Emerging research on school-based suicide prevention programs for at-risk youth, described in Chapter 8, demonstrates increased self-efficacy and decreased suicidality in program participants.

Locus of Control

Another area within cognitive psychology, "learned helplessness," recently expanded to include studies on hopelessness and suicidality. Briefly, the learned helplessness paradigm shows that exposure to uncontrollable stress results in long-term passivity, or the belief that other stressors are also out of an individual's control, *and* exposure to uncontrollable stressors specifically elicits neuroendocrine stress responses (see Chapter 4) and psychological distress (Frankenhaeuser, 1982; Grossi et al., 1998; Hyyppa, 1987; Maier and Seligman, 1976; Seligman, 1975). Explanatory, or attributional style describes how people assign meaning to positive and negative life events by attributing them either to stable (long-lasting), pervasive (global), and internal causes, or to unstable, specific, and external causes (see Weishaar and Beck, 1990). Meta-analyses of studies from the 1980s and early 1990s show a relationship between attributional style and depression in children and adults across psychiatric diagnoses. Specifically, attributing negative life events to internal, stable, global causes while explaining positive life events via external, unstable, specific causes increases self-reported and clinical depression (Gladstone and Kaslow, 1995; Joiner and Wagner, 1995; Sweeney et al., 1986). The reformulation of the learned helplessness model (Abramson et al., 1978) combines helplessness expectancies with depression, hopelessness, and suicidality (see Abramson et al., 2000 for a review). A number of prospective studies and one using path analysis (Abramson et al., 1998; Bonner and Rich, 1991; Hankin et al., 2001; Joiner and Rudd, 1995; Yang and Clum, 2000) have demonstrated that a negative explanatory style interacts with stressful life events to predict hopelessness and suicidality in youth and adults. The aforementioned interventions to teach optimism specifically target attributional style, and follow-up evaluation has demonstrated sustained changes in children's style a number of years after program participation

(Gillham and Reivich, 1999). No study to date, however, has investigated how changing attributional style affects suicidality.

Coping Style and Affect Regulation

Coping and emotion regulation styles refer to how individuals manage stressful conditions or events (actively or passively) and how they regulate their own emotional, physiological, behavioral, and cognitive reactions to stress (Lazarus and Folkman, 1984). Coping styles contribute to physical (see IOM, 2001) and mental health following stressors or trauma (e.g., Beaton et al., 1999; Benight et al., 1999a; Boeschen et al., 2001; Sandler et al., 1994; Schnyder et al., 2001). Specifically, active coping styles such as planning, engaging problems, and seeking social support, and cognitive reinterpretation coping (finding meaning and benefit from adverse events) appear to decrease symptoms of psychological disorder and attenuate hypothalamic-pituitary-adrenal responses to stress (e.g., Antoni et al., 2001; Benight et al., 1999a; Cruess et al., 2000b; Taylor et al., 2000). Likewise, religious coping positively influences physical and mental health (see Chapter 6). Maladaptive coping styles, however, generally correlate with negative outcomes and are such a cardinal feature of suicidal individuals that some have suggested including measures for these variables in assessment tools for suicidality (Shneidman, 1992; Yufit and Bongar, 1992).

Suicidologists consistently find ineffective coping styles for mood and impulse regulation and interpersonal problem-solving among suicidal individuals (for reviews, see Catanzaro, 2000; Weishaar and Beck, 1990). Suicidal individuals use fewer active coping strategies and more avoidant (passive) coping styles such as suppression and blame (Amir et al., 1999; Asarnow et al., 1987; Horesh et al., 1996; Josepho and Plutchik, 1994). Compared to other psychiatric patients, suicidal patients are also less likely to use cognitive coping strategies to de-emphasize the importance of a negative outcome or stressor (Horesh et al., 1996; Kotler et al., 1993). Impulsive problem-solving style and difficulty regulating mood is related to increased rates of suicide attempts (Brent and Kolko, 1990; Catanzaro, 2000). For some suicidal individuals, these inadequate coping styles appear during depressive episodes (are state-dependent); for others, especially those with personality disorders or alcoholism, these skills deficits are characteristics or traits of the individual (Linehan et al., 1987; Weishaar and Beck, 1990).

Many psychotherapeutic interventions target coping and emotion regulation skills (see Chapter 7). Coping skills are also relatively easy to target in school-based primary prevention, with many such programs showing good mental health outcomes (Durlak, 1997; Durlak and Wells, 1997; NRC, 2002). Chapter 8 describes school-based coping skills training programs that appear to reduce youth suicide. Longitudinal studies of children at risk for behavioral and mental health problems reveal that effective problem-solving skills correlate with positive outcomes in adulthood (Felsman and Vaillant, 1987; Rutter and Quinton, 1984; Werner, 1995).

The psychological variables reviewed in this section interact with each other and with environmental and biological factors in their influence on suicidality. Yet these attributes have not been broadly addressed in an integrated way. Coping, attributional style, and self-efficacy beliefs have largely been studied separately from hopelessness and suicidality. As described in Chapter 8, recent suicide prevention programs across the world have incorporated skills training and efficacy enhancement into their efforts, and evaluation of such interventions should yield critical information about the relationship between these variables and suicide.

Temperament and Personality

Research shows that mental health and the experience of stress is confounded with aspects of temperament and personality—individuals higher in emotionality report more negative life events and daily stresses than individuals lower in emotionality (Aldwin et al., 1989). One longitudinal study of older men found that personality characteristics accounted for 25 percent of the variance in mental health (Levenson et al., 1988). Classic studies linking certain personality types high in hostility, anger, stress, and anxiety to a greater susceptibility to coronary heart disease (for review, see IOM, 2001), along with evidence showing that subjective, rather than objective, life stress predicts suicidal outcomes among depressed patients (Malone et al., 2000) highlight the importance of disentangling the relationships between temperament, personality, stress and suicide. Chapter 5 provides a developmental perspective on how stress can affect psychology, but the converse also needs to be better understood. The various personalities and temperaments of individuals may necessitate different treatment, intervention, and prevention strategies for suicidality.

Two temperament types, impulsive/aggressive and depressive/withdrawn, are highly associated with suicide in adults (Kotler et al., 2001; Plutchik, 1995) and in adolescents (Apter et al., 1995; Brent et al., 1994). A cluster analysis of personality traits (Rudd et al., 2000) revealed that three clusters of personality traits describe 97 percent of suicidal psychiatric patients:

- Negativistic, avoidant
- Negativistic, avoidant, and dependent
- Negativistic, avoidant, and antisocial

The first two overlapped with depressive/withdrawn temperament while the third overlapped with impulsive/aggressive temperament.

Among the impulsive/aggressive types, suicide often occurs in the absence of an affective disorder (Apter et al., 1995; 1991). Individuals with irritable/aggressive temperaments have increased risk of violence and suicide. Suicide among this group is associated with antisocial personality traits, impulsiveness, uncontrolled emotions, high novelty-seeking, alcohol and substance abuse, and histories of childhood adversity, including sexual abuse (Fergusson et al., 2000; Verona and Patrick, 2000).

Impulsivity (Eaves et al., 2000) and related sensation-seeking (Hur and Bouchard, 1997) show partial heritability related to physiological markers such as the Lewis red blood cell phenotype (Harburg et al., 1982), and a significant but modest association with the gene for a receptor of the brain chemical norepinephrine, the adrenergic alpha 2A receptor (Comings et al., 2000). Alterations in the serotonin system have also been implicated in studies of impulsivity's relationship to aggression and suicide (Goldston, 2001; Lesch and Merschdorf, 2000; Mann et al., 2001; Verona and Patrick, 2000, see also Chapter 4).

Animal analog studies show that genetic strains with greater novelty-seeking/impulsivity are more susceptible to environmental insults (Piazza et al., 1991; 1993; 1996), with consequent increases in self-administration of addictive substances (Piazza et al., 1991; 1993; 1996). Other animal studies demonstrate that genetic influences on aggressive behavior interact with rearing environment, and that aggressive behavior and defeat experiences alter serotonin levels, future behavior, and genetic expression in the brain (Miczek et al., 2001; 1994; Nikulina et al., 1998; 1999; van Erp and Miczek, 2000). Such studies may provide models of how genetic and neurobiological aspects of impulsive/aggressive temperament interact with environmental factors to increase risks for suicide (see also Chapter 4).

The depressive/withdrawn personality traits are also termed "neuroticism." This temperament is highly correlated with negative affect, poor regulation of emotions, and high anxiety, as well as suicide (Catanzaro, 2000; Goldsmith et al., 1990). High neuroticism was found linked with increased suicide attempts in a 21-year, prospective, study of 1265 children in New Zealand (Fergusson et al., 2000). Like those individuals at risk for suicide with the irritable/aggressive traits, those with high neuroticism who attempted suicide were also more likely to have experienced childhood trauma, including abuse and inadequate relationships with caretakers (see Chapter 5).

Temperament emerges as an important feature in long-term studies of resiliency (Rutter and Quinton, 1984; Werner, 1995; 1996). Temperament interacts in cumulative ways with the environment. For example, Holahan and Moos (1990) found that personality characteristics function as protective factors under high stress, primarily by influencing coping style. The temperament of an infant also evokes different responses from caregivers, creating either positive or negative social experiences for the child. These experiences cumulate as differential social resources throughout childhood and adolescence (Werner, 1996). Youth with psychological problems or psychiatric disorders are at greater risk for behavior-dependent adverse life events, thereby increasing exposure to stressors and trauma, which in turn affects personality development, thus creating a cyclical pathway of greater psychopathology (Ge and Conger, 1999; Sandberg et al., 1998).

Temperament and personality emerge early in life and remain relatively stable over the life-course, and thus may be less easily modifiable than other psychological variables. However, given that their effects on stress and health are often mediated by other cognitive mechanisms such as coping and explanatory style, opportunities for intervention do exist. Constructive strategies to interrupt the pathway leading from pre-existing disposition to self-destructive behavior can be taught. For example, teaching specific strategies for coping with stress have proven successful (Antoni et al., 2000; Linehan et al., 1991, see also Chapter 7).

Knowledge of personality traits and temperament and the psychological variables discussed above needs to be integrated with what is known about stress response and suicidal outcomes in order to design appropriate interventions. Longitudinal life-course studies can help to foster more in-depth knowledge of the role of personality in the development of suicidality over a person's life.

Psychic Pain

Psychic pain represents a particular risk factor for suicide that deserves special comment. One of the founders of suicide theory and research, Edwin Schneidman, wrote about the state of perturbation he observed in highly suicidal individuals (1971; 1984; 1992). He later termed this state "psychache" (Shneidman, 1993), a state of psychic pain that an individual experiences as intolerable and resistant to any efforts to produce relief. Indicators of acute suicidality (see Chapter 7) such as severe anxiety, depression, and agitation may overlap with this state of pain. As described in Chapter 1, psychic pain may be an overarching description of the experiential/phenomenological state that leads an individual to seek death through suicide as an escape.

A study by Malone and colleagues (2000) found that subjective reports of depression and distress more strongly predict suicide than objective measures. Kovacs et al. (1975) report that 56 percent of suicidal patients wanted to commit suicide to escape their psychic pain. Those reporting this motive had high levels of hopelessness. Those who did not report psychic pain as their reason for suicide were more often motivated by a desire to manipulate and control others, and were less likely to exhibit hopelessness. Suicidal ideation and attempts in depressed patients are highly correlated with affective factors such as sadness and crying spells and with cognitive factors like self-hate, and not as strongly with somatic symptoms of depression (Beck and Lester, 1973; Beck et al., 1973; Lester and Beck, 1977). Furthermore, suicidal behavior among those with borderline personality disorder, for example, often represents a strategy to regulate psychic pain (see Catanzaro, 2000).

In depression, this faith in deliverance, in ultimate restoration is absent. The pain is unrelenting, and what makes the condition intolerable is the foreknowledge that no remedy will come—not in a day, an hour, a month, or a minute. If there is mild relief, one knows that it is only temporary; more pain will follow. It is hopelessness even more than pain that crushes the soul. So the decision-making of daily life involves not, as in normal affairs, shifting from one annoying situation to another less annoying—or from discomfort to relative comfort, or from boredom to activity—but moving from pain to pain . . . . And this results in a striking experience—one which I have called, borrowing military terminology, the situation of the walking wounded. For in virtually any other serious sickness, a patient who felt similar devastation would be lying flat in bed, possibly sedated and hooked up to the tubes and wires of life-support systems, but at the very least in a posture of repose and in an isolated setting. His invalidism would be necessary, unquestioned and honorably attained. However, the sufferer from depression has no such option and therefore finds himself, like a walking casualty of war, thrust into the most intolerable social and family situations. There he must, despite the anguish devouring his brain, present a face approximating the one that is associated with ordinary events and companionship. He must try to utter small talk, and be responsive to questions, and knowingly nod and frown and, God help him, even smile (Styron, Darkness Visible: A Memoir of Madness, 1990:62–63).

Life satisfaction, existential and spiritual well-being, and/or beliefs that one can survive and resolve the pain without resorting to suicide are protective against suicide and suicidality (Bonner and Rich, 1991; Ellis and Smith, 1991; Koivumaa-Honkanen et al., 2001; Malone et al., 2000, see also Chapter 6). Positive coping self-efficacy beliefs can directly reduce psychic distress (e.g., Benight et al., 1999b; Catanzaro and Mearns, 1999). Self-efficacy enhancement can be provided through a number of psychotherapeutic approaches such as mastery experiences, verbal persuasion, and modeling/teaching. Studies examining phenomenological and neuroscience variables (e.g., social cognitive neuroscience) have been neglected, but some researchers suggest such integrative studies would be useful for prevention (e.g., Beskow et al., 1999).

FINDINGS

• Approximately 50 percent of those who complete suicides are not in treatment, despite that the vast majority are suffering from psychiatric disorders. Those that are in treatment are often inadequately medicated, insufficiently followed after acute treatment, and/or do not adhere to treatment plans.

Adequate training is essential so that primary care physicians and specialty care physicians understand the appropriate doses of psychopharmacological medications to prescribe and how to follow up to ensure adherence.

• Suicide most commonly is associated with a diagnosis of depression. Recent research has increasingly established anxiety disorders and borderline personality disorder as significantly elevating suicide risk. Comorbidity of psychiatric disorders and/or substance abuse is common and further increases suicide risk. About 90 percent of suicides are associated with mental illness, but over 95 percent of those afflicted never even attempt suicide.

Additional research, especially prospective, longitudinal, and ecological-transactional research, is necessary to understand the etiological pathways to suicide and what identifies those who are at risk.

• About one fourth of all suicides in the U.S. are individuals with alcohol use disorders. Alcohol inebriation is indicated in up to 64 percent of suicide attempts. Abuse of illicit substances also is associated with a significant increase in suicide rate.

Alcohol and substance abuse are important risk factors for suicide and should be heeded by physicians as indicators of potential for suicide.

- Alcohol or substance use disorder, conduct disorder, and impulsivity/sensation-seeking often co-occur and represent particular suicide risk for youth.

The evidence regarding the links between suicide and aggression/impulsivity is growing. This relationship requires additional attention, particularly regarding its developmental etiology.

- Hopelessness is related to suicidality across age, diagnoses, and severity of disorder, yet the field lacks research on the pathways to hopelessness, interrelationships between hopelessness and other psychological aspects of suicide risk, and on the specific effects of reducing hopelessness on suicide. Effective treatments exist for reducing hopelessness.

Clinical trials are needed on the specific effects of reducing hopelessness on suicide.

- Optimism and coping skills enhance both mental and physical health. Research suggests that these can be taught. The opportunity for building resilience through modification of coping and cognitive styles appears potent, but effects of such interventions on suicidality remains largely untested.

Evaluation of mental health promotion programs is needed on the efficacy of reducing suicide via resilience enhancement.

REFERENCES

Abramson LY, Alloy LB, Hogan ME, Whitehouse WG, Cornette M, Akhavan S, Chiara A. 1998. Suicidality and cognitive vulnerability to depression among college students: A prospective study. *Journal of Adolescence*, 21(4): 473-487.

Abramson LY, Alloy LB, Hogan ME, Whitehouse WG, Gibb BE, Hankin BL, Cornette MM. 2000. The hopelessness theory of suicidality. In: Joiner TE, Rudd MD, Editors. *Suicide Science: Expanding the Boundaries.* (pp. 17-32). Norwell, MA: Kluwer Academic Publishers.

Abramson LY, Seligman MEP, Teasdale JD. 1978. Learned helplessness in humans: Critique and reformulation. *Journal of Abnormal Psychology*, 87: 49-74.

Ahrens B, Haug HJ. 1996. Suicidality in hospitalized patients with a primary diagnosis of personality disorder. *Crisis*, 17(2): 59-63.

Alda M. 1997. Bipolar disorder: From families to genes. *Canadian Journal of Psychiatry*, 42(4): 378-487.

Aldwin CM, Levenson MR, Spiro A 3rd, Bosse R. 1989. Does emotionality predict stress? Findings from the normative aging study. *Journal of Personality and Social Psychology*, 56(4): 618-624.

Allgulander C. 2000. Psychiatric aspects of suicidal behaviour: Anxiety disorders. In: Hawton K, van Heeringen K, Editors. *The International Handbook of Suicide and Attempted Suicide.* (pp. 179-192). Chichester, UK: John Wiley and Sons.

Allgulander C, Lavori PW. 1991. Excess mortality among 3302 patients with 'pure' anxiety neurosis. *Archives of General Psychiatry*, 48(7): 599-602.

Alvarez A. 1971/1990. *The Savage God: A Study of Suicide.* New York: W.W. Norton.

Amador XF, Friedman JH, Kasapis C, Yale SA, Flaum M, Gorman JM. 1996. Suicidal behavior in schizophrenia and its relationship to awareness of illness. *American Journal of Psychiatry*, 153(9): 1185-1188.

Ames A, Molinari V. 1994. Prevalence of personality disorders in community-living elderly. *Journal of Geriatric Psychiatry and Neurology*, 7(3): 189-194.

Amir M, Kaplan Z, Efroni R, Kotler M. 1999. Suicide risk and coping styles in posttraumatic stress disorder patients. *Psychotherapy and Psychosomatics*, 68(2): 76-81.

Antoni MH, Cruess S, Cruess DG, Kumar M, Lutgendorf S, Ironson G, Dettmer E, Williams J, Klimas N, Fletcher MA, Schneiderman N. 2000. Cognitive-behavioral stress management reduces distress and 24-hour urinary free cortisol output among symptomatic HIV-infected gay men. *Annals of Behavioral Medicine*, 22(1): 29-37.

Antoni MH, Lehman JM, Klibourn KM, Boyers AE, Culver JL, Alferi SM, Yount SE, McGregor BA, Arena PL, Harris SD, Price AA, Carver CS. 2001. Cognitive-behavioral stress management intervention decreases the prevalence of depression and enhances benefit finding among women under treatment for early-stage breast cancer. *Health Psychology*, 20(1): 20-32.

APA (American Psychiatric Association). 1994. *The Diagnostic and Statistical Manual of Mental Disorders.* 4th ed. Washington, DC.

Appels A. 1997. Depression and coronary heart disease: Observations and questions. *Journal of Psychosomatic Research*, 43(5): 443-452.

Appleby L. 2000. Prevention of suicide in psychiatric patients. In: Hawton K, van Heeringen K, Editors. *The International Handbook of Suicide and Attempted Suicide.* (pp. 617-630). Chichester, UK: John Wiley and Sons.

Apter A, Gothelf D, Orbach I, Weizman R, Ratzoni G, Har-Even D, Tyano S. 1995. Correlation of suicidal and violent behavior in different diagnostic categories in hospitalized adolescent patients. *Journal of American Academy of Child and Adolescent Psychiatry*, 34(7): 912-918.

Apter A, Kotler M, Sevy S, Plutchik R, Brown SL, Foster H, Hillbrand M, Korn ML, van Praag HM. 1991. Correlates of risk of suicide in violent and nonviolent psychiatric patients. *American Journal of Psychiatry*, 148(7): 883-887.

Asarnow JR, Carlson GA, Guthrie D. 1987. Coping strategies, self-perceptions, hopelessness, and perceived family environments in depressed and suicidal children. *Journal of Consulting and Clinical Psychology*, 55(3): 361-366.

Bailer J, Brauer W, Rey ER. 1996. Premorbid adjustment as predictor of outcome in schizophrenia: results of a prospective study. *Acta Psychiatrica Scandinavica*, 93(5): 368-377.

Bandura A. 1982. Self-efficacy mechanism in human agency. *American Psychologist*, 37(2): 122-147.

Bandura A. 1988. Self-efficacy conception of anxiety. *Anxiety Research*, 1(2): 77-98.

Bandura A. 1991. Social cognitive theory of self-regulation. *Organizational Behavior and Human Decision Processes*, 50(2): 248-287.

Bandura A. 1992. Self-efficacy mechanism in psychobiologic functioning. In: Schwarzer R, Editor. *Self-Efficacy: Thought Control of Action.* (pp. 355-394). Washington, DC: Hemisphere Publishing Corp.

Bandura A, Cioffi D, Taylor C, Barr, Brouillard ME. 1988. Perceived self-efficacy in coping with cognitive stressors and opioid activation. *Journal of Personality and Social Psychology*, 55(3): 479-488.

Bandura A, Taylor CB, Williams SL, Mefford IN, Barchas JD. 1985. Catecholamine secretion as a function of perceived coping self-efficacy. *Journal of Consulting and Clinical Psychology*, 53(3): 406-414.

Bayley R. 1996. First person account: Schizophrenia. *Schizophrenia Bulletin*, 22: 727-729.

Beaton R, Murphy S, Johnson C, Pike K, Corneil W. 1999. Coping responses and posttraumatic stress symptomatology in urban fire service personnel. *Journal of Traumatic Stress,* 12(2): 293-308.

Bechtold DW. 1988. Cluster suicide in American Indian adolescents. *American Indian and Alaska Native Mental Health Research,* 1(3): 26-35.

Beck AT. 1986. Hopelessness as a predictor of eventual suicide. *Annals of the New York Academy of Sciences,* 487: 90-96.

Beck AT, Brown G, Berchick RJ, Stewart BL, Steer RA. 1990. Relationship between hopelessness and ultimate suicide: A replication with psychiatric outpatients. *American Journal of Psychiatry,* 147(2): 190-195.

Beck AT, Brown G, Steer RA. 1989. Prediction of eventual suicide in psychiatric inpatients by clinical ratings of hopelessness. *Journal of Consulting and Clinical Psychology,* 57(2): 309-310.

Beck AT, Kovacs M, Weissman A. 1975. Hopelessness and suicidal behavior. An overview. *Journal of the American Medical Association,* 234(11): 1146-1149.

Beck AT, Lester D. 1973. Components of depression in attempted suicides. *Journal of Psychology,* 85: 257-260.

Beck AT, Lester D, Albert N. 1973. Suicidal wishes and symptoms of depression. *Psychological Reports,* 33(3): 770.

Beck AT, Steer RA, Beck JS, Newman CF. 1993. Hopelessness, depression, suicidal ideation, and clinical diagnosis of depression. *Suicide and Life-Threatening Behavior,* 23(2): 139-145.

Beck AT, Steer RA, Kovacs M, Garrison B. 1985. Hopelessness and eventual suicide: A 10-year prospective study of patients hospitalized with suicidal ideation. *American Journal of Psychiatry,* 142(5): 559-563.

Beck AT, Steer RA, McElroy MG. 1982. Relationships of hopelessness, depression and previous suicide attempts to suicidal ideation in alcoholics. *Journal of Studies on Alcohol,* 43(9): 1042-1046.

Beck AT, Weissman A, Kovacs M. 1976. Alcoholism, hopelessness and suicidal behavior. *Journal of Studies on Alcohol,* 37(1): 66-77.

Beck AT, Weissman A, Lester D, Trexler L. 1974. The measurement of pessimism: The hopelessness scale. *Journal of Consulting and Clinical Psychology,* 42(6): 861-865.

Beck AT, Weissman A, Lester D, Trexler L. 1976. Classification of suicidal behaviors. II. Dimensions of suicidal intent. *Archives of General Psychiatry,* 33(7): 835-837.

Bender DS, Dolan RT, Skodol AE, Sanislow CA, Dyck IR, McGlashan TH, Shea MT, Zanarini MC, Oldham JM, Gunderson JG. 2001. Treatment utilization by patients with personality disorders. *American Journal of Psychiatry,* 158(2): 295-302.

Benight CC, Antoni MH, Kilbourn K, Ironson G, Kumar MA, Fletcher MA, Redwine L, Baum A, Schneiderman N. 1997. Coping self-efficacy buffers psychological and physiological disturbances in HIV-infected men following a natural disaster. *Health Psychology,* 16(3): 248-255.

Benight CC, Flores J, Tashiro T. 2001. Bereavement coping self-efficacy in cancer widows. *Death Studies,* 25(2): 97-125.

Benight CC, Ironson G, Klebe K, Carver C, Wynings C, Burnett K, Greenwood D, Baum A, Scheiderman N. 1999a. Conservation of resources and coping self-efficacy predicting distress following a natural disaster: A causal model analysis where the environment meets the mind. *Anxiety, Stress, and Coping,* 12: 107-126.

Benight CC, Swift E, Sanger J, Smith A, Zeppelin D. 1999b. Coping self-efficacy as a mediator of distress following a natural disaster. *Journal of Applied Social Psychology,* 29(12): 2443-2464.

Berenson CK. 1998. Frequently missed diagnoses in adolescent psychiatry. *Psychiatric Clinics of North America,* 21(4): 917-926.

Beskow J, Kerkhof A, Kokkola A, Uutela A. 1999. *Suicide Prevention in Finland 1986-1996: External Evaluation by an International Peer Group*. Helsinki: Ministry of Social Affairs and Health.

Bhatia SC, Khan MH, Mediratta RP, Sharma A. 1987. High risk suicide factors across cultures. *International Journal of Social Psychiatry*, 33(3): 226-236.

Blackwood DH, Visscher PM, Muir WJ. 2001. Genetic studies of bipolar affective disorder in large families. *British Journal of Psychiatry*, 41 (Suppl): S134-S136.

Block J, Block JH, Keyes S. 1988. Longitudinally foretelling drug usage in adolescence: Early childhood personality and environmental precursors. *Child Development*, 59(2): 336-355.

Boeschen LE, Koss MP, Figueredo AJ, Coan JA. 2001. Experiential avoidance and posttraumatic stress disorder: A cognitive mediational model of rape recovery. *Journal of Aggression, Maltreatment and Trauma*, 4(2): 211-245.

Bonner RL, Rich AR. 1991. Predicting vulnerability to hopelessness. A longitudinal analysis. *Journal of Nervous and Mental Disease*, 179(1): 29-32.

Bornstein RF, Klein DN, Mallon JC, Slater JF. 1988. Schizotypal personality disorder in an outpatient population: Incidence and clinical characteristics. *Journal of Clinical Psychology*, 44(3): 322-325.

Borst SR, Noam GG. 1989. Suicidality and psychopathology in hospitalized children and adolescents. *Acta Paedopsychiatrica*, 52(3): 165-175.

Bostwick JM, Pankratz VS. 2000. Affective disorders and suicide risk: A reexamination. *American Journal of Psychiatry*, 157(12): 1925-1932.

Brady KT, Sonne SC. 1995. The relationship between substance abuse and bipolar disorder. *Journal of Clinical Psychiatry*, 56 (Supp 13): 19-24.

Breier A, Astrachan BM. 1984. Characterization of schizophrenic patients who commit suicide. *American Journal of Psychiatry*, 141(2): 206-209.

Brent DA, Holder D, Kolko D, Birmaher B, Baugher M, Roth C, Iyengar S, Johnson BA. 1997. A clinical psychotherapy trial for adolescent depression comparing cognitive, family, and supportive therapy. *Archives of General Psychiatry*, 54(9): 877-885.

Brent DA, Johnson BA, Perper J, Connolly J, Bridge J, Bartle S, Rather C. 1994. Personality disorder, personality traits, impulsive violence, and completed suicide in adolescents. *Journal of the American Academy of Child and Adolescent Psychiatry*, 33(8): 1080-1086.

Brent DA, Kolko DJ. 1990. The assessment and treatment of children and adolescents at risk for suicide. In: Blumenthal SJ, Kupfer DJ, Editors. *Suicide Over the Life Cycle: Risk Factors, Assessment, and Treatment of Suicidal Patients*. (pp. 253-302). Washington, DC: American Psychiatric Press.

Brent DA, Kolko DJ, Allan MJ, Brown RV. 1990. Suicidality in affectively disordered adolescent inpatients. *Journal of the American Academy of Child and Adolescent Psychiatry*, 29(4): 586-593.

Brent DA, Kolko DJ, Birmaher B, Baugher M, Bridge J. 1999. A clinical trial for adolescent depression: Predictors of additional treatment in the acute and follow-up phases of the trial. *Journal of the American Academy of Child and Adolescent Psychiatry*, 38(3): 263-270; discussion 270-271.

Brent DA, Kolko DJ, Birmaher B, Baugher M, Bridge J, Roth C, Holder D. 1998. Predictors of treatment efficacy in a clinical trial of three psychosocial treatments for adolescent depression. *Journal of the American Academy of Child and Adolescent Psychiatry*, 37(9): 906-914.

Brent DA, Perper JA, Allman CJ. 1987. Alcohol, firearms, and suicide among youth: Temporal trends in Allegheny County, Pennsylvania, 1960 to 1983. *Journal of the American Medical Association*, 257(24): 3369-3372.

Brent DA, Perper JA, Moritz G, Allman C, Friend A, Roth C, Schweers J, Balach L, Baugher M. 1993. Psychiatric risk factors for adolescent suicide: A case-control study. *Journal of the American Academy of Child and Adolescent Psychiatry*, 32(3): 521-529.

Brissette I, Scheier MF, Carver CS. 2002. The role of optimism in social network development, coping, and psychological adjustment during a life transition. *Journal of Personality and Social Psychology*, 82(1): 102-111.

Brodsky BS, Malone KM, Ellis SP, Dulit RA, Mann JJ. 1997. Characteristics of borderline personality disorder associated with suicidal behavior. *American Journal of Psychiatry*, 154(12): 1715-1719.

Bromet EJ, Schwartz JE, Fennig S, Geller L, Jandorf L, Kovasznay B, Lavelle J, Miller A, Pato C, Ram R, et al. 1992. The epidemiology of psychosis: The Suffolk County Mental Health Project. *Schizophrenia Bulletin*, 18(2): 243-255.

Brown GR, Anderson B. 1991. Psychiatric morbidity in adult inpatients with childhood histories of sexual and physical abuse. *American Journal of Psychiatry*, 148(1): 55-61.

Caldwell CB, Gottesman II. 1990. Schizophrenics kill themselves too: A review of risk factors for suicide. *Schizophrenia Bulletin*, 16(4): 571-589.

Caldwell CB, Gottesman II. 1992. Schizophrenia—a high-risk factor for suicide: Clues to risk reduction. *Suicide and Life-Threatening Behavior*, 22(4): 479-493.

Catanzaro SJ. 2000. Mood regulation and suicidal behavior. In: Joiner TE, Rudd DM, Editors. *Suicide Science: Expanding the Boundaries.* (pp. 81-103). Norwell, MA: Kluwer Academic Publishers.

Catanzaro SJ, Mearns J. 1999. Mood-related expectancy, emotional experience, and coping behavior. Kirsch I, Editor. *How Expectancies Shape Experience.* (pp. 67-91). Washington, DC: American Psychological Association.

Chochinov HM, Wilson KG, Enns M, Lander S. 1998. Depression, hopelessness, and suicidal ideation in the terminally ill. *Psychosomatics*, 39(4): 366-370.

Chu J. 1999. Trauma and suicide. In: Jacobs DG, Editor. *The Harvard Medical School Guide to Suicide Assessment and Intervention.* (pp. 332-354). San Francisco: Jossey-Bass Publishers.

Cohen BJ, Nestadt G, Samuels JF, Romanoski AJ, McHugh PR, Rabins PV. 1994. Personality disorder in later life: A community study. *British Journal of Psychiatry*, 165(4): 493-499.

Cole DA. 1989. Psychopathology of adolescent suicide: Hopelessness, coping beliefs, and depression. *Journal of Abnormal Psychology*, 98(3): 248-255.

Comings DE, Johnson JP, Gonzalez NS, Huss M, Saucier G, McGue M, MacMurray J. 2000. Association between the adrenergic alpha 2A receptor gene (ADRA2A) and measures of irritability, hostility, impulsivity and memory in normal subjects. *Psychiatric Genetics*, 10(1): 39-42.

Conwell Y, Brent D. 1995. Suicide and aging. I: Patterns of psychiatric diagnosis. *International Psychogeriatrics*, 7(2): 149-164.

Conwell Y, Duberstein PR, Cox C, Herrmann JH, Forbes NT, Caine ED. 1996. Relationships of age and axis I diagnoses in victims of completed suicide: A psychological autopsy study. *American Journal of Psychiatry*, 153(8): 1001-1008.

Corbitt EM, Malone KM, Haas GL, Mann JJ. 1996. Suicidal behavior in patients with major depression and comorbid personality disorders. *Journal of Affective Disorders*, 39(1): 61-72.

Cruess DG, Antoni MH, Kumar M, Schneiderman N. 2000a. Reductions in salivary cortisol are associated with mood improvement during relaxation training among HIV-seropositive men. *Journal of Behavioral Medicine*, 23(2): 107-122.

Cruess DG, Antoni MH, McGregor BA, Kilbourn KM, Boyers AE, Alferi SM, Carver CS, Kumar M. 2000b. Cognitive-behavioral stress management reduces serum cortisol by enhancing benefit finding among women being treated for early stage breast cancer. *Psychosomatic Medicine*, 62(3): 304-308.

Davis T, Gunderson JG, Myers M. 1999. Borderline personality disorder. In: Jacobs DG, Editor. *The Harvard Medical School Guide to Suicide Assessment and Intervention.* (pp. 311-331). San Francisco: Jossey-Bass Publishers.

De Hert M, Peuskens J. 2000. Psychiatric aspects of suicidal behaviour: Schizophrenia. In: Hawton K, van Heeringen K, Editors. *The International Handbook of Suicide and Attempted Suicide.* (pp. 121-134). Chichester, UK: John Wiley and Sons.

Dieserud G, Roysamb E, Ekeberg O, Kraft P. 2001. Toward an integrative model of suicide attempt: A cognitive psychological approach. *Suicide and Life-Threatening Behavior,* 31(2): 153-168.

Dingman CW, McGlashan TH. 1986. Discriminating characteristics of suicides. Chestnut Lodge follow-up sample including patients with affective disorder, schizophrenia and schizoaffective disorder. *Acta Psychiatrica Scandinavica,* 74(1): 91-97.

Drake RE, Gates C, Cotton PG, Whitaker A. 1984. Suicide among schizophrenics. Who is at risk? *Journal of Nervous and Mental Disease,* 172(10): 613-617.

Drake RE, Gates C, Whitaker A, Cotton PG. 1985. Suicide among schizophrenics: A review. *Comprehensive Psychiatry,* 26(1): 90-100.

Duberstein PR, Conwell Y, Caine ED. 1993. Interpersonal stressors, substance abuse, and suicide. *Journal of Nervous and Mental Disease,* 181(2): 80-85.

Dubo ED, Zanarini MC, Lewis RE, Williams AA. 1997. Childhood antecedents of self-destructiveness in borderline personality disorder. *Canadian Journal of Psychiatry,* 42(1): 63-69.

Dunner DL, Gershon ES, Goodwin FK. 1976. Heritable factors in the severity of affective illness. *Biological Psychiatry,* 11(1): 31-42.

Durlak JA. 1997. Primary prevention programs in schools. *Advances in Clinical Child Psychology,* 283-318.

Durlak JA, Wells AM. 1997. Primary prevention mental health programs for children and adolescents: A meta-analytic review. *American Journal of Community Psychology,* 25(2): 115-152.

Eaves L, Rutter M, Silberg JL, Shillady L, Maes H, Pickles A. 2000. Genetic and environmental causes of covariation in interview assessments of disruptive behavior in child and adolescent twins. *Behavior Genetics,* 30(4): 321-334.

Ellis JB, Smith PC. 1991. Spiritual well-being, social desirability and reasons for living: Is there a connection? *International Journal of Social Psychiatry,* 37(1): 57-63.

Evans J, Williams JM, O'Loughlin S, Howells K. 1992. Autobiographical memory and problem-solving strategies of parasuicide patients. *Psychological Medicine,* 22(2): 399-405.

Falloon IR, Talbot RE. 1981. Persistent auditory hallucinations: Coping mechanisms and implications for management. *Psychological Medicine,* 11(2): 329-339.

Feehan M, McGee R, Williams SM. 1993. Mental health disorders from age 15 to age 18 years. *Journal of the American Academy of Child and Adolescent Psychiatry,* 32(6): 1118-1126.

Felsman JK, Vaillant GE. 1987. Resilient children as adults: A 40-year study. In: James AE, Cohler BJ, Editors. *The Invulnerable Child.* (pp. 289-314). New York: Guilford Press.

Fennig S, Putnam K, Bromet EJ, Galambos N. 1995. Gender, premorbid characteristics and negative symptoms in schizophrenia. *Acta Psychiatrica Scandinavica,* 92(3): 173-177.

Fenton WS, McGlashan TH, Victor BJ, Blyler CR. 1997. Symptoms, subtype, and suicidality in patients with schizophrenia spectrum disorders. *American Journal of Psychiatry,* 154(2): 199-204.

Fergusson DM, Lynskey MT. 1996. Adolescent resiliency to family adversity. *Journal of Child Psychology and Psychiatry and Allied Disciplines,* 37(3): 281-292.

Fergusson DM, Woodward LJ, Horwood LJ. 2000. Risk factors and life processes associated with the onset of suicidal behaviour during adolescence and early adulthood. *Psychological Medicine,* 30(1): 23-39.

Figueroa E, Silk KR. 1997. Biological implications of childhood sexual abuse in borderline personality disorder. *Journal of Personality Disorders*, 11(1): 71-92.

Flavin DK, Franklin JE, Frances RJ. 1990. Substance abuse and suicidal behavior. In: Blumenthal SJ, Kupfer DJ, Editors. *Suicide Over the Life Cycle: Risk Factors, Assessment, and Treatment of Suicidal Patients*. (pp. 177-204). Washington, DC: American Psychiatric Press.

Ford AB, Rushforth NB, Rushforth N, Hirsch CS, Adelson L. 1979. Violent death in a metropolitan county: II. Changing patterns in suicides (1959-1974). *American Journal of Public Health*, 69(5): 459-464.

Foster T, Gillespie K, McClelland R. 1997. Mental disorders and suicide in Northern Ireland. *British Journal of Psychiatry*, 170: 447-452.

Fowler RC, Rich CL, Young D. 1986. San Diego Suicide Study. II. Substance abuse in young cases. *Archives of General Psychiatry*, 43(10): 962-965.

Frances A, Fyer M, Clarkin J. 1986. Personality and suicide. *Annals of the New York Academy of Sciences*, 487: 281-293.

Frankenhaeuser M. 1982. Challenge-control interaction as reflected in sympathetic-adrenal and pituitary-adrenal activity: Comparison between the sexes. *Scandinavian Journal of Psychology*, Suppl 1: 158-164.

Friedman RC, Aronoff MS, Clarkin JF, Corn R, Hurt SW. 1983. History of suicidal behavior in depressed borderline inpatients. *American Journal of Psychiatry*, 140(8): 1023-1026.

Funahashi T, Ibuki Y, Domon Y, Nishimura T, Akehashi D, Sugiura H. 2000. A clinical study on suicide among schizophrenics. *Psychiatry and Clinical Neurosciences*, 54(2): 173-179.

Fyer MR, Frances AJ, Sullivan T, Hurt SW, Clarkin J. 1988. Suicide attempts in patients with borderline personality disorder. *American Journal of Psychiatry*, 145(6): 737-739.

Gardner DL, Cowdry RW. 1985. Suicidal and parasuicidal behavior in borderline personality disorder. *Psychiatric Clinics of North America*, 8(2): 389-403.

Garland M, Hickey D, Corvin A, Golden J, Fitzpatrick P, Cunningham S, Walsh N. 2000. Total serum cholesterol in relation to psychological correlates in parasuicide. *British Journal of Psychiatry*, 177: 77-83.

Garvey MJ, Spoden F. 1980. Suicide attempts in antisocial personality disorder. *Comprehensive Psychiatry*, 21(2): 146-149.

Ge X, Conger RD. 1999. Adjustment problems and emerging personality characteristics from early to late adolescence. *American Journal of Community Psychology*, 27(3): 429-459.

Gillham JE, Reivich KJ. 1999. Prevention of depressive symptoms in school children: A research update. *Psychological Science*, 10(5): 461-462.

Gillham JE, Reivich KJ, Jaycox LH, Seligman MEP. 1995. Prevention of depressive symptoms in schoolchildren: Two-year follow-up. *Psychological Science*, 6(6): 343-351.

Gladstone TR, Kaslow NJ. 1995. Depression and attributions in children and adolescents: A meta-analytic review. *Journal of Abnormal Child Psychology*, 23(5): 597-606.

Glantz MD, Sloboda Z. 1999. Analysis and reconceptualization of resilience. In: Glantz MD, Johnson JL, Editors. *Resilience and Development: Positive Life Adaptations*. (pp. 109-128). New York: Kluwer Academic/Plenum Publishers.

Goldberg DP, Lecrubier Y. 1996. Form and frequency of mental disorders across centres. In: Ustun TN, Sartorius N, Editors. *Mental Illness in General Health Care: An International Study*. (pp. 323-334).: John Wiley and Sons.

Goldman S, Beardslee WR. 1999. Suicide in children and adolescents. In: Jacobs DG, Editor. *The Harvard Medical School Guide to Suicide Assessment and Intervention*. (pp. 417-442). San Francisco: Jossey-Bass Publishers.

Goldsmith HH, Lemery KS. 2000. Linking temperamental fearfulness and anxiety symptoms: A behavior-genetic perspective. *Biological Psychiatry*, 48(12): 1199-1209.

Goldsmith SJ, Fryer M, Frances A. 1990. Personality and suicide. In: Blumenthal SJ, Kupfer DJ, Editors. *Suicide Over the Life Cycle: Risk Factors, Assessment, and Treatment of Suicidal Patients.* (pp. 155-176). Washington, DC: American Psychiatric Press.

Goldston DB. 2001. Issues in measurement of suicide risk factors in youth. Workshop presentation at the Institute of Medicine's Workshop on Risk Factors for Suicide, March 14, 2001. Summary available in: Institute of Medicine. *Risk Factors for Suicide: Summary of a Workshop.* (pp. 5-7). Washington, DC: National Academy Press.

Goldston DB, Daniel SS, Reboussin BA, Reboussin DM, Frazier PH, Harris AE. 2001. Cognitive risk factors and suicide attempts among formerly hospitalized adolescents: A prospective naturalistic study. *Journal of the American Academy of Child and Adolescent Psychiatry,* 40(1): 91-99.

Goodman RA, Istre GR, Jordan FB, Herndon JL, Kelaghan J. 1991. Alcohol and fatal injuries in Oklahoma. *Journal of Studies on Alcohol,* 52(2): 156-161.

Goodwin FK, Jamison KR. 1990. *Manic-Depressive Illness.* New York: Oxford University Press.

Gorman JM, Coplan JD. 1996. Comorbidity of depression and panic disorder. *Journal of Clinical Psychiatry,* 57 (Suppl 10): 34-41; discussion 42-43.

Green BL, Rodgers A. 2001. Determinants of social support among low-income mothers: A longitudinal analysis. *American Journal of Community Psychology,* 29(3): 419-441.

Green MA, Curtis GC. 1988. Personality disorders in panic patients: Response to termination of antipanic medication. *Journal of Personality Disorders,* 2: 303-314.

Grossi G, Ahs A, Lundberg U. 1998. Psychological correlates of salivary cortisol secretion among unemployed men and women. *Integrative Physiological and Behavioral Science,* 33(3): 249-263.

Gunderson JG, Sabo AN. 1993. The phenomenological and conceptual interface between borderline personality disorder and PTSD. *American Journal of Psychiatry,* 150(1): 19-27.

Guze SB, Robins E. 1970. Suicide and primary affective disorders. *British Journal of Psychiatry,* 117(539): 437-438.

Hagnell O, Lanke J, Rorsman B. 1981. Suicide rates in the Lundby study: Mental illness as a risk factor for suicide. *Neuropsychobiology,* 7(5): 248-253.

Hankin BL, Abramson LY, Siler M. 2001. A prospective test of the hopelessness theory of depression in adolescence. *Cognitive Therapy and Research,* 25(5): 607-632.

Harburg E, Gleibermann L, Gershowitz H, Ozgoren F, Kulik CL. 1982. Twelve blood markers and measures of temperament. *British Journal of Psychiatry,* 140: 401-409.

Harkavy-Friedman JM, Restifo K, Malaspina D, Kaufmann CA, Amador XF, Yale SA, Gorman JM. 1999. Suicidal behavior in schizophrenia: Characteristics of individuals who had and had not attempted suicide. *American Journal of Psychiatry,* 156(8): 1276-1278.

Harrington R, Kerfoot M, Dyer E, McNiven F, Gill J, Harrington V, Woodham A, Byford S. 1998. Randomized trial of a home-based family intervention for children who have deliberately poisoned themselves. *Journal of the American Academy of Child and Adolescent Psychiatry,* 37(5): 512-518.

Harris EC, Barraclough B. 1997. Suicide as an outcome for mental disorders. A meta-analysis. *British Journal of Psychiatry,* 170: 205-228.

Harris EC, Barraclough B. 1998. Excess mortality of mental disorder. *British Journal of Psychiatry,* 173: 11-53.

Hayward L, Zubrick SR, Silburn S. 1992. Blood alcohol levels in suicide cases. *Journal of Epidemiology and Community Health,* 46(3): 256-260.

Heila H, Isometsa ET, Henriksson MM, Heikkinen ME, Marttunen MJ, Lönnqvist JK. 1997. Suicide and schizophrenia: A nationwide psychological autopsy study on age- and sex-specific clinical characteristics of 92 suicide victims with schizophrenia. *American Journal of Psychiatry,* 154(9): 1235-1242.

108

REDUCING SUICIDE

Heila H, Isometsa ET, Henriksson MM, Heikkinen ME, Marttunen MJ, Lönnqvist JK. 1998. Antecedents of suicide in people with schizophrenia. *British Journal of Psychiatry*, 173: 330-333.

Heim C, Nemeroff CB. 2001. The role of childhood trauma in the neurobiology of mood and anxiety disorders: Preclinical and clinical studies. *Biological Psychiatry*, 49(12): 1023-1039.

Heim C, Owens MJ, Plotsky PM, Nemeroff CB. 1997. Persistent changes in corticotropin-releasing factor systems due to early life stress: Relationship to the pathophysiology of major depression and post-traumatic stress disorder. *Psychopharmacology Bulletin*, 33(2): 185-192.

Hellerstein D, Frosch W, Koenigsberg HW. 1987. The clinical significance of command hallucinations. *American Journal of Psychiatry*, 144(2): 219-221.

Henriksson MM, Aro HM, Marttunen MJ, Heikkinen ME, Isometsa ET, Kuoppasalmi KI, Lönnqvist JK. 1993. Mental disorders and comorbidity in suicide. *American Journal of Psychiatry*, 150(6): 935-940.

Hlady WG, Middaugh JP. 1988. Suicides in Alaska: Firearms and alcohol. *American Journal of Public Health*, 78(2): 179-180.

Holahan CJ, Moos RH. 1990. Life stressors, resistance factors, and improved psychological functioning: An extension of the stress resistance paradigm. *Journal of Personality and Social Psychology*, 58(5): 909-917.

Horesh N, Rolnick T, Iancu I, Dannon P, Lepkifker E, Apter A, Kotler M. 1996. Coping styles and suicide risk. *Acta Psychiatrica Scandinavica*, 93(6): 489-493.

Hur YM, Bouchard TJ Jr. 1997. The genetic correlation between impulsivity and sensation seeking traits. *Behavioral Genetics*, 27(5): 455-463.

Hyyppa MT. 1987. Psychoendocrine aspects of coping with distress. *Annals of Clinical Research*, 19(2): 78-82.

IOM (Institute of Medicine). 2001. *Health and Behavior: The Interplay of Biological, Behavioral, and Societal Influences*. Washington, DC: National Academy Press.

Isometsa ET, Henriksson MM, Aro HM, Lönnqvist JK. 1994. Suicide in bipolar disorder in Finland. *American Journal of Psychiatry*, 151(7): 1020-1024.

Isometsa ET, Henriksson MM, Heikkinen ME, Aro HM, Marttunen MJ, Kuoppasalmi KI, Lönnqvist JK. 1996. Suicide among subjects with personality disorders. *Amreican Journal of Psychiatry*, 153(5): 667-673.

Jaycox LH, Reivich KJ, Gillham J, Seligman ME. 1994. Prevention of depressive symptoms in school children. *Behaviour Research and Therapy*, 32(8): 801-816.

Jenike MA, Baer L, Minichiello WE, Schwartz CE, Carey RJ Jr. 1986. Concomitant obsessive-compulsive disorder and schizotypal personality disorder. *American Journal of Psychiatry*, 143(4): 530-532.

Joffe RT, Regan JJ. 1989. Personality and suicidal behavior in depressed patients. *Comprehensive Psychiatry*, 30(2): 157-160.

Joiner TE Jr, Rudd MD. 1995. Negative attributional style for interpersonal events and the occurrence of severe interpersonal disruptions as predictors of self-reported suicidal ideation. *Suicide and Life-Threatening Behavior*, 25(2): 297-304.

Joiner TE Jr, Steer RA, Abramson LY, Alloy LB, Metalsky GI, Schmidt NB. 2001a. Hopelessness depression as a distinct dimension of depressive symptoms among clinical and non-clinical samples. *Behaviour Research and Therapy*, 39(5): 523-536.

Joiner TE Jr, Voelz ZR, Rudd MD. 2001b. For suicidal young adults with comorbid depressive and anxiety disorders, probem-solving treatment may be better than treatment as usual. *Professional Psychology—Research & Practice*, 32(3): 278-282.

Joiner TE Jr, Wagner KD. 1995. Attribution style and depression in children and adolescents: A meta-analytic review. *Clinical Psychology Review*, 15(8): 777-798.

Josepho SA, Plutchik R. 1994. Stress, coping, and suicide risk in psychiatric inpatients. *Suicide and Life-Threatening Behavior*, 24(1): 48-57.

Joyce P, Beautrais A, Mulder R. 1994. The prevalence of mental disorder in individuals who suicide and attempt suicide. In: Kelleher M, Editor. *Divergent Perspectives on Suicidal Behavior*. Cork: Fifth European Symposium on Suicide.

Kaplan HB. 1999. Toward an understanding of resilience: A critical review of definitions and models. In: Glantz MD, Johnson JL, Editors. *Resilience and Development: Positive Life Adaptations*. (pp. 17-84). New York: Kluwer Academic/Plenum Publishers.

Keilp JG, Sackeim HA, Brodsky BS, Oquendo MA, Malone KM, Mann JJ. 2001. Neuropsychological dysfunction in depressed suicide attempters. *American Journal of Psychiatry*, 158(5): 735-741.

Keller MB, Hanks DL. 1995. Anxiety symptom relief in depression treatment outcomes. *Journal of Clinical Psychiatry*, 56 (Suppl 6): 22-29.

Kendall RE. 1983. Alcohol and suicide. *Substance and Alcohol Actions/Misuse*, 4(2-3): 121-127.

Kessler RC. 2000. Posttraumatic stress disorder: The burden to the individual and to society. *Journal of Clinical Psychiatry*, 61 (Suppl 5): 4-12; discussion 13-14.

Kessler RC, Borges G, Walters EE. 1999. Prevalence of and risk factors for lifetime suicide attempts in the National Comorbidity Survey. *Archives of General Psychiatry*, 56(7): 617-626.

Kessler RC, McGonagle KA, Zhao S, Nelson CB, Hughes M, Eshleman S, Wittchen HU, Kendler KS. 1994. Lifetime and 12-month prevalence of DSM-III-R psychiatric disorders in the United States. Results from the National Comorbidity Survey. *Archives of General Psychiatry*, 51(1): 8-19.

Kessler RC, Sonnega A, Bromet E, Hughes M, Nelson CB. 1995. Posttraumatic stress disorder in the National Comorbidity Survey. *Archives of General Psychiatry*, 52(12): 1048-1060.

King CA, Hill EM, Naylor M, Evans T, Shain B. 1993. Alcohol consumption in relation to other predictors of suicidality among adolescent inpatient girls. *Journal of the American Academy of Child and Adolescent Psychiatry*, 32(1): 82-88.

Klatsky AL, Friedman GD, Siegelaub AB. 1981. Alcohol and mortality. A ten-year Kaiser-Permanente experience. *Annals of Internal Medicine*, 95(2): 139-145.

Klerman GL, Weissman MM. 1989. Increasing rates of depression. *Journal of the American Medical Association*, 261(15): 2229-2235.

Koenig HG, Cohen HJ, George LK, Hays JC, Larson DB, Blazer DG. 1997. Attendance at religious services, interleukin-6, and other biological parameters of immune function in older adults. *International Journal of Psychiatry in Medicine*, 27(3): 233-250.

Koerner K, Linehan MM. 2000. Research on dialectical behavior therapy for patients with borderline personality disorder. *Psychiatric Clinics of North America*, 23(1): 151-167.

Koivumaa-Honkanen H, Honkanen R, Viinamaki H, Heikkila K, Kaprio J, Koskenvuo M. 2001. Life satisfaction and suicide: A 20-year follow-up study. *American Journal of Psychiatry*, 158(3): 433-439.

Kotler M, Finkelstein G, Molcho A, Botsis AJ, Plutchik R, Brown SL, van Praag HM. 1993. Correlates of suicide and violence risk in an inpatient population: Coping styles and social support. *Psychiatry Research*, 47(3): 281-290.

Kotler M, Iancu I, Efroni R, Amir M. 2001. Anger, impulsivity, social support, and suicide risk in patients with posttraumatic stress disorder. *Journal of Nervous and Mental Disease*, 189(3): 162-167.

Kovacs M, Beck AT, Weissman A. 1975. The use of suicidal motives in the psychotherapy of attempted suicides. *American Journal of Psychotherapy*, 29(3): 363-368.

Kroll P, Ryan C. 1983. The schizotypal personality on an alcohol treatment unit. *Comprehensive Psychiatry*, 24(3): 262-270.

Kumpfer KL. 1999. Factors and processes contributing to resilience: The resilience framework. In: Glantz MD, Johnson JL, Editors. *Resilience and Development: Positive Life Adaptations.* (pp. 179-224). New York: Kluwer Academic/Plenum Publishers.

Landmark J, Cernovsky ZZ, Merskey H. 1987. Correlates of suicide attempts and ideation in schizophrenia. *British Journal of Psychiatry,* 151: 18-20.

Lazarus R, Folkman S. 1984. *Stress, Appraisal and Coping.* New York: Springer.

Lerner MS, Clum GA. 1990. Treatment of suicide ideators: A problem-solving approach. *Behavior Therapy,* 21(4): 403-411.

Lesage AD, Boyer R, Grunberg F, Vanier C, Morissette R, Menard-Buteau C, Loyer M. 1994. Suicide and mental disorders: A case-control study of young men. *American Journal of Psychiatry,* 151(7): 1063-1068.

Lesch KP, Merschdorf U. 2000. Impulsivity, aggression, and serotonin: A molecular psychobiological perspective. *Behavioral Sciences and the Law,* 18(5): 581-604.

Lesperance F, Frasure-Smith N. 2000. Depression in patients with cardiac disease: A practical review. *Journal of Psychosomatic Research,* 48(4-5): 379-391.

Lester D. 1995. The association between alcohol consumption and suicide and homicide rates: A study of 13 nations. *Alcohol and Alcoholism,* 30(4): 465-468.

Lester D, Beck AT. 1977. Suicidal wishes and depression in suicidal ideators: A comparison with attempted suicides. *Journal of Clinical Psychology,* 33(1): 92-94.

Levenson MR, Aldwin CM, Bosse R, Spiro A 3rd. 1988. Emotionality and mental health: Longitudinal findings from the normative aging study. *Journal of Abnormal Psychology,* 97(1): 94-96.

Liebowitz MR. 1993. Functional classification of anxiety-panic. *International Clinical Psychopharmacology,* 8 (Suppl 1): 47-52.

Linehan MM, Armstrong HE, Suarez A, Allmon D, Heard HL. 1991. Cognitive-behavioral treatment of chronically parasuicidal borderline patients. *Archives of General Psychiatry,* 48(12): 1060-1064.

Linehan MM, Camper P, Chiles JA, Strosahl K, et al. 1987. Interpersonal problem solving and parasuicide. *Cognitive Therapy and Research,* 11(1): 1-12.

Linehan MM, Goodstein JL, Nielsen SL, Chiles JA. 1983. Reasons for staying alive when you are thinking of killing yourself: The reasons for living inventory. *Journal of Consulting and Clinical Psychology,* 51(2): 276-286.

Linehan MM, Rizvi SL, Welch SS, Page B. 2000. Psychiatric aspects of suicidal behavior: Personality disorders. In: Hawton K, van Heeringen K, Editors. *The International Handbook of Suicide and Attempted Suicide.* (pp. 147-178). Chichester, UK: John Wiley and Sons.

Lönnqvist JK. 2000. Psychiatric aspects of suicidal behaviour: Depression. Hawton K, van Heeringen K, Editors. *The International Handbook of Suicide and Attempted Suicide.* (pp. 107-120). Chichester, UK: John Wiley and Sons.

Magee WJ, Eaton WW, Wittchen HU, McGonagle KA, Kessler RC. 1996. Agoraphobia, simple phobia, and social phobia in the National Comorbidity Survey. *Archives of General Psychiatry,* 53(2): 159-168.

Maier SF, Seligman MEP. 1976. Learned helplessness: Theory and evidence. *Journal of Experimental Psychology: General,* 105: 3-46.

Makela P. 1996. Alcohol consumption and suicide mortality by age among Finnish men, 1950–1991. *Addiction,* 91(1): 101-112.

Malone KM, Oquendo MA, Haas GL, Ellis SP, Li S, Mann JJ. 2000. Protective factors against suicidal acts in major depression: Reasons for living. *American Journal of Psychiatry,* 157(7): 1084-1088.

Mann JJ, Brent DA, Arango V. 2001. The neurobiology and genetics of suicide and attempted suicide: A focus on the serotonergic system. *Neuropsychopharmacology,* 24(5): 467-477.

Mann JJ, Waternaux C, Haas GL, Malone KM. 1999. Toward a clinical model of suicidal behavior in psychiatric patients. *American Journal of Psychiatry*, 156(2): 181-189.

Marcus SC, Olfson M, Pincus HA, Shear MK, Zarin DA. 1997. Self-reported anxiety, general medical conditions, and disability bed days. *American Journal of Psychiatry*, 154(12): 1766-1768.

May PA. 1995. Adolescent suicide in the West. *Second Bi-Regional Adolescent Suicide Prevention Conference*. Washington, DC: US DHHS, Health Resources and Services Administration, Maternal and Child Health Bureau.

May PA, Van Winkle NW, Williams MB, McFelley PJ, DeBruyn LM, Serna P. In press. Alcohol and suicide death among American Indians of New Mexico: 1980–1998. *Suicide and Life-Threatening Behavior*.

Mayfield DG, Montgomery D. 1972. Alcoholism, alcohol intoxication, and suicide attempts. *Archives of General Psychiatry*, 27(3): 349-353.

Medhus A. 1975. Mortality among female alcoholics. *Scandanavian Journal of Social Medicine*, 3(3): 111-115.

Merikangas KR, Mehta RL, Molnar BE, Walters EE, Swendsen JD, Aguilar-Gaziola S, Bijl R, Borges G, Caraveo-Anduaga JJ, DeWit DJ, Kolody B, Vega WA, Wittchen HU, Kessler RC. 1998. Comorbidity of substance use disorders with mood and anxiety disorders: Results of the International Consortium in Psychiatric Epidemiology. *Addictive Behaviors*, 23(6): 893-907.

Merrill J, Milner G, Owens J, Vale A. 1992. Alcohol and attempted suicide. *British Journal of Addiction*, 87(1): 83-89.

Miczek KA, Maxson SC, Fish EW, Faccidomo S. 2001. Aggressive behavioral phenotypes in mice. *Behavioural Brain Research*, 125(1-2): 167-181.

Miczek KA, Weerts E, Haney M, Tidey J. 1994. Neurobiological mechanisms controlling aggression: Preclinical developments for pharmacotherapeutic interventions. *Neuroscience and Biobehavioral Reviews*, 18(1): 97-110.

Miles CP. 1977. Conditions predisposing to suicide: A review. *Journal of Nervous and Mental Disease*, 164(4): 231-246.

Minkoff K, Bergman E, Beck AT, Beck R. 1973. Hopelessness, depression, and attempted suicide. *American Journal of Psychiatry*, 130(4): 455-459.

Mirin SM, Weiss RD. 1986. Affective illness in substance abusers. *Psychiatric Clinics of North America*, 9(3): 503-514.

Modestin J, Oberson B, Erni T. 1997. Possible correlates of DSM-III-R personality disorders. *Acta Psychiatrica Scandinavica*, 96(6): 424-430.

Mohr WK. 2001. Bipolar disorder in children. *Journal of Psychosocial Nursing and Mental Health Services*, 39(3): 12-23.

Molnar BE, Berkman LF, Buka SL. 2001. Psychopathology, childhood sexual abuse and other childhood adversities: Relative links to subsequent suicidal behaviour in the US. *Psychological Medicine*, 31(6): 965-977.

Mortensen PB, Juel K. 1993. Mortality and causes of death in first admitted schizophrenic patients. *British Journal of Psychiatry*, 163: 183-189.

Murphy GE. 1992. *Suicide in Alcoholism*. New York: Oxford University Press.

Murphy GE. 2000. Psychiatric aspects of suicidal behavior: Substance abuse. In: Hawton K., Van Heeringen K, Editors. *International Handbook of Suicide and Attempted Suicide*. (pp. 135-146). Chichester, UK: John Wiley and Sons.

Murphy GE, Armstrong JW Jr, Hermele SL, Fischer JR, Clendenin WW. 1979. Suicide and alcoholism. Interpersonal loss confirmed as a predictor. *Archives of General Psychiatry*, 36(1): 65-69.

Murphy GE, Robins E. 1967. Social factors in suicide. *Journal of the American Medical Association*, 199: 303-308.

Murphy SL, Rounsaville BJ, Eyre S, Kleber HD. 1983. Suicide attempts in treated opiate addicts. *Comprehensive Psychiatry*, 24(1): 79-89.

Nakamura MM, Overall JE, Hollister LE, Radcliffe E. 1983. Factors affecting outcome of depressive symptoms in alcoholics. *Alcoholism, Clinical and Experimental Research*, 7(2): 188-193.

Narrow WE. unpublished. *One-Year Prevalence of Mental Disorders, Excluding Substance Use Disorders, in the U.S.: NIMH ECA Prospective Data. Population Estimates Based on U.S. Census Estimated Residential Population Age 18 and Over on July 1, 1998.* Cited on NIMH website at: http://www.nimh.nih.gov/ publicat/numbers.cfm [accessed December 20, 2001].

Neeleman J, Farrell M. 1997. Suicide and substance misuse. *British Journal of Psychiatry*, 171: 303-304.

Nelson FL, Farberow NL, Litman RE. 1988. Youth suicide in California: A comparative study of perceived causes and interventions. *Community Mental Health Journal*, 24(1): 31-42.

Nemeroff CB. 1996. The corticotropin-releasing factor (CRF) hypothesis of depression: New findings and new directions. *Molecular Psychiatry*, 1(4): 336-342.

NIAAA (National Institute on Alcohol Abuse and Alcoholism). 2001. *Quick Facts.* [Online]. Available: http://www.niaaa.nih.gov/databases/qf.htm [accessed December 20, 2001].

Nikulina EM, Hammer RP Jr, Miczek KA, Kream RM. 1999. Social defeat stress increases expression of mu-opioid receptor mRNA in rat ventral tegmental area. *Neuroreport*, 10(14): 3015-3019.

Nikulina EM, Marchand JE, Kream RM, Miczek KA. 1998. Behavioral sensitization to cocaine after a brief social stress is accompanied by changes in fos expression in the murine brainstem. *Brain Research*, 810(1-2): 200-210.

Nolen-Hoeksema S, Girgus JS, Seligman ME. 1992. Predictors and consequences of childhood depressive symptoms: A 5-year longitudinal study. *Journal of Abnormal Psychology*, 101(3): 405-422.

Norstrom T. 1988. Alcohol and suicide in Scandinavia. *British Journal of Addiction*, 83(5): 553-559.

NRC (National Research Council). 2002. Eccles J, Gootman JA, Editors. *Community Programs to Promote Youth Development.* Washington, DC: National Academy Press.

Nyman AK, Jonsson H. 1986. Patterns of self-destructive behaviour in schizophrenia. *Acta Psychiatrica Scandinavica*, 73(3): 252-262.

Ottoson H, Bodlund O, Ekselius L, Grann M, von Knorring L, Kullgren G, Lindstroem E, Soederberg S. 1998. DSM-IV and ICD-10 personality disorders: A comparison of a self-report questionnaire (DIP-Q) with a structured interview. *European Psychiatry*, 13: 246-253.

Page RM, Allen O, Moore L, Hewitt C. 1993. Co-occurrence of substance use and loneliness as a risk factor for adolescent hopelessness. *Journal of School Health*, 63(2): 104-108.

Paris J. 1998. Does childhood trauma cause personality disorders in adults? *Canadian Journal of Psychiatry*, 43(2): 148-153.

Paris J, Nowlis D, Brown R. 1989. Predictors of suicide in borderline personality disorder. *Canadian Journal of Psychiatry*, 34(1): 8-9.

Peuskens J, De Hert M, Cosyns P, Pieters G, Theys P, Vermote R. 1997. Suicide in young schizophrenic patients during and after inpatient treatment. *International Journal of Mental Health*, 25(4): 39-44.

Pfohl B, Stangl D, Zimmerman M. 1984. The implications of DSM-III personality disorders for patients with major depression. *Journal of Affective Disorders*, 7(3-4): 309-318.

PHS (Public Health Service). 2001. *National Strategy for Suicide Prevention: Goals and Objectives for Action.* Rockville, MD: U.S. Department of Health and Human Services.

Piazza PV, Deroche V, Deminiere JM, Maccari S, Le Moal M, Simon H. 1993. Corticosterone in the range of stress-induced levels possesses reinforcing properties: Implications for sensation-seeking behaviors. *Proceedings of the National Academy of Sciences*, 90(24): 11738-11742.

Piazza PV, Maccari S, Deminiere JM, Le Moal M, Mormede P, Simon H. 1991. Corticosterone levels determine individual vulnerability to amphetamine self-administration. *Proceedings of the National Academy of Sciences*, 88(6): 2088-2092.

Piazza PV, Rouge-Pont F, Deroche V, Maccari S, Simon H, Le Moal M. 1996. Glucocorticoids have state-dependent stimulant effects on the mesencephalic dopaminergic transmission. *Proceedings of the National Academy of Sciences*, 93(16): 8716-8720.

Pilkonis PA, Frank E. 1988. Personality pathology in recurrent depression: Nature, prevalence, and relationship to treatment response. *American Journal of Psychiatry*, 145(4): 435-441.

Plutchik R. 1995. Outward and inward directed aggressiveness: The interaction between violence and suicidality. *Pharmacopsychiatry*, 28 (Suppl 2): 47-57.

Poldrugo F, Forti B. 1988. Personality disorders and alcoholism treatment outcome. *Drug and Alcohol Dependence*, 21(3): 171-176.

Pollock LR, Williams J, Mark G. 2001. Effective problem solving in suicide attempters depends on specific autobiographical recall. *Suicide and Life-Threatening Behavior*, 31(4): 386-396.

Porsteinsson A, Duberstein PR, Conwell Y, Cox C, Forbes N, Caine ED. 1997. Suicide and alcoholism. Distinguishing alcoholic patients with and without comorbid drug abuse. *American Journal on Addictions*, 6(4): 304-310.

Poussaint AF, Alexander A. 2000. *Lay My Burden Down: Unraveling Suicide and the Mental Health Crisis Among African-Americans*. Boston: Beacon Press.

Proulx F, Lesage AD, Grunberg F. 1997. One hundred in-patient suicides. *British Journal of Psychiatry*, 171: 247-250.

Qin P, Agerbo E, Westergard-Nielsen N, Eriksson T, Mortensen PB. 2000. Gender differences in risk factors for suicide in Denmark. *British Journal of Psychiatry*, 177: 546-550.

Radomsky ED, Haas GL, Mann JJ, Sweeney JA. 1999. Suicidal behavior in patients with schizophrenia and other psychotic disorders. *American Journal of Psychiatry*, 156(10): 1590-1595.

Range LM, Penton SR. 1994. Hope, hopelessness, and suicidality in college students. *Psychological Reports*, 75(1, Part 2): 456-458.

Regier DA, Farmer ME, Rae DS, Myers JK, Kramer M, Robins LN, George LK, Karno M, Locke BZ. 1993a. One-month prevalence of mental disorders in the United States and sociodemographic characteristics: The Epidemiologic Catchment Area study. *Acta Psychiatrica Scandinavica*, 88(1): 35-47.

Regier DA, Narrow WE, Rae DS, Manderscheid RW, Locke BZ, Goodwin FK. 1993b. The de facto US mental and addictive disorders service system. Epidemiologic catchment area prospective 1-year prevalence rates of disorders and services. *Archives of General Psychiatry*, 50(2): 85-94.

Regier DA, Rae DS, Narrow WE, Kaelber CT, Schatzberg AF. 1998. Prevalence of anxiety disorders and their comorbidity with mood and addictive disorders. *British Journal of Psychiatry*, Suppl(34): 24-28.

Reich JH. 1988. DSM-III personality disorders and the outcome of treated panic disorder. *American Journal of Psychiatry*, 145(9): 1149-1152.

Rich CL, Fowler RC, Fogarty LA, Young D. 1988. San Diego Suicide Study. III. Relationships between diagnoses and stressors. *Archives of General Psychiatry*, 45(6): 589-592.

Rich CL, Runeson BS. 1992. Similarities in diagnostic comorbidity between suicide among young people in Sweden and the United States. *Acta Psychiatrica Scandinavica*, 86(5): 335-339.

Rich CL, Young D, Fowler RC. 1986. San Diego suicide study. I. Young vs old subjects. *Archives of General Psychiatry*, 43(6): 577-582.

Rifai AH, George CJ, Stack JA, Mann JJ, Reynolds CF 3rd. 1994. Hopelessness in suicide attempters after acute treatment of major depression in late life. *American Journal of Psychiatry*, 151(11): 1687-1690.

Rihmer Z, Barsi J, Arato M, Demeter E. 1990. Suicide in subtypes of primary major depression. *Journal of Affective Disorders*, 18(3): 221-225.

Robins E, Murphy GE, Wilkinson RHJr, Gassner S, Kayes J. 1959. Some clinical considerations in the prevention of suicide based on a study of 134 successful suicides. *American Journal of Public Health*, 49: 888-899.

Robins L, Regier DA. 1991. *Psychiatric Disorders in America: The Epidemiologic Catchment Area Study*. New York: The Free Press.

Roizen J. 1982. Estimating alcohol involvement in serious events. In: National Institute on Alcohol Abuse and Alcoholism. *Alcohol Consumption and Related Problems. Alcohol and Health Monograph No. 1.* (pp. 179-219). Washington, DC: U.S. Government Printing Office. DHHS Pub. No. (ADM) 82-1190.

Rossau CD, Mortensen PB. 1997. Risk factors for suicide in patients with schizophrenia: nested case-control study. *British Journal of Psychiatry*, 171: 355-359.

Roy A. 1982. Suicide in chronic schizophrenia. *British Journal of Psychiatry*, 141: 171-177.

Roy A. 1990. Relationship between depression and suicidal behaviour in schizophrenia. In: Delisi LE, Editor. *Depression and Schizophrenia*. Washington, DC: American Psychiatric Press.

Roy A, Draper R. 1995. Suicide among psychiatric hospital in-patients. *Psychological Medicine*, 25(1): 199-202.

Roy A, Linnoila M. 1986. Alcoholism and suicide. *Suicide and Life-Threatening Behavior*, 16(2): 244-273.

Roy A, Mazonson A, Pickar D. 1984. Attempted suicide in chronic schizophrenia. *British Journal of Psychiatry*, 144: 303-306.

Roy-Byrne PP, Post RM, Hambrick DD, Leverich GS, Rosoff AS. 1988. Suicide and course of illness in major affective disorder. *Journal of Affective Disorders*, 15(1): 1-8.

Rudd MD, Ellis TE, Rajab MH, Wehrly T. 2000. Personality types and suicidal behavior: An exploratory study. *Suicide and Life-Threatening Behavior*, 30(3): 199-212.

Rutter M, Quinton D. 1984. Parental psychiatric disorder: Effects on children. *Psychological Medicine*, 14(4): 853-880.

Saarinen PI, Lehtonen J, Lönnqvist J. 1999. Suicide risk in schizophrenia: An analysis of 17 consecutive suicides. *Schizophrenia Bulletin*, 25(3): 533-542.

SAMHSA (Substance Abuse and Mental Health Services Administration). 1999. *National Household Survey on Drug Abuse.* [Online]. Available: http://www.samhsa.gov/oas/nhsda.htm [accessed December 20, 2001].

Sandberg S, McGuinness D, Hillary C, Rutter M. 1998. Independence of childhood life events and chronic adversities: A comparison of two patient groups and controls. *Journal of the American Academy of Child and Adolescent Psychiatry*, 37(7): 728-735.

Sandler IN, Tein J, West SG. 1994. Coping, stress, and the psychological symptoms of children of divorce: A cross-sectional and longitudinal study. *Child Development*, 65(6): 1744-1763.

Scheier MF, Carver CS. 1992. Effects of optimism on psychological and physical well-being: Theoretical overview and empirical update. *Cognitive Therapy and Research*, 16(2): 201-228.

Scheier MF, Weintraub JK, Carver CS. 1986. Coping with stress: Divergent strategies of optimists and pessimists. *Journal of Personality and Social Psychology*, 51(6): 1257-1264.

Schmidt NB, Woolaway-Bickel K, Bates M. 2000. Suicide and panic disorder: Integration of the literature and new findings. In: Joiner TE, Rudd MD, Editors. *Suicide Science: Expanding the Boundaries*. (pp. 117-136). Norwell, MA: Kluwer Academic Publishers.

Schnyder U, Moergeli H, Klaghofer R, Buddeberg C. 2001. Incidence and prediction of posttraumatic stress disorder symptoms in severely injured accident victims. *American Journal of Psychiatry*, 158(4): 594-599.

Seligman ME. 1975. *Helplessness*. San Francisco: Freeman.

Shaffer D. 1988. The epidemiology of teen suicide: An examination of risk factors. *Journal of Clinical Psychiatry*, 49 (Suppl): 36-41.

Shaffer D, Fisher P, Dulcan MK, Davies M, Piacentini J, Schwab-Stone ME, Lahey BB, Bourdon K, Jensen PS, Bird HR, Canino G, Regier DA. 1996. The NIMH Diagnostic Interview Schedule for Children version 2.3 (DISC-2.3): Description, acceptability, prevalence rates, and performance in the MECA study. *Journal of American Academy of Child and Adolescent Psychiatry*, 35(7): 865-877.

Shafii M, Carrigan S, Whittinghill JR, Derrick A. 1985. Psychological autopsy of completed suicide in children and adolescents. *American Journal of Psychiatry*, 142(9): 1061-1064.

Shen Y, Zhang W, Wang Y, Zhang A, et al. 1992. Epidemiological survey on alcohol dependence in populations of four occupations in nine cities of China: I. Methodology and prevalence. [Chinese]. *Chinese Mental Health Journal*, 6(3): 112-115.

Shneidman ES. 1971. Perturbation and lethality as precursors of suicide in a gifted group. *Life-Threatening Behavior*, 1(1): 23-45.

Shneidman ES. 1984. Aphorisms of suicide and some implications for psychotherapy. *American Journal of Psychotherapy*, 38(3): 319-328.

Shneidman ES. 1992. What do suicides have in common? Summary of the psychological approach. In: Bongar BM, Editor. *Suicide: Guidelines for Assessment, Management, and Treatment*. (pp. 3-15). New York: Oxford University Press.

Shneidman ES. 1993. Suicide as psychache. *Journal of Nervous and Mental Disease*, 181: 147-149.

Sidley GL, Whitaker K, Calam RM, Wells A. 1997. The relationship between problem-solving and autobiographical memory in parasuicide patients. *Behavioural and Cognitive Psychotherapy*, 25(2): 195-202.

Simon GE, Von Korff M. 1998. Suicide mortality among patients treated for depression in an insured population. *American Journal of Epidemiology*, 147(2): 155-160.

Smith SM, Goodman RA, Thacker SB, Burton AH, Parsons JE, Hudson P. 1989. Alcohol and fatal injuries: Temporal patterns. *American Journal of Preventive Medicine*, 5(5): 296-302.

Soloff PH, Lis JA, Kelly T, Cornelius J, Ulrich R. 1994a. Risk factors for suicidal behavior in borderline personality disorder. *American Journal of Psychiatry*, 151(9): 1316-1323.

Soloff PH, Lis JA, Kelly T, Cornelius J, Ulrich R. 1994b. Self-mutilation and suicidal behavior in borderline personality disorder. *Journal of Personality Disorders*, 8(4): 257-267.

Stallone F, Dunner DL, Ahearn J, Fieve RR. 1980. Statistical predictions of suicide in depressives. *Comprehensive Psychiatry*, 21(5): 381-387.

Startup M, Heard H, Swales M, Jones B, Williams JMG, Jones RSP. 2001. Autobiographical memory and parasuicide in borderline personality disorder. *British Journal of Clinical Psychology*, 40(2): 113-120.

Stone M, Hurt S, Stone D. 1987. The PI 500: Long-term follow-up of Borderline inpatients meeting DSM-III criteria I. Global Outcome. *Journal of Personality Disorders*, 1: 291-298.

Strosahl K, Chiles JA, Linehan M. 1992. Prediction of suicide intent in hospitalized parasuicides: Reasons for living, hopelessness, and depression. *Comprehensive Psychiatry*, 33(6): 366-373.

Styron W. 1990. *Darkness Visible: A Memoir of Madness*. New York: Random House.

Suominen K, Henriksson M, Suokas J, Isometsa E, Ostamo A, Lönnqvist J. 1996. Mental disorders and comorbidity in attempted suicide. *Acta Psychiatrica Scandinavica*, 94(4): 234-240.

Swartz M, Blazer D, George L, Winfield I. 1990. Estimating the prevalence of borderline personality disorder in the community. *Journal of Personality Disorders,* 4(3): 257-272.

Sweeney PD, Anderson K, Bailey S. 1986. Attributional style in depression: A meta-analytic review. *Journal of Personality and Social Psychology,* 50(5): 974-991.

Tamerin JS, Mendelson JH. 1969. The psychodynamics of chronic inebriation: Observations of alcoholics during the process of drinking in an experimental group setting. *American Journal of Psychiatry,* 125(7): 886-899.

Taylor SE, Kemeny ME, Reed GM, Bower JE, Gruenewald TL. 2000. Psychological resources, positive illusions, and health. *American Psychologist,* 55(1): 99-109.

The Gallup Organization. 2001. *Percent Who Drink Beverage Alcohol by Gender, 1939-1999.* [Online]. Available: http://www.niaaa.nih.gov/databases/dkpat1.txt [accessed December 20, 2001].

Tsuang MT, Woolson RF, Fleming JA. 1980. Premature deaths in schizophrenia and affective disorders. An analysis of survival curves and variables affecting the shortened survival. *Archives of General Psychiatry,* 37(9): 979-983.

Turner RM. 1987. The effect of personality disorder diagnosis on the outcome of social anxiety symptom reduction. *Journal of Personality Disorders,* 1: 136-143.

Ucok A, Karaveli D, Kundakci T, Yazici O. 1998. Comorbidity of personality disorders with bipolar mood disorders. *Comprehensive Psychiatry,* 39(2): 72-74.

United Nations. 1996. *Prevention of Suicide: Guidelines for the Formulation and Implementation of National Strategies.* New York: United Nations.

Vaillant GE. 1966. A twelve-year follow-up of New York narcotic addicts. I. The relation of treatment to outcome. *American Journal of Psychiatry,* 122(7): 727-737.

Vaillant GE, Blumenthal SJ. 1990. Introduction—Suicide over the life cycle: Risk factors and life-span development. In: Blumenthal SJ, Kupfer DJ, Editors. *Suicide Over the Life Cycle: Risk Factors, Assessment, and Treatment of Suicidal Patients.* (pp. 1-14). Washington, DC: American Psychiatric Press.

van der Kolk BA. 1996. The body keeps score: Approaches to the psychobiology of post-traumatic stress disorder. In: van der Kolk BA, McFarlane AC, Weisaeth L, Editors. *Traumatic Stress: The Effects of Overwhelming Experience on Mind, Body, and Society.* (pp. 214-241). New York: Guilford Press.

van der Kolk BA, Perry JC, Herman JL. 1991. Childhood origins of self-destructive behavior. *American Journal Psychiatry,* 148(12): 1665-1671.

van Erp AM, Miczek KA. 2000. Aggressive behavior, increased accumbal dopamine, and decreased cortical serotonin in rats. *Journal of Neuroscience,* 20(24): 9320-9325.

Van Gastel A, Schotte C, Maes M. 1997. The prediction of suicidal intent in depressed patients. *Acta Psychiatrica Scandinavica,* 96(4): 254-259.

Verona E, Patrick CJ. 2000. Suicide risk in externalizing syndromes: Temperamental and neurobiological underpinnings. In: Joiner TE, Rudd DM, Editors. *Suicide Science: Expanding the Boundaries.* (pp. 137-173). Norwell, MA: Kluwer Academic Publishing.

Ward JA. 1984. Preventive implications of a Native Indian mental health program: Focus on suicide and violent death. *Journal of Preventive Psychiatry,* 2(4): 371-385.

Wasserman D, Varnik A. 2001. Perestroika in the former USSR: History's most effective suicide-preventive programme for men. In: Wasserman D, Editor. *Suicide: An Unnecessary Death.* (pp. 253-257). London: Martin Dunitz Ltd.

Wasserman D, Varnik A, Dankowicz M. 1998. Regional differences in the distribution of suicide in the former Soviet Union during perestroika, 1984–1990. *Acta Psychiatrica Scandinavica Supplement,* 394: 5-12.

Wasserman IM. 1992. The impact of epidemic, war, prohibition and media on suicide: United States, 1910–1920. *Suicide and Life-Threatening Behavior,* 22(2): 240-254.

Weeke A. 1979. Causes of death in manic-depressives. In: Schou M, Strömgren E, Editors. *Origin, Prevention and Treatment of Affective Disorders.* (pp. 289-299). London: Academic Press.

Weishaar ME, Beck AT. 1990. Cognitive approaches to understanding and treating suicidal behavior. In: Blumenthal SJ, Kupfer DJ, Editors. *Suicide Over the Life Cycle: Risk Factors, Assessment, and Treatment of Suicidal Patients.* (pp. 469-498). Washington, DC: American Psychiatric Press.

Weiss RD, Hufford MR. 1999. Substance abuse and suicide. In: Jacobs DG, Editor. *The Harvard Medical School Guide to Suicide Assessment and Intervention.* (pp. 300-310). San Francisco: Jossey-Bass Publishers.

Weissman MM. 1993. The epidemiology of personality disorders: A 1990 update. *Journal of Personality Disorders, Supplement,* Spring: 44-62.

Weissman MM, Bland RC, Canino GJ, Faravelli C, Greenwald S, Hwu HG, Joyce PR, Karam EG, Lee CK, Lellouch J, Lepine JP, Newman SC, Oakley-Browne MA, Rubio-Stipec M, Wells JE, Wickramaratne PJ, Wittchen HU, Yeh EK. 1997. The cross-national epidemiology of panic disorder. *Archives of General Psychiatry,* 54(4): 305-309.

Weissman MM, Klerman GL, Markowitz JS, Ouellette R. 1989. Suicidal ideation and suicide attempts in panic disorder and attacks. *New England Journal of Medicine,* 321(18): 1209-1214.

Weissman MM, Leaf PJ, Tischler GL, Blazer DG, Karno M, Bruce ML, Florio LP. 1988. Affective disorders in five United States communities. *Psychological Medicine,* 18(1): 141-153.

Welte JW, Abel EL, Wieczorek W. 1988. The role of alcohol in suicides in Erie County, NY, 1972–84. *Public Health Reports,* 103(6): 648-652.

Werner EE. 1995. Resilience in development. *Current Directions in Psychological Science,* 4(3): 81-85.

Werner EE. 1996. Vulnerable but invincible: High risk children from birth to adulthood. *European Child and Adolescent Psychiatry,* 5 (Suppl 1): 47-51.

Werner EE, Smith RS. Journeys from Childhood to Midlife: Risk, Resilience, and Recovery. 2001. Ithaca, NY: Cornell University Press.

Westermeyer JF, Harrow M, Marengo JT. 1991. Risk for suicide in schizophrenia and other psychotic and nonpsychotic disorders. *Journal of Nervous and Mental Disease,* 179(5): 259-266.

WHO (World Health Organization). 1999. *Violence Prevention: An Important Element of a Health-Promoting School.* WHO/SCHOOLS/98.3, WHO/HPR/HEP/98.2. Geneva: World Health Organization WHO Information Series on School Health.

Wiersma D, Nienhuis FJ, Slooff CJ, Giel R. 1998. Natural course of schizophrenic disorders: A 15-year followup of a Dutch incidence cohort. *Schizophrenia Bulletin,* 24(1): 75-85.

Winokur G, Tsuang M. 1975. The Iowa 500: Suicide in mania, depression, and schizophrenia. *American Journal of Psychiatry,* 132(6): 650-651.

Wyman PA, Sandler I, Wolchik S, Nelson K. 2000. Resilience as cumulative competence promotion and stress protection: Theory and intervention. In: Cicchetti D, Rappaport J, Sandler I, Weissberg RP, Editors. *The Promotion of Wellness in Children and Adolescents.* (pp. 133-184). Washington, DC: Child Welfare League of America.

Wyman PA, Cowen EL, Work WC, Kerley JH. 1993. The role of children's future expectations in self-esteem functioning and adjustment to life stress: A prospective study of urban at-risk children. *Development and Psychopathology,* 5(4): 649-661.

Yang B, Clum GA. 2000. Childhood stress leads to later suicidality via its effect on cognitive functioning. *Suicide and Life-Threatening Behavior,* 30(3): 183-198.

Yufit RI, Bongar B. 1992. Suicide, stress, and coping with life cycle events. In: Maris RW, Berman AL, Editors. *Assessment and Prediction of Suicide.* New York: Guilford Press.

Zanarini MC, Frankenburg FR, Khera GS, Bleichmar J. 2001. Treatment histories of borderline inpatients. *Comprehensive Psychiatry,* 42(2): 144-150.

Zheng D, Macera CA, Croft JB, Giles WH, Davis D, Scott WK. 1997. Major depression and all-cause mortality among white adults in the United States. *Annals of Epidemiology,* 7(3): 213-218.

What I had begun to discover is that, mysteriously and in ways that are totally remote from normal experience, the gray drizzle of horror induced by depression takes on the quality of physical pain. But it is not an immediately identifiable pain, like that of a broken limb. It may be more accurate to say that despair, owing to some evil trick played upon the sick brain by the inhabiting psyche, comes to resemble the diabolical discomfort of being imprisoned in a fiercely overheated room. And because no breeze stirs this caldron, because there is no escape from this smothering confinement, it is entirely natural that the victim begins to think ceaselessly of oblivion.

—WILLIAM STYRON
Darkness Visible: A Memoir of Madness

4

Biological Factors

Suicide is the outcome of a complex set of factors that are reflected in the neurobiology of the suicidal individual. As discussed in more detail in Chapter 3, current data indicate that mental disorders are present in over 90 percent of suicides in Western society, and many of these disorders are associated with biological changes. Many other factors correlated with suicidality also have well-described biological aspects, including predisposing personality traits such as aggression and impulsivity, effects of acute and chronic stress, impact of trauma, gender, substance or alcohol abuse, and age, as discussed in Chapters 3 and 5.

The biological correlates of suicidality are studied in attempt survivors and in postmortem tissue from those who have completed suicide. Postmortem studies of suicide victims are complicated by other influences on the brain that must be taken into account such as prior medications, substances of abuse and/or self-poisoning, consequences of the suicide-related trauma and injury especially to the head, and postmortem delay prior to preservation of brain tissue samples.

This chapter starts with the physiological stress system, a common pathway for response to acute and cumulative physical and psychological stressors. This is followed by discussion of neurochemical findings in suicide. The chapter concludes with a discussion of what is known about the genetics of suicidal behaviors.

120   REDUCING SUICIDE

THE PHYSIOLOGICAL STRESS SYSTEM

The hypothalamic-pituitary-adrenal (HPA) axis is one of the body's major systems modulating physiological responses to actual, anticipated, or perceived harm, and is a major component of adaptation to stresses of all types. The HPA axis functioning reflects acute, chronic, and developmental stressors and trauma. The influence of long-term stressors on the HPA axis is reviewed in a recent IOM report on the links between health and behavior (IOM, 2001). Briefly, acute stress activates the HPA axis and increases levels of glucocorticoids—a family of hormones that mediates stress. Adaptation to chronic stress activates a negative feedback loop that causes: (1) decreased resting glucocorticoid levels, (2) decreased glucocorticoid secretion in response to subsequent stress, (3) increased density of glucocorticoid receptors in the hippocampus (Sapolsky et al., 1984; Yehuda et al., 1991). Chapter 5 provides a detailed description of the role early adverse experiences play in HPA axis functioning and how this may reflect a physiological mechanism for socioenvironmental influences on psychopathology. Dysregulation of the HPA axis has been found to be significantly associated with severe affective disorders (e.g., Plotsky et al., 1998) and with post-traumatic stress disorder (e.g., van der Kolk, 1996), although findings suggest that this dysregulation may take different forms for specific disorders (Yehuda et al., 1991). Irregularities in HPA axis function also appear to correlate with suicide regardless of psychiatric diagnosis, as described below.

Links between corticosteroids and suicide have been proposed for many years. In the late 1960s it was first noted that urinary 17-hydroxycorticosteroids were elevated in patients who completed suicide (Bunney et al., 1969; Fawcett and Bunney, 1967). Subsequently, several other cases were published (Krieger, 1970), although not all reports were in concurrence (Levy and Hansen, 1969). Other postmortem findings implicated an overactive HPA axis with suicide: individuals who died from suicide were reported to have enlarged adrenal glands compared to controls who died from other violence (Dorovini-Zis and Zis, 1987; Szigethy et al., 1994). Increased levels of corticotropin-releasing factor (CRF) in the cerebrospinal fluid (Arató et al., 1989; Brunner and Bronisch, 1999) and fewer binding sites for CRF in the frontal cortex (Nemeroff et al., 1988) in victims of suicide suggested HPA axis hyperactivity. In patients who had attempted suicide, levels of corticotropin-releasing hormone (CRH), another component of the HPA axis feedback loop, were noted to be lower than other psychiatric patients in cerebrospinal fluid (Brunner et al., 2001; Träskman-Bendz et al., 1992) and in plasma (Westrin et al., 1999), a pattern associated with chronic stress.

A depressed cortisol release following challenge with a corticosteroid, dexamethasone, represents a normal HPA axis response. Non-suppression of cortisol after dexamethasone is interpreted as a consequence of hyperactive HPA axis. This "dexamethasone suppression test" (DST) has been evaluated with suicidal patients. The results have been mixed and subject of some controversy. A number of studies have indicated that abnormal DST results and changes in daily rhythms of stress hormone release correlate with recent suicide attempts independently of psychiatric diagnosis (Banki et al., 1984; Lopez-Ibor et al., 1985; Pfeffer et al., 1991; Targum et al., 1983). Other studies, however, have failed to demonstrate this relationship between DST non-suppression and suicide attempt (Brown et al., 1986). In contrast, strikingly more consistent results have been obtained for the association of an abnormal DST response with completed suicide. Several studies have suggested that non-suppression of cortisol in the DST is a good predictor of future suicide. Carroll et al. (1980) evaluated 250 patients with melancholy. Only about half of them were nonsuppressors but all of the 5 subsequent patients who completed suicide were in this group. Similarly, Coryell and Schlesser (1981) tested 205 patients with unipolar depression and found that 45.8 percent had abnormal DST results but all four suicides were nonsuppressors. Norman et al. (1990) compared 13 depressed inpatients who subsequently completed suicide with 25 attemptors of suicide and 28 non-attemptors from the same inpatient population. While the DST nonsuppression rate was similar for the latter two groups, it was significantly higher for those who competed suicide. A meta-analysis by Lester (1992) supported the conclusion that the DST nonsuppression was more prevalent among those who completed suicide. A more recent study by Coryell and Schlesser (2001) demonstrated dramatic predictive ability of the DST. Seventy-eight inpatients with major depressive disorder or schizoaffective disorder were under assessment between 1978 and 1981 and followed for up to 15 years. Of the 78 patients, 32 had abnormal DST results upon admission to the hospital. Of the 32 patients, 26.8 percent eventually completed suicide; in comparison, only 2.9 percent of those with normal DST responses completed suicide.

The mechanism by which the HPA axis influences suicidal behavior is not yet established. Various researchers investigating the pathophysiology of suicide have summarized findings that integrate HPA hyperfunction with disturbances in serotonin function (Lopez et al., 1997; Yehuda et al., 1988). As described below, serotonin function also appears associated with suicide. Evidence suggests a reciprocal relationship between the serotonergic system and the HPA axis. Activation of serotonergic pathways or administration of agents that increase the activation of serotonin receptors elicit increases in plasma cortisol (Calogero et al., 1990; Dinan, 1996; Fuller, 1990; Matheson et al., 1997a; 1997b; Meltzer et al., 1984; Owens et al., 1990). Conversely, serotonin receptors are inhibited by glucocorticoids (Chaouloff, 1995). The link between the two systems is supported in part by the observation that chronic administration of antidepressants can reverse the overactivity of the HPA axis in animal pre-clinical models (Lopez et al., 1997). Van Praag (1996; 2001) proposes that a subtype of depression, anxiety/aggression-driven depression, is correlated with a sustained overproduction of cortisol, resulting in impaired 5-HT synthesis, and reduced 5-HT_{1a} receptor sensitivity leading to susceptibility to stress induction of depression. He proposed that CRH antagonists would be helpful in such cases. On the other hand, Duval et al. (2001) found that the effectiveness of d-fenfluramine, a specific serotonin reuptake inhibitor, did not correlate with the basal or post-DST cortisol levels, suggesting limited functional links between the two systems in suicidal patients. Evidence does suggest that chronic stress of adverse rearing can lead to both low central serotonin responsivity in primates and in humans (Pine et al., 1997) and to HPA axis dysregulation (see Chapter 5) (Higley and Linnoila, 1997).

NEUROCHEMISTRY

The monoamines, particularly dopamine, norepinephrine, and serotonin, have been the focus of much of the research on mental disorders. Changes in these neurotransmitters appear to mediate the effect of the currently utilized psychotropic medications. These neurochemicals show significant changes in various neuropsychiatric disorders. While observable changes in these systems do not necessarily imply causality, they can offer opportunities for developing or improving interventions. A recently developed class of anti-depressants and anti-anxiety drugs, namely, selective serotonin reuptake inhibitors or SSRIs, work through the serotonin system. A wealth of evidence points to reduced serotonergic and altered noradrenergic function in the brains of suicide victims (both attempters and completers). This section summarizes studies on the serotonergic and noradrenergic systems associated with suicide and touches on the limited data on opiate, GABA, and other systems. Although for clarity, this chapter describes these neurochemical systems separately, the reader is reminded that the various systems are interactive and specific changes must be integrated to understand the comprehensive neurobiological effects.

The Serotonergic System

The serotonergic system is complex. Serotonergic pathways are profuse with major projections arising in the median and dorsal raphe nuclei and contacting thousands of cortical neurons. There are more than one dozen types of serotonin receptors, including at least two auto receptor[1] populations. This section will review the evidence concerning changes in brain and cerebrospinal fluid levels of serotonin and its metabolites, and changes in a few of the serotonin receptors.

Brain Levels

Initial studies of the serotonergic system in suicide victims reported modestly low levels of brainstem serotonin and/or its metabolite 5-hydroxyindoleacetic acid (5-HIAA). The original assessments were methodologically limited. First, postmortem assays do not distinguish where the neurotransmitter was localized at the time of death and consequently, its functional importance. Second, serotonin and 5-HIAA levels drop rapidly after death. About a 70 percent loss of serotonin occurs after death and removal of the brain to the freezer prior to assay. This means that group differences must be detected in the residual 30 percent of the serotonin or metabolite. Nevertheless, most studies found low serotonin or 5-HIAA in the brainstem of suicides (Table 4-1). Only three of nine studies found low 5-HIAA levels, and no studies found low 5-HT in the prefrontal cortex (Table 4-1). Four of six studies of other brain regions also reported low serotonin or 5-HIAA (not shown). Postmortem interval differences do not appear to explain discrepancies in the literature (Arango and Mann, 1992), probably because most of the decline in indolamine levels occurs in the first 2 hours postmortem and all published studies of suicide victims have a longer postmortem delay.

Low serotonin or serotonin turnover in suicide appears to be confined to some brain regions. This may reflect the limitations of the assay methodology, which might not be sufficiently sensitive to measure the lower concentrations of serotonin and 5-HIAA in areas that contain less than the brainstem. Alternatively, there may be a regional localization of changes in serotonin levels or turnover, such that serotonin and 5-HIAA in the terminal fields are altered in some areas and not others. That conclusion is consistent with receptor mapping studies by Arango et al. (1995) and Mann et al. (2000).

The reduction in serotonin or 5-HIAA in the brainstem of suicide victims is independent of diagnostic category (Mann et al., 1989),with a similar degree of reduction seen in patients with depression, schizophre-

---

[1]Auto receptors are found on the cells releasing the chemical, and are involved in regulating further release.

TABLE 4-1 Serotonin and 5-HIAA in the Brainstem and Cerebral
Cortex of Suicide Victims *versus* Controls

	Brainstem		Cerebral Cortex	
Study	Serotonin	5-HIAA	Serotonin	5-HIAA
Shaw, Camps, and Eccleston (1967)	↓ 19%[a]	—	—	—
Bourne et al. (1968)	NC	↓ 28%[a]	—	—
Paré, Yeung, Price, and Stacey (1969)	↓ 11%[a]	NC	—	—
Lloyd, Farley, Deck, and Hornykiewicz (1974)	↓ 30%[a]	NC	—	—
Beskow, Gottfries, Roos, and Winblad (1976)	NC	↓ 30%[a]	—	↓ 43%[a]
Cochran, Robins, and Grote (1976)	NC	—	NC	—
Owen et al. (1983)	—	—	—	↓ 71%
Crow et al. (1984)	—	—	—	↓ 25%
Korpi et al. (1986)	NC	NC	NC	NC
Owen et al. (1986)	—	—	—	—
Arató et al. (1987)	—	—	NC	NC
Cheetham et al. (1989)	—	—	NC	NC
Ohmori, Arora, and Meltzer (1992)	—	—	—	NC
Mann et al. (1996a)	—	—	NC	NC
Arranz et al. (1997)	—	—	NC	NC

[a]Indicates a statistically significant difference.
NC No change was detected between groups.

SOURCE: Adapted from Mann et al., 1996c with permission of American Psychiatric Publishing, Inc.

nia, personality disorders, and alcoholism. Thus, serotonergic impairment appears related to suicide independently of psychiatric diagnosis.

CSF Levels

Serotonin metabolite (5-HIAA) levels in cerebrospinal fluid (CSF) are a strong correlate of current and future suicidal behavior. For those with a history of a suicide attempt, 5-HIAA levels are low across diagnoses of depression, schizophrenia, or personality disorders compared to psychiatrically matched control groups (16 of 22 studies, Table 4-2). Careful analyses of the studies that did not find low CSF 5-HIAA levels in association with suicidal behavior suggest that certain types of mood disorders (e.g., bipolar disorder) may be exceptions to the correlation (Roy-Byrne et al., 1983; Secunda et al., 1986; Vestergaard et al., 1978). One study, for example, found low CSF 5-HIAA levels in association with suicidal behavior in unipolar but not in bipolar depressed patients (Ågren, 1980).

However, another study in which the depressed group was comprised of about 50 percent bipolar cases observed low CSF 5-HIAA in the attempters across diagnostic groups (Banki and Arató, 1983). Distinctions based on diagnosis still require additional evaluations. Low CSF 5-HIAA is not just a correlate of suicidal behavior, but also

TABLE 4-2 CSF 5-HIAA and Suicidal Behavior in Major Depression

Study	Findings in CSF 5-HIAA Attempters vs. Nonattempters
Åsberg, Träskman, and Thoren (1976b)	Low CSF 5-HIAA predicted 22% suicide rate in 1 year
Åsberg, Thoren, Träskman, Bertilsson, and Ringberger (1976a)	↓ 40% of attempters had low CSF 5-HIAA vs. 15% of nonattempters
Vestergaard et al. (1978)	No difference
Ågren (1980)	Seriousness of intent of worst suicide attempt; negative correlation with CSF 5-HIAA in unipolar but not bipolar depression
Träskman, Åsberg, Bertilsson, and Sjostrand (1981)	CSF 5-HIAA ↓ in violent attempters and ↓ in nonviolent attempters
Banki and Arató (1983)	↓ in attempters; ↓ 37% in violent vs. nonviolent attempters and violent attempters vs. nonattempters
Palaniappan, Ramachandran, and Somasundaram (1983)	CSF 5-HIAA ↓ in attempters
Roy-Byrne et al. (1983)	No difference
Ågren and Niklasson (1986)	CSF 5-HIAA ↓ 12% in attempters (p=0.07)
Edman, Åsberg, Levander, and Schalling (1986)	CSF 5-HIAA ↓ in attempters
Secunda et al. (1986)	No difference
van Praag (1986)	CSF 5-HIAA ↓ (probenecid) in attempters
Peabody et al. (1987)	CSF 5-HIAA correlated with HAM-D
Nordin (1988)	No correlation with suicidal thoughts
Westenberg and Verhoeven (1988)	No difference
Jones et al. (1990)	CSF 5-HIAA ↓ in attempters
Lopez-Ibor, Lana, and Saiz-Ruiz (1990)	Low CSF 5-HIAA group had more attempters
Roy et al. (1990)	CSF 5-HIAA 22% ↓ in attempters vs. nonattempters but nonsignificant
Nordström et al. (1994)	Low CSF 5-HIAA predicted future suicide
Mann et al. (1992)	Only high planned suicide attempters had lower CSF 5-HIAA
Mann et al. (1996b)	Reduced in higher lethality attempters
Mann and Malone (1997)	Negative correlation with most lethal lifetime attempt

SOURCE: Adapted from Mann et al., 1996b with permission of Elsevier Science.

a predictor. Low CSF 5-HIAA predicts a higher rate of future suicidal acts, as well as the maximal seriousness of suicidal acts in the lifetime of the individual. More lethal suicide attempts are associated with low CSF 5-HIAA (Malone et al., 1996).

The evidence suggests that serotonin mediates inhibition of impulsive action. Low function of the serotonergic systems may predispose individuals to suicidal and other potentially harmful impulsive acts. Animal and human studies link low serotonin function to impulsive aggression. Impulsive aggression but not planned or predatory aggression correlates with low CSF 5-HIAA (Lidberg et al., 1985; Linnoila et al., 1983; Virkkunen et al., 1989a; Virkkunen et al., 1989b; Virkkunen et al., 1987) suggesting that impulsivity plays a role in suicide attempters and predicting a negative correlation of impulsivity and CSF 5-HIAA. Non-human primate studies find such a relationship between impulsivity and CSF 5-HIAA (Higley et al., 1996). On the other hand, no link has been consistently demonstrated between CSF 5-HIAA and depressed mood or hopelessness.

Serotonergic Assessment in Suicide Attempters

To assess the role of the serotonergic system in suicide attempters, researchers can measure the release of prolactin following administration of fenfluramine (see previous section in this chapter). This works because fenfluramine causes the release of serotonin and inhibits its reuptake. Serotonin in turn evokes the release of prolactin into the blood stream. One caveat with this measurement is that endogenous dopaminergic activity may also modulate the prolactin responses to fenfluramine and dopamine has been associated with depression (Kapur and Mann, 1992).

A blunted prolactin response appears to be associated with a history of suicide attempt (Coccaro et al., 1989; Correa et al., 2000; Malone et al., 1996; Mann et al., 1995; see Newman et al., 1998 for review). Coccaro et al. (1989) found a blunted prolactin response in patients with a personality disorder or major depression characterized by suicidal acts compared to similar patients without a history of suicide attempt. Lopez-lbor et al. (1988), however, did not find this correlation of reduced prolactin response with suicide attempts in patients with major depression, though they did find a relationship with severity of the diagnosis. Similarly Mann et al. (1995) found that significantly more (78 percent) of the younger depression cases had a blunted prolactin response compared to only 29 percent of the older group. These younger depressed people were also distinguished from the older group in clinical characteristics including higher frequency of comorbid borderline personality disorder, younger age at onset of the depression, greater lethal intentions for recent suicide attempts, and twice the level of hopelessness. Other factors may impact these findings: O'Keane et al. (1992) found blunted prolactin responses compared to placebo in antisocial personality disorder.

Serotonin Receptors: SERT

The most studied serotonin receptor in suicidal behavior is the serotonin transporter (SERT). Many studies have suggested that the number of serotonin transporter binding sites is low in suicide victims. Methodological complexities such as the ligand used in the experiments have created some uncertainty about the interpretation of the data.

Furthermore, the changes in binding may be specific to certain brain regions. Gross-Isseroff et al. (1989) found strong regional differences in the binding of the 5-HT receptor ligand ^{3}H-imipramine in suicide victims. Suicide-related decreases in SERT binding may be localized to the ventrolateral prefrontal cortex (Arango et al., 1995; Mann et al., 2000) as evidenced by studies on the binding of ^{3}H-cyanoimipramine, another 5-HT receptor ligand. Earlier studies (Arató et al., 1987; Arató et al., 1991; Crow et al., 1984; Stanley et al., 1982) found low ^{3}H-imipramine binding in the dorsal prefrontal cortex of suicide victims that may reflect fewer SERT sites. Studies of other brain regions are limited, but one preliminary report indicates low brainstem SERT binding (Lloyd et al., 1974).

Serotonin Receptors: 5-HT$_{2A}$

Binding to the 5-HT$_{2A}$ receptor, a major postsynaptic receptor for serotonin may be greater in suicide victims. Several studies (Arango et al., 1990; Arora and Meltzer, 1989; Hrdina et al., 1993; Laruelle et al., 1993; Mann et al., 1986; Stanley and Mann, 1983) have demonstrated high ligand (either ^{3}H-spiroperidol or ^{3}H-ketanserin) binding to the 5-HT$_{2A}$ receptor in prefrontal cortex of suicide victims. Pandey and colleagues (2002) reported that there was greater 5-HT$_{2A}$ receptor protein and mRNA gene expression in the brains of teenage suicide victims than in matched normal controls. It should be noted, however, that the field is not in consensus on these findings; seven published studies have found no alteration in 5-HT$_{2A}$ binding (Arranz et al., 1994; Cheetham et al., 1988; Crow et al., 1984; Gross-Isseroff et al., 1990a; Lowther et al., 1994; Owen et al., 1983; 1986).

The changes in binding to the 5-HT$_{2A}$ receptor are found to be greater in prefrontal cortex than in temporal cortex (Arango et al., 1990). Like SERT, regional differences are evident for this postsynaptic receptor's change with suicide. Further work is needed to map the distribution of change in 5-HT$_{2A}$ receptors in suicide victims throughout the prefrontal cortex as well as in other cortical brain regions. 5-HT$_{2A}$ receptor binding in suicide victims may be linked to more violent methods of suicide since the studies reporting increases (Arango et al., 1990; Arora and Meltzer, 1989; Hrdina et al., 1993; Laruelle et al., 1993; Mann et al., 1986; Stanley and Mann, 1983) had greater representation of violent deaths than the others (Arranz et al., 1994; Cheetham et al., 1988; Crow et al., 1984; Gross-Isseroff et al., 1990a; Lowther et al., 1994; Owen et al., 1983; 1986).

Several other factors may influence the outcomes of these analyses. Psychotropic medication may down-regulate 5-HT$_{2A}$ receptors (Yates et al., 1990), and potentially obscure or reverse the up-regulation related to suicide. The presence or absence of a depressive illness may also be relevant (Yates et al., 1990); high 5-HT$_{2A}$ receptor number may be associated with the presence of a depressive illness independent of suicide risk.

Serotonin Receptors: 5HT$_{1A}$

Another major cortical postsynaptic serotonin receptor is the 5-HT$_{1A}$ receptor. Two studies reported an increase in 5-HT$_{1A}$ binding in suicide victims (Arango et al., 1995; Joyce et al., 1993) and four did not (Brodsky et al., 1997; Dillon et al., 1991; Matsubara et al., 1991; Stockmeier et al., 1997). Arango et al. (1995) and Joyce et al. (1993) found the increase in 5-HT$_{1A}$ binding to be confined to discrete brain regions. Corticosteroids can mediate stress effects via mineralocorticoid (MR) and glucocorticoid (GR) receptors on hippocampal 5-HT$_{1A}$ receptors (Lopez et al., 1998). Stress elevates glucocorticoid levels and downregulates hippocampal 5-HT$_{1A}$ receptors in rodents. Suicide victims have low levels of MR and 5-HT$_{1A}$ mRNA in the hippocampus, an effect consistent with stress (Lopez et al., 1998).

Serotonin Receptors: Others

Few studies are published of 5-HT$_{1B}$, 5-HT$_{2C}$, and 5-HT$_{1D}$ receptors in suicide victims (Arranz et al., 1994). Lowther et al. (1997) reported an increase in 5-HT$_{1D}$ binding in globus pallidus, but not in putamen, parietal or prefrontal cortex of violent suicide victims. Huang et al. (1999) did not find any alteration in 5-HT$_{1B}$ binding in prefrontal cortex. More work needs to be done mapping these receptor changes.

The Noradrenergic System

Altered brain noradrenergic transmission also appears to be associated with suicidal behavior. Postmortem studies performed to date have sought to examine the noradrenergic system in brain by: measuring the concentration of norepinephrine (NE) or its metabolites in brain tissue, morphometric studies of noradrenergic neurons, measurement of tyrosine hydroxylase (the rate-limiting enzyme for NE synthesis), and assaying NE receptor subtypes. Alterations in noradrenergic neurotransmission in suicide are suggested based on a variety of findings, including changes in neurotransmitter indices in postmortem brain tissue and comparable findings *in vivo*.

Arango and colleagues (1996) found 23 percent fewer noradrenergic locus ceruleus[2] neurons in the brain of completed suicides. Klimek et al. (1997) found fewer NE transporter sites in the LC. Ordway and colleagues reported high binding to α_2-adrenergic receptors (1994b) and more tyrosine hydroxylase protein (1994a) in the LC of suicide victims, and a low concentration of NE in the LC (1994b). The latter two observations are consistent with animal studies of stress-induced reductions in NE levels in the LC due to release and compensatory increases in tyrosine hydroxylase activity. Arango and colleagues' finding of fewer noradrenergic neurons may reflect low functional reserve and a greater susceptibility to depletion of NE by stress-induced release. Arango et al. (1993) and Manchon et al. (1987) found more NE in cortex and hippocampus, respectively.

Evidence from neurotransmitter or metabolite concentrations in the cerebrospinal fluid (CSF) is less convincing, with a minority (Ågren, 1980; Ågren, 1982) of studies finding low concentrations of the norepinephrine metabolite 3-methoxy, 4-hydroxyphenyl glycol (MHPG) in suicide attempters (Brown et al., 1982; Pickar et al., 1986; Roy et al., 1985; Roy et al., 1989; Secunda et al., 1986; Träskman et al., 1981). Low urinary excretion of the metabolite MHPG in suicide attempters provides some further indirect evidence of low NE turnover (Ågren, 1980; Ågren, 1982). High binding to β-adrenergic receptors in the cerebral cortex in suicide victims compared to controls has been reported by some investigators (Arango et al., 1990; Biegon and Israeli, 1988; Mann et al., 1986) but not by others (De Paermentier et al., 1990; Little et al., 1993; Stockmeier and Meltzer, 1991). α_1-Adrenergic and/or α_2-adrenergic receptor binding in suicide victims in cerebral cortex have been reported to be increased (Arango et al., 1993; Callado et al., 1998; Gonzalez et al., 1994; Meana and Garcia-Sevilla, 1987) or decreased (Gross-Isseroff et al., 1990b). Taken together, these studies suggest altered noradrenergic neurotransmission is associated with suicidal behavior, perhaps reflecting a stress response that exhausts the noradrenergic system.

---

[2]Norepinephrine-producing cells originate in the locus ceruleus.

Other Neurochemical Pathways

Other neurotransmitter systems may or may not be modified in suicide. Cholinergic receptor binding (ligand: ^{3}H-ZNB) appears unaltered (Stanley, 1984). μ-Opioid receptor binding appears increased in prefrontal cortex and caudate but not thalamus (Gabilondo et al., 1995). CRH binding to prefrontal cortex is reduced (Nemeroff et al., 1988). $GABA_B$ sites in the prefrontal cortex, temporal cortex, and hippocampus are reported to be unchanged (Cross et al., 1988), whereas benzodiazepine binding is increased in suicides (Manchon et al., 1987). Palmer et al. (1994) report no change in the NMDA receptor, but Nowak et al. (1995) found altered NMDA binding in the prefrontal cortex as indicated by a decrease in high affinity binding of the ligand ^{3}H-CGP-39653.

Several studies have found changes in postsynaptic signal transduction pathways in suicide. The phosphoinositide and protein kinase C signaling systems are second messenger systems for serotonin as well as other neurotransmitters. Cowburn et al. (1994) reported low basal, GTPγS and forskolin-stimulated adenylyl cyclase activity in the cortex of suicide victims. Levels of one isoform of the α-subunit of the G-protein (Gsα-s) were reduced in suicides. Pacheco et al. (1996) reported that GTPγS stimulation of phosphoinositide hydrolysis was reduced by 30 percent in suicides. Pandey et al. (1997) found reduced protein kinase C binding of ^{3}H-phorbol dibutyrate in prefrontal cortex of teen suicides. Furthermore, the phosphoinositide-specific enzyme phospholipase C (PLC) was found to be abnormal in adolescent suicide victims (Pandey et al., 1999) but not in adults (Pandey, 2001). The contribution of these biological pathways deserved further analysis for their contribution to the pathophysiology of suicide.

GENETIC FACTORS

Similar to most complex conditions, such as obesity (Boutin and Froguel, 2001), hypertension (Higaki et al., 2001), and coronary artery disease (Winkelmann and Hager, 2000), there is growing evidence that genetic factors are related to liability for suicidal behavior. A clinical phenotype of suicide and suicidal behavior shows genetic liability from two sources. One is a genetic liability to mental illness, and the second to impulsive aggression. When both liabilities converge, the risk for suicidal behavior is particularly high. Candidate gene studies suggest that polymorphisms in serotonergic genes may be related to both alterations in serotonin function and to suicidal behavior, although the effects of individual candidate genes are small and may vary depending on psychiatric disorder, sex, and ethnicity. Since the heritability of liability to suicidal behavior appears to be on the order of 30–50 percent, family-environmental causes for suicidal behavior, such as abuse, must also be considered, as both independent factors and those that may interact with genetic vulnerability. Environmental influences are evidenced by the large shifts in rates of youth suicide in the United States and other Westernized countries over the last 20 years although the genetic makeup of the population has not changed appreciably over this short period of time.

The majority of those who complete and attempt suicide have evidence of at least one, and often more, major mental illness (see Chapter 3). The most common disorders associated with suicide and suicidal behavior are mood disorders, alcohol and substance abuse, and schizophrenia, all of which are familial disorders, which, on the basis of adoption and twin studies, have a strong genetic component (Cooper, 2001; McGuffin and Katz, 1989; McGuffin et al., 1991). Therefore, one set of genetic factors influencing suicide comprises those that predispose to the mental disorders that are associated with suicide (e.g., McGuffin and Katz, 1989).

However, the liability to mental disorder is not synonymous with the liability to suicide. For, while the majority of those who attempt and complete suicide have at least one mental illness, the converse is far from true—a very low proportion of mentally ill persons eventually kill themselves, and the majority never make as much as one suicide attempt (e.g., Bostwick and Pankratz, 2000; Murphy and Wetzel, 1990; Pokorny, 1983). One hypothesis, first advanced several decades ago, is that there are additional genetic factors relevant to suicide and suicidal behavior, perhaps related to a liability to impulsive behavior and aggression (Kety, 1986). The convergence of a mental disorder and aggression is associated with the greatest risk for suicidal behavior. Several studies have shown that mood disordered individuals with impulsive aggression are at much greater risk for suicidal behavior than are those without this trait (Mann et al., 1999). Furthermore, impulsive aggression contributes more to suicide and suicidal behavior in younger individuals (Conwell and Brent, 1995; Rich et al., 1986) than more mature adults.

Familial Aggregation of Suicidal Behavior

Even when suicidal behavior is familial, non genetic explanations must be considered. First, suicidal behavior in a relative can serve as a behavioral model for a family member, making imitation more likely to occur in subsequent generations. Second, there may be other familial factors that increase the liability to suicide such as parental psychopathology, lack of support, discord, and even frank abuse.

As discussed in Chapter 8, media presentation of suicide and suicidal behavior can result in imitation and contagion. This effect is most prominent in adolescents and young adults (Gould and Shaffer, 1986; Phillips, 1974; Phillips and Carstensen, 1986; Schmidtke and Hafner, 1988). However, some evidence from adoption studies suggests that imitation is unlikely to explain all familial transmission because suicides in biological relatives unknown to the adoptee increase his or her risk (Schulsinger et al., 1979). Two other studies examining familial concordance between suicide attempts, one looking at twin pairs of attempts, and the other at parent–child pairs has found wide variability in the timing of the pairs of attempts, not consistent with imitation (Brent et al., in press; Statham et al., 1998).

Family discord impacts suicidal behavior, particularly among adolescents (Brent et al., 1994; Kosky et al., 1986; Kosky et al., 1990; Taylor and Stansfeld, 1984) (see Chapters 5 and 6). However, it is unclear to what extent family discord is the cause or consequence of other difficulties that may lead to suicide. Both sexual and physical abuse (see Chapter 5) have been associated with suicidal behavior (Brent et al., 1999; Brown et al., 1999; Fergusson et al., 1996; Kaplan et al., 1997; Renaud et al., 1999) as well as changes in central serotonin metabolism.

> I see now that I had been incubating this death far longer than I recognized at the time. When I was a child, both my parents had half-heartedly put their heads in the gas oven. Or so they claimed. It seemed to me then a rather splendid gesture, though shrouded in mystery, a little area of veiled intensity, revealed only by hints and unexplained, swiftly suppressed outbursts. It was something hidden, attractive and not for the children, like sex. But it was also something that undoubtedly did happen to grownups. However hysterical or comic the behavior involved—and to a child it seemed more ludicrous than tragic to place your head in the greasy gas oven, like the Sunday roast joint— suicide was a fact, a subject that couldn't be denied; it was something, however awful, that people did. When my own time came, I did not have to discover it for myself (Alvarez, The Savage God: A Study of Suicide, 1971/ 1990: 291-292).

It is difficult to know how genetics and abuse interact in their influence on suicide. First, abuse is more likely to occur in the presence of parental depression and substance abuse (Chaffin et al., 1996). Second, abusing parents have a greater rate of impulsive control disorders, including suicide attempt (Roberts and Hawton, 1980). Third, abuse may bring about conditions that interact with pre-existing genetic vulnerablities for other risk factors such as depression or substance abuse (c.f., Silberg et al., 1999). Finally, there is evidence that some effects of sexual abuse may be transmitted across generations, since non-abused children of sexually abused parents have increased suicidal behaviors (Brent et al., in press). Additional research is needed to sort out these issues.

Genetic Assessments

Several lines of evidence point to a link between genetic inheritance and risk of suicide. The following sections describe some of that evidence that derives from adoption studies, twin studies, family studies, candidate genes, and a new microarray approach.

Adoption Studies

Schulsinger et al. (1979) conducted a record linkage study among Danish adoptees, and found that the rate of suicide in the biological relatives of adoptees who had completed suicide was 6-fold higher than the rate in the biological relatives of living adoptees. There was no elevation of the rate of suicide in the adoptive relatives. This study strongly supports a genetic component to suicide, although it is less informative on exactly what is being transmitted—psychopathology or some other liability. It also argues against imitation.

A second adoption study examined the risk of suicide in the biological and adoptive relatives of adoptee probands who had a mood disorder (Wender et al., 1986). Interestingly, the highest rate of suicide was in the biological relatives of those probands with a diagnosis of "affect reaction," which roughly corresponds to borderline personality disorder. This rate (7.6 percent) was almost 3 times higher than the rate of suicide in the biological relatives of those with unipolar depression (2.2 percent), suggesting that the familial transmission of suicidal behavior might be more closely related to the transmission of difficulty with regulation of affect and impulses than mood disorder *per se*. An analysis of this study (Abbar et al., 1996) concluded that the genetic susceptibility to suicide was transmitted independently of the transmission of personality disorder.

Twin Studies

Juel-Nielsen and Videbech (1970) showed that monozygotic (identical) twins showed greater concordance for suicide than did dizygotic (fraternal) twins. Roy and colleagues (1991) updated these results, reviewed the world literature of case reports of twin suicides, and again found a much higher concordance for suicide among monozygotic than dizygotic twins (11.3 percent vs. 1.8 percent), consistent with a genetic etiology, most likely polygenic. In a subsequent study, Roy et al. (1995)

showed a high concordance of attempted suicide in a surviving twin with suicide in monozygotic twins (38 percent), but not in dizygotic co-twins (0 percent[3]). A large Australian study of almost 3000 twin pairs confirmed these findings (Statham et al., 1998). If a monozygotic twin attempted suicide, his/her co-twin had a 17.5-fold increased risk of having made an attempt. In controlling for other risk factors for suicide, such as mood disorder, substance abuse, trauma, personality problems, and life events, a family history of a suicide attempt still conveyed a 4-fold increased risk for the co-twin making an attempt. All studies of suicide in twins discussed here were carried out in twins who were raised together, with ostensibly a shared environment, thereby controlling for environmental effects. To date, there are no published findings for suicide for twins raised apart, which is another way to examine this issue. The attempts among twins did not cluster in time, making imitation a less likely explanation.

In this study, genetic modeling showed that 45 percent of the variance for suicidal thoughts and behavior was genetic, which suggests a continuity between ideation and attempt (Statham et al., 1998). Glowinski et al. (2001) studied 3416 Missouri female adolescent twins and found that genetic and shared environmental influences together accounted for 35 percent to 75 percent of the variance in risk. The twin/cotwin suicide attempt odds ratio was 5.6 (95 percent confidence interval [CI] 1.75–17.8) for monozygotic twins and 4.0 (95 percent CI 1.1–14.7) for dizygotic twins after controlling for other psychiatric risk factors.

Family Studies

Several family studies have compared the risk for suicide or suicide attempt in the first degree relatives of individuals who have completed suicide, compared to the rate among relatives of control probands. Although the methodology varies to some degree, the results consistently point to a 4-fold increase in risk among relatives of suicide probands compared to the relatives of controls. Tsuang (1983) reported that the rates of suicide in the relatives of patients who completed suicide were higher than the rates among the relatives of patients who did not complete suicide. This suggests that something other than mental disorder is being transmitted to increase the familial transmission of suicide. Similarly, Egeland and Sussex (1985) found that the rate of suicide in the pedigrees of the Old Order Amish showed a marked degree of clustering

---

[3]This very low rate may be due to reporting bias.

of suicide that could not be explained by the clustering of mood disorder alone (see also Chapter 6).

Several studies also show that the families of suicide attempters display an increased risk of suicidal behavior. The methodology varies significantly in this set of studies from chart review (Garfinkel et al., 1982; Roy, 1983; Roy, 2000) to family history (Linkowski et al., 1985; Malone et al., 1995), to formal family history study with direct interview of several first degree relatives (Bridge et al., 1997; Johnson et al., 1998; Pfeffer et al., 1994). The median odds ratio of these studies was around 4. Some report that the greater the lethality of the attempt, the greater the familial incidence of suicide (Garfinkel et al., 1982; but see Johnson et al., 1998; Linkowski et al., 1985; Mitterauer, 1990; Papadimitriou et al., 1991).

Candidate Gene Studies

Candidate gene studies compare the prevalence of different genetic variants (polymorphisms) of specific genes in cases of suicide or suicidal behavior to controls. The choice of candidate genes to examine in studying the etiology of suicide is guided by findings described earlier in the chapter regarding changes in serotonin metabolites and receptors in suicide victims and attempters. It is becoming evident, for example, that levels of 5-HIAA in CSF are under genetic control (about 40 percent of the variance is genetic; Clarke et al., 1995; Higley et al., 1994). Consequently, variation in genes related to the serotonergic system are important candidates. Those relating to the responsivity to serotonin include tryptophan hydroxylase (Manuck et al., 1999), the serotonin transporter promoter regions (Lesch et al., 1996), or the monoamine oxidase-A promoter regions (Manuck et al., 2000). Genes related to the serotonin transporter, $5HT_{1A}$, $5HT_{2A}$, and $5HT_{1B}$ are also candidates. These candidate genes will be reviewed in the following sections.

TPH. Trytophan hydroxylase (TPH) is the rate-limiting enzyme in the synthesis of serotonin. Most of the studies consider one of two polymorphisms, A779C and A218C, which have been reported to be in tight disequilibrium (i.e., tightly linked genetically). Several studies linked low CSF 5-HIAA to the 779C allele especially in males (Jonsson et al., 1997; Nielsen et al., 1998) but not to A218C (Mann et al., 1997; Nielsen et al., 1998). The A218C allele has been linked to changes in serotonin functioning in a study done by Mannuc and colleagues (1999). Studies comparing suicide completers to controls found no association between the A218C polymorphism and suicide (Bennett et al., 2000; Du et al., 2000b; Ono et al., 2000; Turecki et al., 2001), but suggested a relationship between the A779C allele and suicide (Bennett et al., 2000; Roy et al., 2001). The current research does not support a stronger relationship for either of these alleles compared to the other, and overall differences in research findings are likely more indicative of differences in the populations studied.

In alcoholic offenders an association between the 779C allele and suicide attempt was reported, with multiple attempts related to the number of C alleles (Nielsen et al., 1994). In addition, several studies report an association between the 218C allele and suicide attempt in non-mood-disordered individuals (Nielsen et al., 1998; Paik et al., 2000; Rotondo et al., 1999). In mood-disordered patients compared to healthy controls (Abbar et al., 2001; Bellivier et al., 1998; Tsai et al., 1999) and attempters compared to mood-disordered controls (Mann et al., 1997; Tsai et al., 1999), the A218 Allele was associated significantly with suicide attempt. The association was stronger for violent suicide attempt, especially if there was a history of depression (Abbar et al., 2001), with a dose response of the number of A alleles in one study (Abbar et al., 2001; Mann et al., 1997).

In a study of community volunteers, an association between impulsive aggressive traits and the A218 form of the TPH allele was reported, particularly in men (Manuck et al., 1999). Mann et al. (1997) reported an association between borderline personality disorder and the A218 polymorphism. In a small series of males with personality disorders, New et al. (1998) reported an association between the 218C allele and impulsive aggression.

Serotonin transporter studies. The serotonin transporter has two allelic variants in the promoter regions, a short (S) form and a long (L) form. Exposure to a serotonin agonist activates less transcription of the S than the L form (Greenberg et al., 1999). Comparing suicide victims to controls revealed an association between the L allele and depressed suicides (Du et al., 2000b), between the L allele and depression but not suicide (Mann et al., 2000), and between the S allele and violent suicide (Bondy et al., 2000). Others found no associations (Roy et al., 2001; Turecki et al., 1999). Family based studies on attempts demonstrated a relationship with the S allele, particularly for violent attempts in mood disordered (Bellivier et al., 2000) and alcoholic samples (Gorwood et al., 2000). There was a dose response between the number of S alleles and suicide attempt in those alcoholics with comorbid depression, with no relationship between the number of S alleles and attempts in those alcoholics without depression. On the other hand, Zalsman et al. (2001) reported that the L allele was associated with high measures of aggression. However, Geijer et al. (2000), in a comparison of a diagnostically mixed sample of attempters to healthy controls, found no association.

HT2A studies. Studies of suicidal behavior and the HTR2A receptor have examined three polymorphisms—T102C, His 452Tyr, and A1438G. Comparisons of suicide victims to controls (Du et al., 1999; Turecki et al., 1999) revealed no relationship between HTR2A polymorphisms (His452Tyr for Du et al., 1999; T102C in both studies, A1438G for Turecki et al., 1999). Turecki et al. (1999) found some functional significance of the 102T/1438A haplotype, which was associated with increased 5HT2A receptor binding. Most studies comparing suicide attempters to controls also demonstrated no effect (Geijer et al., 2000; Kunugi et al., 1999; Tsai et al., 1999). One study did report an association between suicide attempt and the 102C form of the allele (Zhang et al., 1997).

MAOA studies. In a study of community volunteers, Manuck et al. (2000) identified 4 haplotypes of monoamine oxidase-A (MAOA) and found an association between the 2-3 haplotype[4] and impulsive aggression in men. This haplotype was also associated with an altered response to the fenfluramine challenge test. The relationship of these genetic variants to suicide attempt has not yet been studied.

Methodological issues. To date, while some trends are evident in the results for candidate genes, inconsistencies in the literature exist. Differences in diagnostic makeup may have accounted for differences in results. For example, many of the TPH studies that examined attempts in non-affectively-disordered samples found associations with the 779C or 218C allele, where studies in mood disordered samples tended to find associations with the A218 allele. In this linked set of polymorphisms, some studies find an association with the A and some with the C allele. The inconsistency is hard to explain—it could be due to sex differences, diagnostic differences, or design differences, or it could be that both polarities of the allele, under different circumstances, predispose to a suicide attempt. The association of the S allele in the serotonin transporter promoter region to suicide attempt in alcoholics was strongly influenced by the presence or absence of a history of major depression (Gorwood et al., 2000). Some studies used "healthy" controls, although screening for "healthy" ranged from an extensive psychiatric interview to asking subjects whether they had ever had any psychiatric difficulties. Other studies used diagnostically matched controls. By controlling for diagnosis, one can detect genes above and beyond those related to disorder that may account for suicidal behavior.

---

[4]A haplotype is a combination of alleles that tend to be inherited together.

Characterization of the sample by other behavioral characteristics may have a critical impact on results. For example, in the study of Nielsen et al. (1998), a differentiation was made on the basis of whether an offender was "impulsive" or "non-impulsive." This turned out to be a critical differentiation since the associations were found to be much stronger in the impulsive sub-group. This differentiation was made on the basis of the most recent crime, so that a person could actually be reclassified from impulsive to non-impulsive, which goes against the view that impulsivity is a trait characteristic. Most studies did not ascertain Axis II conditions, except Mann et al. (1997) who did find a significant association between borderline personality disorder and TPH.

A related issue is that there may be an "endophenotype" associated with suicidal behavior, namely impulsive aggression, yet most studies did not assess this, even though it appeared to be related to both TPH, polymorphisms of the serotonin transporter, and MAOA (Manuck et al., 1999; Manuck et al., 2000; New et al., 1998; Zalsman et al., 2001).

Sex differences. It would be surprising if genetic effects were not moderated by gender. In fact, the functional significance of TPH polymorphisms appears to be different in males and females, with a more profound effect on central serotonin metabolism in men (Jonsson et al., 1997; Manuck et al., 1999). The relationship between impulsive aggression and TPH A218C appears to be moderated by sex (Manuck et al., 1999), as do relationships between other personality measures and polymorphisms of the serotonin transporter (Du et al., 2000a). Inconsistencies between studies of suicide and suicide attempt could be explained in part by differences in the sex composition of the groups. Sex effects need to be considered in these analyses.

Ethnic differences. Ethnic differences are also an important consideration, and may explain how studies in clinically similar samples might differ (e.g., a positive study in depressed Caucasians [Mann et al., 1997] versus a negative one in Japanese mood-disordered patients [Kunugi et al., 1999]). Particularly when studying haplotypes, there are likely to be significant ethnic differences, with a finding that alleles are tightly linked in a Caucasian sample, but not in a Japanese one (Ono et al., 2000; Turecki et al., 2001).

Screening Expressed Genes

It has been hypothesized that a separate unique set of expressed genes could be associated with suicidal behavior and that the interaction of these genes with depressive or schizophrenic genes may be necessary for the expression of the suicidal phenotype. Whole genome scans of depressed and schizophrenic patients have revealed areas on the human genome containing genes that contribute to the depressive and/or schizophrenic phenotype. In the past for example, candidate genes implicated by our understanding of the pathophysiology of these diseased states or by their location in regions identified by whole genome scans have been investigated. So far, this has been a tedious and relatively unproductive approach in that researchers have only been able to evaluate one gene at a time. Previous technical limitations have severely hindered efforts to study the level and pattern of expression of many brain genes simultaneously in different regions. However, recent technological developments have dramatically altered the scientific landscape and made it possible, for the first time, to use microarray technology in postmortem brain tissue to screen 10,000 to 15,000 genes in one experiment.

The microarray technology involves the extraction of mRNA from brain regions of interest, construction of mRNA expression arrays following PCR amplification and purification of DNA clones, hybridization of labeled cDNA tissue to the array, and the quantification of the arrays. The arrays, which are an inch or so square and contain elements identifying up to 15,000 genes, can be robotically printed or obtained commercially. These arrays can be labeled with fluor dyes and the differential expression of the genes between patient and control tissue can be detected with lasers. A large number of genes can be screened for differential expressions between patient and control tissue, thus identifying new candidate genes.

A research strategy involves (1) identifying regions of interest in postmortem brain tissue and individually matched controls, (2) performing high density microarray analysis comparing the relative levels of gene transcripts in patients and controls, (3) analyzing gene expression profiling with cluster analysis and data mining tools, (4) evaluating selected mRNAs with real time quantitative polymerase chain reaction (PCR) and in situ hybridization mapping, and (5) repeating analyses of additional cohorts for each disease or condition. In the future, evidence from three bodies of data may converge to signal the relevance of specific identified genes. A gene of major interest could have (1) been identified as over- or underexpressed in suicidal patients versus controls, (2) occurred in a region of the genome identified as a "hotspot" in suicidal patients by whole genome scans; (3) occurred in brain regions and cell types compatible with our understanding of the pathophysiology of suicide. Possible experiments to attempt to identify a set of genes unique to suicide might involve scientists investigating brain tissue from a cohort of major depressive disorder patients with and without suicidal behavior, bipolar affective disorder patients with and without suicidal behavior, and schizophrenic patients with and without suicidal behavior. In this design, diseased states remain constant while suicidal behavior varies. It should be emphasized that identified genes associated with suicide may or may not be causative, but may be vulnerability genes, or downstream modulating genes. Nevertheless, this technology will provide important candidate genes for future interaction with the pharmaceutical industry in the development of novel therapeutic compounds and could make important contributions to our understanding of the pathophysiology of suicide.

FINDINGS

• Dysregulation of one of the body's primary stress response systems, the hypothalamic-pituitary-adrenal (HPA) axis, appears associated with suicidality across psychiatric diagnoses. Such HPA axis dysfunction often develops following adverse developmental experiences and traumatic or chronic stress; HPA axis dysregulation is also implicated in the development of some mental disorders. Although screening for abnormal HPA axis function seems promising for predicting eventual suicide, it does not consistently predict acute suicidal behavior.

The utility of assessing HPA axis function as a physiological screening tool for suicide risk should be explored. Longitudinal, prospective studies of the influence of HPA axis function on suicidality are needed. Medical and psychosocial treatments that attenuate HPA dysregulation should be further developed and tested for their efficacy in reducing suicide.

• Neurobiological research on suicide has revealed significant changes in the serotonergic systems. Low levels of serotonin and/or its metabolite have been found in the brains and cerebrospinal fluid of serious suicide attempters and/or those who complete suicide; abnormalities in serotonin receptors have also been found in those who complete suicide. Studies suggest that impaired serotonin function specifically influences suicidality via increased impulsive aggression. Other neurotransmitter systems, especially noradrenergic function, also show alterations with suicidal behavior. Neurochemical changes appear to be specific to certain brain regions. Brain mapping techniques provide a valuable tool for determining biological markers for suicide.

• Studies find evidence of genetic influences on suicidality via familial aggregation of suicide, high suicide rates among adoptees whose biological families have elevated rates, and high concordance of suicide among identical vs. fraternal twins. This line of research represents a still-developing area of suicidology; no studies of suicide in identical twins raised apart has been conducted, for example, and much remains un-known about non-genetic familial transmission of suicide.

Biological predictors of suicidal behavior should be sought through brain mapping studies. Prospective, rather than cross-sectional studies, are crucial. Analyses *in vivo* would allow the examination of changes over time to elucidate response to treatment and remission from episodes of mental illness. Moreover, brain mapping studies may help to identify individuals at risk for suicidal behavior.

• Genetic factors are strongly related to liability for suicidal behavior, accounting for 30–50 percent of the variance. The genetic liability may be linked to the heritability of mental illness and/or impulsive aggression. However, family, cultural, and other environmental factors must be considered as independent factors. Family studies have shown that offspring of suicide attempters are much more likely to engage in suicidal behavior. Factors that increase the likelihood of transmission of suicidal behavior include the transmission of impulsive aggression and sexual abuse from parent to child. Therefore, offspring of parents who have made suicide attempts are at high risk for suicidal behavior and may inform us about the mechanisms of familial transmission, both genetic and non-genetic.

Prospective studies of populations at high risk for the onset of suicidal behavior, such as the offspring of suicide completers or attempters, can allow for studies of neurobiologic, genetic, and non-genetic factors that predict the onset of suicidal behavior.

Genetic markers that have functional significance and correlate with impulsive aggression and suicidal behavior cross-sectionally may have the potential to identify individuals at risk and help pinpoint treatment.

• Adoption studies, twin studies, and family studies are effective approaches to elucidate the genetic liability for suicide and to assess both genetic and non-genetic influences. Candidate gene analyses suggest the genetic targets that influence suicidal behavior. New microarray technology can aid researchers in identifying genetic variations between suicidal and non-suicidal individuals. These approaches hold great promise for elucidating the risk factors for suicide and providing tools for its assessment, treatment and prevention.

Future research using these approaches should be pursued. Twin studies of suicidal behavior should examine familial transmission through genetic and non-genetic pathways and explore associations with both mental disorders and impulsive aggression to shed light on the genetic antecedents of suicidal behavior.

Candidate gene approaches should be used to (a) study multiple genes, e.g., along the serotonin pathway; (b) examine candidate genes in greater depth, through direct sequencing and haplotype analyses; (c) examine candidate gene associations with related quantitative traits (endophenotypes) and should (d) use statistical approaches that fully exploit case control designs, and at the same time control for overdispersion (genetically related subjects), using, for example, the methods of genomic control or excess haplotype sharing extension.[5]

Genetic samples from psychiatric populations can provide valuable information. To get the most from genetic analyses, all psychiatric genetic studies should also gather information about suicidal behavior, including lethality, intent, and age of onset of first attempt. Existing samples of DNA on psychiatric populations should be studied to examine the relationship between genetic markers and suicidal behavior. Genetic isolates (i.e., populations that have had few or no new genes added from outsiders for many generations) with a high rate of suicide and suicidal behavior should be identified for linkage studies.

---

[5]Genomic control is a type of analysis of candidate gene data where one can control for the amount of overdispersion by genotypic "null genes" that are thought not to be involved with the disorder. If those null genes show a relationship to the disorder, that suggests overdispersion rather than a true relationship to the disease. Excess haplotype sharing means that a great extent of genetic material is shared in common. This would be rare and unlikely to be due to chance.

REFERENCES

Abbar M, Courtet P, Bellivier F, Leboyer M, Boulenger JP, Castelhau D, Ferreira M, Lambercy C, Mouthon D, Paoloni-Giacobino A, Vessaz M, Malafosse A, Buresi C. 2001. Suicide attempts and the tryptophan hydroxylase gene. *Molecular Psychiatry*, 6(3): 268-273.

Abbar M, Courtet P, Malafosse A, Castelnau D. 1996. Epidemiologic and molecular genetic of suicidal behavior. *L'Encephale*, 22 (Spec No 4): 19-24.

Ågren H. 1980. Symptom patterns in unipolar and bipolar depression correlating with monoamine metabolites in the cerebrospinal fluid: II. Suicide. *Psychiatry Research*, 3(2): 225-236.

Ågren H. 1982. Depressive symptom patterns and urinary MHPG excretion. *Psychiatry Research*, 6(2): 185-196.

Ågren H, Niklasson F. 1986. Suicidal potential in depression: Focus on CSF monoamine and purine metabolites. *Psychopharmacology Bulletin*, 22(3): 656-660.

Alvarez A. 1971/1990. *The Savage God: A Study of Suicide*. New York: W.W. Norton.

Arango V, Ernsberger P, Marzuk PM, Chen JS, Tierney H, Stanley M, Reis DJ, Mann JJ. 1990. Autoradiographic demonstration of increased serotonin 5-HT2 and beta-adrenergic receptor binding sites in the brain of suicide victims. *Archives of General Psychiatry*, 47(11): 1038-1047.

Arango V, Ernsberger P, Sved AF, Mann JJ. 1993. Quantitative autoradiography of alpha 1- and alpha 2-adrenergic receptors in the cerebral cortex of controls and suicide victims. *Brain Research*, 630(1-2): 271-282.

Arango V, Mann JJ. 1992. Relevance of serotonergic postmortem studies to suicidal behavior. *International Review of Psychiatry*, 4: 131-140.

Arango V, Underwood MD, Gubbi AV, Mann JJ. 1995. Localized alterations in pre- and postsynaptic serotonin binding sites in the ventrolateral prefrontal cortex of suicide victims. *Brain Research*, 688(1-2): 121-133.

Arango V, Underwood MD, Mann JJ. 1996. Fewer pigmented locus coeruleus neurons in suicide victims: Preliminary results. *Biological Psychiatry*, 39(2): 112-120.

Arató M, Banki CM, Bissette G, Nemeroff CB. 1989. Elevated CSF CRF in suicide victims. *Biological Psychiatry*, 25(3): 355-359.

Arató M, Tekes K, Tothfalusi L, Magyar K, Palkovits M, Demeter E, Falus A. 1987. Serotonergic split brain and suicide. *Psychiatry Research*, 21(4): 355-356.

Arató M, Tekes K, Tothfalusi L, Magyar K, Palkovits M, Frecska E, Falus A, MacCrimmon DJ. 1991. Reversed hemispheric asymmetry of imipramine binding in suicide victims. *Biological Psychiatry*, 29(7): 699-702.

Arora RC, Meltzer HY. 1989. 3H-imipramine binding in the frontal cortex of suicides. *Psychiatry Research*, 30(2): 125-135.

Arranz B, Blennow K, Eriksson A, Mansson JE, Marcusson J. 1997. Serotonergic, noradrenergic, and dopaminergic measures in suicide brains. *Biological Psychiatry*, 41(10): 1000-1009.

Arranz B, Eriksson A, Mellerup E, Plenge P, Marcusson J. 1994. Brain 5-HT1A, 5-HT1D, and 5-HT2 receptors in suicide victims. *Biological Psychiatry*, 35(7): 457-463.

Åsberg M, Thoren P, Träskman L, Bertilsson L, Ringberger V. 1976a. "Serotonin depression"—a biochemical subgroup within the affective disorders? *Science*, 191: 470-480.

Åsberg M, Träskman L, Thoren P. 1976b. 5-HIAA in the cerebrospinal fluid. A biochemical suicide predictor? *Archives of General Psychiatry*, 33(10): 1193-1197.

Banki CM, Arató M. 1983. Amine metabolites and neuroendocrine responses related to depression and suicide. *Journal of Affective Disorders*, 5(3): 223-232.

Banki CM, Arató M, Papp Z, Kurcz M. 1984. Biochemical markers in suicidal patients. Investigations with cerebrospinal fluid amine metabolites and neuroendocrine tests. *Journal of Affective Disorders*, 6(3-4): 341-350.

Bellivier F, Leboyer M, Courtet P, Buresi C, Beaufils B, Samolyk D, Allilaire JF, Feingold J, Mallet J, Malafosse A. 1998. Association between the tryptophan hydroxylase gene and manic-depressive illness. *Archives of General Psychiatry*, 55(1): 33-37.

Bellivier F, Szoke A, Henry C, Lacoste J, Bottos C, Nosten-Bertrand M, Hardy P, Rouillon F, Launay JM, Laplanche JL, Leboyer M. 2000. Possible association between serotonin transporter gene polymorphism and violent suicidal behavior in mood disorders. *Biological Psychiatry*, 48(4): 319-322.

Bennett PJ, McMahon WM, Watabe J, Achilles J, Bacon M, Coon H, Grey T, Keller T, Tate D, Tcaciuc I, Workman J, Gray D. 2000. Tryptophan hydroxylase polymorphisms in suicide victims. *Psychiatric Genetics*, 10(1): 13-17.

Beskow J, Gottfries CG, Roos BE, Winblad B. 1976. Determination of monoamine and monoamine metabolites in the human brain: Post mortem studies in a group of suicides and in a control group. *Acta Psychiatrica Scandinavica*, 53(1): 7-20.

Biegon A, Israeli M. 1988. Regionally selective increases in beta-adrenergic receptor density in the brains of suicide victims. *Brain Research*, 442(1): 199-203.

Bondy B, Erfurth A, de Jonge S, Kruger M, Meyer H. 2000. Possible association of the short allele of the serotonin transporter promoter gene polymorphism (5-HTTLPR) with violent suicide. *Molecular Psychiatry*, 5: 193-195.

Bostwick JM, Pankratz VS. 2000. Affective disorders and suicide risk: A reexamination. *American Journal of Psychiatry*, 157(12): 1925-1932.

Bourne HR, Bunney WE Jr, Colburn RW, Davis JM, Davis JN, Shaw DM, Coppen AJ. 1968. Noradrenaline, 5-hydroxytryptamine, and 5-hydroxyindoleacetic acid in hindbrains of suicidal patients. *Lancet*, 2(7572): 805-808.

Boutin P, Froguel P. 2001. Genetics of human obesity. *Best Practice and Research. Clinical Endocrinology and Metabolism*, 15(3): 391-404.

Brent DA, Baugher M, Bridge J, Chen T, Chiappetta L. 1999. Age- and sex-related risk factors for adolescent suicide. *Journal of the American Academy of Child and Adolescent Psychiatry*, 38(12): 1497-1505.

Brent DA, Oquendo MA, Birmaher B, Greenhill L, Kolko DJ, Stanley B, Zelazny J, Brodsky BS, Bridge J, Ellis SP, Salazar O, Mann JJ. in press. Familial pathways to early-onset suicide attempts: A high-risk study. *Archives of General Psychiatry*.

Brent DA, Perper JA, Moritz G, Liotus L, Schweers J, Balach L, Roth C. 1994. Familial risk factors for adolescent suicide: A case-control study. *Acta Psychiatrica Scandinavica*, 89(1): 52-58.

Bridge JA, Brent DA, Johnson BA, Connolly J. 1997. Familial aggregation of psychiatric disorders in a community sample of adolescents. *Journal of the American Academy of Child and Adolescent Psychiatry*, 36(5): 628-636.

Brodsky BS, Malone KM, Ellis SP, Dulit RA, Mann JJ. 1997. Characteristics of borderline personality disorder associated with suicidal behavior. *American Journal of Psychiatry*, 154(12): 1715-1719.

Brown GL, Ebert MH, Goyer PF, Jimerson DC, Klein WJ, Bunney WE, Goodwin FK. 1982. Aggression, suicide, and serotonin: Relationships to CSF amine metabolites. *American Journal of Psychiatry*, 139(6): 741-746.

Brown J, Cohen P, Johnson JG, Smailes EM. 1999. Childhood abuse and neglect: Specificity of effects on adolescent and young adult depression and suicidality. *Journal of the American Academy of Child and Adolescent Psychiatry*, 38(12): 1490-1496.

Brown RP, Mason B, Stoll P, Brizer D, Kocsis J, Stokes PE, Mann JJ. 1986. Adrenocortical function and suicidal behavior in depressive disorders. *Psychiatry Research*, 17(4): 317-323.

Brunner J, Bronisch T. 1999. Neurobiological correlates of suicidal behavior. *Fortschritte Der Neurologie-Psychiatrie*, 67(9): 391-412.

Brunner J, Stalla GK, Stalla J, Uhr M, Grabner A, Wetter TC, Bronisch T. 2001. Decreased corticotropin-releasing hormone (CRH) concentrations in the cerebrospinal fluid of eucortisolemic suicide attempters. *Journal of Psychiatry Research*, 35(1): 1-9.

Bunney WE Jr, Fawcett JA, Davis JM, Gifford S. 1969. Further evaluation of urinary 17-hydroxycorticosteroids in suicidal patients. *Archives of General Psychiatry*, 21(2): 138-150.

Callado LF, Meana JJ, Grijalba B, Pazos A, Sastre M, Garcia-Sevilla JA. 1998. Selective increase of alpha2A-adrenoceptor agonist binding sites in brains of depressed suicide victims. *Journal of Neurochemistry*, 70(3): 1114-1123.

Calogero AE, Bagdy G, Szemeredi K, Tartaglia ME, Gold PW, Chrousos GP. 1990. Mechanisms of serotonin receptor agonist-induced activation of the hypothalamic-pituitary-adrenal axis in the rat. *Endocrinology*, 126(4): 1888-1894.

Carroll BJ, Greden JF, Feinberg M. 1980. Suicide, neuroendocrine dysfunction and CSF 5-HIAA concentrations in depression. In: Angrist B, Editor. *Recent Advances in Neuropsychopharmacology: Proceedings of the 12th CINP Congress.* (pp. 307-313). Oxford, UK: Pergamon Press.

Chaffin M, Kelleher K, Hollenberg J. 1996. Onset of physical abuse and neglect: Psychiatric, substance abuse, and social risk factors from prospective community data. *Child Abuse and Neglect*, 20(3): 191-203.

Chaouloff F. 1995. Regulation of 5-HT receptors by corticosteroids: Where do we stand? *Fundamental and Clinical Pharmacology*, 9(3): 219-233.

Cheetham SC, Crompton MR, Czudek C, Horton RW, Katona CL, Reynolds GP. 1989. Serotonin concentrations and turnover in brains of depressed suicides. *Brain Research*, 502(2): 332-340.

Cheetham SC, Crompton MR, Katona CL, Horton RW. 1988. Brain 5-HT2 receptor binding sites in depressed suicide victims. *Brain Research*, 443(1-2): 272-280.

Clarke AS, Kammerer CM, George KP, Kupfer DJ, McKinney WT, Spence MA, Kraemer GW. 1995. Evidence for heritability of biogenic amine levels in the cerebrospinal fluid of rhesus monkeys. *Biological Psychiatry*, 38(9): 572-577.

Coccaro EF, Siever LJ, Klar HM, Maurer G, Cochrane K, Cooper TB, Mohs RC, Davis KL. 1989. Serotonergic studies in patients with affective and personality disorders. Correlates with suicidal and impulsive aggressive behavior. *Archives of General Psychiatry*, 46(7): 587-599.

Cochran E, Robins E, Grote S. 1976. Regional serotonin levels in brain: A comparison of depressive suicides and alcoholic suicides with controls. *Biological Psychiatry*, 11(3): 283-294.

Conwell Y, Brent D. 1995. Suicide and aging. I: Patterns of psychiatric diagnosis. *International Psychogeriatrics*, 7(2): 149-164.

Cooper B. 2001. Nature, nurture and mental disorder: Old concepts in the new millennium. *British Journal of Psychiatry. Supplement*, 40: S91-S101.

Correa H, Duval F, Mokrani M, Bailey P, Tremeau F, Staner L, Diep TS, Hode Y, Crocq MA, Macher JP. 2000. Prolactin response to D-fenfluramine and suicidal behavior in depressed patients. *Psychiatry Research*, 93(3): 189-199.

Coryell W, Schlesser M. 2001. The dexamethasone suppression test and suicide prediction. *American Journal of Psychiatry*, 158(5): 748-753.

Coryell W, Schlesser MA. 1981. Suicide and the dexamethasone suppression test in unipolar depression. *American Journal of Psychiatry*, 138(8): 1120-1121.

Cowburn RF, Marcusson JO, Eriksson A, Wiehager B, O'Neill C. 1994. Adenylyl cyclase activity and G-protein subunit levels in postmortem frontal cortex of suicide victims. *Brain Research*, 633(1-2): 297-304.

Cross JA, Cheetham SC, Crompton MR, Katona CL, Horton RW. 1988. Brain GABAB binding sites in depressed suicide victims. *Psychiatry Research*, 26(2): 119-129.

Crow TJ, Cross AJ, Cooper SJ, Deakin JFW, Ferrier IN, Johnson JA, Joseph MH, Owen F, Poulter M, Lofthouse R, Corsellis JAN, Chambers DR, Blessed G, Perry EK, Perry RH, Tomlinson BE. 1984. Neurotransmitter receptors and monoamine metabolites in the brains of patients with Alzheimer-type dementia and depression, and suicides. *Neuropharmacology*, 23(12B): 1561-1569.

De Paermentier F, Cheetham SC, Crompton MR, Katona CL, Horton RW. 1990. Brain beta-adrenoceptor binding sites in antidepressant-free depressed suicide victims. *Brain Research*, 525(1): 71-77.

Dillon KA, Gross-Isseroff R, Israeli M, Biegon A. 1991. Autoradiographic analysis of serotonin 5-HT1A receptor binding in the human brain postmortem: Effects of age and alcohol. *Brain Research*, 554(1-2): 56-64.

Dinan TG. 1996. Serotonin and the regulation of hypothalamic-pituitary-adrenal axis function. *Life Sciences*, 58(20): 1683-1694.

Dorovini-Zis K, Zis AP. 1987. Increased adrenal weight in victims of violent suicide. *American Journal of Psychiatry*, 144(9): 1214-1215.

Du L, Bakish D, Hrdina PD. 2000a. Gender differences in association between serotonin transporter gene polymorphism and personality traits. *Psychiatric Genetics*, 10(4): 159-164.

Du L, Bakish D, Lapierre YD, Ravindran AV, Hrdina PD. 2000b. Association of polymorphism of serotonin 2A receptor gene with suicidal ideation in major depressive disorder. *American Journal of Medical Genetics*, 96(1): 56-60.

Du L, Faludi G, Palkovits M, Demeter E, Bakish D, Lapierre YD, Sotonyi P, Hrdina PD. 1999. Frequency of long allele in serotonin transporter gene is increased in depressed suicide victims. *Biological Psychiatry*, 46(2): 196-201.

Duval F, Mokrani MC, Correa H, Bailey P, Valdebenito M, Monreal J, Crocq MA, Macher JP. 2001. Lack of effect of HPA axis hyperactivity on hormonal responses to d-fenfluramine in major depressed patients: Implications for pathogenesis of suicidal behaviour. *Psychoneuroendocrinology*, 26(5): 521-537.

Edman G, Åsberg M, Levander S, Schalling D. 1986. Skin conductance habituation and cerebrospinal fluid 5-hydroxyindoleacetic acid in suicidal patients. *Archives of General Psychiatry*, 43(6): 586-592.

Egeland JA, Sussex JN. 1985. Suicide and family loading for affective disorders. *Journal of the American Medical Association*, 254(7): 915-918.

Fawcett JA, Bunney WE Jr. 1967. Pituitary adrenal function and depression. An outline for research. *Archives of General Psychiatry*, 16(5): 517-535.

Fergusson DM, Horwood LJ, Lynskey MT. 1996. Childhood sexual abuse and psychiatric disorder in young adulthood: II. Psychiatric outcomes of childhood sexual abuse. *Journal of the American Academy of Child and Adolescent Psychiatry*, 35(10): 1365-1374.

Fuller RW. 1990. Serotonin receptors and neuroendocrine responses. *Neuropsychopharmacology*, 3(5-6): 495-502.

Gabilondo AM, Meana JJ, Garcia-Sevilla JA. 1995. Increased density of mu-opioid receptors in the postmortem brain of suicide victims. *Brain Research*, 682(1-2): 245-250.

Garfinkel BD, Froese A, Hood J. 1982. Suicide attempts in children and adolescents. *American Journal of Psychiatry*, 139(10): 1257-1261.

Geijer T, Frisch A, Persson ML, Wasserman D, Rockah R, Michaelovsky E, Apter A, Jonsson EG, Nothen MM, Weizman A. 2000. Search for association between suicide attempt and serotonergic polymorphisms. *Psychiatric Genetics*, 10(1): 19-26.

Glowinski AL, Bucholz KK, Nelson EC, Fu Q, Madden PA, Reich W, Heath AC. 2001. Suicide attempts in an adolescent female twin sample. *Journal of the American Academy of Child and Adolescent Psychiatry*, 40(11): 1300-1307.

Gonzalez AM, Pascual J, Meana JJ, Barturen F, del Arco C, Pazos A, Garcia-Sevilla JA. 1994. Autoradiographic demonstration of increased alpha 2-adrenoceptor agonist binding sites in the hippocampus and frontal cortex of depressed suicide victims. *Journal of Neurochemistry*, 63(1): 256-265.

Gorwood P, Batel P, Ades J, Hamon M, Boni C. 2000. Serotonin transporter gene polymorphisms, alcoholism, and suicidal behavior. *Biological Psychiatry*, 48(4): 259-264.

Gould MS, Shaffer D. 1986. The impact of suicide in television movies. Evidence of imitation. *New England Journal of Medicine*, 315(11): 690-694.

Greenberg BD, Tolliver TJ, Huang SJ, Li Q, Bengel D, Murphy DL. 1999. Genetic variation in the serotonin transporter promoter region affects serotonin uptake in human blood platelets. *American Journal of Medical Genetics*, 88(1): 83-87.

Gross-Isseroff R, Dillon KA, Fieldust SJ, Biegon A. 1990b. Autoradiographic analysis of alpha 1-noradrenergic receptors in the human brain postmortem. Effect of suicide. *Archives of General Psychiatry*, 47(11): 1049-1053.

Gross-Isseroff R, Israeli M, Biegon A. 1989. Autoradiographic analysis of tritiated imipramine binding in the human brain post mortem: Effects of suicide. *Archives of General Psychiatry*, 46(3): 237-241.

Gross-Isseroff R, Salama D, Israeli M, Biegon A. 1990a. Autoradiographic analysis of [3H]ketanserin binding in the human brain postmortem: Effect of suicide. *Brain Research*, 507(2): 208-215.

Higaki J, Katsuya T, Morishita R, Ogihara T. 2001. Symposium on the etiology of hypertension-summarizing studies in 20th century. 1. Hypertension and genes. *Internal Medicine*, 40(2): 144-147.

Higley JD, Linnoila M. 1997. Low central nervous system serotonergic activity is traitlike and correlates with impulsive behavior. A nonhuman primate model investigating genetic and environmental influences on neurotransmission. *Annals of the New York Academy of Sciences*, 836: 39-56.

Higley JD, Linnoila M, Suomi S. 1994. Ethological contributions. In: Hersen M, Ammerman RT, Sisson LA, Editors. *Handbook of Aggressive and Destructive Behavior in Psychiatric Patients*. (pp. 17-32). New York: Plenum Press.

Higley JD, Mehlman PT, Poland RE, Taub DM, Vickers J, Suomi SJ, Linnoila M. 1996. CSF testosterone and 5-HIAA correlate with different types of aggressive behaviors. *Biological Psychiatry*, 40(11): 1067-1082.

Hrdina PD, Demeter E, Vu TB, Sotonyi P, Palkovits M. 1993. 5-HT uptake sites and 5-HT2 receptors in brain of antidepressant-free suicide victims/depressives: Increase in 5-HT2 sites in cortex and amygdala. *Brain Research*, 614(1-2): 37-44.

Huang YY, Grailhe R, Arango V, Hen R, Mann JJ. 1999. Relationship of psychopathology to the human serotonin1B genotype and receptor binding kinetics in postmortem brain tissue. *Neuropsychopharmacology*, 21(2): 238-246.

IOM (Institute of Medicine). 2001. *Health and Behavior: The Interplay of Biological, Behavioral, and Societal Influences*. Washington, DC: National Academy Press.

Johnson BA, Brent DA, Bridge J, Connolly J. 1998. The familial aggregation of adolescent suicide attempts. *Acta Psychiatrica Scandinavica*, 97(1): 18-24.

Jones JS, Stanley B, Mann JJ, Frances AJ, Guido JR, Träskman-Bendz L, Winchel R, Brown RP, Stanley M. 1990. CSF 5-HIAA and HVA concentrations in elderly depressed patients who attempted suicide. *American Journal of Psychiatry*, 147(9): 1225-1227.

Jonsson EG, Goldman D, Spurlock G, Gustavsson JP, Nielsen DA, Linnoila M, Owen MJ, Sedvall GC. 1997. Tryptophan hydroxylase and catechol-O-methyltransferase gene polymorphisms: Relationships to monoamine metabolite concentrations in CSF of healthy volunteers. *European Archives of Psychiatry and Clinical Neuroscience*, 247(6): 297-302.

Joyce JN, Shane A, Lexow N, Winokur A, Casanova MF, Kleinman JE. 1993. Serotonin uptake sites and serotonin receptors are altered in the limbic system of schizophrenics. *Neuropsychopharmacology*, 8(4): 315-336.

Juel-Nielsen N, Videbech T. 1970. A twin study of suicide. *Acta Geneticae Medicae Et Gemellologiae*, 19(1): 307-310.

Kaplan SJ, Pelcovitz D, Salzinger S, Mandel FS, Weiner M. 1997. Adolescent physical abuse and suicide attempts. *Journal of the American Academy of Child and Adolescent Psychiatry*, 36(6): 799-808.

Kapur S, Mann JJ. 1992. Role of the dopaminergic system in depression. *Biological Psychiatry*, 32(1): 1-17.

Kety SS. 1986. Genetic factors in suicide. In: Roy A, Editor. *Suicide*. (pp. 41-45). Baltimore, MD: Williams and Wilkins.

Klimek V, Stockmeier C, Overholser J, Meltzer HY, Kalka S, Dilley G, Ordway GA. 1997. Reduced levels of norepinephrine transporters in the locus coeruleus in major depression. *Journal of Neuroscience*, 17(21): 8451-8458.

Korpi ER, Kleinman JE, Goodman SI, Phillips I, DeLisi LE, Linnoila M, Wyatt RJ. 1986. Serotonin and 5-hydroxyindoleacetic acid in brains of suicide victims. Comparison in chronic schizophrenic patients with suicide as cause of death. *Archives of General Psychiatry*, 43(6): 594-600.

Kosky R, Silburn S, Zubrick S. 1986. Symptomatic depression and suicidal ideation. A comparative study with 628 children. *Journal of Nervous and Mental Disease*, 174(9): 523-528.

Kosky R, Silburn S, Zubrick SR. 1990. Are children and adolescents who have suicidal thoughts different from those who attempt suicide? *Journal of Nervous and Mental Disease*, 178(1): 38-43.

Krieger G. 1970. Biochemical predictors of suicide. *Diseases of the Nervous System*, 31(7): 478-582.

Kunugi H, Ishida S, Kato T, Sakai T, Tatsumi M, Hirose T, Nanko S. 1999. No evidence for an association of polymorphisms of the tryptophan hydroxylase gene with affective disorders or attempted suicide among Japanese patients. *American Journal of Psychiatry*, 156(5): 774-776.

Laruelle M, Abi-Dargham A, Casanova MF, Toti R, Weinberger DR, Kleinman JE. 1993. Selective abnormalities of prefrontal serotonergic receptors in schizophrenia. A postmortem study. *Archives of General Psychiatry*, 50(10): 810-818.

Lesch KP, Bengel D, Heils A, Sabol SZ, Greenberg BD, Petri S, Benjamin J, Muller CR, Hamer DH, Murphy DL. 1996. Association of anxiety-related traits with a polymorphism in the serotonin transporter gene regulatory region. *Science*, 274(5292): 1527-1531.

Lester D. 1992. The dexamethasone suppression test as an indicator of suicide: A meta-analysis. *Pharmacopsychiatry*, 25(6): 265-270.

Levy B, Hansen E. 1969. Failure of the urinary test for suicide potential. Analysis of urinary 17-OHCS steroid findings prior to suicide in two patients. *Archives of General Psychiatry*, 20(4): 415-418.

Lidberg L, Tuck JR, Asberg M, Scalia-Tomba GP, Bertilsson L. 1985. Homicide, suicide and CSF 5-HIAA. *Acta Psychiatrica Scandinavica*, 71(3): 230-236.

Linkowski P, de Maertelaer V, Mendlewicz J. 1985. Suicidal behavior in major depressive illness. *Acta Psychiatrica Scandinavica*, 72: 233-238.

Linnoila M, Virkkunen M, Scheinin M, Nuutila A, Rimon R, Goodwin FK. 1983. Low cerebrospinal fluid 5-hydroxyindoleacetic acid concentration differentiates impulsive from nonimpulsive violent behavior. *Life Sciences*, 33(26): 2609-2614.

Little KY, Clark TB, Ranc J, Duncan GE. 1993. Beta-adrenergic receptor binding in frontal cortex from suicide victims. *Biological Psychiatry*, 34(9): 596-605.

Lloyd KG, Farley IJ, Deck JH, Hornykiewicz O. 1974. Serotonin and 5-hydroxyindoleacetic acid in discrete areas of the brainstem of suicide victims and control patients. *Advances in Biochemical Psychopharmacology*, 11(0): 387-397.

Lopez-Ibor JJ Jr, Lana F, Saiz-Ruiz J. 1990. Impulsive suicidal behavior and serotonin. *Actas Luso Españolas De Neurologia Psiquiatria y Ciencias Afines*, 18(5): 316-325.

Lopez-Ibor JJ Jr, Saiz-Ruiz J, Iglesias LM. 1988. The fenfluramine challenge test in the affective spectrum: A possible marker of endogeneity and severity. *Pharmacopsychiatry*, 21(1): 9-14.

Lopez-Ibor JJ Jr, Saiz-Ruiz J, Perez de los Cobos JC. 1985. Biological correlations of suicide and aggressivity in major depressions (with melancholia): 5-hydroxyindoleacetic acid and cortisol in cerebral spinal fluid, dexamethasone suppression test and therapeutic response to 5-hydroxytryptophan. *Neuropsychobiology*, 14(2): 67-74.

Lopez JF, Chalmers DT, Little KY, Watson SJ. 1998. A.E. Bennett Research Award. Regulation of serotonin1A, glucocorticoid, and mineralocorticoid receptor in rat and human hippocampus: Implications for the neurobiology of depression. *Biological Psychiatry*, 43(8): 547-573.

Lopez JF, Vazquez DM, Chalmers DT, Watson SJ. 1997. Regulation of 5-HT receptors and the hypothalamic-pituitary-adrenal axis: Implications for the neurobiology of suicide. *Annals of the New York Academy of Sciences*, 836: 106-134.

Lowther S, De Paermentier F, Crompton MR, Katona CL, Horton RW. 1994. Brain 5-HT2 receptors in suicide victims: Violence of death, depression and effects of antidepressant treatment. *Brain Research*, 642(1-2): 281-289.

Lowther S, Katona CL, Crompton MR, Horton RW. 1997. 5-HT1D and 5-HT1E/1F binding sites in depressed suicides: Increased 5- HT1D binding in globus pallidus but not cortex. *Molecular Psychiatry*, 2(4): 314-321.

Malone KM, Corbitt EM, Li S, Mann JJ. 1996. Prolactin response to fenfluramine and suicide attempt lethality in major depression. *British Journal of Psychiatry*, 168(3): 324-329.

Malone KM, Haas GL, Sweeney JA, Mann JJ. 1995. Major depression and the risk of attempted suicide. *Journal of Affective Disorders*, 34: 173-185.

Manchon M, Kopp N, Rouzioux JJ, Lecestre D, Deluermoz S, Miachon S. 1987. Benzodiazepine receptor and neurotransmitter studies in the brain of suicides. *Life Sciences*, 41(24): 2623-2630.

Mann JJ, Arango V, Marzuk PM, Theccanat S, Reis DJ. 1989. Evidence for the 5-HT hypothesis of suicide. A review of post-mortem studies. *British Journal of Psychiatry. Supplement*, (8): 7-14.

Mann JJ, Henteleff RA, Lagattuta TF, Perper JA, Li S, Arango V. 1996a. Lower 3H-paroxetine binding in cerebral cortex of suicide victims is partly due to fewer high affinity, nontransporter sites. *Journal of Neural Transmission*, 103(11): 1337-1350.

Mann JJ, Huang YY, Underwood MD, Kassir SA, Oppenheim S, Kelly TM, Dwork AJ, Arango V. 2000. A serotonin transporter gene promoter polymorphism (5-HTTLPR) and prefrontal cortical binding in major depression and suicide. *Archives of General Psychiatry*, 57(8): 729-738.

Mann JJ, Malone KM. 1997. Cerebrospinal fluid amines and higher-lethality suicide attempts in depressed inpatients. *Biological Psychiatry*, 41(2): 162-171.

Mann JJ, Malone KM, Nielsen DA, Goldman D, Erdos J, Gelernter J. 1997. Possible association of a polymorphism of the tryptophan hydroxylase gene with suicidal behavior in depressed patients. *American Journal of Psychiatry*, 154(10): 1451-1453.

Mann JJ, Malone KM, Psych MR, Sweeney JA, Brown RP, Linnoila M, Stanley B, Stanley M. 1996b. Attempted suicide characteristics and cerebrospinal fluid amine metabolites in depressed inpatients. *Neuropsychopharmacology*, 15(6): 576-586.

Mann JJ, McBride PA, Brown RP, Linnoila M, Leon AC, DeMeo M, Mieczkowski T, Myers JE, Stanley M. 1992. Relationship between central and peripheral serotonin indexes in depressed and suicidal psychiatric inpatients. *Archives of General Psychiatry*, 49(6): 442-446.

Mann JJ, McBride PA, Malone KM, DeMeo M, Keilp J. 1995. Blunted serotonergic responsivity in depressed inpatients. *Neuropsychopharmacology*, 13(1): 53-64.

Mann JJ, Stanley M, McBride PA, McEwen BS. 1986. Increased serotonin2 and beta-adrenergic receptor binding in the frontal cortices of suicide victims. *Archives of General Psychiatry*, 43(10): 954-959.

Mann JJ, Underwood MD, Arango V. 1996c. Postmortem studies of suicide victims. In: Watson SJ, Editor. *Biology of Schizophrenia and Affective Disease.* (pp. 197-221). Washington, DC: American Psychiatric Press.

Mann JJ, Waternaux C, Haas GL, Malone KM. 1999. Toward a clinical model of suicidal behavior in psychiatric patients. *American Journal of Psychiatry*, 156(2): 181-189.

Manuck SB, Flory JD, Ferrell RE, Dent KM, Mann JJ, Muldoon MF. 1999. Aggression and anger-related traits associated with a polymorphism of the tryptophan hydroxylase gene. *Biological Psychiatry*, 45(5): 603-614.

Manuck SB, Flory JD, Ferrell RE, Mann JJ, Muldoon MF. 2000. A regulatory polymorphism of the monoamine oxidase-A gene may be associated with variability in aggression, impulsivity, and central nervous system serotonergic responsivity. *Psychiatry Research*, 95(1): 9-23.

Matheson GK, Knowles A, Gage D, Michel C, Guthrie D, Bauer C, Blackbourne J, Weinzapfel D. 1997a. Modification of hypothalamic-pituitary-adrenocortical activity by serotonergic agents in the rat. *Pharmacology*, 55(2): 59-65.

Matheson GK, Knowles A, Guthrie D, Gage D, Weinzapfel D, Blackbourne J. 1997b. Actions of serotonergic agents on hypothalamic-pituitary-adrenal axis activity in the rat. *General Pharmacology*, 29(5): 823-828.

Matsubara S, Arora RC, Meltzer HY. 1991. Serotonergic measures in suicide brain: 5-HT1A binding sites in frontal cortex of suicide victims. *Journal of Neural Transmission. General Section*, 85(3): 181-194.

McGuffin P, Katz R. 1989. The genetics of depression and manic-depressive disorder. *British Journal of Psychiatry*, 155: 294-304.

McGuffin P, Katz R, Rutherford J. 1991. Nature, nurture and depression: A twin study. *Psychological Med*, 21(2): 329-335.

Meana JJ, Garcia-Sevilla JA. 1987. Increased alpha 2-adrenoceptor density in the frontal cortex of depressed suicide victims. *Journal of Neural Transmission*, 70(3-4): 377-381.

Meltzer HY, Umberkoman-Wiita B, Robertson A, Tricou BJ, Lowy M, Perline R. 1984. Effect of 5-hydroxytryptophan on serum cortisol levels in major affective disorders. I. Enhanced response in depression and mania. *Archives of General Psychiatry*, 41(4): 366-374.

Mitterauer B. 1990. A contribution to the discussion of the role of the genetic factor in suicide, based on five studies in an epidemiologically defined area (Province of Salzburg, Austria). *Comprehensive Psychiatry*, 31(6): 557-565.

Murphy GE, Wetzel RD. 1990. The lifetime risk of suicide in alcoholism. *Archives of General Psychiatry*, 47(4): 383-392.

Nemeroff CB, Owens MJ, Bissette G, Andorn AC, Stanley M. 1988. Reduced corticotropin releasing factor binding sites in the frontal cortex of suicide victims. *Archives of General Psychiatry*, 45(6): 577-579.

New AS, Gelernter J, Yovell Y, Trestman RL, Nielsen DA, Silverman J, Mitropoulou V, Siever LJ. 1998. Tryptophan hydroxylase genotype is associated with impulsive-aggression measures: A preliminary study. *American Journal of Medical Genetics*, 81(1): 13-17.

Newman ME, Shapira B, Lerer B. 1998. Evaluation of central serotonergic function in affective and related disorders by the fenfluramine challenge test: A critical review. *International Journal of Neuropsychopharmcology*, 1(1): 49-69.

Nielsen DA, Goldman D, Virkkunen M, Tokola R, Rawlings R, Linnoila M. 1994. Suicidality and 5-hydroxyindoleacetic acid concentration associated with a tryptophan hydroxylase polymorphism. *Archives of General Psychiatry*, 51(1): 34-38.

Nielsen DA, Virkkunen M, Lappalainen J, Eggert M, Brown GL, Long JC, Goldman D, Linnoila M. 1998. A tryptophan hydroxylase gene marker for suicidality and alcoholism. *Archives of General Psychiatry*, 55(7): 593-602.

Nordin C. 1988. Relationships between clinical symptoms and monoamine metabolite concentrations in biochemically defined subgroups of depressed patients. *Acta Psychiatrica Scandinavica*, 78(6): 720-729.

Nordström P, Samuelsson M, Asberg M, Träskman-Bendz L, Aberg-Wistedt A, Nordin C, Bertilsson L. 1994. CSF 5-HIAA predicts suicide risk after attempted suicide. *Suicide and Life-Threatening Behavior*, 24(1): 1-9.

Norman WH, Brown WA, Miller IW, Keitner GI, Overholser JC. 1990. The dexamethasone suppression test and completed suicide. *Acta Psychiatrica Scandinavica*, 81(2): 120-125.

Nowak G, Ordway GA, Paul IA. 1995. Alterations in the N-methyl-D-aspartate (NMDA) receptor complex in the frontal cortex of suicide victims. *Brain Research*, 675(1-2): 157-164.

O'Keane V, Moloney E, O'Neill H, O'Connor A, Smith C, Dinan TG. 1992. Blunted prolactin responses to d-fenfluramine in sociopathy. Evidence for subsensitivity of central serotonergic function. *British Journal of Psychiatry*, 160: 643-646.

Ohmori T, Arora RC, Meltzer HY. 1992. Serotonergic measures in suicide brain: The concentration of 5-HIAA, HVA, and tryptophan in frontal cortex of suicide victims. *Biological Psychiatry*, 32(1): 57-71.

Ono H, Shirakawa O, Nishiguchi N, Nishimura A, Nushida H, Ueno Y, Maeda K. 2000. Tryptophan hydroxylase gene polymorphisms are not associated with suicide. *American Journal of Medical Genetics*, 96(6): 861-863.

Ordway GA, Smith KS, Haycock JW. 1994a. Elevated tyrosine hydroxylase in the locus coeruleus of suicide victims. *Journal of Neurochemistry*, 62(2): 680-685.

Ordway GA, Widdowson PS, Smith KS, Halaris A. 1994b. Agonist binding to alpha 2-adrenoceptors is elevated in the locus coeruleus from victims of suicide. *Journal of Neurochemistry*, 63(2): 617-624.

Owen F, Chambers DR, Cooper SJ, Crow TJ, Johnson JA, Lofthouse R, Poulter M. 1986. Serotonergic mechanisms in brains of suicide victims. *Brain Research*, 362(1): 185-188.

Owen F, Cross AJ, Crow TJ, Deakin JF, Ferrier IN, Lofthouse R, Poulter M. 1983. Brain 5-HT-2 receptors and suicide. *Lancet*, 2(8361): 1256.

Owens MJ, Edwards E, Nemeroff CB. 1990. Effects of 5-HT1A receptor agonists on hypothalamo-pituitary-adrenal axis activity and corticotropin-releasing factor containing neurons in the rat brain. *European Journal of Pharmacology*, 190(1-2): 113-122.

Pacheco MA, Stockmeier C, Meltzer HY, Overholser JC, Dilley GE, Jope RS. 1996. Alterations in phosphoinositide signaling and G-protein levels in depressed suicide brain. *Brain Research*, 723(1-2): 37-45.

Paik I, Toh K, Kim J, Lee C. 2000. TPH gene may be associated with suicidal behavior, but not with schizophrenia in the Korean population. *Human Heredity*, 50(6): 365-369.

Palaniappan V, Ramachandran V, Somasundaram O. 1983. Suicidal ideation and biogenic amines in depression. *Indian Journal of Psychiatry*, 25(4): 286-292.

Palmer AM, Burns MA, Arango V, Mann JJ. 1994. Similar effects of glycine, zinc and an oxidizing agent on [3H] dizocilpine binding to the N-methyl-D-aspartate receptor in neocortical tissue from suicide victims and controls. *Journal of Neural Transmission. General Section*, 96(1): 1-8.

Pandey GN. 2001. Neurobiology of teenage and adult suicide: Possible biological markers for identification of suicidal patients. Workshop presentation at the Institute of Medicine's Workshop on Risk Factors for Suicide, March 14, 2001. Summary available in: Institute of Medicine. *Risk Factors for Suicide: Summary of a Workshop.* (pp. 10-11). Washington, DC: National Academy Press.

Pandey GN, Dwivedi Y, Pandey SC, Conley RR, Roberts RC, Tamminga CA. 1997. Protein kinase C in the postmortem brain of teenage suicide victims. *Neuroscience Letters*, 228(2): 111-114.

Pandey GN, Dwivedi Y, Pandey SC, Teas SS, Conley RR, Roberts RC, Tamminga CA. 1999. Low phosphoinositide-specific phospholipase C activity and expression of phospholipase C beta1 protein in the prefrontal cortex of teenage suicide subjects. *American Journal of Psychiatry*, 156(12): 1895-1901.

Pandey GN, Dwivedi Y, Rizavi HS, Ren X, Pandey SC, Pesold C, Roberts RC, Conley RR, Tamminga CA. 2002. Higher expression of serotonin 5-HT(2A) receptors in the postmortem brains of teenage suicide victims. *American Journal of Psychiatry*, 159(3): 419-429.

Papadimitriou GN, Linkowski P, Delarbre C, Mendlewicz J. 1991. Suicide on the paternal and maternal sides of depressed patients with a lifetime history of attempted suicide. *Acta Psychiatrica Scandinavica*, 83(6): 417-419.

Paré CM, Yeung DP, Price K, Stacey RS. 1969. 5-hydroxytryptamine, noradrenaline, and dopamine in brainstem, hypothalamus, and caudate nucleus of controls and of patients committing suicide by coal-gas poisoning. *Lancet*, 2(7612): 133-135.

Peabody CA, Faull KF, King RJ, Whiteford HA, Barchas JD, Berger PA. 1987. CSF amine metabolites and depression. *Psychiatry Research*, 21(1): 1-7.

Pfeffer CR, Normandin L, Kakuma T. 1994. Suicidal children grow up: Suicidal behavior and psychiatric disorders among relatives. *Journal of the American Academy of Child and Adolescent Psychiatry*, 33(8): 1087-1097.

Pfeffer CR, Stokes P, Shindledecker R. 1991. Suicidal behavior and hypothalamic-pituitary-adrenocortical axis indices in child psychiatric inpatients. *Biological Psychiatry*, 29(9): 909-917.

Phillips DP. 1974. The influence of suggestion on suicide: Substantive and theoretical implications of the Werther effect. *American Sociological Review*, 39(3): 340-354.

Phillips DP, Carstensen LL. 1986. Clustering of teenage suicides after television news stories about suicide. *New England Journal of Medicine*, 315(11): 685-689.

Pickar D, Roy A, Breier A, Doran A, Wolkowitz O, Colison J, Ågren H. 1986. Suicide and aggression in schizophrenia. Neurobiologic correlates. *Annals of the New York Academy of Sciences*, 487: 189-196.

Pine DS, Coplan JD, Wasserman GA, Miller LS, Fried JE, Davies M, Cooper TB, Greenhill L, Shaffer D, Parsons B. 1997. Neuroendocrine response to fenfluramine challenge in boys. Associations with aggressive behavior and adverse rearing. *Archives of General Psychiatry*, 54(9): 839-846.

Plotsky PM, Owens MJ, Nemeroff CB. 1998. Psychoneuroendocrinology of depression. Hypothalamic-pituitary-adrenal axis. *Psychiatric Clinics of North America*, 21(2): 293-307.

Pokorny AD. 1983. Prediction of suicide in psychiatric patients. Report of a prospective study. *Archives of General Psychiatry*, 40(3): 249-257.

Renaud J, Brent DA, Birmaher B, Chiappetta L, Bridge J. 1999. Suicide in adolescents with disruptive disorders. *Journal of the American Academy of Child and Adolescent Psychiatry*, 38(7): 846-851.

Rich CL, Young D, Fowler RC. 1986. San Diego suicide study. I. Young vs old subjects. *Archives of General Psychiatry*, 43(6): 577-582.

Roberts J, Hawton K. 1980. Child abuse and attempted suicide. *British Journal of Psychiatry*, 137: 319-323.

Rotondo A, Schuebel K, Bergen A, Aragon R, Virkkunen M, Linnoila M, Goldman D, Nielsen D. 1999. Identification of four variants in the tryptophan hydroxylase promoter and association to behavior. *Molecular Psychiatry*, 4(4): 360-368.

Roy A. 1983. Family history of suicide. *Archives of General Psychiatry*, 40(9): 971-974.

Roy A. 2000. Relation of family history of suicide to suicide attempts in alcoholics. *American Journal of Psychiatry*, 157(12): 2050-2051.

Roy A, Lamparski D, De Jong J, Adinoff B, Ravitz B, George DT, Nutt D, Linnoila M. 1990. Cerebrospinal fluid monoamine metabolites in alcoholic patients who attempt suicide. *Acta Psychiatrica Scandinavica*, 81(1): 58-61.

Roy A, Ninan P, Mazonson A, Pickar D, Van Kammen D, Linnoila M, Paul SM. 1985. CSF monoamine metabolites in chronic schizophrenic patients who attempt suicide. *Psychological Medicine*, 15(2): 335-340.

Roy A, Pickar D, De Jong J, Karoum F, Linnoila M. 1989. Suicidal behavior in depression: Relationship to noradrenergic function. *Biological Psychiatry*, 25(3): 341-350.

Roy A, Rylander G, Forslund K, Asberg M, Mazzanti CM, Goldman D, Nielsen DA. 2001. Excess tryptophan hydroxylase 17 779C allele in surviving cotwins of monozygotic twin suicide victims. *Neuropsychobiology*, 43(4): 233-236.

Roy A, Segal NL, Centerwall BS, Robinette CD. 1991. Suicide in twins. *Archives of General Psychiatry*, 48(1): 29-32.

Roy A, Segal NL, Sarchiapone M. 1995. Attempted suicide among living co-twins of twin suicide victims. *American Journal of Psychiatry*, 152(7): 1075-1076.

Roy-Byrne P, Post RM, Rubinow DR, Linnoila M, Savard R, Davis D. 1983. CSF 5HIAA and personal and family history of suicide in affectively ill patients: A negative study. *Psychiatry Research*, 10(4): 263-274.

Sapolsky RM, Krey LC, McEwen BS. 1984. Stress down-regulates corticosterone receptors in a site-specific manner in the brain. *Endocrinology*, 114(1): 287-292.

Schmidtke A, Hafner H. 1988. The Werther effect after television films: New evidence for an old hypothesis. *Psychological Medicine*, 18(3): 665-676.

Schulsinger F, Kety SS, Rosenthal D, Wender PH. 1979. A family study of suicide. In: Schou M, Strömgren E, Editors. *Origin, Prevention and Treatment of Affective Disorders*. (pp. 277-287). London: Academic Press.

Secunda SK, Cross CK, Koslow S, Katz MM, Kocsis J, Maas JW, Landis H. 1986. Biochemistry and suicidal behavior in depressed patients. *Biological Psychiatry*, 21(8-9): 756-767.

Shaw DM, Camps FE, Eccleston EG. 1967. 5-Hydroxytryptamine in the hind-brain of depressive suicides. *British Journal of Psychiatry*, 113(505): 1407-1411.

Silberg JL, Pickles A, Rutter M, Hewitt J, Simonoff E, Maes H, Carbonneau R, Murrelle L, Foley D, Eaves L. 1999. The influence of genetic factors and life stress on depression among adolescent girls. *Archives of General Psychiatry*, 56(3): 225-232.

Stanley M. 1984. Cholinergic receptor binding in the frontal cortex of suicide victims. *American Journal of Psychiatry*, 141(11): 1432-1436.

Stanley M, Mann JJ. 1983. Increased serotonin-2 binding sites in frontal cortex of suicide victims. *Lancet*, 1(8318): 214-216.

Stanley M, Virgilio J, Gershon S. 1982. Tritiated imipramine binding sites are decreased in the frontal cortex of suicides. *Science*, 216(4552): 1337-1339.

Statham DJ, Heath AC, Madden PA, Bucholz KK, Bierut L, Dinwiddie SH, Slutske WS, Dunne MP, Martin NG. 1998. Suicidal behaviour: An epidemiological and genetic study. *Psychological Medicine*, 28(4): 839-855.

Stockmeier CA, Dilley GE, Shapiro LA, Overholser JC, Thompson PA, Meltzer HY. 1997. Serotonin receptors in suicide victims with major depression. *Neuropsychopharmacology*, 16(2): 162-173.

Stockmeier CA, Meltzer HY. 1991. Beta-adrenergic receptor binding in frontal cortex of suicide victims. *Biological Psychiatry*, 29(2): 183-191.

Styron W. 1990. *Darkness Visible: A Memoir of Madness*. New York: Random House.

Szigethy E, Conwell Y, Forbes NT, Cox C, Caine ED. 1994. Adrenal weight and morphology in victims of completed suicide. *Biological Psychiatry*, 36(6): 374-380.

Targum SD, Rosen L, Capodanno AE. 1983. The dexamethasone suppression test in suicidal patients with unipolar depression. *American Journal of Psychiatry*, 140(7): 877-879.

Taylor EA, Stansfeld SA. 1984. Children who poison themselves. I. A clinical comparison with psychiatric controls. *British Journal of Psychiatry*, 145: 127-132.

Träskman-Bendz L, Ekman R, Regnell G, Ohman R. 1992. HPA-related CSF neuropeptides in suicide attempters. *European Neuropsychopharmacology*, 2(2): 99-106.

Träskman L, Åsberg M, Bertilsson L, Sjostrand L. 1981. Monoamine metabolites in CSF and suicidal behavior. *Archives of General Psychiatry*, 38(6): 631-636.

Tsai SJ, Hong CJ, Wang YC. 1999. Tryptophan hydroxylase gene polymorphism (A218C) and suicidal behaviors. *Neuroreport*, 10(18): 3773-3775.

Tsuang MT. 1983. Risk of suicide in the relatives of schizophrenics, manics, depressives, and controls. *Journal of Clinical Psychiatry*, 44(11): 396-400.

Turecki G, Briere R, Dewar K, Antonetti T, Lesage AD, Seguin M, Chawky N, Vanier C, Alda M, Joober R, Benkelfat C, Rouleau GA. 1999. Prediction of level of serotonin 2A receptor binding by serotonin receptor 2A genetic variation in postmortem brain samples from subjects who did or did not commit suicide. *American Journal of Psychiatry*, 156(9): 1456-1458.

Turecki G, Zhu Z, Tzenova J, Lesage A, Seguin M, Tousignant M, Chawky N, Vanier C, Lipp O, Alda M, Joober R, Benkelfat C, Rouleau GA. 2001. TPH and suicidal behavior: A study in suicide completers. *Molecular Psychiatry*, 6(1): 98-102.

van der Kolk BA. 1996. The body keeps score: Approaches to the psychobiology of post-traumatic stress disorder. In: van der Kolk BA, McFarlane AC, Weisaeth L, Editors. *Traumatic Stress: The Effects of Overwhelming Experience on Mind, Body, and Society*. (pp. 214-241). New York: Guilford Press.

van Praag HM. 1986. Indoleamines in depression and suicide. *Progress in Brain Research*, 65: 59-71.

van Praag HM. 1996. Faulty cortisol/serotonin interplay. Psychopathological and biological characterisation of a new, hypothetical depression subtype (SeCA depression). *Psychiatry Research*, 65(3): 143-157.

van Praag HM. 2001. Anxiety/aggression–driven depression. A paradigm of functionalization and verticalization of psychiatric diagnosis. *Progress in Neuropsychopharmacology and Biological Psychiatry*, 25(4): 893-924.

Vestergaard P, Sorensen T, Hoppe E, Rafaelsen OJ, Yates CM, Nicolaou N. 1978. Biogenic amine metabolites in cerebrospinal fluid of patients with affective disorders. *Acta Psychiatrica Scandinavica*, 58(1): 88-96.

Virkkunen M, De Jong J, Bartko J, Goodwin FK, Linnoila M. 1989a. Relationship of psychobiological variables to recidivism in violent offenders and impulsive fire setters. A follow-up study. *Archives of General Psychiatry*, 46(7): 600-603.

Virkkunen M, De Jong J, Bartko J, Linnoila M. 1989b. Psychobiological concomitants of history of suicide attempts among violent offenders and impulsive fire setters. *Archives of General Psychiatry*, 46(7): 604-606.

Virkkunen M, Nuutila A, Goodwin FK, Linnoila M. 1987. Cerebrospinal fluid monoamine metabolite levels in male arsonists. *Archives of General Psychiatry*, 44(3): 241-247.

Wender PH, Kety SS, Rosenthal D, Schulsinger F, Ortmann J, Lunde I. 1986. Psychiatric disorders in the biological and adoptive families of adopted individuals with affective disorders. *Archives of General Psychiatry*, 43(10): 923-929.

Westenberg HG, Verhoeven WM. 1988. CSF monoamine metabolites in patients and controls: support for a bimodal distribution in major affective disorders. *Acta Psychiatrica Scandinavica*, 78(5): 541-549.

Westrin A, Ekman R, Träskman-Bendz L. 1999. Alterations of corticotropin releasing hormone (CRH) and neuropeptide Y (NPY) plasma levels in mood disorder patients with a recent suicide attempt. *European Neuropsychopharmacology*, 9(3): 205-211.

Winkelmann BR, Hager J. 2000. Genetic variation in coronary heart disease and myocardial infarction: Methodological overview and clinical evidence. *Pharmacogenomics*, 1(1): 73-94.

Yates M, Leake A, Candy JM, Fairbairn AF, McKeith IG, Ferrier IN. 1990. 5HT2 receptor changes in major depression. *Biological Psychiatry*, 27(5): 489-496.

Yehuda R, Giller EL, Southwick SM, Lowy MT, Mason JW. 1991. Hypothalamic-pituitary-adrenal dysfunction in posttraumatic stress disorder. *Biological Psychiatry*, 30(10): 1031-1048.

Yehuda R, Southwick SM, Ostroff RB, Mason JW, Giller E Jr. 1988. Neuroendocrine aspects of suicidal behavior. *Endocrinology and Metabolism Clinics of North America*, 17(1): 83-102.

Zalsman G, Frisch A, Bromberg M, Gelernter J, Michaelovsky E, Campino A, Erlich Z, Tyano S, Apter A, Weizman A. 2001. Family-based association study of serotonin transporter promoter in suicidal adolescents: No association with suicidality but possible role in violence traits. *American Journal of Medical Genetics*, 105(3): 239-245.

Zhang HY, Ishigaki T, Tani K, Chen K, Shih JC, Miyasato K, Ohara K, Ohara K. 1997. Serotonin2A receptor gene polymorphism in mood disorders. *Biological Psychiatry*, 41(7): 768-773.

In a Time

In a time of secret wooing
Today prepares tomorrow's ruin
Left knows not what right is doing
My heart is torn asunder.

In a time of furtive sighs
Sweet hellos and sad goodbyes
Half-truths told and entire lies
My conscience echoes thunder

In a time when kingdoms come
Joy is brief as summer's fun
Happiness, its race has run
Then pain stalks in to plunder.

—MAYA ANGELOU

5

Childhood Trauma

With the long maturation process in humans comes a prolonged period of vulnerability to developmental trauma. Events occurring during development can have profound and lasting impact on functioning and the brain. For the unwanted outcome of suicide, there appear to be at least two pathways through which developmental events can change risk. First, a large body of research describes the impact of developmental events, including childhood trauma, on the occurrence and severity of the mental and substance abuse disorders that increase suicide risk. Secondly, childhood trauma has emerged as a strong and independent risk factor for suicidal behavior in adolescents and adults (Browne and Finkelhor, 1986; Paolucci et al., 2001; Santa Mina and Gallop, 1998). Therefore, understanding childhood trauma and its psychobiological effects has the potential to illuminate the pathway of causation from early trauma to later suicide. With this understanding comes a lengthy, often years-long, opportunity for targeted intervention, both to prevent childhood trauma from taking place and to minimize its impact if it has occurred. Currently, delivery of appropriate intervention and prevention is hampered by numerous obstacles. These include problems in the responsible educational, legal and medical systems, the stigma of mental illness, and limited knowledge among the public about the importance of early emotional development. For additional discussion, see the Surgeon General's Conference Report on Children's Mental Health (PHS, 2000).

This chapter describes major advances in understanding the relationships between childhood trauma and suicidality. The chapter focuses on recent population-based studies that redress long-standing methodological limitations that have hitherto cast doubt on the veracity of early trauma as a causative factor in suicidality (for review, see Wagner, 1997). It also describes the biological, cognitive, behavioral, and emotional responses to trauma that may lead to psychopathology and later suicidality. These responses occur against the backdrop of development, which is marked by dramatic changes and emergent functions. Trauma during childhood can disrupt psychological and biological development, as manifested by developmental delays or enduring changes in the anatomy and physiology of the brain (Cicchetti and Toth, 1995; De Bellis, 2001; Glaser, 2000; Heim and Nemeroff, 2001). The impact of trauma on the brain's stress response systems can make children more vulnerable to later stressful events and to the onset of psychopathology. Childhood trauma can also cause earlier onset of psychopathology and suicidality and lead to a cascade of other life events, each of which increase the risk for suicidality.

The relatively new field of developmental traumatology attempts to integrate knowledge from disparate fields of developmental psychopathology, developmental neuroscience, and stress and trauma research (De Bellis, 2001). Developmental traumatology benefits from a solid base of biological, behavioral, and psychological research on the effects of trauma. The integration of many disciplines, involving both human and animal evidence, holds enormous potential for tracing the developmental pathways culminating in mental illness or suicidal behavior.

This chapter begins with the range of childhood traumas and their prevalence. It then presents the evidence for childhood trauma as a risk factor for later suicidality. Childhood sexual abuse emerges as such a strong risk factor that the next section covers its quantitative contribution to the extent of suicide nationwide. From there, the chapter deals with the more immediate effects of childhood trauma on children's biological, psychological, and social functioning. It then covers the relationship between trauma and psychopathology. Finally, the chapter covers possible pathways from childhood trauma to suicidality and how they can be interrupted through prevention and treatment.

SCOPE AND DEFINITIONS

This chapter covers many types of childhood traumas. The list in Table 5-1 includes the more extreme forms of trauma that have traditionally been grouped together under the term "maltreatment": physical abuse, sexual abuse,[1] neglect, and psychological maltreatment (NRC,

---

[1]Unless specified further, child sexual abuse refers to a range of behaviors from genital touching and fondling to penetration.

TABLE 5-1 Types of Childhood Trauma

Physical abuse by adults or peers
Sexual abuse by adults or peers
Neglect
Psychological maltreatment
Witnessing violence, especially against the mother
Family members with substance use, mental disorders, suicidality
Family members who have been incarcerated
Loss or separation from parents[a]
Childhood socio-economic disadvantage[a]

[a]Not covered by Felitti et al., 1998, but found significant other studies of suicide attempts or completion (Cheng et al., 2000; Fergusson et al., 2000b).

1993). The list also includes other types of trauma, such as witnessing family violence, parental loss, or other serious family adversities. In keeping with the epidemiological literature, childhood traumas do not include "stressful life events," which are generally defined as the breakdown of a close relationship, interpersonal conflict with parents or friends, school- or work-related difficulties, and legal or disciplinary crises.

Sexual and physical abuse have the strongest relationship to suicidality, but there are several reasons for this chapter's broad focus on many types of childhood trauma. (1) They are similar in violating the child's home environment as a safe haven and in compromising parents' roles as physical and emotional care takers (Margolin and Gordis, 2000). (2) Children are often exposed to more than one type of trauma (Felitti et al., 1998; McGee et al., 1995). For example, one-third to one-half of neglected children witness domestic violence (De Bellis, 2001), and child neglect frequently occurs in association with maternal depression (Glaser, 2000). Furthermore, about one-third of abused adults report *both* physical and sexual abuse as children (McCauley et al., 1997). (3) Despite the range of trauma types, there are finite ways for biological stress systems to respond, and finite categories of mental disorders associated with trauma (anxiety, mood, and personality disorders, see later section) (De Bellis, 2001). (4) Recent epidemiological research indicates that the adverse, long-term health impact of trauma may be cumulative, irrespective of trauma category. The greater the number of past traumas, the greater the health problems (Felitti et al., 1998; see later section).

160

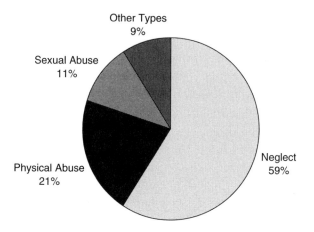

FIGURE 5-1 Types of Child Maltreatment. Source: US DHHS, 2001a.

Prevalence of Childhood Trauma

National surveillance of child maltreatment is conducted annually through the National Child Abuse and Neglect Data System (NCANDS).[2] In 1999, an estimated 826,000 children in the U.S. were maltreated (US DHHS, 2001a). The majority of victims (58.4 percent) suffered neglect, 21 percent suffered physical abuse, and 11 percent suffered sexual abuse (Figure 5-1). The remainder were victimized by other types of maltreatment including medical neglect, abandonment, threats of harm, and congenital drug addiction. The overall child victimization rate for 1999 was 11.8 per 1,000, with only small gender differences.[3] Trends can be established by comparing this figure to annual figures dating back to 1990, when national surveillance began. The rate in 1990—at 13.4 per 1000—climbed by 1993 to a peak of 15.3 per 1000, and then gradually declined to 1999 (Figure 5-2). These rates are based on official records of children who come to the attention of child protective services.

Rates of physical and sexual abuse are much higher when measured in surveys of parents or victims. Surveys of parents find self-reported rates of child physical abuse that are 5–11 times higher than rates from official records (reviewed in Margolin and Gordis, 2000). In terms of cumulative prevalence, two recent community-based surveys of large

[2]The national data collection and analysis is a consequence of the Child Abuse Prevention and Treatment Act of 1988.
[3]The rate was 12.2 per 1000 female and 10.8 per 1000 male children (US DHHS, 2001a).

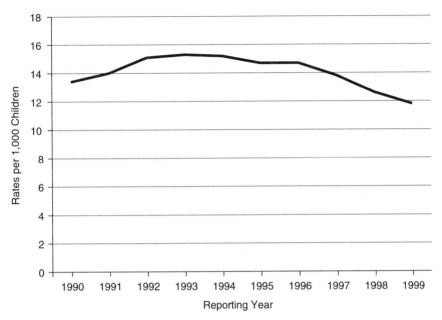

FIGURE 5-2 Victimization Rates, 1990–1999. Source: US DHHS, 2001a.

samples of adult primary care patients found 22–32 percent of them to report *ever* experiencing physical or sexual abuse during childhood or adolescence (Felitti et al., 1998; McCauley et al., 1997). While neither study asked subjects about the identity of the perpetrator (e.g., parent, other adult, peer), another study of high school girls (grades 9–12) explicitly asked about victimization by dating partners. In this population-based survey, about 20 percent of girls reported having ever been physically and/or sexually abused by a dating partner (Silverman et al., 2001). Traumas arising within the household are also common: about 26 percent of adults reported having grown up in a household[4] with substance abuse, 19 percent with mental illness, 12.5 percent with violence against their mother, and 3.4 percent with a household member being incarcerated (Felitti et al., 1998).

According to official crime statistics,[5] about 30 per 1000 children (ages 12–17) report being victims of serious violent crimes of rape, robbery, and

---

[4]The household adversity could have affected a parent or other adult (Felitti et al., 1998).
[5]The National Crime Victimization Survey.

aggravated assault in 1996—a rate that is almost two times higher than the adult rate (Snyder and Sickmund, 1999). Victimization rates are highest for American Indians and roughly equivalent for Whites and African Americans. Most of these crimes are perpetrated by friends and acquaintances rather than by relatives (11 percent of the total). Bearing witness to community violence is very common in inner city neighborhoods, with estimates of one-third or more of children and adolescents being exposed (for review, see Margolin and Gordis, 2000).

Altogether, these disparate statistics on the prevalence of various forms of trauma indicate that, by adulthood, past traumatic exposure is widespread. In one large study, about 52 percent of adults report having ever been exposed to at least one type of childhood trauma covered in this chapter (Felitti et al., 1998).

Methodological Issues

The study of childhood trauma is beset by methodological limitations (NRC, 1993). These limitations have implications for efforts to understand the relationship between early childhood trauma and later suicidal behavior. The first area of limitation concerns estimates of the incidence and prevalence of childhood trauma. There are two general sources of information about the magnitude of the problem and the relationship of child trauma to other health outcomes: official records; and self-report by victims/survivors and/or their caregivers and parents. Official report statistics are compiled annually from mandated reporters, most commonly social service, education, law enforcement, and medical personnel as well as non-mandated categories of persons including neighbors, kin, and friends. Official statistics cover several types of reportable trauma: neglect, physical and sexual abuse, psychological maltreatment, medical neglect, and miscellaneous types of abuse. Official records are thought to underreport and underestimate the magnitude of child maltreatment because generally only the more severe and "substantiated"[6] cases are reported to local and state authorities, which in turn report their findings to the federal government. Some states include cases that are "indicated," or those cases about which there is a high level of suspicion but insufficient evidence for adjudication by child protection professionals.

The other source of information about the magnitude of child maltreatment—self-reports by victims/survivors—is essential because of underestimation by official records. In a large national sample of more than

---

[6]Substantiated cases are those determined by the child protection agency to be valid based on state law or on policy.

2000 adolescents, more than 80 percent of abuse victims did not report the abuse to *anyone* (Edgardh and Ormstad, 2000). All self-reporting is vulnerable to bias, with particular concern for reports elicited years after events. Some studies have suggested that recall of childhood abuse varies with psychological adjustment (e.g., Falsetti and Resnick, 2000), while others have not found an association (Fergusson et al., 2000a; Robins et al., 1985). Examining this issue in a population-based, longitudinal, prospective study with repeated measures of child abuse self-reports, Fergusson and colleagues (2000a) discovered about a 50 percent rate of forgetting and/or not reporting documented abuse during assessments. They found that lack of recall did not vary with psychiatric diagnosis or suicidality. Other available data on reporting bias of childhood abuse also consistently indicates that abuse is significantly *under-reported*, with, depending on measures used, 40–60 percent lack of recall for documented cases of maltreatment (Fergusson et al., 2000a; Widom and Shepard, 1996; Widom, 1997; Williams, 1994). The reasons are complex, including forgetting (usually if the victim was less than 5 years old), stigma and embarrassment, relationship to the perpetrator, nature of the abusive or traumatic incident, and sensitivity of the survey or interview measures (see for example Kessler, 2000; Williams, 1994).

Another concern about self-reports, particularly with sexual abuse, regards repression of memories as a means of self-protection, with later recovery in adulthood. Repression could lead to either false positive or false negative reporting, but the evidence for repression appears to be controversial (Berliner and Williams, 1994; Loftus et al., 1998). There are no data to indicate what percentage of "recovered memories" are inaccurate, but data indicate 47–95 percent of recovered memories of non-bizarre child abuse are confirmed, and only 1–3 percent of bizarre abuse memories are confirmed (Bowman, 1996a; Bowman, 1996b). A recent study demonstrated that 74 percent of both always recalled and recovered memories could be confirmed from a legal point of view (Dahlenberg, 1996). The aforementioned analysis of longitudinal data by Fergusson's team (Fergusson et al., 2000a) further suggests that forgetting and later recall of childhood abuse represents a common phenomenon not associated with psychopathology, though they could not distinguish between active repression and simple forgetting. These investigators caution that recall bias obscures true prevalence rates of child maltreatment, though it does not, it appears, significantly alter estimates of relative risk of child abuse for subsequent psychological disorders.

A second limitation in the current research on childhood abuse is the use of inconsistent and imprecise definitions of maltreatment (NRC, 1993). Definitions may vary among mandated reporters, both within and across agencies, localities, and states, thereby affecting official reporting statistics in unknown directions. Definitions also vary across research studies, making comparability problematic. Studies attempting to link child maltreatment and suicide, then, might misestimate the relationship based on the definition of child maltreatment employed.

The third limitation is instrumentation. Previous reports by the National Research Council have commented on the lack of reliability and validity testing of self-report instruments (NRC, 1993). However, recently published studies have begun to address this problem (e.g., Bremner et al., 2000; Straus et al., 1998).

A fourth limitation is that child maltreatment questions are often excluded from larger studies and epidemiological surveys of children, representing significant missed opportunities. The reasons for the exclusion is that identifying victims triggers responsibility to report potentially illegal activity and to provide them with care and treatment (NRC, 1993). Ethical dilemmas and mandated reporting laws have thus constrained research seeking to question children directly about maltreatment (Black and Ponirakis, 2000; King and Churchill, 2000; Knight et al., 2000; NRC, 1993). Most studies have therefore relied on convenience and clinical samples of adults that restrict the generalizability of the results, making recent nationally representative (e.g., Molnar et al., 2001a) and population-based child samples (e.g., Fergusson et al., 2000b) critical.

Finally, the bulk of research on child maltreatment's role in suicidality employs cross-sectional, retrospective designs generally incapable of establishing variables as causative (see Wagner, 1997) Researchers are therefore increasingly using pathway analyses and controlling for possible confounding variables (e.g., Brent et al., in press; Fergusson et al., 2000b; Yang and Clum, 2000). All of these methodological limitations must be kept in mind in attempts to link childhood trauma to health outcomes, including suicidality.

CHILDHOOD TRAUMA AS A RISK FACTOR FOR SUICIDALITY

Childhood trauma, especially child sexual abuse, has been identified as a strong risk factor for suicidality. A large body of national and international evidence supports the relationship, including many recent studies from the United States, Sweden, New Zealand, and Australia.

An earlier review of about 20 studies, published between 1988 and 1998, assessed the evidence for physical or sexual abuse in relation to suicide attempts (Santa Mina and Gallop, 1998). The review concluded that, despite methodological limitations, there was robust evidence linking childhood sexual and physical abuse and suicidal behavior. The odds ratios from these studies ranged from 1.3 to 25, indicating that adults with a past history of abuse were up to 25 times more likely than adults without a past history to attempt suicide.

Child sexual abuse, in particular, was examined in a meta-analysis of 37 studies published between 1981 and 1995 (Paolucci et al., 2001). The total number of subjects was more than 25,000. The unweighted and weighted effect sizes of child sexual abuse on suicide were 0.64 and 0.44,[7] confirming a substantial link between child sexual abuse and suicide (defined as suicidal ideation or a suicide attempt).

A spate of recent, well-designed studies, including prospective studies, add to this body of evidence (Table 5-2). Virtually all studies found a significant relationship, with odds ratios ranging from about 2 to 10. These odds ratios were derived from prevalences of about 21–34 percent of participants having a past history of abuse or neglect and making a suicide attempt versus about 4–9 percent of participants without a history of abuse or neglect making an attempt (Brown et al., 1999; Fergusson et al., 2000b; Molnar et al., 2001a). The only negative study in Table 5-2 was restricted to physical abuse in children ages 9–17 (Flisher et al., 1997). The difference may be explained by study subjects being younger and by suicide attempts being ascertained only for the previous 6 months. Most other studies record *any* past suicide attempt.

Beyond maltreatment, other childhood adversities have been studied in relation to suicide attempts, but the associations are generally not as strong. Significant associations from large, population-based studies have been found for parental psychopathology (especially depression) or substance use disorders, parental suicide, and family socioeconomic adversity (Fergusson et al., 2000b; Molnar et al., 2001a). Other family factors, while also significantly associated with suicide attempts, were not found by Fergusson and colleagues (2000b) to be independent predictors: parental history of alcoholism/alcohol problems; parental changes due to separation/divorce, death, remarriage and reconciliation; parental history of illicit drug use; and parental history of criminal offending. Nevertheless, these other types of family traumas have a cumulative effect on suicide attempts and independent associations with psychopathology, as explained in later sections.

It is important to point out that the studies in Table 5-2 measure suicide attempts as opposed to suicide completion. The psychological autopsy method used for studying suicide victims cannot readily ascertain physical or sexual abuse because family members and friends are generally reluctant to disclose, or lack knowledge of, the abuse. The sole

---

[7]Weighting based on study sample size.

TABLE 5-2 Child Trauma as a Risk Factor for Attempted Suicide: Recent Large, Controlled Studies

Citation	No. Subjects	Odds Ratio for Suicide Attempts	
Prospective, Population- or Community-based Studies			
Silverman et al., 1996	375	Physical abuse	8^a
		Sexual abuse	14.4^a
Brown et al., 1999	776	Sexual abuse	5.71^b
		Physical abuse	1.79^b
		Neglect	1.42^b
Fergusson et al., 2000a	1265	Sexual abuse	7.9
		Physical abuse	5.41
Cross-sectional, Population- or Community-based Studies			
Molnar et al., 2001a	5877 Ages 15-54	Rape and molestation	3-11
Silverman et al., 2001	2186 Girls	Intimate partner violence^d	8.6
Dinwiddie et al., 2000	5995 twins Adults	Sexual abuse	7.07-7.74
Edgardh and Ormstad, 2000	1943 Age 17	Sexual abuse	4.36-9.28
Flisher et al., 1997	665 Ages 9-17	Physical abuse	Not significant^e
Cross-sectional, Community-based Primary Care			
Felitti et al., 1998	9508 Adults	1-4 or more categories of adverse childhood exposures^d	1.8-12.2
McCauley et al., 1997	1931 Women	Physical or sexual abuse	3.7^c

^{a}Females only. Findings for physically abused males were non-significant, and males were not assessed for suicide attempts and sexual abuse because too few males were affected.

^{b}After controlling for other factors. Neglect and physical abuse were not significant, as confidence intervals included 1.0.

^{c}Crude prevalence ratio reported by study.

^{d}1999 only; Intimate partner violence= physical and/or sexual.

Adverse childhood exposures refers to psychological, physical, or sexual abuse; violence against mother; or living with household members who were substance abusers, mentally ill or suicidal, or ever imprisoned.

^{e}Suicide attempts in the past 6 months only.

suicide completer study to have included a measure of past abuse found very large odds ratios of 11.7–49.3 for suicide by adolescents (Brent et al., 1999). These odds ratios were derived from prevalences of 30–42 percent of suicides having an abuse history versus about 2.5 percent of matched controls without a history of abuse. Abuse history, obtained as part of a life events inventory, was collected from about half of subjects and all of controls (n=131). Thus, this study of suicide victims confirms studies of suicide attempters on the importance of abuse as a risk factor.

> Daniel, an 18-year-old college freshman, was the eldest of three children. Throughout his childhood, Daniel was physically beaten by his alcoholic father. . . . At the age of 13, Daniel chose to live with his divorcing mother while his two siblings stayed with the father. . . . The family was bitterly divided and his father refused to pay his mother any alimony. [He] earned . . . an academic scholarship at a local university. In the summer prior to his freshman year, Daniel's mother was diagnosed as having inoperable stomach cancer and she died one month prior to Daniel's starting college. . . . His Thanksgiving visit to his father's home was a disaster. Daniel returned to school a day early. On the night of his return, Daniel called his father and during an argument on the phone, shot himself in the head with a revolver he had apparently taken from his father's home. Daniel's last words to his father prior to the fatal gunshot were "I hate me and I hate you—it's time for the big payback, Dad. . . ." (Berman & Jobes, Adolescent Suicide: Assessment and Intervention, 1991: 40-41).

CHILDHOOD SEXUAL ABUSE AND POPULATION ATTRIBUTABLE RISK FOR SUICIDE

Child sexual abuse carries the highest risk of a suicide attempt compared with other types of childhood maltreatment (Table 5-2). For example, Brown and colleagues (1999) found that sexual abuse carried higher odds ratios for a suicide attempt than did physical abuse or neglect, after controlling for other contextual factors. Child sexual abuse also carried the highest odds ratio for suicide attempts in a prospective, population-based study in New Zealand (Fergusson et al., 2000b). Sexual abuse also carried an extremely high risk (OR=30.3) for *repeated* suicide attempts in adolescents (Brown et al., 1999).

Based on the strength of childhood sexual abuse as a risk factor, several population-based studies calculated the percentage of suicide attempts that are attributable to child sexual abuse, i.e., the population attributable risk (PAR). The PAR for child sexual abuse was 9–20 percent of suicide attempts (Brown et al., 1999; Fergusson et al., 1996; Molnar et al., 2001a). This means that, independent of psychopathology and other known risk factors, child sexual abuse accounts for 9–20 percent of suicide attempts in adults. The study by Molnar and colleagues (2001a), from the National Comorbidity Survey, is especially significant because it is nationally representative of the U.S. population. Their analysis of serious suicide attempts revealed a PAR from child sexual abuse of 9–12 percent, and a PAR from mental disorders of 70–80 percent. The latter figure means that 70–80 percent of suicide attempts are associated with mental disorders.

On the basis of their findings, Molnar and colleagues suggested that a substantial proportion of suicide risk is missed by sole reliance on the presence of psychopathology. This point is discussed again later in the chapter.

MODIFYING FACTORS

Gender

Until recently, gender effects were not found to modify child sexual abuse as a risk factor for suicide. A meta-analysis, covering studies from 1981–1995, did not find a gender effect in the impact of child sexual abuse on suicidality (Paolucci et al., 2001). Nevertheless, two more recent and large population-based studies (Edgardh and Ormstad, 2000; Molnar et al., 2001a) found that child sexual abuse placed males at greater risk for suicide attempts. These two studies were consistent in finding odds that were 4–11 times higher among males and 2–4 times higher among females. While another large, population-based study did not find a gender effect (Dinwiddie et al., 2000), the odds ratios for both males and females hovered around 7, a figure in the mid-range of the other population based studies. It also found the population prevalence of child sexual abuse to be somewhat lower than other studies.[8] Thus, the newer body of evidence suggests that once sexual abuse occurs, males appear to be at higher risk of suicide attempts, but findings are not uniform.

For other types of childhood trauma, gender effects have not been reported in large, population-based studies. In a clinical sample of alcoholic inpatients (n=802), physical abuse displayed a gender effect: suicide attempts were significantly associated with physical abuse in men, but not in women (Windle et al., 1995).

---

[8]In general, the prevalence of child sexual abuse is higher for females (12-17 percent) than for males (5-8 percent) (Gorey and Leslie, 1997; Molnar et al., 2001b).

Age of Onset

For child sexual abuse, there is no established relationship between age of onset of the abuse and suicidality. A meta-analysis of studies published between 1981 and 1995 did not find an effect (Paolucci et al., 2001). Two more recent studies produced mixed results. Davidson and colleagues (1996) studied 2918 adults as part of the Epidemiological Catchment Area Study. In their community-based sample, they found a striking effect in women when the abuse occurred before 16 years of age. These women were three to four times more likely to have attempted suicide compared with women who were 16 years or older. A study of 251 psychiatric outpatients found an effect for the age of onset of child sexual abuse (higher prevalences of suicide attempts from 0 to 12), but the effect disappeared when the investigators controlled for abusive experiences in adulthood (Kaplan et al., 1995).[9] The age of onset of suicide (rather than the abuse) is profoundly affected by childhood sexual abuse (see "pathways" section).

Investigating relationships between age of onset of the abuse and later suicide attempts is beset by methodological problems. The largest problem is differential recall: sexual abuse victims younger than age 7 are significantly less likely than victims older than age 7 to recall a previously documented sexual abuse (Williams, 1994). Other problems are differential methods of inquiry, victim self-perceptions, and regional differences (Carlin et al., 1994; Davidson et al., 1996). For traumas other than child sexual abuse, age of onset effects have generally not been investigated in community- or population-based studies.

Dose-Response Relationships

Research has established that the severity of childhood trauma is associated with a greater likelihood of suicide. The relationship is sometimes characterized as a "dose–response" relationship wherein response varies according to "dose." Dose in the context of childhood trauma can be measured in a variety of ways, such as by duration of trauma, relationship of the perpetrator to the victim, penetration (for child sexual abuse), or number of incidents or adversities. Research conducted over the decade of 1988 to 1998 generally reveals a stronger relationship between childhood trauma and suicide when the trauma has been of long duration, the perpetrator has been known to the victim, and when force and penetration have taken place (Santa Mina and Gallop, 1998).

---

[9]Kaplan et al. (1995) was not included in the meta-analysis by Paolucci et al. (2001).

More recent research has extended these findings. Cumulative risks from both physical and sexual abuse for suicide attempts have been found in studies of high school girls (Silverman et al., 2001) and African American women (Kaslow et al., 2000). A nationally representative study found that suicide attempts were more prevalent in adults with five or more childhood adversities, including child sexual abuse, physical abuse, psychological abuse, and parental suicide or psychopathology (Molnar et al., 2001a).

The most ambitious study of cumulative effects of childhood trauma was performed by Felitti and colleagues (1998). A survey asking about major types of childhood trauma was sent to 13,494 adults who also completed a standardized primary care evaluation at a San Diego HMO. Childhood traumas referred to physical and sexual abuse, neglect, as well as most other traumas listed in Table 5-1. The number of childhood traumas was found to have a dose–response relationship with suicide attempts (Table 5-3). With four or more traumas, for example, adults had 12 times the likelihood of a suicide attempt, a likelihood that was far greater than that associated with fewer traumas. Moreover, the number of traumas had a dose–response relationship with several disease conditions, including ischemic heart disease, cancer, and chronic bronchitis or emphysema.

BIOPSYCHOSOCIAL EFFECTS OF CHILDHOOD TRAUMA

Childhood trauma induces immediate biological, psychological, and behavioral effects, some of which can be persist for long periods. This section, while not exhaustive, offers a portrait of these effects. How they relate to later suicidality is discussed in a later section.

TABLE 5-3 Childhood Traumas and Adjusted Odds of a Suicide Attempt

Number of Traumas[a]	Adjusted[b] Odds Ratio of Ever Attempting Suicide
0	1.0
1	1.8
2	3.0
3	6.6
4 or more	12.2

[a]Listed in Table 5-1.
[b]Adjusted for age, gender, race, and educational attainment.

SOURCE: Felitti et al., 1998.

Biological Effects

Over the last decade, a new avenue of research has established that biological changes are induced by exposure to severe childhood trauma. There have been two major areas of focus: the hypothalamic-pituitary-adrenal axis (HPA) and brain development (for reviews, see De Bellis, 2001; Glaser, 2000; Heim and Nemeroff, 2001). The observed biological changes may underlie the pronounced cognitive, social, and behavioral effects that are discussed in later sections.

Hypothalamic-Pituitary-Adrenal (HPA) Axis

Children exposed to trauma are likely to have disturbances in arousal, increased startle response, sleep disturbance, and cardiovascular regulation (Perry et al., 1995). Studies in adults and animal models suggest long-term hyper-arousal as a result of childhood trauma (De Bellis, 2001; Heim and Nemeroff, 2001; Kendall-Tackett, 2000). Alterations in arousal reflect dysfunction of the HPA axis.

The HPA axis is the body's frontline system for responding to stress (for review, see Stratakis and Chrousos, 1995). Corticotropin releasing factor (CRF), a neurotransmitter and neurohormone, orchestrates the cascading components of this axis. When a stressor is encountered, the brain registers its presence through the sensory system and relays the information to nucleus in the brain known as the amygdala. If the amygdala interprets the stressor as a serious threat, it releases CRF, which stimulates, through direct and indirect pathways, two other brain centers—the locus coeruleus and the hypothalamus. The former then releases catecholamines (norepinephrine, dopamine, epinephrine) which, in turn, activate the sympathetic nervous system. The hallmarks of sympathetic activation are a sudden surge in heart rate, blood pressure, breathing, and metabolic activity. The hypothalamus, when stimulated by CRF, releases even more CRF, which activates the pituitary. Pituitary activation causes the release of adrenocorticotrophic hormone (ACTH), which migrates to the adrenal gland. There it stimulates the release of cortisol, a hormone with widespread actions on the brain and the rest of the body.

Many of the biochemicals activated throughout the HPA axis have been studied in relation to childhood trauma exposure. Researchers strive to find biological markers that may explain the symptoms and behaviors associated with exposure to severe stressors. Separately, HPA alterations have long been known to cause emotional, cognitive, and behavioral effects, as evidenced by patients with Cushing's disease and Addison's disease.

Studies of childhood trauma have focused on abused children with depression, PTSD, or symptoms thereof. Studies suggest a dysregulation of the HPA axis after children's exposure to severe stress. The persistence of HPA dysregulation is not fully known, yet indications are that HPA dysregulation can last up to at least 5 years (De Bellis et al., 1994a; Goenjian et al., 1996; Putnam and Trickett, 1997). While findings are not always consistent and studies are difficult to perform, there is an expanding literature on children, adults with past childhood abuse, and on animal models (for review, see Heim and Nemeroff, 2001).

Altered activity of the HPA axis in children has been found in several studies focusing on cortisol and catecholamine levels. Studies of traumatized children with depression found lower salivary cortisol in the morning and a rise, rather than an expected reduction, in cortisol by evening (Hart et al., 1996; Kaufman, 1991). Elevations in urinary norepinephrine were found in neglected children with depression (Queiroz et al., 1991). A pilot study of sexually abused girls found elevated 24-hour catecholamine excretion (De Bellis et al., 1994b). A larger study of maltreated children with PTSD, mostly from sexual abuse, were found to have elevated levels of 24-hour urinary free cortisol, dopamine, and norepinephrine (De Bellis et al., 1999a). The degree of elevation was correlated with duration of the trauma and with severity of symptoms. Elevated cortisol and catecholamine levels are also found in adult women who were sexually abused as children (Lemieux and Coe, 1995). On the other hand, cortisol is lowered in adults with PTSD from combat or Holocaust exposure (Yehuda, 2000).

There are other indications of HPA dysregulation. One finding was increased ACTH response to CRF challenge in depressed children undergoing current abuse (Kaufman et al., 1997). The opposite had been found in children with *past* trauma studied several *years* after the abuse had been disclosed (De Bellis et al., 1994a). The difference may be from individual variability or from short-term effects versus long-term adaptations of the HPA axis. Lastly, dysfunctions of the serotonin system, which has interactions with the HPA axis, have been found in abused children (Kaufman et al., 1998). For discussion of the association between HPA axis and serotonergic system functioning and suicide, see Chapter 4.

Brain Development

Significant alterations in the anatomy and physiology of the developing brain are proposed to result from childhood trauma. Some of the observed changes in brain development may be produced by chronically elevated catecholamine and cortisol levels, possibly through their effects on neuron metabolism or death, neurogenesis or migration patterns, and delays in myelination (reviewed by De Bellis, 2001).

Indications of abnormal cortical and limbic system[10] development come from symptom self-reports by adults with past sexual or physical abuse (Teicher et al., 1993). The symptom findings were followed up with EEG studies which found that children hospitalized from physical or sexual abuse had left hemisphere deficits (Ito et al., 1998; Ito et al., 1993). The significance of these findings is unclear, but researchers speculate that early abuse may impede hemispheric integration and the establishment of normal left cortical dominance.

Through brain imaging studies, maltreated children with PTSD were found to have smaller intracranial and cerebral volumes compared with matched controls. Corpus callosum area was smaller, and the size of lateral ventricles was larger (after adjustment for intracranial volume). The reductions in brain volume were positively correlated with age of trauma onset and inversely correlated with duration of abuse (De Bellis et al., 1999b). The size of the hippocampus was slightly increased, in contrast to findings in adults. Adult hippocampal volume is reduced in cases of past physical or sexual abuse (Bremner et al., 1997; Stein et al., 1997). Disparate findings between adults and children may be attributed to differences in methodology, co-morbid substance use, or neuroplasticity (De Bellis et al., 1999b). Finally, preliminary work with MRS spectroscopy suggests that maltreated children with PTSD have heightened neuron metabolism and loss (De Bellis et al., 2000).

Psychosocial and Behavioral Effects

The psychosocial and behavioral consequences of childhood trauma can be severe. Apart from later effects on psychopathology or suicidal behavior, research has established a spectrum of more immediate effects, ranging from low self-esteem to substance use and delinquent behavior (for reviews, see Cicchetti and Toth, 1995; Cicchetti et al., 2000; Margolin and Gordis, 2000; NRC, 1993; Trickett and Putnam, 1998). Most of the research literature deals with maltreatment. Yet maltreatment often occurs within the context of many other childhood traumas, such as parental psychopathology, violence (domestic and community), and household substance abuse. Researchers have gravitated to the view that it is very difficult to disentangle the effects of one trauma from another (Margolin and Gordis, 2000). Overall, studies have found that multiple, rather than individual, traumas are tied to a broad range of difficulties in childhood

---

[10]The limbic system, which regulates emotions and emotional memories, includes the amygdala, hypothalamus, hippocampus, and pre-frontal cerebral cortex.

and adolescence, including compromised socioemotional and cognitive development, psychopathology (see later section) and participation in criminal behavior (Cicchetti et al., 2000; Felitti et al., 1998; Glaser, 2000).

A common theme is the failure of traumatized children to self-regulate their mood and behavior (De Bellis, 2001). Another major theme is the importance of a developmental perspective—that the consequences of trauma vary according to intensity and form at distinct developmental stages. Also key are moderating variables such as the quality of family and social relations and child characteristics, such as cognitive style and temperament (see Chapter 3, Margolin and Gordis, 2000; NRC, 1993). Yet it is worth underscoring that a significant proportion of maltreated children—by some estimates between 20–49 percent after child sexual abuse—do not display noticeable symptoms[11] (Kendall-Tackett et al., 1993; NRC, 1993; Stevenson, 1999). Protective factors include high intelligence and scholastic achievement, paternal care or support, connection to other competent adults, internal locus of control and social skills (Lynskey and Fergusson, 1997; NRC, 1993; Tiet et al., 1998). Further discussion of individual-level protective factors can be found in Chapter 3, and societal-level protective factors in Chapter 6. The following sections are meant to be illustrative rather than comprehensive about the adverse effects of childhood trauma.

Cognitive and Psychological Effects

Lower self-esteem is a major cognitive effect of several types of childhood trauma. It has been found after sexual abuse, physical abuse, neglect, and exposure to parental psychopathology (for reviews, see Kendall-Tackett et al., 1993; Margolin and Gordis, 2000; Yang and Clum, 1996). Lower self-esteem can persist into adulthood. A large study of women with past physical or sexual abuse found them to be three times more likely to have lower self-esteem than women without a history (McCauley et al., 1997). In separate studies, including longitudinal studies, low self-esteem has been found to be a long-term predictor of suicidal behavior (Yang and Clum, 1996).

Poorer school performance has also been found after many types of trauma, but the effect is strongest for childhood neglect (Margolin and Gordis, 2000). For child sexual abuse, a meta-analysis found a relatively weak effect size of .19 for poor academic achievement (Paolucci et al.,

---

[11]The reasons for lack of symptoms may relate to insufficient follow-up time and insufficient sensitivity of measurement (Kendall-Tackett et al., 1993).

2001). Maltreatment is associated with delays in verbal intelligence and social processing deficits (NRC, 1993; Stevenson, 1999).

Other cognitive outcomes of childhood trauma have received somewhat less attention. Maltreatment is associated with hopelessness (Allen and Tarnowski, 1989) and an external locus of control (the perception that external events control the outcome) (Barahal et al., 1981; Brown et al., 1998). External locus of control is also associated with parental divorce (Guidubaldi et al., 1987). Exposure to marital violence is associated with children having extreme approaches to problem solving (Rosenberg, 1987). All of these cognitive factors are, in separate studies, related to suicidal behavior (Yang and Clum, 1996). Hopelessness, in particular, is a powerful risk factor for suicidality (see Chapter 3).

There also has been attention to the role of cognitive appraisal as contributing to symptoms or outcomes of childhood trauma. A negative attributional style, including self-blame, is associated with increased depression symptoms after sexual abuse (for review, see Spaccarelli, 1994). An avoidant coping strategy (i.e., denial or avoidance of the abuse) by adolescent victims or adult survivors tends to increase the likelihood of developing symptoms after sexual abuse (Spaccarelli, 1994). Similar findings concerning cognitive and psychological mechanisms that may contribute to suicidal outcomes point to the importance of understanding the role of pre-existing psychological traits in shaping responses to stress and trauma (see Chapter 3).

Social and Behavioral Effects

Among the key consequences of childhood maltreatment are impaired social attachments. More than 70 percent of maltreated children display insecure attachments with caregivers, which often assume a disorganized/disoriented pattern. The research literature suggests that attachment problems with caregivers generalize to potentially life-long patterns of maladaptive interpersonal relationships (Cicchetti and Toth, 1995; Cicchetti et al., 2000).

Maltreatment of children and adolescents is also associated with poor peer relationships, social isolation, and poorer social skills (Cicchetti et al., 2000; Margolin and Gordis, 2000; NRC, 1993). For example, in a large, community-based study of children and adolescents, physical abuse in particular was strongly associated with poor social competence and impairment of social functioning, even after controlling for psychopathology (Flisher et al., 1997).

Behavior patterns are also affected, especially in relation to the type of trauma. Physical abuse leads to more aggression and other externalizing behaviors than does sexual abuse or neglect. Community violence exposure is also associated with aggressive behavior, as is verbal aggression by parents (Margolin and Gordis, 2000; Vissing et al., 1991). Sexual abuse leads to more internalizing childhood behaviors, including fear and withdrawn behavior (for reviews, see Brown and Anderson, 1991; Grilo et al., 1999; Kendall-Tackett et al., 1993; Margolin and Gordis, 2000; NRC, 1993; Taussig and Litrownik, 1997). As they mature into adolescence and adulthood, children who are sexually abused may display inappropriate sexual behaviors. A meta-analysis found a strong effect size (d=.6) for child sexual abuse on sexual promiscuity (defined as early involvement in sexual activity and/or prostitution, Paolucci et al., 2001).

Childhood maltreatment is also associated with use of alcohol and drugs (Felitti et al., 1998; NRC, 1993; Silverman et al., 2001), as well as with substance use disorders (see later section). Many believe that substance use is initiated in the teen years as a coping device to temper symptoms of anxiety, depression, and the effects of dysregulated stress symptoms (De Bellis, 2001). Victims of child maltreatment are also at risk for delinquency and running away (NRC, 1993; Wolfe et al., 2001). Although a link between childhood maltreatment and serious violence[12] has been proposed, a recent Surgeon General report found only a small effect size (r<.20) for a relationship between the two (US DHHS, 2001b).

Intergenerational Transmission of Childhood Trauma

The effects of child maltreatment and its relationship to suicide are compounded by the intergenerational transmission of abusive parenting. A recent two-site study by Brent and colleagues (in press) found a 6-fold increased risk of suicide attempts among offspring of suicide attempters versus non-attempters, and that the familial transmission was more likely if the attempting parent had been sexually abused as a child. Thus, abuse is not only a risk factor for suicide for those abused as children, but also for their subsequent children.

While early assumptions about the inevitability of intergenerational transmission have been discounted, the experience of abuse in childhood is one of the most commonly agreed upon risk factors for subsequent abusive parenting (Kaufman and Zigler, 1987; NRC, 1993). The variability in transmission, however, provides an opportunity to examine protective factors that break this cycle. These include effective therapeutic intervention either in childhood or adulthood, the presence of significant others, and insight into one's own childhood experience of abuse (e.g., Egeland et al., 1988). Prevention of child maltreatment and treatment of its victims/

---

[12]Serious violence refers to aggravated assault, forcible rape, robbery, and homicide.

survivors can break the cycle of abusive parenting and be considered a preventive measure for suicidal behavior.

CHILDHOOD TRAUMA AS A RISK FACTOR FOR PSYCHOPATHOLOGY

Childhood trauma is a risk factor for the onset of psychopathology. Child sexual abuse and physical abuse have been the most intensively studied. They are associated with wide-ranging categories of mental disorders or symptomatology (for reviews, see Kendall-Tackett et al., 1993; Margolin and Gordis, 2000; NRC, 1993). About 40–50 percent of abuse victims develop at least two disorders by age 21 (Silverman et al., 1996). The most common outcomes of sexual or physical abuse are depression and post-traumatic stress disorder (PTSD). A meta-analysis of 37 studies of child sexual abuse, published between 1981–1995, found robust effect sizes for depression (d=0.44) and PTSD (d=0.40) (Paolucci et al., 2001). Most studies in this meta-analysis were conducted in clinical populations, but more recent studies feature population or community samples. After exposure to sexual abuse *or* physical abuse, about one-third to one-half of children prospectively develop PTSD (Silverman et al., 1996; Widom, 1999). Similar proportions of exposed children or adolescents prospectively develop depression (Brown et al., 1999; Fergusson et al., 1996; Silverman et al., 1996). PTSD or depression can persist from childhood into young adulthood (Brown et al., 1999; Fergusson et al., 1996; McCauley et al., 1997; Silverman et al., 1996; Widom, 1999).

Other outcomes of child sexual or physical abuse, from population or community studies, are substance use disorders (Dinwiddie et al., 2000; Fergusson et al., 1996; Kendler et al., 2000; Molnar et al., 2001b; Silverman et al., 1996; Widom et al., 1995; Wilsnack et al., 1997) and conduct disorder (Fergusson et al., 1996; Flisher et al., 1997; McLeer et al., 1998). Anti-social personality disorder and borderline personality disorder are also associated with childhood physical or sexual abuse (Brown and Anderson, 1991; Horwitz et al., 2001; Luntz and Widom, 1994; Silverman et al., 1996; van der Kolk et al., 1991).

Given the wide range of possible psychiatric outcomes, one study of child sexual abuse provides an indication of their relative likelihood. In a cohort of 1019 young adults (18 years old), the study found that adjusted odds ratios[13] were greatest for conduct disorder, substance use disorders,

---

[13]In comparison to young people not exposed to childhood sexual abuse, after adjustment for social, family, and contextual factors that are associated with child sexual abuse and increased risk of disorder.

anxiety disorder, and major depression (Fergusson et al., 1996). Furthermore, the study estimated the population attributable risk (PAR) for each disorder—namely, the percentage of cases of each disorder that are attributable to child sexual abuse. It found PARs ranging from 9.3 to 18.5 percent, depending on the disorder (Table 5-4). The largest was for conduct disorder: more than 18 percent of cases of conduct disorder would have been eliminated if sexual abuse had not occurred.

Other childhood traumas, apart from sexual or physical abuse, are associated with psychopathology, but the evidence is more limited. Exposure to domestic violence or community violence (as witness or victim) are associated with onset of PTSD and depression (for review, see Margolin and Gordis, 2000). Childhood neglect is associated with PTSD (Widom, 1999), a highly important finding given that neglect is the most common type of childhood maltreatment. Childhood neglect, however, does not appear to be significantly related to depressive disorders (Brown et al., 1999). Parental loss is associated with the development of depression, anxiety disorders, PTSD, and substance disorders (Agid et al., 1999; Kendler et al., 1992; Widom, 1999).

Studies of childhood trauma rarely investigate more than two types of trauma. An exception is the National Comorbidity Survey (Kessler et al., 1997), which found that childhood adversities exert multiplicative effects on the onset of psychopathology. Another noteworthy exception is a large study of primary care patients (n=13,494) by Felitti and coworkers

TABLE 5-4 Childhood Sexual Abuse and Psychopathology

Outcome[a]	Adjusted Odds Ratio[b]	Estimated Population Attributable Risk For CSA[c]
Major depression	5.4	14.0 %
Anxiety disorder	3.2	13.3%
Conduct disorder	11.9	18.5%
Alcohol abuse/dependence	2.7	9.3%
Other substance abuse/dependence	6.6	10.8%
Suicide attempt	5.0	19.5%

[a]Assessed by the Composite International Diagnostic Interview (CIDI) and by the Self-Report Delinquency Instrument (SRDI, for conduct disorder).
[b]Intercourse (Attempted/Completed) only, in comparison with no history of CSA after adjustment for covariates.
[c]CSA=Child Sexual Abuse, defined as non-contact sexual abuse, contact, and intercourse.

SOURCE: Fergusson et al., 1996.

(1998). They found a graded relationship between the number of child-hood traumas (Table 5-3) and alcoholism, drug abuse, and depressed mood. Similarly, they found a graded relationship with physical disorders, such as severe obesity, cancer, stroke, and chronic bronchitis or emphysema. This study's findings in relation to suicide attempts were discussed in an earlier section.

PATHWAYS TO SUICIDALITY

The preceding sections spotlight the grim and sometimes enduring impact of childhood trauma, especially sexual abuse and physical abuse, on mental health. Yet most studies are not suited to illuminating the pathways to suicidality. They examine the immediate or short-term effects of trauma in children, typically through a cross-sectional design, or they look much later, at adult populations, to retrospectively assess risk factors. This means that there is knowledge about the beginning and later stages, but not the complex pathways linking the two. Furthermore, most studies are not population- or community-based. Finally, and perhaps most importantly, there have been few attempts to study how the process unfolds by *integration* of known biological, psychological, and behavioral sequelae of trauma.

The best insight into pathways to suicidality comes from a small body of longitudinal studies (Brown et al., 1999; Fergusson et al., 2000b; Silverman et al., 1996) and a nationally representative, cross-sectional United States study of adults from the National Comorbidity Survey (Molnar et al., 2001a). What emerges from these studies is that childhood trauma induces a range of effects that, over time, can coalesce into diagnosable mental disorders, suicidal ideation, and suicide attempts by adolescence and young adulthood. The underlying mechanisms are not known. The timing of these events is difficult to discern, even from longitudinal studies, because survey questions about physical and sexual abuse are, for legal and ethical reasons, not usually asked until study subjects reach age 18.

One analysis of timing is from the National Comorbidity Survey, which is representative of the United States population (Molnar et al., 2001a). This retrospective, cross-sectional study dealt with child sexual abuse and suicidality. The mean age of onset of sexual abuse was 9 years for females and 11 years for males. The mean age of onset of a mental disorder was 16–17 years. The probability of the first suicide attempt came at an earlier age if the victim of sexual abuse also met criteria for any lifetime mental disorder. This group attempted suicide in adolescence, 8–12 years *before* those who had been sexually abused *but did not develop a disorder. This finding suggests that detection of both sexual abuse and psychopa-*

thology is critical in adolescence because of the greater likelihood of earlier suicide attempts.

The most comprehensive longitudinal study of suicide pathways was conducted in New Zealand (Fergusson et al., 2000b). It focused on a cohort of 1265 children studied over the course of 21 years. The study sought to determine the extent to which social background, personality factors, mental illness, stressful life events, and childhood trauma contribute to suicide attempts.[14] The childhood traumas (occurring before 16 years) were most of those covered by this chapter: sexual abuse, physical abuse, attachment to parents, caregiver separation/divorce or death, and parental substance abuse. Applying a proportional hazards model, three of the six predictors of suicide attempts at age 21 were related to childhood adversities: (1) child sexual abuse, (2) parental alcoholism, (3) low attachment to parents. The other three predictors were lower family SES and two child personality factors (neuroticism and novelty-seeking). The investigators then used a time dynamic model to account for the roles of mental illness and stressful life events in suicide attempts. *This model found that none of the childhood traumas predicted suicide attempts independent of mental illness and stressful life events in adolescence.* The study concluded that the effects of childhood traumas were completely mediated by mental illness and stressful life events. It suggested that the causal chain begins with childhood adversity, which increases the risk of suicide by increasing young people's vulnerability to later mental health problems and stressful life events. In other words, both mental illness and exposure to stressful life events mediated the effect of childhood trauma on suicidality (Fergusson et al., 2000b).

The New Zealand study's finding on child sexual abuse was not consistent with a finding from the U.S. National Comorbidity Survey. The major debate centered on whether psychopathology *completely* mediates the relationship between child sexual abuse and suicidal attempts, or whether child sexual abuse, by itself, without the presence of psychopathology, confers an independent risk (after controlling for confounding factors). These questions have important implications for prevention. If child sexual abuse is an independent predictor, then victims should be targeted for prevention programs, regardless of whether they have psychopathology.

In the United States study, Molnar and colleagues (2001a) found that, while the *majority* of suicide attempts were attributed to prior mental disorders, a significant percentage of suicide attempts occurred in the absence of psychopathology. The investigators suggested that methodological differences may explain the discrepancy with the New Zealand

---

[14]Findings not presented for suicidal ideation.

study. On the basis of their findings, the United States investigators suggested that a substantial proportion of suicide risk would be overlooked by sole reliance on the presence of psychopathology. They recommend screening and prevention efforts targeted at people with a history of child sexual abuse. Their findings about earlier onset of suicide attempts for those with past abuse and a current mental disorder point to the importance of early screening for both child sexual abuse and psychopathology.

Several models of pathways from childhood trauma to suicidality have been developed. A cognitive model was developed by Yang and Clum (1996). It sought to identify which cognitive factors were common to two previously unrelated sets of evidence: studies of the cognitive consequences of many types of childhood trauma, and studies of cognitive risk factors for suicidality (discussed in Chapter 3). The cognitive factors which were linked to both sets of evidence were found to be low self-esteem, external locus of control, field dependence, poor problem solving skills, and hopelessness. The investigators proposed and then later tested the role of these cognitive factors as mediators between early adverse events and high levels of suicidal ideation in a sample of college students (Yang and Clum, 2000). Using structural equation analyses, the study found childhood adverse events had a direct impact on cognitive deficits, which, in turn, strongly affected suicidal ideation. Since childhood traumas had an only mildly direct relationship to suicidal ideation, the study found support for the importance of cognitive factors as mediators between trauma and suicidal ideation. While the study was not of suicide attempts and was based on a unrepresentative sample, it is pioneering in its attempts to develop a cognitive pathway from childhood trauma to suicidality.

A behavioral model has been developed by Felitti and colleagues (1998) on the basis of their large study showing strong and graded relationships between many types of childhood trauma and a spectrum of symptoms and risk factors for premature death, including attempted suicide (see earlier sections). Stressing the cumulative nature of childhood traumas, the researchers proposed that adverse childhood experiences lead to social, emotional, and cognitive impairments, which, in turn, triggers the adoption of health-risk behaviors, such as substance use. Health-risk behaviors, originally adopted as a means of coping with childhood trauma, become counterproductive and heighten the later probability of suicidality (or premature death from heart disease and lung cancer).

One of the few models to integrate biology and behavior has been proposed by De Bellis (2001). Drawing on his studies of the biological effects of trauma, De Bellis places central importance on persistent dysfunction of the HPA axis, which underlies chronic PTSD symptoms, especially hyperarousal. De Bellis proposes that hyperaroused stress systems affect brain development, ushering in a failure to self-regulate emotion and behavior, especially upon exposure to other traumas or to stressful life events. This failure to regulate emotion and behavior underlies a range of behavioral outcomes: externalizing behavior, internalizing behavior, as well as cognitive and learning disorders. By early to middle childhood, these problem behaviors can lead to chronic PTSD, depression, attention-deficit disorders, and poor school performance. These can progress to, or be accompanied by, conduct disorder or substance abuse by adolescence and personality disorders by adulthood.

These models represent a milestone in attempting to integrate the wide-ranging short-term and long-term effects of childhood trauma. They form an important departure point for integrative neuroscience research to examine biological, psychological, and behavioral measures and their interactions. What makes this line of research even more challenging is that trauma can occur at distinct stages of development. There is likely to be a diversity of pathways from childhood trauma to suicidality, any of which can by determined by (or interrupted by) a host of risk and protective factors prior to, during, or after trauma exposure (Cicchetti et al., 2000; Fergusson et al., 2000b). These risk and protective factors can arise in the individual (e.g., genes, age, gender, temperament), family, school, peer group, or community (US DHHS, 1999).

PREVENTION/INTERVENTION

In the United States, the health and welfare of children are protected by multiple institutions: schools, the health care system, and the legal system. According to the Surgeon General's Conference Report on Children's Mental Health (PHS, 2000), these systems have been largely ineffective at improving the health of our children. The prevalence of serious emotional disturbances is no different in younger versus older children and has failed to change over the last 20 years (PHS, 2000). The Surgeon General's Report goes on to suggest that integration of these systems, along with home and community care, would enhance timely recognition of children at risk, and therefore enable delivery of data-based interventions prior to any further developmental costs (PHS, 2000). Given the impact of child abuse on risk of suicide, such an integration of services would likely have positive repercussions for this important outcome, as well.

Family-oriented programs are effective in the prevention of child abuse. A meta-analysis found a weighted effect size of .41, meaning that programs were effective by comparison with control/comparison groups. The greater the level or frequency of intervention, the more successful the program in preventing child abuse (MacLeod and Nelson, 2000). One of the most prominent programs is a home visitation program by nurses targeted to high risk mothers during pregnancy and infancy (almost 25 visits). A 15-year follow-up of a home visitation program with a randomized controlled design found lower incidence of verified reports of childhood abuse and neglect in comparison with families in comparison group (Olds et al., 1997). Since social supports significantly influence the intergenerational cycle of child abuse (Egeland et al., 1988), intervention programs that offer support to high-risk children and their families can be of great benefit in terms of providing protective functions and promoting positive outcomes (Berrueta-Clement, 1984; Consortium for Longitudinal Studies, 1983; Copple et al., 1987; Price et al., 1988).

Individuals with a history of child abuse may require alternative approaches to standard treatment. Holmes (1995) found that within a group of adults being treated for depression and anxiety, a history of child abuse was the main determinant of treatment effectiveness. However, while the various psychological treatments were very effective for patients without a history of abuse, they were ineffective for those with a history of abuse. Consequently, Stevenson (1999: 92) points out that "the assumption that treatments found to be effective in general are also likely to be of greatest benefit to victims of maltreatment needs to be treated with caution." Yet the controlled clinical trials conducted thus far have found that cognitive-behavioral therapy for child sexual abuse, in particular, is effective at reducing symptoms of anxiety and depression, both risk factors for suicide, in children. These trials included treatment of non-offending parents (Cohen and Mannarino, 1996; 1998; Deblinger and Heflin, 1996; King et al., 2000).

The American Academy of Pediatrics recommends universal screening of adolescents for sexual victimization (AAP, 2001). While there appears to be no formal study of pediatrician practices, it is believed that universal screening is not done as frequently or consistently as it should be (Personal communication, D.W. Kaplan, University of Colorado, October 11, 2001).

FINDINGS

• Childhood traumas are highly prevalent in the population and elevate suicide risk. While childhood abuse increases the risk for development of mental disorders, it also may be a risk factor for suicide independent of psychopathology. Of the many types of childhood trauma, childhood sexual abuse is the strongest and most independent risk factor for suicide attempts, accounting for 9–20 percent of suicide attempts.

• Exposure to trauma can affect the developing brain with potentially lifelong alterations in the physiological stress response system and cognitive development. Childhood trauma also has psychological and behavioral effects, including low self-esteem, poor attachments to caregivers, and substance use, all of which are associated with suicide.

The study of childhood trauma and its relationship to suicide offers a powerful opportunity for integrative neuroscience research. Interdisciplinary research that weaves together biological, cognitive, and social effects of trauma has the potential to elucidate the complex pathways from childhood trauma to mental illness and/or suicidality and thereby elucidate multiple possibilities for intervention.

• Early adversity increases the likelihood of developing mental illnesses associated with suicide risk, such as substance use, posttraumatic stress disorder, and depression. Understanding the precise pathways from childhood trauma to suicidality has been hampered by the paucity of longitudinal, population-based studies and the legal and ethical difficulties of asking children and adolescents about childhood sexual and physical abuse.

The field requires longitudinal, inter-sectoral research to reveal post-trauma protective factors and processes and effective means of intervention and prevention across the life span. Including measures of suicidality in follow-up studies of child abuse prevention programs would yield invaluable information for suicide reduction strategies.

• Early treatment for child abuse survivors and early family-based interventions to reduce child abuse are expected to reduce suicide.

Society has a large window of opportunity to treat identified victims of childhood trauma in order to minimize the likelihood of psychopathology and suicidality. The development of biological, social, or cognitive markers to identify children at greatest risk for adverse effects could enhance targeted prevention/intervention efforts.

REFERENCES

AAP (American Academy of Pediatrics, Committee on Adolescence). 2001. Care of the adolescent sexual assault victim. *Pediatrics*, 107(6): 1476-1479.
Agid O, Shapira B, Zislin J, Ritsner M, Hanin B, Murad H, Troudart T, Bloch M, Heresco-Levy U, Lerer B. 1999. Environment and vulnerability to major psychiatric illness: A case control study of early parental loss in major depression, bipolar disorder and schizophrenia. *Molecular Psychiatry*, 4(2): 163-172.

Allen DM, Tarnowski KJ. 1989. Depressive characteristics of physically abused children. *Journal of Abnormal Child Psychology*, 17(1): 1-11.

Barahal RM, Waterman J, Martin HP. 1981. The social cognitive development of abused children. *Journal of Consulting and Clinical Psychology*, 49(4): 508-516.

Berliner L, Williams LM. 1994. Memories of child sexual abuse: A reponse to Lindsay and Read. *Applied Cognitive Psychology*, 8(4): 379-387.

Berman AL, Jobes DA. 1991. *Adolescent Suicide: Assessment and Intervention*. Washington, DC: American Psychological Association.

Berrueta-Clement JR. 1984. *Changed Lives: The Effects of the Perry Preschool Program on Youths Through Age 19*. Ypsilanti, MI: High/Scope Press.

Black MM, Ponirakis A. 2000. Computer-administered interviews with children about maltreatment: Methodological, developmental and ethical issues. *Journal of Interpersonal Violence*, 15(7): 682-695.

Bowman ES. 1996a. Delayed memories of child abuse: Part I: An overview of research findings on forgetting, remembering, and corroborating trauma. *Dissociation: Progress in the Dissociative Disorders*, 9(4): 221-231.

Bowman ES. 1996b. Delayed memories of child abuse: Part II: An overview of research findings relevant to understanding their reliability and suggestibility. *Dissociation: Progress in the Dissociative Disorders*, 9(4): 232-243.

Bremner JD, Randall P, Vermetten E, Staib L, Bronen RA, Mazure C, Capelli S, McCarthy G, Innis RB, Charney DS. 1997. Magnetic resonance imaging-based measurement of hippocampal volume in posttraumatic stress disorder related to childhood physical and sexual abuse—a preliminary report. *Biological Psychiatry*, 41(1): 23-32.

Bremner JD, Vermetten E, Mazure CM. 2000. Development and preliminary psychometric properties of an instrument for the measurement of childhood trauma: The Early Trauma Inventory. *Depression and Anxiety*, 12(1): 1-12.

Brent DA, Baugher M, Bridge J, Chen T, Chiappetta L. 1999. Age- and sex-related risk factors for adolescent suicide. *Journal of the American Academy of Child and Adolescent Psychiatry*, 38(12): 1497-1505.

Brent DA, Oquendo MA, Birmaher B, Greenhill L, Kolko DJ, Stanley B, Zelazny J, Brodsky BS, Bridge J, Ellis SP, Salazar O, Mann JJ. in press. Familial pathways to early-onset suicide attempts: A high-risk study. *Archives of General Psychiatry*.

Brown GR, Anderson B. 1991. Psychiatric morbidity in adult inpatients with childhood histories of sexual and physical abuse. *American Journal of Psychiatry*, 148(1): 55-61.

Brown J, Cohen P, Johnson JG, Salzinger S. 1998. A longitudinal analysis of risk factors for child maltreatment: Findings of a 17-year prospective study of officially recorded and self-reported child abuse and neglect. *Child Abuse and Neglect*, 22(11): 1065-1078.

Brown J, Cohen P, Johnson JG, Smailes EM. 1999. Childhood abuse and neglect: Specificity of effects on adolescent and young adult depression and suicidality. *Journal of the American Academy of Child and Adolescent Psychiatry*, 38(12): 1490-1496.

Browne A, Finkelhor D. 1986. Impact of child sexual abuse: A review of the research. *Psychological Bulletin*, 99(1): 66-77.

Carlin AS, Kemper K, Ward NG, Sowell H, Gustafson B, Stevens N. 1994. The effect of differences in objective and subjective definitions of childhood physical abuse on estimates of its incidence and relationship to psychopathology. *Child Abuse and Neglect*, 18(5): 393-399.

Cheng AT, Chen TH, Chen CC, Jenkins R. 2000. Psychosocial and psychiatric risk factors for suicide. Case-control psychological autopsy study. *Br J Psychiatry*, 177: 360-5.

Cicchetti D, Toth SL. 1995. A developmental psychopathology perspective on child abuse and neglect. *Journal of the American Academy of Child and Adolescent Psychiatry*, 34(5): 541-565.

Cicchetti D, Toth SL, Rogosch FA. 2000. The development of psychological wellness in maltreated children. In: Cicchetti D, Rappaport J, Sandler I, Weissberg RP, Editors. *The Promotion of Wellness in Children and Adolescents.* (pp. 395-426). Washington, DC: Child Welfare League of America, Inc.

Cohen JA, Mannarino AP. 1996. Factors that mediate treatment outcome of sexually abused preschool children. *Journal of the American Academy of Child and Adolescent Psychiatry,* 35(10): 1402-1410.

Cohen JA, Mannarino AP. 1998. Factors that mediate treatment outcome of sexually abused preschool children: Six- and 12-month follow-up. *Journal of the American Academy of Child and Adolescent Psychiatry,* 37(1): 44-51.

Consortium for Longitudinal Studies. 1983. *As the Twig Is Bent—Lasting Effects of Preschool Programs.* Hillsdale, NJ: Lawrence Erlbaum Associates.

Copple C, Cline MG, Smith AN. 1987. *Path to the Future: Long-Term Effects of Head Start in the Philadelphia School District.* U.S. Department of Health and Human Services, Office of Human Development Services, Administration for Children, Youth and Families, Head Start Bureau.

Dahlenberg CJ. 1996. Accuracy, timing and circumstances of disclosure in therapy in recovered and continuous memories of abuse. *Journal of Psychiatry and the Law,* 24: 229-275.

Davidson JR, Hughes DC, George LK, Blazer DG. 1996. The association of sexual assault and attempted suicide within the community. *Archives of General Psychiatry,* 53(6): 550-555.

De Bellis MD. 2001. Developmental traumatology: The psychobiological development of maltreated children and its implications for research, treatment, and policy. *Development and Psychopathology,* 13(3): 539-564.

De Bellis MD, Baum AS, Birmaher B, Keshavan MS, Eccard CH, Boring AM, Jenkins FJ, Ryan ND. 1999a. A.E. Bennett Research Award. Developmental traumatology. Part I: Biological stress systems. *Biological Psychiatry,* 45(10): 1259-1270.

De Bellis MD, Chrousos GP, Dorn LD, Burke L, Helmers K, Kling MA, Trickett PK, Putnam FW. 1994a. Hypothalamic-pituitary-adrenal axis dysregulation in sexually abused girls. *Journal of Clinical Endocrinology and Metabolism,* 78(2): 249-255.

De Bellis MD, Keshavan MS, Clark DB, Casey BJ, Giedd JN, Boring AM, Frustaci K, Ryan ND. 1999b. A.E. Bennett Research Award. Developmental traumatology. Part II: Brain development. *Biological Psychiatry,* 45(10): 1271-1284.

De Bellis MD, Keshavan MS, Spencer S, Hall J. 2000. N-Acetylaspartate concentration in the anterior cingulate of maltreated children and adolescents with PTSD. *American Journal of Psychiatry,* 157(7): 1175-1177.

De Bellis MD, Lefter L, Trickett PK, Putnam FW Jr. 1994b. Urinary catecholamine excretion in sexually abused girls. *Journal of the American Academy of Child and Adolescent Psychiatry,* 33(3): 320-327.

Deblinger E, Heflin AH. 1996. *Treating Sexually Abused Children and Their Nonoffending Parents: A Cognitive Behavioral Approach.* Thousand Oaks, CA: Sage Publications.

Dinwiddie S, Heath AC, Dunne MP, Bucholz KK, Madden PA, Slutske WS, Bierut LJ, Statham DB, Martin NG. 2000. Early sexual abuse and lifetime psychopathology: A co-twin-control study. *Psychological Med,* 30(1): 41-52.

Edgardh K, Ormstad K. 2000. Prevalence and characteristics of sexual abuse in a national sample of Swedish seventeen-year-old boys and girls. *Acta Paediatrica,* 89(3): 310-319.

Egeland B, Jacobvitz D, Sroufe LA. 1988. Breaking the cycle of abuse. *Child Development,* 59(4): 1080-1088.

Falsetti SA, Resnick HS. 2000. Treatment of PTSD using cognitive and cognitive behavioral therapies. *Journal of Cognitive Psychotherapy,* 14(3): 261-285.

Felitti VJ, Anda RF, Nordenberg D, Williamson DF, Spitz AM, Edwards V, Koss MP, Marks JS. 1998. Relationship of childhood abuse and household dysfunction to many of the leading causes of death in adults. The Adverse Childhood Experiences (ACE) Study. *American Journal of Preventive Medicine*, 14(4): 245-258.

Fergusson DM, Horwood LJ, Lynskey MT. 1996. Childhood sexual abuse and psychiatric disorder in young adulthood: II. Psychiatric outcomes of childhood sexual abuse. *Journal of the American Academy of Child and Adolescent Psychiatry*, 35(10): 1365-1374.

Fergusson DM, Horwood LJ, Woodward LJ. 2000a. The stability of child abuse reports: A longitudinal study of the reporting behaviour of young adults. *Psychological Medicine*, 30(3): 529-544.

Fergusson DM, Woodward LJ, Horwood LJ. 2000b. Risk factors and life processes associated with the onset of suicidal behaviour during adolescence and early adulthood. *Psychological Medicine*, 30(1): 23-39.

Flisher AJ, Kramer RA, Hoven CW, Greenwald S, Alegria M, Bird HR, Canino G, Connell R, Moore RE. 1997. Psychosocial characteristics of physically abused children and adolescents. *Journal of the American Academy of Child and Adolescent Psychiatry*, 36(1): 123-131.

Glaser D. 2000. Child abuse and neglect and the brain—a review. *Journal of Child Psychology and Psychiatry*, 41(1): 97-116.

Goenjian AK, Yehuda R, Pynoos RS, Steinberg AM, Tashjian M, Yang RK, Najarian LM, Fairbanks LA. 1996. Basal cortisol, dexamethasone suppression of cortisol, and MHPG in adolescents after the 1988 earthquake in Armenia. *American Journal of Psychiatry*, 153(7): 929-934.

Gorey KM, Leslie DR. 1997. The prevalence of child sexual abuse: Integrative review adjustment for potential response and measurement biases. *Child Abuse and Neglect*, 21(4): 391-398.

Grilo CM, Sanislow CA, Fehon DC, Lipschitz DS, Martino S, McGlashan TH. 1999. Correlates of suicide risk in adolescent inpatients who report a history of childhood abuse. *Comprehensive Psychiatry*, 40(6): 422-428.

Guidubaldi J, Perry JD, Natashi BK. 1987. Growing up in a divorced family: Initial and long-term perspectives on children's adjustment. *Applied Social Psychology Annual*, 7: 202-237.

Hart J, Gunnar M, Cicchetti D. 1996. Altered neuroendocrine activity in maltreated children related to symptoms of depression. *Development and Psychopathology*, 8(1): 201-214.

Heim C, Nemeroff CB. 2001. The role of childhood trauma in the neurobiology of mood and anxiety disorders: Preclinical and clinical studies. *Biological Psychiatry*, 49(12): 1023-1039.

Holmes TR. 1995. A history of childhood abuse as a predictor variable: Implications for outcome research. *Research on Social Work Practice*, 5(3): 297-308.

Horwitz AV, Widom CS, McLaughlin J, White HR. 2001. The impact of childhood abuse and neglect on adult mental health: A prospective study. *Journal of Health and Social Behavior*, 42(2): 184-201.

Ito Y, Teicher MH, Glod CA, Ackerman E. 1998. Preliminary evidence for aberrant cortical development in abused children: A quantitative EEG study. *Journal of Neuropsychiatry and Clinical Neuroscience*, 10(3): 298-307.

Ito Y, Teicher MH, Glod CA, Harper D, Magnus E, Gelbard HA. 1993. Increased prevalence of electrophysiological abnormalities in children with psychological, physical, and sexual abuse. *Journal of Neuropsychiatry and Clinical Neuroscience*, 5(4): 401-408.

Kaplan ML, Asnis GM, Lipschitz DS, Chorney P. 1995. Suicidal behavior and abuse in psychiatric outpatients. *Comprehensive Psychiatry*, 36(3): 229-235.

Kaslow NJ, Thompson MP, Brooks AE, Twomey HB. 2000. Ratings of family functioning of suicidal and nonsuicidal African American women. *Journal of Family Psychology*, 14(4): 585-599.

Kaufman J. 1991. Depressive disorders in maltreated children. *Journal of the American Academy of Child and Adolescent Psychiatry*, 30(2): 257-265.

Kaufman J, Birmaher B, Perel J, Dahl RE, Moreci P, Nelson B, Wells W, Ryan ND. 1997. The corticotropin-releasing hormone challenge in depressed abused, depressed nonabused, and normal control children. *Biological Psychiatry*, 42(8): 669-679.

Kaufman J, Birmaher B, Perel J, Dahl RE, Stull S, Brent D, Trubnick L, al-Shabbout M, Ryan ND. 1998. Serotonergic functioning in depressed abused children: Clinical and familial correlates. *Biological Psychiatry*, 44(10): 973-981.

Kaufman J, Zigler E. 1987. Do abused children become abusive parents? *American Journal of Orthopsychiatry*, 57(2): 186-192.

Kendall-Tackett KA. 2000. Physiological correlates of childhood abuse: chronic hyperarousal in PTSD, depression, and irritable bowel syndrome. *Child Abuse and Neglect*, 24(6): 799-810.

Kendall-Tackett KA, Williams LM, Finkelhor D. 1993. Impact of sexual abuse on children: A review and synthesis of recent empirical studies. *Psychological Bulletin*, 113(1): 164-180.

Kendler KS, Bulik CM, Silberg J, Hettema JM, Myers J, Prescott CA. 2000. Childhood sexual abuse and adult psychiatric and substance use disorders in women: An epidemiological and cotwin control analysis. *Archives of General Psychiatry*, 57(10): 953-959.

Kendler KS, Neale MC, Kessler RC, Heath AC, Eaves LJ. 1992. Childhood parental loss and adult psychopathology in women. A twin study perspective. *Archives of General Psychiatry*, 49(2): 109-116.

Kessler RC. 2000. Posttraumatic stress disorder: The burden to the individual and to society. *Journal of Clinical Psychiatry*, 61 (Suppl 5): 4-12; discussion 13-14.

Kessler RC, Davis CG, Kendler KS. 1997. Childhood adversity and adult psychiatric disorder in the US National Comorbidity Survey. *Psychological Medicine*, 27(5): 1101-1119.

King NJ, Tonge BJ, Mullen P, Myerson N, Heyne D, Rollings S, Martin R, Ollendick TH. 2000. Treating sexually abused children with posttraumatic stress symptoms: A randomized clinical trial. *Journal of the American Academy of Child and Adolescent Psychiatry*, 39(11): 1347-1355.

King NMP, Churchill LR. 2000. Ethical principles guiding research on child and adolescent subjects. *Journal of Interpersonal Violence*, 15(7): 710-724.

Knight ED, Runyan DK, Dubowitz H, Brandford C, Kotch J, Litrownik A, Hunter W. 2000. Methodological and ethical challenges associated with child self-report of maltreatment: Solutions implemented by the LongSCAN consortium. *Journal of Interpersonal Violence*, 15(7): 760-775.

Lemieux AM, Coe CL. 1995. Abuse-related posttraumatic stress disorder: Evidence for chronic neuroendocrine activation in women. *Psychosomatic Medicine*, 57(2): 105-115.

Loftus E, Joslyn S, Polage D. 1998. Repression: A mistaken impression? *Development and Psychopathology*, 10(4): 781-792.

Luntz BK, Widom CS. 1994. Antisocial personality disorder in abused and neglected children grown up. *American Journal of Psychiatry*, 151(5): 670-674.

Lynskey MT, Fergusson DM. 1997. Factors protecting against the development of adjustment difficulties in young adults exposed to childhood sexual abuse. *Child Abuse and Neglect*, 21(12): 1177-1190.

MacLeod J, Nelson G. 2000. Programs for the promotion of family wellness and the prevention of child maltreatment: A meta-analytic review. *Child Abuse and Neglect*, 24(9): 1127-1149.

Margolin G, Gordis EB. 2000. The effects of family and community violence on children. *Annual Review of Psychology*, 51: 445-479.

McCauley J, Kern DE, Kolodner K, Dill L, Schroeder AF, DeChant HK, Ryden J, Derogatis LR, Bass EB. 1997. Clinical characteristics of women with a history of childhood abuse: Unhealed wounds. *Journal of the American Medical Association*, 277(17): 1362-1368.

Mcgee RA, Wolfe DA, Yuen SA, Wilson SK, Carnochan J. 1995. The measurement of maltreatment: A comparison of approaches. *Child Abuse and Neglect*, 19(2): 233-249.

McLeer SV, Dixon JF, Henry D, Ruggiero K, Escovitz K, Niedda T, Scholle R. 1998. Psychopathology in non-clinically referred sexually abused children. *Journal of the American Academy of Child and Adolescent Psychiatry*, 37(12): 1326-1333.

Molnar BE, Berkman LF, Buka SL. 2001a. Psychopathology, childhood sexual abuse and other childhood adversities: Relative links to subsequent suicidal behaviour in the US. *Psychological Medicine*, 31(6): 965-977.

Molnar BE, Buka SL, Kessler RC. 2001b. Child sexual abuse and subsequent psychopathology: Results from the National Comorbidity Survey. *American Journal of Public Health*, 91(5): 753-760.

NRC (National Research Council). 1993. *Understanding Child Abuse and Neglect*. Washington, DC: National Academy Press.

Olds DL, Eckenrode J, Henderson CR Jr, Kitzman H, Powers J, Cole R, Sidora K, Morris P, Pettitt LM, Luckey D. 1997. Long-term effects of home visitation on maternal life course and child abuse and neglect. Fifteen-year follow-up of a randomized trial. *Journal of the American Medical Association*, 278(8): 637-643.

Paolucci EO, Genuis ML, Violato C. 2001. A meta-analysis of the published research on the effects of child sexual abuse. *Journal of Psychology*, 135(1): 17-36.

Perry BD, Pollard RA, Blakley TL, Baker WL, Vigilante D. 1995. Childhood trauma, the neurobiology of adaptation, and "use-dependent" development of the brain: How "states" become "traits." *Infant Mental Health Journal*, 16(4): 271-291.

PHS (Public Health Service). 2000. *Report of the Surgeon General's Conference on Children's Mental Health: A National Action Agenda*. Rockville, MD: U.S. Department of Health and Human Services.

Price RH, Cowen EL, Lorion RP, Ramos-McKay J, Editors. 1988. *Fourteen Ounces of Prevention: A Casebook for Practitioners*. Washington, DC: American Psychological Association.

Putnam FW, Trickett PK. 1997. Psychobiological effects of sexual abuse. A longitudinal study. *Annals of the New York Academy of Sciences*, 821: 150-159.

Queiroz EA, Lombardi AB, Furtado CR, Peixoto CC, Soares TA, Fabre ZL, Basques JC, Fernandes ML, Lippi JR. 1991. Biochemical correlate of depression in children. *Arquivos De Neuro-Psiquiatria*, 49(4): 418-425.

Robins LN, Schoenberg SP, Holmes SJ, Ratcliff KS, Benham A, Works J. 1985. Early home environment and retrospective recall: A test for concordance between siblings with and without psychiatric disorders. *American Journal of Orthopsychiatry*, 55(1): 27-41.

Rosenberg MS. 1987. Children of battered women: The effects of witnessing violence on their social problem-solving abilities. *Behavior Therapist*, 10(4): 85-89.

Santa Mina EE, Gallop RM. 1998. Childhood sexual and physical abuse and adult self-harm and suicidal behaviour: A literature review. *Canadian Journal of Psychiatry*, 43(8): 793-800.

Silverman AB, Reinherz HZ, Giaconia RM. 1996. The long-term sequelae of child and adolescent abuse: A longitudinal community study. *Child Abuse and Neglect*, 20(8): 709-723.

Silverman JG, Raj A, Mucci LA, Hathaway JE. 2001. Dating violence against adolescent girls and associated substance use, unhealthy weight control, sexual risk behavior, pregnancy, and suicidality. *Journal of the American Medical Association*, 286(5): 572-579.

Snyder HN, Sickmund M. 1999. *Juvenile Offenders and Victims: 1999 National Report.* Washington, DC: Office of Juvenile Justice and Delinquency Prevention.

Spaccarelli S. 1994. Stress, appraisal, and coping in child sexual abuse: A theoretical and empirical review. *Psychological Bulletin,* 116(2): 340-362.

Stein MB, Koverola C, Hanna C, Torchia MG, McClarty B. 1997. Hippocampal volume in women victimized by childhood sexual abuse. *Psychological Medicine,* 27(4): 951-959.

Stevenson J. 1999. The treatment of the long-term sequelae of child abuse. *Journal of Child Psychology and Psychiatry,* 40(1): 89-111.

Stratakis CA, Chrousos GP. 1995. Neuroendocrinology and pathophysiology of the stress system. *Annals of the New York Academy of Sciences,* 771: 1-18.

Straus MA, Hamby SL, Finkelhor D, Moore DW, Runyan D. 1998. Identification of child maltreatment with the Parent-Child Conflict Tactics Scales: Development and psychometric data for a national sample of American parents. *Child Abuse and Neglect,* 22(4): 249-270.

Taussig HN, Litrownik AJ. 1997. Self- and other-directed destructive behaviors: Assessment and relationship to type of abuse. *Child Maltreatment,* Vol 2(2): 172-182.

Teicher MH, Glod CA, Surrey J, Swett C. 1993. Early childhood abuse and limbic system ratings in adult psychiatric outpatients. *Journal of Neuropsychiatry and Clinical Neuroscience,* 5(3): 301-306.

Tiet QQ, Bird HR, Davies M, Hoven C, Cohen P, Jensen PS, Goodman S. 1998. Adverse life events and resilience. *Journal of the American Academy of Child and Adolescent Psychiatry,* 37(11): 1191-1200.

Trickett PK, Putnam FW. 1998. Developmental consequences of child sexual abuse. In: Trickett PK, Schellenbach CJ, Editors. *Violence Against Children in the Family and the Community.* (pp. 39-57). Washington, DC: American Psychological Association.

US DHHS (U.S. Department of Health and Human Services). 1999. *Mental Health: A Report of the Surgeon General.* Rockville, MD: U.S. Department of Health and Human Services, Substance Abuse and Mental Health Services Administration, Center for Mental Health Services, National Institutes of Health, National Institute of Mental Health.

US DHHS (U.S. Department of Health and Human Services). 2001a. *Child Maltreatment 1999.* Washington, DC: U.S. Government Printing Office.

US DHHS (U.S. Department of Health and Human Services). 2001b. *Youth Violence: A Report of the Surgeon General.* Rockville, MD: U.S. Department of Health and Human Services, Centers for Disease Control and Prevention, National Center for Injury Prevention and Control, Substance Abuse and Mental Health Services Administration, Center for Mental Health Services, National Institutes of Health, National Institute of Mental Health.

van der Kolk BA, Perry JC, Herman JL. 1991. Childhood origins of self-destructive behavior. *American Journal Psychiatry,* 148(12): 1665-1671.

Vissing YM, Straus MA, Gelles RJ, Harrop JW. 1991. Verbal aggression by parents and psychosocial problems of children. *Child Abuse and Neglect,* 15(3): 223-238.

Wagner BM. 1997. Family risk factors for child and adolescent suicidal behavior. *Psychological Bulletin,* 121(2): 246-298.

Widom CS. 1999. Posttraumatic stress disorder in abused and neglected children grown up. *American Journal of Psychiatry,* 156(8): 1223-1229.

Widom CS, Ireland T, Glynn PJ. 1995. Alcohol abuse in abused and neglected children followed-up: Are they at increased risk? *Journal of Studies on Alcohol,* 56(2): 207-217.

Widom CS, Shepard RL. 1996. Accuracy of adult recollections of childhood victimization, Part 1: Childhood physical abuse. *Psychological Assessment,* 8(4): 412-421.

Widom CSMS. 1997. Accuracy of adult recollections of childhood victimization, Part 2: Childhood sexual abuse. *Psychological Assessment.* 9(1): 34-46.

Williams LM. 1994. Recall of childhood trauma: A prospective study of women's memories of child sexual abuse. *Journal of Consulting and Clinical Psychology*, 62(6): 1167-1176.

Wilsnack SC, Vogeltanz ND, Klassen AD, Harris TR. 1997. Childhood sexual abuse and women's substance abuse: National survey findings. *Journal of Studies on Alcohol*, 58(3): 264-271.

Windle M, Windle RC, Scheidt DM, Miller GB. 1995. Physical and sexual abuse and associated mental disorders among alcoholic inpatients. *American Journal of Psychiatry*, 152(9): 1322-1328.

Wolfe DA, Scott K, Wekerle C, Pittman AL. 2001. Child maltreatment: Risk of adjustment problems and dating violence in adolescence. *Journal of the American Academy of Child and Adolescent Psychiatry*, 40(3): 282-289.

Yang B, Clum GA. 1996. Effects of early negative life experiences on cognitive functioning and risk for suicide: A review. *Clinical Psychology Review*, 16(3): 177-195.

Yang B, Clum GA. 2000. Childhood stress leads to later suicidality via its effect on cognitive functioning. *Suicide and Life-Threatening Behavior*, 30(3): 183-198.

Yehuda R. 2000. Biology of posttraumatic stress disorder. *Journal of Clinical Psychiatry*, 61 (Suppl 7): 14-21.

Life is what I want; dutifulness is also what I want. If I cannot have both, I would rather take dutifulness than life.

—MENCIUS (VI.A.10)

6

Society and Culture

Suicide carries a social and moral meaning in all societies. At both the individual and population levels, the suicide rate has long been understood to correlate with cultural, social, political, and economic forces (Giddens, 1964). Suicide is not everywhere linked with pathology but represents a culturally recognized solution to certain situations. As such, understanding suicide and attempting risk prevention requires an understanding of how suicide varies with these forces and how it relates to individual, group and contextual experiences.

Society and culture play an enormous role in dictating how people respond to and view mental health and suicide. Culture influences the way in which we define and experience mental health and mental illness, our ability to access care and the nature of the care we seek, the quality of the interaction between provider and patient in the health care system, and our response to intervention and treatment. This has important implications for treating individuals belonging to different racial, ethnic and cultural groups in the United States, as discussed in detail in the Surgeon General's Report, Mental Health: Culture, Race, and Ethnicity (US DHHS, 2001). Cultural variables have a far-ranging impact on suicide. They shape risk and protective factors as well as the availability and types of treatment that might intervene to lessen suicide. This chapter describes a framework for thinking about the continuum of cultural influences on suicide. Next, it explores the roles of the individual, of geographical location, of society, and of historical perspective on the social factors that impact the risk of suicide. Finally, some of the barriers to a full understanding of social and cultural forces on suicide are described.

FRAMEWORK: A SOCIAL SAFETY NET

Human connections through informal and formal organizations and
the tenor of social change are sources of both distressing and liberating
events. They also are the building blocks of a "safety net" that can push
individuals toward or pull them away from suicide as a "solution" to
their problems. A description of this social safety net originated early in
the history of suicide research and evolved over time (Durkheim, 1897/
1951). As illustrated in Figure 6-1, individuals in crises often find themselves in social and cultural situations where the both the integration (i.e.,
love, comfort, caring, feelings of belonging) and regulation (i.e., obliga-
tions, duties, responsibilities, oversight) are moderate in level. They would
be near the bottom of the net where the bonds to others are able to "catch"
the individual in crises, protecting them from suicide. However, as a
social or cultural group becomes too loosely bound together on either
dimension, individuals facing crises are not provided with bonds of either concern or obligation, are not provided with sufficient support to
deter the resort to suicide as a solution. These circumstances are presented at the front and left-hand side of the social safety net in Figure 6-1.
For example, historically, in the Austro-Hungarian Empire in the nineteenth century, suicide rates have been reported to be correlated with low
levels of social integration (Ausenda et al., 1991). In contemporary times,
individuals in the United Kingdom under age 35 who completed suicide

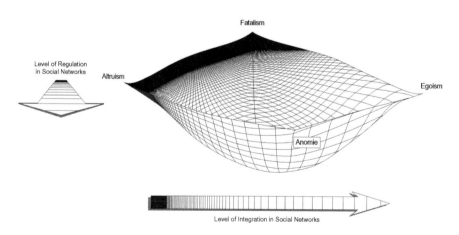

FIGURE 6-1 Networks and the Durkheimian Theory of Suicide. SOURCE: Pescosolido and Levy, 2002. Copyright © 2002. Reprinted with permission from Elsevier Science.

were found to be more "rootless" and have withdrawn socially compared to case-controls (Appleby et al., 1999; see also Trout, 1980, on the general role of social isolation on suicide). Bille-Brahe (1987) attributes the differences between Norway and Denmark's suicide rates to be due to difference in social integration; and in Norway, where the level of integration among young men was reported to be in decline, suicide rates among this groups are increasing. Over time, the doubling of the Irish suicide rate since 1945 appears to be directly related to lower levels of regulation and integration (Swanwick and Clare, 1997).

However, social and cultural groups can also be repressive, stifling, and conducive to suicide. In circumstances where the social group demands 100 percent loyalty and commitment, individuals lose their capacity to decide on options to crises. In these "greedy groups" as Coser and Coser (1979) called them, individuals are called on to demonstrate their commitment to the group and its causes by handing over the power of life and death to the group's needs (See Box 6-1; see right and back side of the social safety net). Under these circumstances, the social network ties of

---

BOX 6-1
Cases of "Altruistic" or "Fatalistic" Suicide: September 11, 2001, Jonestown, and the Branch Davidians

There have been a number of recorded instances of apparently ideologically motivated suicides best explained by understanding the power of the group beliefs over individuals. The terrorists who willingly gave their lives to promote the anti-American cause of the Al-Qaeda terrorist organization; the over 700 individuals in Jonestown, Guyana, who drank cyanide-laced Kool-Aid; and the members of David Koresh's religious group who allegedly set fire to their compound in the face of the federal government's attempt to enter, all represent cases where individuals were expected to give up their lives for the group and its cause. In some cases, there is debate whether these are situations where the attachment to the group was so strong that individuals had handed over their lives willingly (over-integration) or whether there was coercion (over-regulation) involved. Nevertheless, there is no evidence, for example, that the religious extremists who become "martyrs" have a mental illness. Palestinian and Israeli psychiatrists and psychologists who have interviewed "suicide bombers" (recruited or foiled) are impressed with their acceptance of suicide as a highly positive status, a moral status that is elevated by their commitment to a radical religious goal. These are all seen as suicides explained not by individual level decisions or problems but by the power of the social and cultural groups to which individuals belonged (Black, 1990; Maris, 1997; Pescosolido, 1994).

integration and regulation are so dense that the safety net closes up and forms a wall which shatters rather than supports (Pescosolido, 1994). Social and cultural forces that are this strong in their contribution to suicide must be understood fully and considered in risk prevention.

SOCIETY AND CULTURE IN SUICIDE

The social and cultural factors correlated with suicide have been considered at four different levels: individual, geographic, societal, and historical influences. The first, the individual, focuses on the influence of specific events in someone's life and their affiliation with and participation in social groups. An approach at this level assumes that critical life events or circumstances are responsible for suicides. For example, individuals who face divorce, economic strain, or political repression are often characterized as suicide risks. Here, empirical research often relies on the case-control method, comparing at-risk individuals to others, often matched by age and gender. When considering the second level, the focus is on the geographic distributions of suicide, often within countries, and socio-cultural profiles are assessed to see if they contribute to the suicide rate. These studies rely on suicide rates and characteristics of geographical areas. For example, individuals living in areas of low social integration (e.g., high divorce or unemployment rates) have higher risk of suicide. Third, research at the societal level has examined differences in suicide rates cross-nationally. Different countries, having different institutional arrangements, differ significantly with respect to suicide. For example, Northern European societies, especially Finland and Austria, have especially high rates, as do many Eastern European post-Soviet countries (e.g., Hungary and Russia; see Chapter 2, Table 2-1), whose suicide rates reflect a general worsening of health conditions in a time of societal turmoil and crisis with vast economic, political, and social changes. Further, Confucian societies, Japan and China in particular, have comparatively higher suicide rates than other Asian societies. Moreover, the discrepancy between male and female rate of suicide is much smaller for Asian, especially East Asian, societies. At the historical level of analysis, suicide rates are compared over time periods, to examine either short period effects or longer-term trends. Trends can be examined and correlated with changes over time in social and cultural indictors for various societies. Although these studies use very different approaches and consequently are difficult to compare and analyze (see van Egmond and Diekstra, 1990), they do reflect the importance of understanding context and historical period. The following sections will explore many of the social and cultural factors that influence suicide and will draw upon data from these multiple levels.

Family and Other Social Support

Across societies, family attachments influence suicide probability. Some researchers maintain that the family unit is the single most important factor in understanding suicide (e.g., in India, see Gehlot and Nathawat, 1983). However, others demonstrate that economic circumstance of life must also be considered (e.g., Leenaars and Lester, 1995, see also discussion of the interplay of these variables under occupation and suicide). Whatever the societal context, living alone increases the risk of suicide (Allebeck et al., 1987; Drake et al., 1986; Heikkinen et al., 1995). Family and other social support are protective factors, as will be discussed.

> My mother also was wonderful. She cooked meal after meal for me during my long bouts of depression, helped me with my laundry, and helped pay my medical bills. She endured my irritability and boringly bleak moods, drove me to the doctor, took me to pharmacies, and took me shopping. Like a gentle mother cat who picks up a straying kitten by the nape of its neck, she kept her marvelously maternal eyes wide-open, and, if I floundered too far away, she brought me back into a geographic and emotional range of security, food, and protection. Her formidable strength slowly eked its way into my depleted marrowbone. It, coupled with medicine for my brain and superb psychotherapy for my mind, pulled me through day after impossibly hard day (Jamison, An Unquiet Mind: A Memoir of Moods and Madness, 1995: 118–119).

Marital Status

Marital status provides an opportunity to see the convergence of sociodemographic effects on suicide; its influence on suicide rates varies by gender, culture and across the life course. In general, however, across many cultures, marriage is associated with lower overall suicide rates, while divorce and marital separation are associated with increased suicide risk (Allebeck et al., 1987; Charlton, 1995; Heikkinen et al., 1995; Leenaars and Lester, 1999; Lester and Moksony, 1989; Motohashi, 1991; Petronis et al., 1990; Zacharakis et al., 1998). Widowed persons are also more likely to complete suicide (e.g., Heikkinen et al., 1995; Kaprio et al., 1987; Li, 1995; Ross et al., 1990; Zacharakis et al., 1998; Zonda, 1999). Other studies suggest that being single also influences the likelihood of committing suicide (e.g., Charlton, 1995; Heikkinen et al., 1995; Li, 1995; Qin et al.,

2000). Results for suicide attempts and marital status are slightly different. As seen with completions, divorced and single individuals were over-represented among suicide attempters (Schmidtke et al., 1996). However, a study in the Netherlands found the lowest overall rates of attempts were among the widowed (Arensman et al., 1995), perhaps reflecting the lethality of attempts among this cohort (see Chapter 2).

Cultural context provides insight into the role of marital status in suicide. In the United States, Stack (1996) found that among African-Americans, divorce or death of a spouse significantly raised the risk of suicide, but being single did not. The strength of the association between marital status and suicide was less than the effect for whites, which the author suggests is due to stronger family ties.

The impact of marital status also differs for men and women, and varies across the life course. Models that account for gender often have found that divorce increases suicide risk in men only; in women divorce does not seem to exert a strong influence on suicide (e.g., Kposowa, 2000; Pescosolido and Wright, 1990). In Israel, increased divorce rates between 1960 and 1989 were associated with higher suicide rates for men and lower suicide rates for women (Lester, 1997). In contemporary Pakistan, suicides were more prevalent in married than unmarried women (Khan and Reza, 2000). One controlled study (Heikkinen et al., 1995) found that suicides were especially common among never-married men ages 30-39 compared to the general population. Theoretical interpretations of this data frequently echo the suppositions of Durkheim, who proposed that marriage is protective when it is not over- or under-regulating, and provides social integration and support through a strong family network (Durkheim, 1897/1951). For example, reflecting Durkheim's notion that very early marriage for men is "over-regulating," high proportions of never-married populations are related to lower suicide rates among young men (Pescosolido and Wright, 1990).

Although the research in this area is incomplete, these results caution against generalizing on the basis of any single sociodemographic factor. Heikkinen and colleagues (1995) suggest that some of the age-related variations in social factors for suicide may be better explained by mental illness and alcohol abuse. An analysis by Qin and colleagues (2000) supported this theory. Controlling for psychiatric hospitalization, they found that marital status was no longer an independent significant suicide risk factor for women. Other research suggests that the quality of the marital bond may be most important; domestic violence seems to increase risk for suicide ideation and attempts across the world (McCauley et al., 1995; Muelleman et al., 1998; Roberts et al., 1997; WHO, 2001). It has also been suggested that when marital ties represent the only or primary source of social integration and support, the dissolution of the marriage will have an especially strong effect on increasing suicide risk (Pescosolido and Wright, 1990). Integration of individual-level variables is necessary to understand the confluence of these factors.

Parenthood

Being a parent, particularly for mothers, appears to decrease the risk of suicide. In a prospective study of over 900,000 women followed for 15 years, Hoyer and Lund (1993) noted that both having children and the number of children decreased the risk of suicide. Across countries, having a young child appears to be a significant protective factor for women (de Castro and Martins, 1987; Qin et al., 2000). Pregnant women have a lower risk of suicide than women of childbearing age who are not pregnant (Marzuk et al., 1997).

Family Discord and Connectedness

Discord within the family also has an impact on suicide. Increases in the suicide rates in Ireland between 1970 and 1985 were correlated with a general decline in social cohesion as marked by a fall in the marriage rate and rise in the number of separated couples (Kelleher and Daly, 1990). A study in Scotland (Cavanagh et al., 1999) demonstrated that among patients with mental disorders, family conflict increased the risk of suicide by about a factor of 9. The effect of domestic discord also can influence the suicide rate for children and adolescents. Adolescents who had lived in single parent families or who were exposed to parent–child discord were more likely than matched controls to complete suicide (Brent et al., 1994; see also the case of young Canadians, Trovato, 1992). Furthermore, Tedeschi (1999) found that exposure to trauma, such as violence, predicts poor outcomes in children, especially if parental responses are inadequate (Bat-Aion and Levy-Shiff, 1993; Garbarino and Kostelny, 1993) (see also Chapter 5). But if parental physical and mental health are sound, children can do surprisingly well even in the face of terrorism (Freud and Burlingham, 1943; Miller, 1996).

On the other hand, some researchers (Borowsky et al., 2001; Resnick et al., 1997) have noted that perceived parental and family connectedness significantly protected against suicidality for youth. Other studies also demonstrated a protective effect of family connectedness and cohesion on suicidal behavior among American Indian and Alaska Native youth (Borowsky et al., 1999), Mexican American teenagers (Guiao and Esparza, 1995), and a largely white sample of adolescents (Rubenstein et al., 1989).

Social Support

Those who enjoy close relationships with others cope better with various stresses, including bereavement, rape, job loss, and physical illness (Abbey and Andrews, 1985; Perlman and Rook, 1987), and enjoy better psychological and physical health (IOM, 2001; Sarason et al., 1990). Studies have documented that social support can attentuate severity of depression and can speed remission of depression in at-risk groups such as immigrants and the physically ill (Barefoot et al., 2000; Brummett et al., 1998; Shen and Takeuchi, 2001). Studies of youth at risk for adverse outcomes, including suicide, have demonstrated that social support potently buffers the effects of negative life events (Carbonell et al., 1998; O'Grady and Metz, 1987; Vance et al., 1998).

As mentioned above, completed suicide occurs more often in those who are socially isolated and lack supportive family and friendships (e.g., Allebeck et al., 1988; Appleby et al., 1999; Drake et al., 1986). Studies from across sundry countries and ethnic groups show that suicide attempts and ideation among youths and adults correlate with low social support (De Wilde et al., 1994; Eskin, 1995; Hovey, 1999; Hovey, 2000a; Hovey, 2000b; Ponizovsky and Ritsner, 1999), with one study suggesting that perceived social support may account for about half the variance in suicide potential for youth (D'Attilio et al., 1992). Research has demonstrated that social support moderates suicidal ideation and risk of suicide attempts among various racial/ethnic groups, abused youths and adults, those with psychiatric diagnoses, and those facing acculturation stress (Borowsky et al., 1999; Hovey, 1999; Kaslow et al., 1998; Kotler et al., 2001; Nisbet, 1996; Rubenstein et al., 1989; Thompson et al., 2000; Yang and Clum, 1994).

Evidence suggests different mechanisms of support's influence. Social support sometimes represents part of a protective process that increases self-efficacy and thereby reduces suicidal behavior (Thompson et al., 2000). At other times social support more directly reduces suicidality via reducing psychic distress (Schutt et al., 1994). Furthermore, family and friendship support appear to play somewhat different roles in protecting against suicidality (Rubenstein et al., 1989; Veiel et al., 1988); men and woment may differ in use and types of social support (Heikkinen et al., 1994; Mazza and Reynolds, 1998).

Effective treatment for suicidality, whether medical or psychosocial, involves human contact and support (see Chapter 7). Recent suicide prevention programming to increase social support and other positive variables (e.g., Thompson et al., 2000) builds on emerging evidence suggesting a greater ameliorative effect of increasing protective factors than reducing risk (Borowsky et al., 1999; Vance et al., 1998).

Religion and Religiosity

In general, participation in religious activities is a protective factor for suicide. In the United States, areas with higher percentages of individuals without religious affiliation report correspondingly higher suicide rates (Pescosolido and Georgianna, 1989). Annual variation in the suicide rate tends to correlate with annual variation in church attendance (Martin, 1984). Furthermore, older adults (50 or more years of age) who are involved with organized religion are less likely to complete suicide (Nisbet et al., 2000). Similarly, areas in the former Soviet Union with a strong tradition of religion had lower suicide rates from 1965 to 1984 (e.g., the Caucasus and Central Asia; Varnik and Wasserman, 1992).

The protection afforded by religion may have several components. Involvement with religion may provide a social support system through active social networks (see Stack, 1992; Stack and Wasserman, 1992). Suicide may be reduced with religious affiliation because of the proscription against the act (e.g., Ellis and Smith, 1991). Belief structures and spiritualism may also be protective at an individual level as a coping resource (e.g., Conway, 1985-1986; Koenig et al., 1992) and via creating a sense of purpose and hope (see Chapter 3 on these protective factors) (e.g., Herth, 1989; Werner, 1992; 1996).

Religious Affiliation

Historically, studies of Western Europe indicated that those countries or regions within countries that were Catholic as opposed to those that were Protestant had lower suicide rates; this has been proposed to be related to increased social contact and affiliation in practiced Catholicism (Durkheim, 1897/1951; Masaryk, 1970). In the United States, this classic hypothesis also has received empirical support (Breault, 1986; Lester, 2000b). However, unlike much of Europe, the United States has experienced intensive and widespread denominationalism among Protestant groups. While religion continues to be correlated differentially with suicide, it appears that areas with both a greater presence of Catholics and evangelical or conservative types of Protestantism (e.g., Southern Baptist) report lower suicide rates compared to those with higher representation of mainline or institutional Protestantism (e.g., Episcopalian, Unitarian). The presence of Jewish adherents results in a small but inconsistent effect on reducing suicide rates (Pescosolido and Georgianna, 1989). However, the proportion of Islamic adherents does not appear to be related to suicide rates (Lester, 2000a).

This research points to the social ties formed (by volition and obligation) across these different religious groups rather than differences in dogma. This conclusion is further supported by evidence that indicates that in the "historical hubs" of religions (e.g., Lutherans in the Midwest, Jews in the Northeast), the protective effects of religious affiliation are stronger. Conversely, where religious adherents are located outside of these places, the effect of affiliation on suicide (e.g., Jews and Catholics in the South) may produce more suicides. It has been suggested that it is precisely in those places where religions have constructed institutions of assistance and informal communities of support that religion's protective effects are strongest (Pescosolido, 1990).

Studies at the individual level of assessment further explicate the role of religion in reducing risk of suicide. Maris (1981) compared suicide rates among Catholics and Protestants in Chicago between 1966 and 1968. He found that for all age groups and across both sexes, the suicide rate for Protestants was greater than the suicide rate for Catholics. Immigrants to the United States who identified as Catholic report significantly lower lifetime rates of suicide ideation (3.7% vs. 11.8%) and suicide attempts (1.6% vs. 2.6%) than non-Catholic immigrants. Scores on church attendance, perception of religiosity, and influence of religion were negatively associated with suicidal ideation. When sex, marital status, and socioeconomic status were factored in, the perceived influence of the religion item was the strongest significant independent predictor of suicidal ideation. Those individuals who perceived religion to be influential in their lives reported less suicidal ideation, and those individuals who attended church more often reported less suicidal ideation. These findings yielded no support for the notion that affiliation with Catholicsm shows less suicide risk than with other religions, as church attendance rather than religious affiliation accounted for most of the variation in suicide attitudes. These findings do, however, lend support to the notion that religiosity plays a protective role against suicide. Although most studies of religion and suicide have focused on adult samples, some have found that church attendance among youths of various ethnic/racial backgrounds reduces suicide risk, including suicide attempts (Conrad, 1991; Kirmayer et al., 1998; 1996). A large meta-analysis of U.S. adolescent data that controlled for sociodemographic variables indicates that religiousness decreases risk of suicide ideation and attempts in youths (Donahue, 1995).

Religious Beliefs

Actively religious North Americans are much less likely than nonreligious people to abuse drugs and alcohol (associated with suicide), to divorce (associated with suicide), and to complete suicide (Batson et al., 1993; Colasanto and Shriver, 1989). Stack and Lester (1991) found that those individuals who attended church more often reported less approval of suicide as a solution to life's problems. In a study involving 100 college students, Ellis and Smith (1991), using the Reasons for Living Inventory (Linehan et al., 1983) and the Spiritual Well-Being Scale (Paloutzian and Ellison, 1982), found results that strongly indicate a high positive relationship between an individual's religious well-being (faith in God) and that person's moral objections to suicide; existential well-being correlated with adaptive survival and coping beliefs (see Chapter 3). Decades-long study of at-risk individuals has also suggested that religious involvement and beliefs can influence positive outcomes by providing persons with a sense of meaning and purpose (Werner, 1992; 1996).

Several epidemiologic studies have reported lower rates of depression among religious persons, whether healthy or medically ill (Kendler et al., 1997; Kennedy et al., 1996; Koenig et al., 1992; Koenig et al., 1997; Pressman et al., 1990). Koenig et al. (1998) also found that intrinsic religiousness (i.e., religious beliefs representing a person's primary, unifying life motive) significantly increased the speed of remission from depression by 70 percent for every 10-point increase on the Hoge Intrinsic Religiousness scale. These changes were independent of other factors predicted to speed remission, including changing physical health status, religious activity, and social support.

Religious activity has also been found to be protective against suicide risk factors such as alcohol abuse, drug abuse, and anxiety disorder (Braam et al., 1997a; Braam et al., 1997b; Gorsuch, 1995; Koenig et al., 1992; Koenig et al., 1993; Koenig et al., 1994; Pressman et al., 1990). Further, a number of studies provide some evidence that spiritual protective factors (e.g., religious beliefs) may inoculate individuals against stressful life experiences (Conway, 1985-1986; Koenig et al., 1999; McRae, 1984; Pargament, 1990; Pargament et al., 1998; Park and Cohen, 1993; Park et al., 1990). At least one study has found attenuation of immune-inflammatory responses in those who regularly attend religious activities that could not be explained by differences in depression, negative life events, or other covariates (Koenig et al., 1997).

Koenig et al. (1998) noted that using spiritual/religious practices to treat depression and anxiety has been found effective. Propst et al. (1992) found religious therapy resulted in significantly faster recovery from depression when compared with standard secular cognitive-behavioral therapy. Similarly, Azhar et al. (1994) randomized 62 Muslim patients with generalized anxiety disorder to either traditional treatment (supportive therapy and anxiolytic drugs) or traditional treatment plus religious psychotherapy. Religious psychotherapy involved the use of prayer and reading verses of the Holy Koran specific to the person's situation. Patients receiving religious psychotherapy showed significantly more rapid improvement in anxiety symptoms than those receiving traditional therapy. Such studies suggest that being exposed to spiritual protective factors may also provide some protection from some types of mental illness associated with suicide.

Cultural Values and Suicide

In some cultures, suicide is morally acceptable under particular circumstances. Although most Western religions forbid suicide (see Chapter 1), some Eastern religions are more accepting. Among Buddhist monks for example, self-sacrifice for religious reasons can be viewed as an honorable act. During the Vietnam War, Buddhist monks set themselves on fire in protest (Kitagawa, 1989). In Japan, attitudes toward suicide are mixed, but some sanction and even glorify suicide when done for "good" reasons for controlling one's own destiny (Tierney, 1989). The Hindu code of conduct condones suicide for incurable diseases or great misfortune (Weiss, 1994).

Other cultural traditions sanction suicide. For example, in India it is acceptable for a widow to burn herself on her husband's funeral pyre in order to remain connected to her husband rather than to become an outcast in society. The traditional belief is that with this act, a husband and wife will be blessed in paradise and in their subsequent rebirth (Tousignant et al., 1998). In Japan, hara-kiri was a traditional suicide completed by warriors in the feudal era (Andriolo, 1998) and as recently at 1945 army officers completed suicide after the defeat of Japan (Takahashi, 1997). Suicide by hara-kiri, a disembowelment, is slow and painful and considered by some to symbolize exercising power over death (Takahashi, 1997).

Some cultures see suicide as an acceptable option in particular situations. Suicide in Japan may be a culturally acceptable response to disgrace. Furthermore, it is more acceptable to kill one's children along with oneself than to complete suicide alone, leaving the children in others' care (Iga, 1996; Sakuta, 1995). Similarly, in the Pacific region, suicide represents one culturally recognized response to domestic violence (Counts, 1987). Wolf (1975) reports that Chinese women with no children can demonstrate their faithfulness to their husbands through suicide upon their spouse's death.

Clearly, a society's perception of suicide and its cultural traditions can influence the suicide rate. Greater societal stigma against suicide is thought to be protective from suicide, while lesser stigma may increase suicide. Chapter 9 discusses further the ways in which stigma and perceptions of suicide may affect suicide and mental health care in general.

Economic Influences and Socioeconomic Status

Epidemiological analyses reveal that occupation, employment status, and socioeconomic status (SES) affect the risk of suicide. A recent IOM report (2001) describes at length the influence of social factors (including employment and SES) on health in general. Many of the same issues exist when focusing on suicide. Some studies that address these issues for suicide and suicidal behavior are described here.

Occupation

Some professions have higher risk for suicide than others. Physicians and dentists, for example, have elevated suicide rates even after controlling for confounding demographic variables, whereas higher suicide rates for occupational groups such as police officers and manual laborers, may be best explained by the demographics of these subgroups (see Chapter 2). It is interesting that in some northern European countries, rates among physicians show gender differences; women having greater risk than men (in Sweden, see Arnetz et al., 1987; in England and Wales see Charlton, 1995; Hawton et al., 2001; in Finland, see Lindeman et al., 1997; Stefansson and Wicks, 1991). Some suggest that greater access to means among these professions contribute to the higher rates (Pitts et al., 1979). While some find that blue-collar workers are more likely to complete suicide, others find high suicide among professional classes (Kung et al., 1998), confirming earlier theories (e.g., Powell, 1958) suggesting that the risk of suicide is elevated at both ends of the occupational prestige spectrum. Chapter 2 describes recent research on this phenomenon.

Specific influences of occupation-related factors on suicide remain unclear. Mental illness and employment variables influence each other, with mental illness sometimes disrupting employment, and unemployment sometimes exacerbating mental illness. Research has implicated economic strain in marital disruption (e.g., Conger et al., 1990; Kinnunen and Pulkkinen, 1998; Vinokur et al., 1996; White and Rogers, 2000), and Zimmerman (1987) found, for example, that state welfare spending appears to influence suicide rates via increasing income and lowering divorce (see above section on marital status and suicide). The occupation-suicide relationship also demonstrates variability according to ethnic differences. One recent study (Wasserman and Stack, 1999) suggests no difference between Black and White suicide in high-status occupations when controlling demographic factors, whereas Whites evidence greater suicide rates for low-status jobs. South (1984), however, found a positive correlation between diminishing Black-White income gaps and Black suicide rates. Increased income has been shown to increase the risk for attempted suicide in African-American females (Nisbet, 1996). One hypothesis for such relationships (Kirk and Zucker, 1979) posits that as discrimination against Blacks decreases, they are less able to blame external factors/society for life difficulties, and so turn blame inward. Nisbet (1996) contends, however, that observations of income's effects on Black suicide rates most strongly reflect changes in African Americans' social support networks as their socioeconomic status changes.

HEADLINE: Four Ukrainians kill themselves in separate incidents
DATELINE: Kiev

Four Ukrainians ended their lives in Kiev in separate overnight incidents, the Interfax news agency reported Thursday.

The usual suicide rate in the Ukrainian capital is three or four a month, a city spokesman said.

One woman, 76, threw herself from the sixth floor balcony of a hospital where she was undergoing treatment. A man, 74, jumped from his window in an apartment high-rise.

Another retiree ended his life by pouring petrol over his body and setting himself on fire in his own apartment. Firemen responding to the scene were able to douse the blaze, but could not save him.

Though Ukraines economy is slowly improving, retirees are often forced to live on pensions as small as 20 dollars a month, sometimes not paid on time.

A man, 37, hanged himself in his house because of reported business problems.

More than 14,000 Ukrainians commit suicide every year, in a population of around 50 million, the report said.

SOURCE: Deutsche Presse-Agentur, November 23, 2000. Reprinted by permission of Deutsche Presse-Agentur.

Such transactional processes between individual characteristics and environmental contexts underscore the complexity of the issue and the lack of transactional, longitudinal research uncovering the relative contributions to suicide risk of occupational stress, professional milieu, discrimination and acculturation, demographics, and means availability.

Unemployment

Unemployment is clearly associated with increased rates of suicide. In a broad review (Platt, 1984), an analysis of individual and aggregate cross-sectional studies and individual and aggregate longitudinal studies showed that almost all demonstrated a greater rate of suicide and/or suicide attempts with unemployment. This relationship has been documented in many countries, including Canada, Australia, Germany, Italy, Trinidad and Tobago, England and Wales, and Taiwan (Cantor et al., 1995; Chuang and Huang, 1996; Hutchinson and Simeon, 1997; Preti and Miotto, 1999; Saunderson and Langford, 1996; respectively: Trovato, 1992; Weyerer and Wiedenmann, 1995). A recent study in the United States, based on National Longitudinal Mortality Study (Kposowa, 2001), revealed a 2-fold increase in risk of suicide among the unemployed. Some gender differences may exist, as noted by Crombie (1990) in an assessment of suicide across 16 countries (e.g., in: Japan, Goto et al., 1994; the U.S., Kposowa, 2001; England and Wales, Lewis and Sloggett, 1998; Italy, Platt et al., 1992; New Zealand, Rose et al., 1999; Northern Ireland, Snyder, 1992). Within Italian counties, for instance, the influence of unemployment on suicide rates was reported to be greater for men than women (Preti and Miotto, 1999). In the United States, a recent analysis (Kposowa, 2001) suggested that while the relationship is stronger in men within the short-term, when followed for 9 years, unemployed women were actually more vulnerable to suicide than unemployed men.

Increases in national unemployment rates have had a mixed influence on suicide rates. Increased unemployment in Ireland has been credited with increased suicide between 1978 and 1985 (Kelleher and Daly, 1990). On the other hand, unemployment rates did not predict suicide rates in Hong Kong from 1976 to 1992, or in either the United States or Canada from 1950 to 1980 (Leenaars et al., 1993; Lester, 1999). In Japan from 1953 to 1972, the suicide rate for both men and women was positively correlated with unemployment. However, after 1972 and through 1986, the relationship did not hold. This change was hypothesized to reflect larger changes in the global economy as a transition from an industrial to a service economy occurred in Japan as it did in many capitalist societies (Motohashi, 1991).

Socioeconomic Status

A strong predictor of suicide, across levels, time, and countries, is socioeconomic disadvantage. Overall suicide rates appear to be associated with indicators of economic distress (Stack, 2000). For example, suicide rates are highest in low-income areas within Stockholm and across

Sweden as a whole (Ferrada-Noli, 1997; Ferrada-Noli and Asberg, 1997). The same relationship holds true in Canada (Hasselback et al., 1991), Australia (Cantor et al., 1995), and London (Kennedy et al., 1999). In addition, perceptions of individuals' possibilities for earnings (i.e., permanent income) have been implicated in suicide risk (Hamermesh and Soss, 1974). Using individual level data on suicides of men in New Orleans, Breed (1963) documented a link between suicide and indicators of downward mobility, reduced income, and unemployment. In England and Wales, areas characterized by lower social class had higher rates of suicide (Kreitman et al., 1991). Even among those younger than 25, lower social status increased the likelihood of suicide compared to the local population (Hawton et al., 1999).

Similarly, societal-wide economic downturns have been linked to higher suicide rates. For instance in the United States, Wasserman (1984), using a multivariate time-series analysis, found that the average monthly duration of unemployment (1947 to 1977) and the Ayres business index (1910 to 1939) were related to the suicide rate. Pierce (1967) notes that the greatest changes in the economic cycle have been associated with greater increase in the suicide rate.[1] Reflecting the importance of social stratification, as discussed earlier, the greatest increases in the British suicide rate occurred in areas with the greatest absolute increase in social fragmentation and economic deprivation (Whitley et al., 1999). In Japan, Singapore, Taiwan, and Hong Kong following the decline of Asian post-World War II prosperity (La Vecchia et al., 2000; Schmidtke et al., 1999), suicide rates increased. In contrast, in the Nis region of Yugoslavia, the suicide rates dropped between 1987, when the country was economically and politically stable, and 1999, at the peak of the economic and political crisis (14.8/100,000 to 13.8 in males and 6.8 to 3.7 in females). Likewise, the rate in China remained high in its period of greatest economic growth (Chan et al., 2001). Phillips, Liu, and Zhang (1999) suggest that current high rates of suicide in China are related to social changes resulting from economic reforms that were instituted in 1978. These trends in suicide, repeated in many developing societies, suggest the destabilizing effects of current phases of social change spurred by economic shifts and further points to the critical role of the social environment and larger contextual forces.

Economic conditions can affect suicide in other ways as well. Alcohol consumption and marital discord can increase with financial difficulties, which can increase risk of suicide. Relocation of individuals or families can result as a consequence of unemployment or financial strain. The increased stress of breaking social bonds increase suicide risk (Stack, 2000).

---

[1]However, the Depression years saw a drop in the suicide rate from a high of 17 per 1000,000 in 1933 to a low 9.6 in 1944.

Those left behind may also be at increased risk. For example, in China, 100,000,000 economic migrants from rural to urban areas left behind young wives responsible for small children, care of the elderly, and farming. With limited economic support, many of these women complete suicide as a result of the tremendous pressure (Shiang et al., 1998).

The Political System

During time of war, suicide among the population is generally reduced (Lester, 1993; Somasundaram and Rajadurai, 1995). However, political coercion or violence can increase suicide. In the former Soviet Union, areas experiencing sociopolitical oppression (the Baltic states) and forced social change (Russia) had higher suicide rates compared to other regions (Varnik and Wasserman, 1992). While Sri Lanka's Tamils have long experienced a high suicide rate, its majority Sinhalese population experienced a low rate until the start of Civil War two decades ago, when its rate increased greatly (Marecek, 1998; Ratnayeke, 1998; Somasundaram and Rajadurai, 1995). Furthermore, war can promote altruistic suicides. In ancient times in China, for example, those soldiers thought to be particularly brave stepped forward in front of battle lines to complete suicide as a demonstration of the fierceness of their loyalty and determination against invading armies from Central Asia (Lin, 1990; Liu and Li, 1990).

General political activity such as United States presidential elections correlates with decreased suicide rates; researchers suggest that this is a consequence of stronger social integration during these times (Boor, 1981). However (Phillips and Feldman, 1973), this correlation is not supported by all studies (Wasserman, 1983).

The relationship between political, social and economic power and suicide rates is interesting, but direct data is limited. A positive correlation has been observed across 26 nations between male and female suicide rates and women's access to social, economic, and political power (Mayer, 2000). De Castro et al. (1988) showed that in Portugal, the rise of the female independence movement correlated with a significant rise in the female suicide rate, particularly among professional women living in urban areas. This change in the rate may have been mediated through an increase in alcohol use among the professional women subsequent to achieving greater independence. As mentioned in Chapter 2, infrequently-held professional roles (e.g., women entering male-dominated professions) appear to increase suicide risk, though precise pathways of influence remain unknown.

The discussions above regarding occupation/employment and socioeconomic status, and the discussion in Chapter 2 of racial and ethnic differences in suicidality allude to differential social power as reflected by

racial/ethnic and sexual discrimination. The relationship of power to suicide in these contexts is extremely complex; the power a certain group has
on a macro-social level must be disentangled from individuals' perceived
personal and interpersonal control, economic power, and self-perception
of the ability to foster change. Emerging areas of community and cultural
psychology refer to this latter concept as "sociopolitical control," and
have found evidence that sociopolitical control may moderate the relationship between certain risk factors and mental health outcomes (e.g.,
Zimmerman et al., 1999) by contributing to self-esteem and promoting
self-efficacy. Other research shows that lack of power may engender hopelessness and exacerbate stress. Studies that focus on these concepts could
help explicate phenomenological and etiological aspects of suicide among
marginalized and disadvantaged sub-populations.

Community Characteristics: Rural vs. Urban

Consistently, suicide rates are higher in rural areas than in urban
areas (see Chapter 2). In China, the rate is two to five times greater in the
rural regions (Ji et al., 2001; Jianlin, 2000; Phillips et al., 1999; Yip, 2001).
Young Chinese women kill themselves three times more often in rural
areas than in urban areas (Ji et al., 2001). This same trend has also been
documented in young males in Australia (Wilkinson and Gunnell, 2000).
Even among Greek adolescents where the suicide rate is relatively low,
urban areas reported significantly lower suicide rates than rural areas
(Beratis, 1991). In the Ukraine, suicide is also more frequent in rural areas
and in industrially developed regions than in the cities (Kryzhanovskaya
and Pilyagina, 1999). Over time in some countries, the effects of rural–
urban residence are changing. In Japan, for example, the discrepancy
between suicide rates in rural and urban districts increased from 1975 to
1985 but declined in subsequent years (Goto et al., 1994).

Social Changes and Suicide

From the beginnings of the social science study of suicide rates, mas-
sive social change, especially that evidenced by the rise of the industrial
age, has been implicated as a major cause of rising suicide rates (Masaryk,
1970; Porterfield, 1952). Not surprising then, is the recent decrease in
suicide in many Western European countries and the contrasting increase
in Eastern European countries (Sartorius, 1995). The rates in Russia during the post-Soviet era have increased, in keeping with an overall increase
in age-adjusted mortality and morbidity. Age-standardized suicide rates
have almost doubled between 1970 and 1995 in Latvia (Kalediene, 1999).
In the Ukraine, the suicide rate increased by 57 percent between 1988 and

1997 (Kryzhanovskaya and Pilyagina, 1999). However, during Perestroika in Russia (1984 to 1990), suicide rates declined by approximately 32 percent for males and 19 percent for females (Varnik et al., 1998). The decrease in female suicide was the same as seen in the rest of Europe, whereas the male decrease in suicide rate was 3.8 times that observed in other European countries. This large decrease in Russian male suicides coincided with a national, multi-pronged anti-alcoholism campaign over the same period. In this way, social circumstances interacted to provide increased hope for economic prosperity and social freedoms, with significantly reduced access to alcohol, creating a period associated with the greatest decrease in male suicide rates across the globe in the last 20 years (Wasserman and Varnik, 2001).

Suicide rates have declined in the Baltic countries (Estonia, Latvia, and Lithuania) since 1986, which marked the onset of turbulent social change (Varnik et al., 1994). Rancans and colleagues (2001) determined that the rapid swings in the suicide rate in Latvia between 1980 and 1998 could not be explained by the changing employment rate, a sudden drop in the GDP, or a rapid increase in first-time alcohol psychosis. Makinen (2000) concludes that, while suicide and social processes in Eastern Europe during recent periods of social change are clearly linked, there remain complexities regarding the mechanisms and the specific aspects of the social change that may affect suicide rates.

LaVecchi et al. (1994) analyzed World Health Organization data from 1955–1989 for 57 countries and suggested that trends are decreasing in many parts of the less developed world including Latin America and Asia (with the exception of Sri Lanka). Others contend that suicide rates have increased in less developed countries or among particular segments of the population in these countries (Makinen, 1997). For example, the rate of suicide in Sri Lanka has risen from modest levels to one of the highest in the world over the last 50 years (Marecek, 1998). In Singapore, the last 10 years shows a greater disparity in male and female suicide rates. Prior to this time, the gender gap had diminished, and the current discrepancy appears to result from decreasing rates among women rather than any real change in male suicide levels (Parker and Yap, 2001). Micronesia witnessed a spike among adolescents and youth in the 1970s and 1980s. Researchers attributed this "epidemic" to vast social changes associated with modernization and globalization, which resulted in the breakdown of traditional values and practices and the development of "normlessness" or anomie, especially among adolescents (Rubinstein, 1983). In Western Samoa, for example, the rise in suicide rates since 1970 has been hypothesized to result from rising expectations among adolescents in the context of fading opportunities due to Western Samoa's peripheral position in the world economy (Macpherson and Macpherson, 1987). In China, most recent data from the Chinese government for 2000 show a significant fall in suicide rate from 23 per 100,000 to 17 per 100,000.

CHALLENGES

Cross-National Differences: Real or Artifact?

Interpretation of cross-national suicide rates are subject to several limitations. First, different countries may assign different meaning and classification to the acts. Kelleher et al. (1998) report that countries with religious sanctions against suicide were less likely to report their suicide rates to the World Health Organization, and on average, their reported rates were lower than for countries without sanctions.[2] In India, suicide rates may be misrepresented due to traditional and unique cultural practices such as "dowry death," which is a category of deaths of young married women including both homicide and suicide following from intense coercion for payment of unpaid or additional dowry. It may be difficult to differentiate homicide from suicide in the investigation of such deaths (Khan and Ray, 1984; Leslie, 1998). Second, difference among countries may reflect the capacity of the emergency health care system to respond rather than differences in the intent of the individuals. For example, the high rate of suicide among young Chinese women may result from the lethality of available means in the face of limited treatment availability. Women living on farms in China often have ready access to extremely toxic pesticides. It is often not possible to obtain emergency treatment after these chemicals are ingested in an impulsive moment. Thus, cases that might end up as suicide attempts in the United States are fatal in China. Difference in the demographics of suicide attempts and completions between counties may reflect these artifacts of infrastructure rather than psychological or biological differences (Ji et al., 2001). Third, the organization and functioning of medico-legal officials across countries has long been thought to produce artifactual differences even between similar countries such as Britain and Scotland (Barraclough, 1972). Most developing societies lack registries and expertly trained officials to record suicide. Further, there are cross-national differences in the underlying logic of classifications systems. In India, for example, the classification scheme focuses on social stressors rather than psychopathology. In 1997, only 4.9 percent of all suicides were attributed to mental disorders, while other causes were cited for the remaining 95.1 percent (e.g., family problems (18.4 percent), love affairs (3.7 percent), poverty (3.4 percent)) (Gov-

---

[2]It is uncertain whether the rates are low because of the protective effects of religion or because of misrepresentation of cause of death.

ernment of India, 1999). Phillips and colleagues (1999) suggest that the high suicide rates in China might be due to lower deliberate miscalculations of rates there than in other countries where suicide is illegal or can elicit serious consequences for families.

Integrating Approaches

Individual and Aggregate Studies

Studies that integrate the events at an individual level with events at an aggregate level can be extremely valuable to the understanding of suicide risk. These studies are scarce. The few that have been done suggest that contextual level findings do not simply reflect summed individual level effects. For example, in one study in the United States, the influence of social and cultural characteristics at the county level (a lower level of aggregation) was not as strongly associated with suicide rates as at the county group level (a higher level of aggregation; Pescosolido and Mendelsohn, 1986). Theoretical and methodological barriers impede understanding how individuals facing similar personal crises respond differently depending on the social and cultural context in which they live their lives. For example, even with the classic findings regarding religion, it is essential to document whether it is only the Catholics in areas with high representation of Catholics who are "protected" from suicidal risk, whether the social context exerts a protective effect across the region, and whether being a member of a different group results in greater suicidal risk. Appendix A illustrates an approach that can be used to address some of these issues. As described in greater detail there, a breakdown of suicide rate by county shows geographic distributions. Using a spatial distribution of Bayes estimates reveals outliers, that is, counties that are unlike those surrounding them. For example, in the western United States and Alaska where suicide rates are typically high, a few counties have Bayes estimates that are consistent with the national average. Similarly, in the central United States where there is a high concentration of counties with the lowest suicide rates, there are also a few counties that exhibit the highest suicide rates. Identification of these spatial anomalies and examining the particular characteristics that account for them can be a fruitful area for further research.

A Biopsychosocial Understanding

The interactions between social environment and general health are well documented, and it is clear from the evidence that the mechanism goes beyond access to health care or exposure to environmental toxins

(IOM, 2001). Poverty, discrimination, and social isolation are associated with poor health. Links between mental illness and culture, race, and ethnicity also have been described (US DHHS, 1999; US DHHS, 2001). Risk factors are thought to involve everything from genetic variation in metabolism to the adverse effects of poverty and discrimination. These links are likely to extend to suicide, but the evidence is limited.

As described in this report, many factors impact the risk of suicide: social, psychological, and biological. Box 6-2 describes efforts to disentangle the roles of these factors among the Old Order Amish. Mental illness, personality and temperament, societal and individual experiential factors like economic depression, interpersonal loss, societal violence and childhood trauma, and the social context for these experiences are all important to consider in assessment of any individual. Psychic distress may be a common thread across cultures and diagnoses for those who are

---

BOX 6-2
**The Old Order Amish: Interplay of Genetic and
Socio-cultural Factors**

In studying 26 suicides over a 100 year period among the Amish of Pennsylvania, Egeland and Sussex (1985) found that suicides clustered in four primary pedigrees with heavy loading for bipolar, unipolar, and affective illnesses. Yet attempts to verify a specific genetic link have failed (Egeland et al., 1987; Kelsoe et al., 1989). While still cited as evidence for a genetic component for affective disorders and suicide (e.g., Roy, 1993), the specific link for inheritance among the Amish is unresolved. To understand suicide among the Amish, it is important to consider their social and cultural circumstances. While the Amish have rates of bipolar illness similar to the non-Amish population (Egeland et al., 1983), Amish communities have a high level of social integration. Consequently, individuals are at greater risk if their social support networks are affected or if the larger community faces crises. Kraybill et al. (1986) suggest that suicides clustered during times when the community as a whole was under stress from outside social pressure resulting from the modernization of agriculture and schooling. This is further supported by the socio-demographic profiles of the suicides. While the gender distribution (3 males to 1 female) did not vary from the surrounding area, they were predominant among the middle age groups, those most likely to confront the outside pressures. There were no suicides among youth (under 18). Elders (over 59) were also at much lower risk in comparison with the surrounding population. While these findings need to be interpreted cautiously because of the small number of cases, these patterns suggest the utility of and need for integrated biological, genetic, and social/behavioral science research.

suicidal. Despite years of research, we cannot predict who will commit suicide. African-American women, for example, have many risk factors including discrimination, poverty, exposure to violence, etc., but also have one of the lowest suicide rates. Why do some people with such adversity not commit suicide while others do? An understanding of this seemingly paradoxical relationship through biopsychosocial research is critical to the advancement of suicidology. Suicide can only be understood by integrating approaches that have historically remained distinct.

FINDINGS

• Culture strongly influences how individuals view suicide. Cultural values and social structures largely determine the type and degree of both stressors and support, availability of means and access to treatment, and social prescriptions or proscriptions concerning suicidal behavior.

• Across cultures, family cohesion and support acts as a buffer against suicidality; parenthood protects against suicide, particularly for women. Divorced and never-married status generally increases suicide risk, especially among men. Social support and various types of religious involvement and beliefs are protective against suicide.

• Unemployment and low socioeconomic status generally increase suicide risk. Societal-wide economic and social changes also influence the incidence of suicide. Social change can create economic hardship, increase family discord, result in migration or separation of families and friends, increase use of alcohol, etc. Investigation into the complex interaction of the macro-social and individual variables is valuable. Yet there are few studies that integrate the events at an individual level with events at an aggregate level.

The field requires additional research on the interactions of individual and aggregate level variables. Since biological, psychosocial, and sociological factors all amplify or buffer the risk of suicide, future research needs to incorporate interdisciplinary, multi-level approaches. Studies on the interactions of genetics and psychosocial, socio-political, and socioeconomic context, for example, are necessary.

Use of data from developing societies that comprise more than 80 percent of the world's population and look somewhat different than United States data may provide a more representative picture for poor and middle income countries. Contrasts among international suicide data also offer important insights into the influence of cultural/macro-social contexts on suicide.

• Cultures vary in their stigma against suicide, in treatment availability, in classifications of suicide and mental illness, and in the infrastructure for monitoring death by suicide. These differences render cross-national comparisons of suicidal behavior difficult.

New approaches and assessments are needed to ensure that social epidemiological findings are sufficiently powerful in predicting suicide to overcome classification differences that arise from diverse understandings and recording of behaviors that may be considered suicides. In addition, research based on ethnography and other qualitative methods provides greater detail about the setting, conditions, process, and outcome of suicide and should be developed to deepen and make more valid psychological autopsy studies.

REFERENCES

Abbey A, Andrews FM. 1985. Modeling the psychological determinants of life quality. *Social Indicators Research*, 16(1): 1-34.

Allebeck P, Allgulander C, Fisher LD. 1988. Predictors of completed suicide in a cohort of 50,465 young men: Role of personality and deviant behaviour. *British Medical Journal*, 297(6642): 176-178.

Allebeck P, Varla A, Kristjansson E, Wistedt B. 1987. Risk factors for suicide among patients with schizophrenia. *Acta Psychiatrica Scandinavica*, 76(4): 414-419.

Andriolo KR. 1998. Gender and the cultural construction of good and bad suicides. *Suicide and Life-Threatening Behavior*, 28(1): 37-49.

Appleby L, Cooper J, Amos T, Faragher B. 1999. Psychological autopsy study of suicides by people aged under 35. *British Journal of Psychiatry*, 175: 168-174.

Arensman E, Kerkhof AJ, Hengeveld MW, Mulder JD. 1995. Medically treated suicide attempts: A four year monitoring study of the epidemiology in The Netherlands. *Journal of Epidemiology and Community Health*, 49(3): 285-289.

Arnetz BB, Horte LG, Hedberg A, Theorell T, Allander E, Malker H. 1987. Suicide patterns among physicians related to other academics as well as to the general population. Results from a national long-term prospective study and a retrospective study. *Acta Psychiatrica Scandinavica*, 75(2): 139-143.

Ausenda G, Lester D, Yang B. 1991. Social correlates of suicide and homicide in the Austro-Hungarian Empire in the 19th century. *European Archives of Psychiatry and Clinical Neuroscience*, 240(4-5): 301-302.

Azhar MZ, Varma SL, Dharap AS. 1994. Religious psychotherapy in anxiety disorder patients. *Acta Psychiatrica Scandinavica*, 90(1): 1-3.

Barefoot JC, Brummett BH, Helms MJ, Mark DB, Siegler IC, Williams RB. 2000. Depressive symptoms and survival of patients with coronary artery disease. *Psychosomatic Medicine*, 62(6): 790-795.

Barraclough BM. 1972. Are the Scottish and English suicide rates really different? *British Journal of Psychiatry*, 120(556): 267-273.

Bat-Aion N, Levy-Shiff R. 1993. Children in war: Stress and coping reactions under the threat of scud missile attacks and the effect of proximity. In: Leavitt LA, Fox NA, Editors. *The Psychological Effects of War and Violence on Children*. (pp. 143-161). Hillsdale, NJ: Lawrence Erlbaum Associates.

Batson CD, Schoenrade P, Ventis WL. 1993. *Religion and the Individual: A Social-Psychological Perspective*. New York: Oxford University Press.

Beratis S. 1991. Suicide among adolescents in Greece. *British Journal of Psychiatry*, 159: 515-519.

Bille-Brahe U. 1987. Suicide and social integration. A pilot study of the integration levels in Norway and Denmark. *Acta Psychiatrica Scandinavica. Supplement*, 336: 45-62.

Black A Jr. 1990. Jonestown—two faces of suicide: A Durkheimian analysis. *Suicide and Life-Threatening Behavior*, 20(4): 285-306.

Boor M. 1981. Effects of United States presidential elections on suicides and other causes of death. *American Sociological Review*, 46: 616-618.

Borowsky IW, Ireland M, Resnick MD. 2001. Adolescent suicide attempts: Risks and protectors. *Pediatrics*, 107(3): 485-493.

Borowsky IW, Resnick MD, Ireland M, Blum RW. 1999. Suicide attempts among American Indian and Alaska Native youth: Risk and protective factors. *Archives of Pediatrics and Adolescent Medicine*, 153(6): 573-580.

Braam AW, Beekman AT, Deeg DJ, Smit JH, van Tilburg W. 1997a. Religiosity as a protective or prognostic factor of depression in later life: Results from a community survey in The Netherlands. *Acta Psychiatrica Scandinavica*, 96(3): 199-205.

Braam AW, Beekman AT, van Tilburg TG, Deeg DJ, van Tilburg W. 1997b. Religious involvement and depression in older Dutch citizens. *Social Psychiatry and Psychiatric Epidemiology*, 32(5): 284-291.

Breault KD. 1986. Suicide in America: A test of Durkheim's theory of religious and family integration, 1933-1980. *American Journal of Sociology*, 92(3): 628-656.

Breed W. 1963. Occupational mobility and suicide among white males. *American Sociological Review*, 28: 179-188.

Brent DA, Perper JA, Moritz G, Liotus L, Schweers J, Balach L, Roth C. 1994. Familial risk factors for adolescent suicide: A case-control study. *Acta Psychiatrica Scandinavica*, 89(1): 52-58.

Brummett BH, Babyak MA, Barefoot JC, Bosworth HB, Clapp-Channing NE, Siegler IC, Williams RB Jr, Mark DB. 1998. Social support and hostility as predictors of depressive symptoms in cardiac patients one month after hospitalization: A prospective study. *Psychosomatic Medicine*, 60(6): 707-713.

Cantor CH, Slater PJ, Najman JM. 1995. Socioeconomic indices and suicide rate in Queensland. *Australian Journal of Public Health*, 19(4): 417-420.

Carbonell DM, Reinherz HZ, Giaconia RM. 1998. Risk and resilience in late adolescence. *Child and Adolescent Social Work Journal*, 15(4): 251-272.

Cavanagh JT, Owens DG, Johnstone EC. 1999. Life events in suicide and undetermined death in south-east Scotland: A case-control study using the method of psychological autopsy. *Social Psychiatry and Psychiatric Epidemiology*, 34(12): 645-650.

Chan KP, Hung SF, Yip PS. 2001. Suicide in response to changing societies. *Child and Adolescent Psychiatric Clinics of North America*, 10(4): 777-795.

Charlton J. 1995. Trends and patterns in suicide in England and Wales. *International Journal of Epidemiology*, 24 (Suppl 1): S45-S52.

Chuang HL, Huang WC. 1996. A reexamination of "Sociological and economic theories of suicide: A comparison of the U.S.A. and Taiwan". *Social Science and Medicine*, 43(3): 421-423.

Colasanto D, Shriver J. 1989. Mirror of America: Middle-aged face marital crisis. *Gallup Report, No. 284*, 34-38.
Conger RD, Elder GHJ, Lorenz FO, Conger KJ, Simons RL, Whitbeck LB, Huck S, Melby JN. 1990. Linking economic hardship to marital quality and instability. *Journal of Marriage and the Family*, 52(3): 643-656.
Conrad N. 1991. Where do they turn? Social support systems of suicidal high school adolescents. *Journal of Psychosocial Nursing and Mental Health Services*, 29(3): 14-20.
Conway K. 1985-1986. Coping with the stress of medical problems among Black and White elderly. *International Journal of Aging and Human Development*, 21(1): 39-48.
Coser RL, Coser L. 1979. Jonestown as perverse utopia. *Dissent*, 26: 158-163.
Counts DA. 1987. Female suicide and wife abuse: A cross-cultural perspective. *Suicide and Life-Threatening Behavior*, 17(3): 194-204.
Crombie IK. 1990. Can changes in the unemployment rates explain the recent changes in suicide rates in developed countries? *International Journal of Epidemiology*, 19(2): 412-416.
D'Attilio JP, Campbell BM, Lubold P, Jacobson T, Richard JA. 1992. Social support and suicide potential: Preliminary findings for adolescent populations. *Psychological Reports*, 70(1): 76-78.
de Castro EF, Martins I. 1987. The role of female autonomy in suicide among Portuguese women. *Acta Psychiatrica Scandinavica*, 75(4): 337-343.
de Castro EF, Pimenta F, Martins I. 1988. Female independence in Portugal: Effect on suicide rates. *Acta Psychiatrica Scandinavica*, 78(2): 147-155.
De Wilde EJ, Kienhorst CW, Diekstra RF, Wolters WH. 1994. Social support, life events, and behavioral characteristics of psychologically distressed adolescents at high risk for attempting suicide. *Adolescence*, 29(113): 49-60.
Donahue MJ. 1995. Religion and the well-being of adolescents. *Journal of Social Issues*, 51(2): 145-160.
Drake RE, Gates C, Cotton PG. 1986. Suicide among schizophrenics: A comparison of attempters and completed suicides. *British Journal of Psychiatry*, 149: 784-787.
Durkheim E. 1897/1951. Translated by JA Spaulding and G Simpson. *Suicide: A Study in Sociology*. New York: Free Press.
Egeland JA, Gerhard DS, Pauls DL, Sussex JN, Kidd KK, Allen CR, Hostetter AM, Housman DE. 1987. Bipolar affective disorders linked to DNA markers on chromosome 11. *Nature*, 325(6107): 783-787.
Egeland JA, Hostetter AM, Eshleman SK 3rd. 1983. Amish Study, III: The impact of cultural factors on diagnosis of bipolar illness. *American Journal of Psychiatry*, 140(1): 67-71.
Egeland JA, Sussex JN. 1985. Suicide and family loading for affective disorders. *Journal of the American Medical Association*, 254(7): 915-918.
Ellis JB, Smith PC. 1991. Spiritual well-being, social desirability and reasons for living: Is there a connection? *International Journal of Social Psychiatry*, 37(1): 57-63.
Eskin M. 1995. Suicidal behavior as related to social support and assertiveness among Swedish and Turkish high school students: A cross-cultural investigation. *Journal of Clinical Psychology*, 51(2): 158-172.
Ferrada-Noli M. 1997. Social psychological variables in populations contrasted by income and suicide rate: Durkheim revisited. *Psychological Reports*, 81(1): 307-316.
Ferrada-Noli M, Asberg M. 1997. Psychiatric health, ethnicity and socioeconomic factors among suicides in Stockholm. *Psychological Reports*, 81(1): 323-332.
Freud A, Burlingham D. 1943. *War and Children*. New York: International Universities Press.
Garbarino J, Kostelny K. 1993. Children's response to war: What do we know? In: Leavitt LA, Fox NA, Editors. *The Psychological Effects of War and Violence on Children*. (pp. 23-39). Hillsdale, NJ: Lawrence Erlbaum Associates.

Gehlot PS, Nathawat SS. 1983. Suicide and family constellation in India. *American Journal of Psychotherapy*, 37(2): 273-278.

Giddens A. 1964. Suicide, attempted suicide and the suicidal threat. *Man: A Record of Anthropological Science*, 64: 115-116.

Gorsuch RL. 1995. Religious aspects of substance abuse and recovery. *Journal of Social Issues*, 51(65-83).

Goto H, Nakamura H, Miyoshi T. 1994. Epidemiological studies on regional differences in suicide mortality and its correlation with socioeconomic factors. *Tokushima Journal of Experimental Medicine*, 41(3-4): 115-132.

Government of India, National Crime Records Bureau, Ministry of Home Affairs. 1999. *Accidental Death and Suicide in India 1997*.

Guiao IZ, Esparza D. 1995. Suicidality correlates in Mexican American teens. *Issues in Mental Health Nursing*, 16(5): 461-479.

Hamermesh DS, Soss NM. 1974. An economic theory of suicide. *Journal of Political Economy*, 82(1): 83-98.

Hasselback P, Lee KI, Mao Y, Nichol R, Wigle DT. 1991. The relationship of suicide rates to sociodemographic factors in Canadian census divisions. *Canadian Journal of Psychiatry*, 36(9): 655-659.

Hawton K, Clements A, Sakarovitch C, Simkin S, Deeks JJ. 2001. Suicide in doctors: A study of risk according to gender, seniority and specialty in medical practitioners in England and Wales, 1979-1995. *Journal of Epidemiology and Community Health*, 55(5): 296-300.

Hawton K, Houston K, Shepperd R. 1999. Suicide in young people. Study of 174 cases, aged under 25 years, based on coroners' and medical records. *British Journal of Psychiatry*, 175: 271-276.

Heikkinen M, Aro H, Lonnqvist J. 1994. Recent life events, social support and suicide. *Acta Psychiatrica Scandinavica. Supplement*, 377: 65-72.

Heikkinen ME, Isometsa ET, Marttunen MJ, Aro HM, Lonnqvist JK. 1995. Social factors in suicide. *British Journal of Psychiatry*, 167(6): 747-753.

Herth KA. 1989. The relationship between level of hope and level of coping response and other variables in patients with cancer. *Oncology Nursing Forum*, 16(1): 67-72.

Hovey JD. 1999. Moderating influence of social support on suicidal ideation in a sample of Mexican immigrants. *Psychological Reports*, 85(1): 78-79.

Hovey JD. 2000a. Acculturative stress, depression, and suicidal ideation among Central American immigrants. *Suicide and Life-Threatening Behavior*, 30(2): 125-139.

Hovey JD. 2000b. Acculturative stress, depression, and suicidal ideation in Mexican immigrants. *Cultural Diversity and Ethnic Minority Psychology*, 6(2): 134-151.

Hoyer G, Lund E. 1993. Suicide among women related to number of children in marriage. *Archives of General Psychiatry*, 50(2): 134-137.

Hutchinson GA, Simeon DT. 1997. Suicide in Trinidad and Tobago: Associations with measures of social distress. *International Journal of Social Psychiatry*, 43(4): 269-275.

Iga M. 1996. Cultural aspects of suicide: The case of Japanese oyako shinju (parent-child suicide). *Archives of Suicide Research*, 2: 87-102.

IOM (Institute of Medicine). 2001. *Health and Behavior: The Interplay of Biological, Behavioral, and Societal Influences*. Washington, DC: National Academy Press.

Jamison KR. 1995. *An Unquiet Mind: A Memoir of Moods and Madness*. New York: A.A. Knopf.

Ji J, Kleinman A, Becker AE. 2001. Suicide in contemporary China: A review of China's distinctive suicide demographics in their sociocultural context. *Harvard Review of Psychiatry*, 9(1): 1-12.

Jianlin J. 2000. Suicide rates and mental health services in modern China. *Crisis*, 21(3): 118-121.

Kalediene R. 1999. Time trends in suicide mortality in Lithuania. *Acta Psychiatrica Scandinavica*, 99(6): 419-422.

Kaprio J, Koskenvuo M, Rita H. 1987. Mortality after bereavement: A prospective study of 95,647 widowed persons. *American Journal of Public Health*, 77(3): 283-287.

Kaslow NJ, Thompson MP, Meadows LA, Jacobs D, Chance S, Gibb B, Bornstein H, Hollins L, Rashid A, Phillips K. 1998. Factors that mediate and moderate the link between partner abuse and suicidal behavior in African American women. *Journal of Consulting and Clinical Psychology*, 66(3): 533-540.

Kelleher MJ, Chambers D, Corcoran P, Williamson E, Keeley HS. 1998. Religious sanctions and rates of suicide worldwide. *Crisis*, 19(2): 78-86.

Kelleher MJ, Daly M. 1990. Suicide in Cork and Ireland. *British Journal of Psychiatry*, 157: 533-538.

Kelsoe JR, Ginns EI, Egeland JA, Gerhard DS, Goldstein AM, Bale SJ, Pauls DL, Long RT, Kidd KK, Conte G, et al. 1989. Re-evaluation of the linkage relationship between chromosome 11p loci and the gene for bipolar affective disorder in the Old Order Amish. *Nature*, 342(6247): 238-43.

Kendler KS, Gardner CO, Prescott CA. 1997. Religion, psychopathology, and substance use and abuse: A multimeasure, genetic-epidemiologic study. *American Journal of Psychiatry*, 154(3): 322-329.

Kennedy GJ, Kelman HR, Thomas C, Chen J. 1996. The relation of religious preference and practice to depressive symptoms among 1,855 older adults. *Journals of Gerontology. Series B, Psychological Sciences and Social Sciences*, 51(6): P301-P308.

Kennedy HG, Iveson RC, Hill O. 1999. Violence, homicide and suicide: Strong correlation and wide variation across districts. *British Journal of Psychiatry*, 175: 462-466.

Khan MM, Reza H. 2000. The pattern of suicide in Pakistan. *Crisis*, 21(1): 31-35.

Khan MZ, Ray R. 1984. Dowry death. *Indian Journal of Social Work*, 45(3): 303-315.

Kinnunen U, Pulkkinen L. 1998. Linking economic stress to marital quality among Finnish marital couples: Mediator effects. *Journal of Family Issues*, 19(6): 705-724.

Kirk AR, Zucker RA. 1979. Some sociopsychological factors in attempted suicide among urban black males. *Suicide and Life-Threatening Behavior*, 9(2): 76-86.

Kirmayer LJ, Boothroyd LJ, Hodgins S. 1998. Attempted suicide among Inuit youth: Psychosocial correlates and implications for prevention. *Canadian Journal of Psychiatry*, 43(8): 816-822.

Kirmayer LJ, Malus M, Boothroyd LJ. 1996. Suicide attempts among Inuit youth: A community survey of prevalence and risk factors. *Acta Psychiatrica Scandinavica*, 94(1): 8-17.

Kitagawa JM. 1989. Buddhist medical history. In: Sullivan LE, Editor. *Healing and Restoring—Health and Medicine in the World's Religious Traditions*. New York: Macmillan.

Koenig HG, Cohen HJ, Blazer DG, Pieper C, Meador KG, Shelp F, Goli V, DiPasquale B. 1992. Religious coping and depression among elderly, hospitalized medically ill men. *American Journal of Psychiatry*, 149(12): 1693-1700.

Koenig HG, Cohen HJ, George LK, Hays JC, Larson DB, Blazer DG. 1997. Attendance at religious services, interleukin-6, and other biological parameters of immune function in older adults. *International Journal of Psychiatry in Medicine*, 27(3): 233-250.

Koenig HG, Ford S, George LK, Blazer DG, Meador KG. 1993. Religion and anxiety disorder: An examination and comparison of associations in young, middle-aged and elderly adults. *Journal of Anxiety Disorders*, 7: 321-342.

Koenig HG, George LK, Meador KG, Blazer DG, Ford SM. 1994. The relationship between religion and alcoholism in a sample of community dwelling adults. *Hospital and Community Psychiatry*, 45: 225-231.

Koenig HG, George LK, Peterson BL. 1998. Religiosity and remission of depression in medically ill older patients. *American Journal of Psychiatry*, 155(4): 536-542.

Koenig HG, George LK, Siegler IC. 1999. The use of religion and other emotion-regulating coping strategies among older adults. *Gerontologist*, 28: 303-310.

Koenig HG, Hays JC, George LK, Blazer DG, Larson DB, Landerman LR. 1997. Modeling the cross-sectional relationships between religion, physical health, social support, and depressive symptoms. *American Journal of Geriatric Psychiatry*, 5(2): 131-144.

Koenig HG, Larson DB, Weaver AJ. 1998. Research on religion and serious mental illness. *New Directions for Mental Health Services*, 80: 81-95.

Kotler M, Iancu I, Efroni R, Amir M. 2001. Anger, impulsivity, social support, and suicide risk in patients with posttraumatic stress disorder. *Journal of Nervous and Mental Disease*, 189(3): 162-167.

Kposowa AJ. 2000. Marital status and suicide in the National Longitudinal Mortality Study. *Journal of Epidemiology and Community Health*, 54(4): 254-261.

Kposowa AJ. 2001. Unemployment and suicide: A cohort analysis of social factors predicting suicide in the US National Longitudinal Mortality Study. *Psychological Medicine*, 31(1): 127-138.

Kraybill D, Hostetter J, Shaw D. 1986. Suicide patterns in a religious subculture: The Old Order Amish. *International Journal of Moral and Social Studies*, 1: 249-263.

Kreitman N, Carstairs V, Duffy J. 1991. Association of age and social class with suicide among men in Great Britain. *Journal of Epidemiology and Community Health*, 45(3): 195-202.

Kryzhanovskaya L, Pilyagina G. 1999. Suicidal behavior in the Ukraine, 1988–1998. *Crisis*, 20(4): 184-190.

Kung KC, Liu X, Juon HS. 1998. Risk factors for suicide in Caucasians and in African-Americans: A matched case-control study. *Social Psychiatry and Psychiatric Epidemiology*, 33(4): 155-161.

La Vecchia C, Lucchini F, Levi F. 1994. Worldwide trends in suicide mortality, 1955–1989. *Acta Psychiatrica Scandinavica*, 90(1): 53-64.

La Vecchia C, Lucchini F, Levi F, Negri E. 2000. Trends in suicide mortality, 1955-1989: America, Africa, Asia and Oceania. In: Columbus F, Editor. *Advances in Psychology Research, Volume 1*. (pp. 77-109). Huntington, NY: Nova Science Publishers.

Leenaars AA, Lester D. 1995. The changing suicide pattern in Canadian adolescents and youth, compared to their American counterparts. *Adolescence*, 30(119): 539-547.

Leenaars AA, Lester D. 1999. Domestic integration and suicide in the provinces of Canada. *Crisis*, 20(2): 59-63.

Leenaars AA, Yang B, Lester D. 1993. The effect of domestic and economic stress on suicide rates in Canada and the United States. *Journal of Clinical Psychology*, 49(6): 918-921.

Leslie J. 1998. Dowry, 'dowry deaths' and violence against women: A journey of discovery. In: Menski W, Editor. *South Asians and the Dowry Problem*. (pp. 21-35). London: Trentham Books.

Lester D. 1993. The effect of war on suicide rates. A study of France from 1826 to 1913. *European Archives of Psychiatry and Clinical Neuroscience*, 242(4): 248-249.

Lester D. 1997. Domestic social integration and suicide in Israel. *Israel Journal of Psychiatry and Related Sciences*, 34(2): 157-161.

Lester D. 1999. Predicting the time-series suicide and homicide rates in Hong Kong. *Perceptual and Motor Skills*, 89(1): 204.

Lester D. 2000a. Islam and suicide. *Psychological Reports*, 87(2): 692.

Lester D. 2000b. Religious homogeneity and suicide. *Psychological Reports*, 87(3, Part 1): 766.

Lester D, Moksony F. 1989. Ecological correlates of suicide in the United States and Hungary. *Acta Psychiatrica Scandinavica*, 79(5): 498-499.

Lewis G, Sloggett A. 1998. Suicide, deprivation, and unemployment: Record linkage study. *British Medical Journal*, 317(7168): 1283-1286.

Li G. 1995. The interaction effect of bereavement and sex on the risk of suicide in the elderly: An historical cohort study. *Social Science and Medicine*, 40(6): 825-828.

Lin YH. 1990. *The Weight of Mount T'Ai: Patterns of Suicide in Traditional Chinese History and Culture.* Doctoral Dissertation, University of Wisconsin Madison.

Lindeman S, Laara E, Hirvonen J, Lonnqvist J. 1997. Suicide mortality among medical doctors in Finland: Are females more prone to suicide than their male colleagues? *Psychological Medicine*, 27(5): 1219-1222.

Linehan MM, Goodstein JL, Nielsen SL, Chiles JA. 1983. Reasons for staying alive when you are thinking of killing yourself: The reasons for living inventory. *Journal of Consulting and Clinical Psychology*, 51(2): 276-286.

Liu JC, Li YZ. 1990. *Unraveling the Suicide Riddle.* Chengdu, China: Sichuan Publishing House of Science and Technology:3.

Macpherson C, Macpherson L. 1987. Towards an explanation of recent trends in Western Samoa. *Man (New Series)*, 22: 305-330.

Makinen I. 1997. Are there social correlates to suicide? *Social Science and Medicine*, 44(12): 1919-1929.

Makinen IH. 2000. Eastern European transition and suicide mortality. *Social Science and Medicine*, 51(9): 1405-1420.

Marecek J. 1998. Culture, gender, and suicidal behavior in Sri Lanka. *Suicide and Life-Threatening Behavior*, 28(1): 69-81.

Maris RW. 1981. *Pathways to Suicide: A Survey of Self-Destructive Behaviors.* Baltimore: Johns Hopkins University Press.

Maris RW. 1997. Social suicide. *Suicide and Life-Threatening Behavior*, 27(1): 41-49.

Martin WT. 1984. Religiosity and United States suicide rates, 1972-1978. *Journal of Clinical Psychology*, 40(5): 1166-1169.

Marzuk PM, Tardiff K, Leon AC, Hirsch CS, Portera L, Hartwell N, Iqbal MI. 1997. Lower risk of suicide during pregnancy. *American Journal of Psychiatry*, 154(1): 122-123.

Masaryk TG. 1970. *Suicide and the Meaning of Civilization.* Chicago: University of Chicago Press.

Mayer P. 2000. Development, gender equality, and suicide rates. *Psychological Reports*, 87(2): 367-372.

Mazza JJ, Reynolds WM. 1998. A longitudinal investigation of depression, hopelessness, social support, and major and minor life events and their relation to suicidal ideation in adolescents. *Suicide and Life-Threatening Behavior*, 28(4): 358-374.

McCauley J, Kern DE, Kolodner K, Dill L, Schroeder AF, DeChant HK, Ryden J, Bass EB, Derogatis LR. 1995. The "battering syndrome": Prevalence and clinical characteristics of domestic violence in primary care internal medicine practices. *Annals of Internal Medicine*, 123(10): 737-746.

McRae RR. 1984. Situational determinants of coping response: Loss, threat, and challenge. *Journal of Personality and Social Psychology*, 46: 919-928.

Miller KE. 1996. The effects of state terrorism and exile on indigenous Guatemalan refugee children: A mental health assessment and an analysis of children's narratives. *Child Development*, 67(1): 89-106.

Motohashi Y. 1991. Effects of socioeconomic factors on secular trends in suicide in Japan, 1953-86. *Journal of Biosocial Science*, 23(2): 221-227.

Muelleman RL, Lenaghan PA, Pakieser RA. 1998. Nonbattering presentations to the ED of women in physically abusive relationships. *American Journal of Emergency Medicine*, 16(2): 128-131.

Nisbet PA. 1996. Protective factors for suicidal black females. *Suicide and Life-Threatening Behavior*, 26(4): 325-341.

Nisbet PA, Duberstein PR, Conwell Y, Seidlitz L. 2000. The effect of participation in religious activities on suicide versus natural death in adults 50 and older. *Journal of Nervous and Mental Disease*, 188(8): 543-546.

O'Grady D, Metz JR. 1987. Resilience in children at high risk for psychological disorder. *Journal of Pediatric Psychology*, 12(1): 3-23.

Paloutzian RF, Ellison CW. 1982. Loneliness, spiritual well-being and the quality of life. In: Peplau LA, Perlman D, Editors. *Loneliness: A Sourcebook of Current Theory, Research and Therapy.* New York: Wiley.

Pargament KI. 1990. God help me: Towards a theoretical framework of coping for the psychology of religion. *Research in the Scientific Study of Religion*, 2: 195-224.

Pargament KI, Zinnbauer BJ, Scott AB, Butter EM, Zerowin J, Stanik P. 1998. Red flags and religious coping: Identifying some religious warning signs among people in crisis. *Journal of Clinical Psychology*, 54(1): 77-89.

Park C, Cohen LH. 1993. Religious and nonreligious coping with the death of a friend. *Cognitive Therapy and Research*, 17: 561-577.

Park C, Cohen LH, Herb L. 1990. Intrinsic religiousness and religious coping as life stress moderators for Catholics verses Protestants. *Journal of Personality and Social Psychology*, 54: 562-574.

Parker G, Yap HL. 2001. Suicide in Singapore: A changing sex ratio over the last decade. *Singapore Medical Journal*, 42(1): 011-014.

Perlman D, Rook KS. 1987. Social support, social deficits, and the family: Toward the enhancement of well-being. *Applied Social Psychology Annual*, 7: 17-44.

Pescosolido BA. 1990. The social context of religious integration and suicide: Pursuing the network explanation. *Sociological Quarterly*, 31(3): 337-357.

Pescosolido BA. 1994. Bringing Durkheim into the 21st century: A social network approach to unresolved issues in the study of suicide. In: Lester D, Editor. *Emile Durkheim: Le Suicide—100 Years Later.* (pp. 264-295). Philadelphia: The Charles Press.

Pescosolido BA, Georgianna S. 1989. Durkheim, suicide, and religion: Toward a network theory of suicide. *American Sociological Review*, 54(1): 33-48.

Pescosolido BA, Mendelsohn R. 1986. Social causation or social construction of suicide? An investigation into the social organization of official rates. *American Sociological Review*, 51(1): 80-100.

Pescosolido BA, Wright ER. 1990. Suicide and the role of the family over the life course. *Family Perspectives*, 24: 41-58.

Pescosolido B, Levy JA. 2002. The role of social networks in health, illness, disease and healing: The accepting present, the forgotten past, and the dangerous potential for a complacent future. *Social Networks and Health*, 8: 3-25.

Petronis KR, Samuels JF, Moscicki EK, Anthony JC. 1990. An epidemiologic investigation of potential risk factors for suicide attempts. *Social Psychiatry and Psychiatric Epidemiology*, 25(4): 193-199.

Phillips DP, Feldman KA. 1973. A dip in deaths before ceremonial occasions: Some new relationships between social integration and mobility. *American Sociological Review*, 38: 678-696.

Phillips MR, Liu H, Zhang Y. 1999. Suicide and social change in China. *Culture, Medicine and Psychiatry*, 23: 25-50.

Pierce A. 1967. The economic cycle and the social suicide rate. *American Sociological Review*, 32: 457-462.

Pitts FN Jr, Schuller AB, Rich CL, Pitts AF. 1979. Suicide among U.S. women physicians, 1967-1972. *American Journal of Psychiatry*, 136(5): 694-696.

Platt S. 1984. Unemployment and suicidal behaviour: A review of the literature. *Social Science and Medicine*, 19(2): 93-115.

Platt S, Micciolo R, Tansella M. 1992. Suicide and unemployment in Italy: Description, analysis and interpretation of recent trends. *Social Science and Medicine*, 34(11): 1191-1201.

Ponizovsky AM, Ritsner MS. 1999. Suicide ideation among recent immigrants to Israel from the former Soviet Union: An epidemiological survey of prevalence and risk factors. *Suicide and Life-Threatening Behavior*, 29(4): 376-392.

Porterfield AL. 1952. Suicide and crime in folk and secular society. *American Journal of Sociology*, 57: 331-338.

Powell EH. 1958. Occupation, status, and suicide: Toward a redefinition of anomie. *American Sociological Review*, 23: 131-139.

Pressman P, Lyons JS, Larson DB, Strain JJ. 1990. Religious belief, depression, and ambulation status in elderly women with broken hips. *American Journal of Psychiatry*, 147(6): 758-760.

Preti A, Miotto P. 1999. Suicide and unemployment in Italy, 1982-1994. *Journal of Epidemiology and Community Health*, 53(11): 694-701.

Propst LR, Ostrom R, Watkins P, Dean T, Mashburn D. 1992. Comparative efficacy of religious and nonreligious cognitive-behavioral therapy for the treatment of clinical depression in religious individuals. *Journal of Consulting and Clinical Psychology*, 60(1): 94-103.

Qin P, Agerbo E, Westergard-Nielsen N, Eriksson T, Mortensen PB. 2000. Gender differences in risk factors for suicide in Denmark. *British Journal of Psychiatry*, 177: 546-550.

Rancans E, Salander Renberg E, Jacobsson L. 2001. Major demographic, social and economic factors associated to suicide rates in Latvia 1980-98. *Acta Psychiatrica Scandinavica*, 103(4): 275-281.

Ratnayeke L. 1998. Suicide in Sri Lanka. In: Kosky RJ, Eshkevari HS, Editors. *Suicide Prevention: The Global Context.* (pp. 139-142). New York: Plenum Press.

Resnick MD, Bearman PS, Blum RW, Bauman KE, Harris KM, Jones J, Tabor J, Beuhring T, Sieving RE, Shew M, Ireland M, Bearinger LH, Udry JR. 1997. Protecting adolescents from harm. Findings from the National Longitudinal Study on Adolescent Health. *Journal of the American Medical Association*, 278(10): 823-832.

Roberts GL, Lawrence JM, O'Toole BI, Raphael B. 1997. Domestic violence in the Emergency Department: I. Two case-control studies of victims. *General Hospital Psychiatry*, 19(1): 5-11.

Rose J, Hatcher S, Koelmeyer T. 1999. Suicide in Auckland 1989 to 1997. *New Zealand Medical Journal*, 112(1094): 324-326.

Ross RK, Bernstein L, Trent L, Henderson BE, Paganini-Hill A. 1990. A prospective study of risk factors for traumatic deaths in a retirement community. *Preventive Medicine*, 19(3): 323-334.

Roy A. 1993. Genetic and biologic risk factors for suicide in depressive disorders. *Psychiatric Quarterly*, 64(4): 345-58.

Rubenstein JL, Heeren T, Housman D, Rubin C, Stechler G. 1989. Suicidal behavior in "normal" adolescents: Risk and protective factors. *American Journal of Orthopsychiatry*, 59(1): 59-71.

Rubinstein DH. 1983. Epidemic suicide among Micronesian adolescents. *Social Science and Medicine*, 17(10): 657-665.

Sakuta T. 1995. A study of murder followed by suicide. *Medicine and Law*, 14(1-2): 141-153.

Sarason IG, Sarason BR, Pierce GR. 1990. Social support, personality, and performance. *Journal of Applied Sport Psychology*, 2(2): 117-127.

Sartorius N. 1995. Recent changes in suicide rates in selected eastern European and other European countries. *International Psychogeriatrics*, 7(2): 301-308.

Saunderson TR, Langford IH. 1996. A study of the geographical distribution of suicide rates in England and Wales 1989-92 using empirical bayes estimates. *Social Science and Medicine*, 43(4): 489-502.

Schmidtke A, Bille-Brahe U, DeLeo D, Kerkhof A, Bjerke T, Crepet P, Haring C, Hawton K, Lonnqvist J, Michel K, Pommereau X, Querejeta I, Phillipe I, Salander-Renberg E, Temesvary B, Wasserman D, Fricke S, Weinacker B, Sampaio-Faria JG. 1996. Attempted suicide in Europe: rates, trends and sociodemographic characteristics of suicide attempters during the period 1989-1992. Results of the WHO/EURO Multicentre Study on Parasuicide. *Acta Psychiatrica Scandinavica*, 93(5): 327-338.

Schmidtke A, Weinacker B, Apter A, Batt A, Berman A, Bille-Brahe U, Botsis A, De Leo D, Doneux A, Goldney R, Grad O, Haring C, Hawton K, Hjelmeland H, Kelleher M, Kerkhof A, Leenaars A, Lonnqvist J, Michel K, Ostamo A, Salander-Renberg E, Sayil I, Takahashi Y, Van Heeringen C, Vaernik A, Wasserman D. 1999. Suicide rates in the world: Update. *Archives of Suicide Research*, 5(1): 81-89.

Schutt RK, Meschede T, Rierdan J. 1994. Distress, suicidal thoughts, and social support among homeless adults. *Journal of Health and Social Behavior*, 35(2): 134-142.

Shen B-J, Takeuchi DT. 2001. A structural model of acculturation and mental health status among Chinese Americans. *American Journal of Community Psychology*, 29(3): 387-418.

Shiang J, Barron S, Xiao S.Y, Blinn R, Tam W-CC. 1998. Suicide and gender in the people's republic of China, Taiwan, Hong Kong, and Chinese in the US. *Transcultural Psychiatry*, 35(2): 235-251.

Snyder ML. 1992. Unemployment and suicide in Northern Ireland. *Psychological Reports*, 70: 1116-1118.

Somasundaram DJ, Rajadurai S. 1995. War and suicide in northern Sri Lanka. *Acta Psychiatrica Scandinavica*, 91(1): 1-4.

South SJ. 1984. Racial differences in suicide: The effect of economic convergence. *Social Science Quarterly*, 651: 172-180.

Stack S. 1992. Marriage, family, religion, and suicide. In: Maris RW, Berman AL, Maltsberger JT, Yufit RI, Editors. *Assessment and Prediction of Suicide*. (pp. 540-552). New York: The Guilford Press.

Stack S. 1996. The effect of marital integration on African American suicide. *Suicide and Life-Threatening Behavior*, 26(4): 405-414.

Stack S. 2000. Suicide: A 15-year review of the sociological literature. Part I: Cultural and economic factors. *Suicide and Life-Threatening Behavior*, 30(2): 145-162.

Stack S, Lester D. 1991. The effect of religion on suicide ideation. *Social Psychiatry and Psychiatric Epidemiology*, 26(4): 168-170.

Stack S, Wasserman J. 1992. The effect of religion on suicide ideology: An analysis of the networks perspective. *Journal for the Scientific Study of Religion*, 31: 457-466.

Stefansson CG, Wicks S. 1991. Health care occupations and suicide in Sweden 1961-1985. *Social Psychiatry and Psychiatric Epidemiology*, 26(6): 259-264.

Swanwick GR, Clare AW. 1997. Suicide in Ireland 1945-1992: Social correlates. *Irish Medical Journal*, 90(3): 106-108.

Takahashi Y. 1997. Culture and suicide: From a Japanese psychiatrist's perspective. *Suicide and Life-Threatening Behavior*, 27(1): 137-145.

Tedeschi RG. 1999. Violence transformed: Posttraumatic growth in survivors and their societies. *Aggression and Violent Behavior*, 4(3): 319-341.

Thompson EA, Eggert LL, Herting JR. 2000. Mediating effects of an indicated prevention program for reducing youth depression and suicide risk behaviors. *Suicide and Life-Threatening Behavior*, 30(3): 252-271.

Tierney EO. 1989. Health care in contemporary Japanese religions. In: Sullivan LE, Editor. *Healing and Restoring—Health and Medicine in the World's Religious Traditions.* New York: Macmillan.

Tousignant M, Seshadri S, Raj A. 1998. Gender and suicide in India: A multiperspective approach. *Suicide and Life-Threatening Behavior,* 28(1): 50-61.

Trout DL. 1980. The role of social isolation in suicide. *Suicide and Life-Threatening Behavior,* 10(1): 10-23.

Trovato F. 1992. A Durkheimian analysis of youth suicide: Canada, 1971 and 1981. *Suicide and Life-Threatening Behavior,* 22(4): 413-427.

US DHHS (U.S. Department of Health and Human Services). 1999. *Mental Health: A Report of the Surgeon General.* Rockville, MD: U.S. Department of Health and Human Services, Substance Abuse and Mental Health Services Administration, Center for Mental Health Services, National Institutes of Health, National Institute of Mental Health.

US DHHS (U.S. Department of Health and Human Services). 2001. *Mental Health: Culture, Race and Ethnicity—A Supplement to Mental Health: A Report of the Surgeon General.* Rockville, MD: U.S. Department of Health and Human Services, Substance Abuse and Mental Health Services Administration, Center for Mental Health Services, National Institutes of Health, National Institute of Mental Health.

van Egmond M, Diekstra RF. 1990. The predictability of suicidal behavior: The results of a meta-analysis of published studies. *Crisis,* 11(2): 57-84.

Vance JE, Fernandez G, Biber M. 1998. Educational progress in a population of youth with aggression and emotional disturbance: The role of risk and protective factors. *Journal of Emotional and Behavioral Disorders,* 6(4): 214-221.

Varnik A, Wasserman D. 1992. Suicides in the former Soviet republics. *Acta Psychiatrica Scandinavica,* 86(1): 76-78.

Varnik A, Wasserman D, Dankowicz M, Eklund G. 1998. Marked decrease in suicide among men and women in the former USSR during perestroika. *Acta Psychiatrica Scandinavica. Supplement,* 394: 13-19.

Varnik A, Wasserman D, Eklund G. 1994. Suicides in the Baltic countries, 1968-90. *Scandinavian Journal of Social Medicine,* 22(3): 166-169.

Veiel HO, Brill G, Hafner H, Welz R. 1988. The social supports of suicide attempters: The different roles of family and friends. *American Journal of Community Psychology,* 16(6): 839-861.

Vinokur AD, Price RH, Caplan RD. 1996. Hard times and hurtful partners: How financial strain affects depression and relationshipsatisfaction of unemployed persons and their spouses. *Journal of Personality and Social Psychology,* 71(1): 166-179.

Wasserman D, Varnik A. 2001. Perestroika in the former USSR: History's most effective suicide-preventive programme for men. In: Wasserman D, Editor. *Suicide: An Unnecessary Death.* (pp. 253-257). London: Martin Dunitz Ltd.

Wasserman IM. 1983. Political business cycles, presidential elections, and mortality patterns. *American Sociological Review,* 48: 711-720.

Wasserman IM. 1984. The influence of economic business cycles on United States suicide rates. *Suicide and Life-Threatening Behavior,* 14(3): 143-156.

Wasserman IM, Stack S. 1999. The relationship between occupation and suicide among African American males: Ohio, 1989–1991. In: Maris RWBAL, Silverman MM, Editors. *Review of Suicidology 2000.* (pp. 242-251). New York: Guilford Press.

Weiss M. 1994. Hinduism. In: Reich WT, Editor. *Encyclopedia of Bioethics, Volume 2.* New York: Macmillan.

Werner EE. 1992. The children of Kauai: Resiliency and recovery in adolescence and adulthood. *Journal of Adolescent Health,* 13(4): 262-268.

Werner EE. 1996. Vulnerable but invincible: High risk children from birth to adulthood. *European Child and Adolescent Psychiatry*, 5 (Suppl 1): 47-51.

Weyerer S, Wiedenmann A. 1995. Economic factors and the rates of suicide in Germany between 1881 and 1989. *Psychological Reports*, 76: 1331-1341.

White L, Rogers SJ. 2000. Economic circumstances and family outcomes: A review of the 1990s. *Journal of Marriage and the Family*, 62(4): 1035-1051.

Whitley E, Gunnell D, Dorling D, Smith GD. 1999. Ecological study of social fragmentation, poverty, and suicide. *British Medical Journal*, 319(7216): 1034-1037.

WHO (World Health Organization). 2001. *The World Health Report, 2001. Mental Health: New Understanding, New Hope.* Geneva: World Health Organization.

Wilkinson D, Gunnell D. 2000. Youth suicide trends in Australian metropolitan and non-metropolitan areas, 1988–1997. *Australian and New Zealand Journal of Psychiatry*, 34(5): 822-828.

Wolf M. 1975. Women and suicide in China. In: Wolf M, Witke R, Editors. *Women in Chinese Society.* (pp. 111-114). Stanford, CA: Stanford University Press.

Yang B, Clum GA. 1994. Life stress, social support, and problem-solving skills predictive of depressive symptoms, hopelessness, and suicide ideation in an Asian student population: A test of a model. *Suicide and Life-Threatening Behavior*, 24(2): 127-139.

Yip PS. 2001. An epidemiological profile of suicides in Beijing, China. *Suicide and Life-Threatening Behavior*, 31(1): 62-70.

Zacharakis CA, Madianos MG, Papadimitriou GN, Stefanis CN. 1998. Suicide in Greece 1980-1995: Patterns and social factors. *Social Psychiatry and Psychiatric Epidemiology*, 33(10): 471-476.

Zimmerman MA, Ramirez-Valles J, Maton KI. 1999. Resilience among urban African American male adolescets: A study of the protective effects of sociopolitical control on their mental health. *American Journal of Community Psychology*, 27(6):733-751.

Zimmerman SL. 1987. States' public welfare expenditures as predictors of state suicide rates. *Suicide and Life-Threatening Behavior*, 17(4): 271-287.

Zonda T. 1999. Suicide in Nograd County, Hungary, 1970-1994. *Crisis*, 20(2): 64-70.

I like living. I have sometimes been wildly, despairingly, acutely miserable, racked with sorrow, but through it all I still know quite certainly that just to be alive is a grand thing.

—AGATHA CHRISTIE

7

Medical and Psychotherapeutic Interventions

Almost half of the individuals who complete suicide in the United States are diagnosed with a mental disorder and are under treatment by a mental health professional (Conwell et al., 1996; Fawcett et al., 1991; Harris and Barraclough, 1997; Isometsa et al., 1994; Robins et al., 1959). To be able to prevent suicide through treatment and therapy, it is necessary to know when the individual is in immediate danger of dying by suicide. However, existing assessment instruments may help in identifying who is at risk, but do indicate *when* they will be at risk. Further, since certain life events can precipitate suicide in some but not all patients, their predictive value is poor. Many at-risk patients receive medication for mental disorders. But while these medications often reduce the symptoms of these disorders, the effectiveness of such medications to decrease the risk of suicide is unknown. Medications are best delivered in the context of a therapeutic relationship featuring an ongoing and appropriate psychotherapy or counseling, conscientious follow-up, and an overall flexible treatment plan that considers the socio-cultural context of the patient. This chapter addresses issues of assessment, reviews current knowledge about the effectiveness of medications for suicidality, and describes the impact of hospitalization and psychotherapy on suicidality.

ASSESSMENT

Suicide risk is difficult to assess. Individuals making serious suicide attempts may knowingly withhold their intentions (e.g., Apter et al., 2001;

Morrison and Downey, 2000; Negron et al., 1997). No psychological test, clinical technique, or biological marker is sufficiently sensitive and specific to accurately assess short-term prediction of suicide in an individual (Goldstein et al., 1991). A prospective study (Pokorny, 1983) of 4800 consecutive patients at a Veterans Administration hospital used 21 known suicide risk factors to identify 803 patients with increased risk of suicide. Thirty of these identified patients completed suicide during a 5-year follow-up period. But an additional 37 patients than had not been assessed as at-risk also completed suicide. Even an optimal measure with the unrealistically low rate of false-positives and false-negatives (1 percent) would only correctly assess 20 percent of those who complete suicide (MacKinnon and Farberow, 1976). Assessment instruments can be useful tools but are not a substitute for clinical judgement. Nevertheless, assessment is an important component of psychopharmacological and psychotherapeutic interventions.

Assessment Instruments

Whether using a standardized psychological test or interview only, it is important to assess for suicidal symptoms, symptoms of the known risk factors for suicide, and current abilities to cope with acute or chronic stress (Bech et al., 2001). Assessment instruments fall into four broad categories: (1) detection instruments, (2) risk assessment instruments, (3) assessment of clinical characteristics of suicidal behavior, and (4) a miscellaneous category (e.g., compilations, assessment of attitudes around suicide, projective psychological tests[1]). Assessment tools for adults and youths have been extensively reviewed by Brown (2000) and Goldston (2000), respectively.

One of the most widely used and best-evaluated measures is the Scale for Suicide Ideation (SSI) (Beck et al., 1979). It is a 19-item scale, available as interview, self-report, or computer-administered. Only if a person endorses an item indicating intent to complete suicide, is the rest of the scale administered. It has been standardized on both inpatient and outpatient clinical samples. It has also been used in emergency rooms, primary care settings, jails, and in college student samples. A prospective study with almost 7000 patients and an approximately 20-year follow-up with psychiatric outpatients used standardized, structured interviews and standardized assessment measures (Brown et al., 2000). These data were

---

[1]Projective psychological tests use abstract, or non-definitive test stimuli allowing the test subject to project their psychological makeup onto the material.

matched to the National Death Index, and death certificates were obtained for those who had died. Through this process, 49 suicide cases were identified. The average length of follow-up was 10 years, and the average length of time to death was approximately 4.3 years from the baseline interview. Patients who scored above 3 on the SSI were about 6.5 times more likely to complete suicide than patients who scored below this cut-off.

Other scales that have been shown to have some predictive validity include the Beck Hopelessness Scale, Beck Depression Inventory, Beck Anxiety Scale, and the Hamilton Rating Scale for Depression. Measurements of personal contentment, such as Linehan's (1983) Reasons for Living Inventory and Koivumaa-Honkanen and colleagues' (2001) simple life satisfaction measure, also seem to have value in some populations. All of the instruments have their strengths as well as their weaknesses, but there may be no single "best" instrument for all purposes. The choice of instruments depends on the needs of the clinician or researcher, the intended use of the instruments, and an assessment of how an instrument compares to other similar instruments in meeting diagnostic needs. Furthermore, the age, gender, and culture of the suicidal individual must also be considered in choosing assessment scales. Some measures of psychopathology and suicide risk may not be as accurate or appropriate for specific populations, since risk and protective profiles differ across ethnicity, gender, and age. Cognitive measures of mental disorders, for example, may not be as sensitive for ethnic groups that experience psychopathology in more somatic than in cognitive terms (Marsella et al., 1975; Marsella and Yamada, 2000), and culture and developmental stage (e.g., single adolescent *vs.* adult parent) influence such things as reasons for living (see Chan, 1995; Linehan et al., 1983; Osman et al., 1998).

Confounding Factors

Variations in Purpose

Assessment tools differ; there are detection instruments, risk assessment instruments, and instruments for assessing clinical characteristics of suicidal behavior. Each of these groups of instruments is useful for answering certain types of questions, but the use of the wrong instrument may yield insufficient or even misleading information. A risk assessment instrument will not provide information about whether someone is currently suicidal (an issue of detection). A person may score "low" on a risk assessment instrument assessing a particular domain (e.g., hopelessness) while still experiencing suicidal ideation or even having made a recent attempt (Goldston, 2000).

Incomplete Use

Further confounding the use of assessment tools is their misuse. At times, researchers have used one or two items from an assessment scale, when the tools have only been validated in their full form. Studies frequently use just a single item from the Hamilton Depression Scale, a practice which results in a decreased sensitivity of the assessment tool. Complete, standardized suicide assessment measurements are most appropriate in clinical trials.

Population Specificity

Instruments may not have the same predictive utility when used in populations other than those in which they were developed (Meehl and Rosen, 1955). The base rate of risk factors may vary significantly across different populations, so that the same level of a risk factor may have significant predictive utility in some groups, but not others. In addition to base rate differences, risk factors may vary in meaning, salience, and/or presence across groups. The prevalence of risk factors for suicidal behaviors differs in different samples or population groups, just as the base rates of suicidal ideation and suicide attempts differ. Moreover, some instruments may be more appropriate than others for certain age groups, and some instruments may be more "culturally sensitive" than others. For these and other reasons, an instrument that has been demonstrated to be of use in one population may not be as useful with other groups.

Instruments developed with school-based or community samples may not have the same predictive utility in "high-risk" or clinically ascertained samples, and vice versa. Risk factors in a community may not be useful as a predictor of suicidal behavior in higher risk populations. First-time suicide attempters may differ from those who attempt more than once, and predicting first and later attempts may involve different risk factors. Goldston's team (2001) found that hopelessness was a strong predictor of future suicide attempts following hospitalization among adolescents who previously had made at least a single suicide attempt, but hopelessness was not a significant predictor in those without a history of suicide attempt(s).

Distal vs. Proximal Factors

The relationship between vulnerability factors assessed with risk instruments (distal risk factors) and precipitating stresses (proximal risk factors) needs to be better understood. Using instruments focused on identifying groups based on various risk factors may tell us who is at risk, but not when they are at risk. Specific life events may precipitate or provide the occasion for suicidal behavior, but they do not tell us who is likely to make those attempts. The course or persistence of vulnerability factors over time and an individual's reactions to life events and stressors are important influences. To accurately predict suicidal behavior, a better understanding of the interplay between vulnerability factors and stresses is needed.

PSYCHOACTIVE MEDICATIONS

Since 90 percent of suicide occurs in people with mental disorders, it is thought that treating the underlying disorder could reduce suicide risk. For some medications there is evidence that the effects on suicidality may be independent from the effects on the mental disorder. This section reviews the evidence that medications used to treat mental disorders can influence the risk of suicide.

Mood Stabilizers

Mood stabilizers are used to treat bipolar illness. These drugs fall into two major classes. The first is lithium, a naturally occurring salt, which is effective in reducing the manic and depressive symptoms. Another group of medications proven effective for bipolar disorder is the anticonvulsants (e.g., carbamazepine and valproic acid).

Lithium

Evidence suggests that lithium treatment of bipolar disorder significantly reduces suicide rates (Baldessarini et al., 1999). In fact, lithium may have specific anti-suicide effects for people with this disorder since these effects may be *separate* from its antidepressant and antimanic effects. A prospective, randomized controlled clinical trial (Thies-Flechtner et al., 1996) in patients with bipolar illness found that lithium carbonate significantly reduced suicidal acts per patient, relative to patient years. A series of reviews and a meta-analysis of the effect of lithium on suicidality by Tondo and colleagues (Tondo et al., 1997; 1998; 2001) supported the finding that lithium reduced the rate of both suicides and suicide attempts in bipolar patients. The meta-analysis of 12 studies on lithium reported that the risk ratio in favor of a therapeutic lithium effect on suicide is 8.85 (confidence interval=4.14-19.1) (Tondo et al., 2001). This estimate, if correct, would make lithium the most potent therapeutic agent so far identified. However, the protective effects of lithium are not consistent across studies (see Bowden, 2000; Brodersen et al., 2000), and some methodological concerns have been raised (Bowden et al., 2000; Calabrese et al., 2001a; Goodwin, 1999). Some also caution that although the data is mostly positive, the anti-suicidal effect of lithium may not be as strong as originally thought (Bowden et al., 2000).

One of the confounding issues in these studies is the time course of psychopharmacological treatment. Decreased rates of suicide are most pronounced when lithium has been used for a minimum of 2 years (Baldessarini and Tondo, 1999). Rates were reduced only while the patients took lithium; following discontinuation of lithium, the rates began to rise to levels similar to those seen prior to the commencement of lithium. Rapid discontinuation of lithium may lead to a more dramatic increase in rates of suicidal behavior as compared to more gradual discontinuation. Early studies, because of their abrupt discontinuation of lithium, may have increased placebo relapse figures (Bowden et al., 2000). Tondo, Baldessarini and colleagues (Baldessarini and Tondo, 1999; Tondo and Baldessarini, 2000; Baldessarini et al., 1999; Tondo et al., 1997) noted that the latency from onset of bipolar disorder to lithium maintenance in their patients averaged 8.3 years, but that half of the suicidal acts had occurred in the first 7.5 years. Thus, it may be of crucial importance to commence lithium treatment as early as possible in the course of bipolar disorder for patients thought to be at risk for suicidal behavior. It is noteworthy that lithium and clozapine (see below) are both effective in reducing suicidal behavior and both require regular clinic visits and blood tests. This suggests a benefit from regular clinic monitoring.

Nonadherence with medication, particularly lithium, is a critical issue for individuals with bipolar disorder and one of the primary reasons for poor treatment response (Goodwin and Jamison, 1990). Since lithium treatment is associated with an almost 8-fold decreased suicide rate (Tondo and Baldessarini, 2000), this has a serious impact on suicide risk. Research has shown that almost one-half of patients with bipolar disorder are non-adherent to lithium treatment at some point in their lives, and one-third are non-adherent two or more times (Jamison and Akiskal, 1983; Jamison et al., 1979). Younger males within the first year of lithium treatment and those patients who have elevated moods and a history of euphoric manias, especially those who complain about missing the "highs" of their illness, are more likely to be nonadherent (Goodwin and Jamison, 1990). Many people stop taking their medication after being released from the hospital, one of the factors causing significantly increased risk of suicide during this period (see below). Furthermore, clinical research with bipolar populations is very difficult due to poor treatment adherence (Goodwin and Jamison, 1990; Goodwin, 1999; Jamison and Akiskal, 1983; Jamison et al., 1979), and the poor adherence rate makes interpreting results more difficult and the conclusions less powerful in many studies.

Important questions regarding lithium still remain. Greil and colleagues (1996; 1997a; 1997b), in a series of randomized controlled studies with treatment periods of 2.5 years, found that the prophylactic efficacy of lithium on suicidality varied according to the underlying mental disorder. Carbamazepine was more effective than lithium in reducing suicidal behavior in schizoaffective disorder, especially in subgroups with depressive or schizophrenia-like features; in bipolar types it was not superior (Greil et al., 1997a). For unipolar depressed patients, lithium was found to be superior to amitriptyline (Greil et al., 1996), and in bipolar disorder patients, lithium was judged to be superior to carbamazepine (Greil et al., 1997b). Several studies also suggest that bipolar patients with rapid cycling or mixed states are difficult to treat effectively and do not seem to respond as well to lithium (Bowden et al., 2000; Calabrese et al., 2001b; Montgomery et al., 2000). Comorbidities, especially with substance use disorder, also interfere with treatment outcome (Macqueen and Young, 2001; Vestergaard et al., 1998), though comorbidity appears to moderate outcomes via treatment adherence (Calabrese et al., 2001b).

The mechanism of action of lithium is unknown. It has been hypothesized that it exerts antisuicidal effects on aggressive impulsive traits via the serotonergic system or otherwise. Importantly, lithium appears to have a direct effect on suicidal behavior, not simply by reducing the suicidality caused by depressive relapses (Möller, 2001).

Anticonvulsants

The other class of mood stabilizers found to reduce symptoms of bipolar disorder are the anti-convulsants, such as carbamazepine, divalproex, and valproic acid. These medications are recommended for bipolar patients when lithium is not an option, whether due to lithium intolerance or resistance to lithium treatment (Möller, 2001). Valproate is the most commonly prescribed mood stabilizer in the United States, overtaking lithium. However the data are very limited on the efficacy of anticonvulsants to reduce suicidal behavior; only one randomized controlled study was identified in a recent review (Goodwin and Ghaemi, 2000). Thies-Flechtner et al. (1996) conducted a 2.5 year prospective study on 175 inpatients with bipolar disorder. These patients were treated either with carbamazine or with lithium. Of the 6 patients who committed suicide, 4 were taking carbamazine. None were taking lithium at time of death, but one had discontinued lithium. All of the suicide attempts occurred in patients who were taking carbamazine. These data demonstrated a statistically significant benefit of lithium over carbamazine in the prevention of suicide. Because of the frequency with which anticonvulsants are prescribed for bipolar disorder, it is exceptionally important to evaluate their effectiveness compared to lithium for prevention of suicide.

Anti-Psychotic Medications

Anti-psychotic medications, including neuroleptics, may also be effective in the reduction of both suicidal behavior and the overall suicide rate when suicidality is seen as a feature of psychosis in schizophrenia. Particularly compelling evidence exists for the atypical anti-psychotic, clozapine.

Meltzer (1999) found that the mortality rate from suicide was reduced by 80 to 85 percent of the expected rate for schizophrenic patients in a population of treatment-resistant schizophrenic patients treated with clozapine after adjusting for the duration of treatment.

Recently, Meltzer and colleagues (2001) reported that in a multi-centered, randomized clinical trial of 980 patients with schizophrenia or schizoaffective disorder, treatment with clozapine when compared to treatment with olanzapine resulted in significantly fewer suicide attempts and a reduced need for additional medications to control suicidality.

Meltzer and Okayli (1995) reported that clozapine in neuroleptic-resistant psychotic patients, when given as continuation or maintenance pharmacotherapy, was associated with markedly less suicidality. They reported that the number of serious suicide attempts decreased significantly and that this decrease was associated with a reduction in depression and hopelessness. Interestingly, they stated that the beneficial effect occurred independently of the response to the psychosis, so it appears to be more attributable to the effect on depression and hopelessness. Both treatment-responsive and treatment-resistant patients were included, but similar results were obtained in the two groups for both prior suicidal behavior and suicidal behavior on treatment. The suicide attempt rate fell from 25 percent prior to treatment to 3.4 percent after clozapine treatment. The lethality of the suicide attempts was also significantly reduced after clozapine treatment.

Walker and colleagues (1997) reported on data from a national registry of clozapine recipients involving 67,072 current and former clozapine users, linking the data to the National Death Index and the Social Security Administration Death Master Files. They identified 396 deaths in 85,399 person-years for patients ages 10–54 years. Mortality was lower during current clozapine use than during periods of nonuse. The mortality from suicide decreased in current clozapine users by comparison with past users. The investigators confirmed that the principal reason for the reduction in deaths was a decrease in the suicide rate. Using the Texas Department of Mental Health and Mental Retardation database, Reid's research team (1998) found that the annual suicide rate for 30,000 patients with schizophrenia and schizoaffective disorders was 63.1 per 100,000 patients (between 1993 and 1995), approximately five times higher than in the general population. In contrast, only one suicide occurred in 6 years among patients treated with clozapine who were of similar diagnosis, age, and sex (a yearly rate of about 12.7 per 100,000 patients). Similarly, the suicide rate was found to be 15.7 per 100,000 patients per year in all United States patients treated with clozapine based on the clozapine national registry system maintained by Novartis Pharmaceutical Corporation, the United States manufacturer of clozapine. Similar analyses with other novel antipsychotic medications have been initiated, and preliminary results suggest that they may also have some beneficial effect in reducing suicide rates.

Antidepressant Medications

A number of investigators worldwide have recently reviewed outcomes across large populations showing that a decrease in suicides correlates with the increase of antidepressant use in various European countries (Isacsson et al., 1996; Markowitz, 2001; Ohberg et al., 1998; Rich, 1999; Rihmer et al., 1998) and that suicidal behavior correlates with the inadequate prescription of antidepressants (Henriksson et al., 2001; Oquendo et al., 1999). Such population-based changes in the suicide rate may be due to numerous causes in addition to the increase in antidepressant prescriptions, but these findings suggest a benefit from receiving antidepressants which may be related to appropriate treatment of the underlying depression.

Psychological autopsy studies suggest that the rate of adequate treatment with antidepressants of depressed suicide victims is about 6–14 percent, and toxicological analyses indicate the presence of antidepressants and other prescription psychotropics in about 8–17 percent of suicides, with the frequency in men being about half that of women, and in Blacks and Hispanics being half that of Caucasians (Blazer et al., 2000; Isacsson et al., 1999; Marzuk et al., 1995; Rich and Isacsson, 1997). In general, surveys of university teaching hospitals indicate that most depressed outpatients, even in such academic centers, are either not treated or are under-treated with antidepressant medications (Keller et al., 1986; Oquendo et al., 1999). Oquendo and colleagues (1999) showed that this was just as frequent a problem for those depressed patients with a history of suicidal behavior as for those without.

A variation on the epidemiological studies is the examination of the benefits of an educational intervention. Gotland, an island province of Sweden with a population of 58,000, is a single epidemiological catchment area and most treatment is provided by general practitioners (GPs). In a series of papers since 1989, Rutz, Rihmer, and colleagues (Rihmer et al., 1995; Rutz, 2001; Rutz et al., 1989a; Rutz et al., 1989b) reported that educating the Gotland GPs about depression recognition increased the use of antidepressants and lowered suicide rates by 60 percent (see also Chapter 8).

SSRIs

Serotonin reuptake inhibitors (SSRIs) are used to treat depressive symptoms in the affective disorders as well as for symptom relief for those who have other diagnoses, or do not meet the criteria for the major affective disorders. SSRIs have gained great popularity in recent years, with the number of prescriptions increasing both in the United States and in other western nations (Isacsson, 2000; Lawrenson et al., 2000; Sclar et al., 1998). Although the SSRIs reduce depressive symptoms, their potency in reducing suicide is uncertain.

Verkes et al. (1998) found that patients with personality disorders and brief depression, but not major depression, had fewer suicide attempts when treated with paroxetine as compared with placebo. On the other hand, most studies failed to find statistically significant differences in suicide or suicidal behavior with SSRI treatments. Leon et al. (1999) followed 185 patients treated with fluoxetine (from among 643 patients as part of the NIMH Collaborative Depression Study). Using a mixed effects survival analysis, they found a decreased risk of suicide attempts and completions in the fluoxetine group, but this decrease did not achieve statistical significance, perhaps because the patients given fluoxetine were more severely ill than the comparison group before treatment. On the other hand, three meta-analyses failed to show effects of the SSRIs on suicide. Two (Khan et al., 2001; Khan et al., 2000) assessed FDA trials for efficacy and found that the major SSRI antidepressants were not significantly different than placebo with respect to suicides. Another meta-analysis of 17 clinical trials (Beasley et al., 1991) indicated that fluoxetine may reduce suicidal ideation but was not significantly different from either placebo or the tricyclic antidepressants in reducing suicides or attempts.

Several factors may enter into the interpretation of these results. Hirschfeld (2000) pointed out that these studies were time-limited. In addition, they mostly attempted to screen out those at risk for suicide. In most of the clinical studies, the base rate of suicide attempts was too low to determine effectively whether the antidepressant medications reduced the number of suicide attempts or suicides in comparison with placebo (Khan et al., 2001; Khan et al., 2000; Letizia et al., 1996; Montgomery et al., 1994; Tollefson et al., 1993). To a large extent, the low base rate of suicidal acts in most studies was a consequence of the exclusion of suicidal patients for safety reasons (see Chapter 10). Some investigators (Khan et al., 2001; Khan et al., 2000) also note that the increased contact with mental health professionals for both treatment and placebo groups confounds the observed relationships, and could possibly represent a kind of treatment in itself.

As mentioned earlier, however, increasing prescription rates for antidepressants, in particular SSRIs, has correlated with declines in suicide rates observed in a number of countries including Sweden, Finland, Hungary, and the United States (Isacsson, 2000; Ohberg et al., 1998; Rich and Isacsson, 1997; Rihmer et al., 2001). With access to national health data, it was found that with a doubling of the number of SSRI prescriptions, the suicide rate was reduced by 25 percent in Sweden (Isacsson et al., 1992). A similar result was reported in Italy, but the effect was confined almost entirely to females (Barbui et al., 1999). Though these correlations do not determine causality, they suggest the potential for antidepressants, particularly SSRIs, to reduce suicide rates. This is further supported by the findings of psychological autopsies and toxicological analyses that frequently have found that suicide victims with a mood disorder were taking inadequate therapeutic amounts of antidepressants (Blazer et al., 2000; Isacsson et al., 1994; Isacsson et al., 1992; 1997; Marzuk et al., 1995; Ohberg et al., 1996; Rich and Isacsson, 1997).

Tricyclic Antidepressants

The tricyclic antidepressants are effective for the treatment of depressive symptoms. A tricyclic such as amitriptyline may be chosen in cases of suicidality due to its sedative effects, but the high risk of fatal outcome in overdose of tricyclics is a particular concern with regard to suicidal patients. Soloff et al. (1986) found that amitriptyline non-responders made more suicidal communications than placebo non-responders in a group of 29 borderline personality disorder patients.

Other Classes of Antidepressants

In terms of actual suicidal behavior, a prospective long-term, placebo-controlled treatment study of 1141 patients found more suicide attempts, including suicides in the group treated with the norepinephrine reuptake inhibitor maprotiline compared with placebo (Rouillon et al., 1989). While maprotiline was an effective antidepressant, it was associated with increased suicide attempts.

Comparison Studies

Four of 11 randomized controlled clinical studies demonstrated that an SSRI reduced suicidal ideation compared to another antidepressant (usually a tricyclic antidepressant) and to placebo (Eberhard et al., 1988; Gonella et al., 1990; Kasper et al., 1995; Montgomery et al., 1978). Venlafaxine, given in a dose that predominantly inhibits the serotonin transporter, showed greater efficacy compared with a tricyclic after up to six weeks of treatment (Mahapatra and Hackett, 1997). Four of the remaining studies found comparable improvement in suicidal ideation with SSRIs and the reference compound (Judd et al., 1993; Lapierre, 1991; Möller and Steinmeyer, 1994; Tollefson et al., 1993). In a comparison of moclobemide, a reversible monoamine oxidase inhibitor, with the SSRI clomipramine, increased suicidality was seen among the moclobemide group but not among the clomipramine group (Danish University Antidepressant Group, 1993).

Possible Adverse Effects of Antidepressants

Mental illness can be incapacitating, and the possibility exists that as the symptoms lift (because of treatment) individuals become more capable of carrying out plans of violence toward self or others. This has been of great concern in the use of antidepressants. Müller-Oerlinghausen and Berghofer (1999) have described situations where antidepressants increase the risk of suicide in some patients by "energizing patients with preexisting suicidal thoughts or inducing akathisa (increased movement with associated anxiety/agitation)." It has long been known that affective disorders can carry a significant risk of suicide, and that some small number of patients will deteriorate rather than improve after being treated with any antidepressant or will become at an increased risk for suicide associated with abrupt improvement.

Case reports have led some investigators to suggest that there may be a risk of emergent suicidality on SSRIs, in particular, fluoxetine. For example, Teicher and colleagues (1990) observed eight patients with major depression and personality disorders who developed suicidal thoughts and in some cases made attempts as their clinical condition deteriorated and fluoxetine was being increased to the 80 mg dosing range. There were several criticisms of these conclusions, including atypical EEG findings in these patients and the persistent increase in dosage as the patients deteriorated.

Healy and colleagues (1999) have outlined several possible mechanisms by which antidepressant medication may lead to suicide in some depressed patients. These proposed mechanisms include antidepressants simply ameliorating the lethargy and immobility of depression more rapidly than the depressed mood, suicide by overdose of medication, specific actions of antidepressant medication(s), or through side-effects of the antidepressants. Lastly, antidepressants may not be effective, or have yet to exert their therapeutic effects during the first weeks of the regime, hence the risk of suicide has not yet changed. However, the frequency of *emergent* suicidality has been evaluated in controlled treatment studies in mood disorders and non-mood disorders treated with SSRIs (see Montgomery et al., 1995 for paroxetine in depression; see Tollefson et al., 1993 for fluoxetine in depression). Emergent suicidality is more frequent on placebo than with SSRIs. Wheadon et al. (1992) examined fluoxetine in bulimia and found more emergent suicidality with placebo than with fluoxetine.

Marchesi et al. (1998) compared drugs in two different chemical classes of anti-depressant medication, fluoxetine (a serotonin re-uptake inhibitor) versus amitriptyline (a noradrenergic receptor blocker) treatment in 142 patients with major depression. They found no significant differences in measures for "psychic anxiety," "somatic anxiety," "agitation," and "insomnia" and no increase in these measures with fluoxetine treatment. Similar claims of causing a worsening of these symptoms have been made in the course of a number of lawsuits blaming medications and the companies who develop and market them for suicides.

However, a review of emergent suicidality (see Mann et al., 1993; Mann and Kapur, 1991) has found that such reports exist for almost all classes of psychotropics (with no evidence of pharmacological specificity) and there is no consistent temporal or dose relationship. Thus, the case reports are not convincing. It has been hypothesized that this alleged effect is due to the development of akathisia. Although akathisia reports with SSRIs have occurred with or without suicidal behavior, the akathisia-like features are generally less frequent than reported with antipsychotic medications and also milder. Thus, it is not clear that this kind of akathisia-like effect can actually lead to suicidal behavior or, for that matter, violent behavior, in patients receiving SSRIs.

All of the controlled clinical data do not provide evidence of emergent suicidality, even among patients without mood disorders who are receiving SSRIs (Montgomery et al., 1995; Tollefson et al., 1993). There have been no double-blind controlled challenge and re-challenge studies done to confirm the hypothesized emergence of suicidal behavior or ideation in patients receiving SSRIs. There is a case report of individuals re-challenged with a SSRI, but that was not done in a double-blind controlled fashion (Rothschild and Locke, 1991). Thus, the anecdotal evidence at this stage is unsupported by any controlled clinical trial data. A related hypothesized mechanism for explaining the alleged relationship between

SSRIs and suicidality is the induction of anxiety and agitation by SSRIs. Again, controlled studies do not support this suggestion; in fact, they suggest the converse. Controlled studies such as those reported by Sheehan et al. (1992) demonstrate that SSRIs result in an earlier onset of therapeutic effect on somatic anxiety compared with other antidepressants or placebo. Paroxetine is superior to placebo in the treatment of agitation after 4 and 6 weeks of treatment, and superior to the active control after 4 weeks of treatment. Both paroxetine and the active control are more protective against newly emergent agitation compared with placebo. So, there appears to be little evidence of an aggravating effect on anxiety. Controlled studies indicate that drugs like paroxetine seem to have a therapeutic effect and not an aggravating effect on agitation.

Postmarketing surveillance studies have been carried out that bear on this question of emergent suicidality (Inman et al., 1993; Zaninelli and Meister, 1999). Such postmarketing surveys of thousands of patients who received paroxetine found the incidence of reported suicidal behavior attributed to the medication to be so infrequent as to be negligible. Thus, both controlled clinical trials, including large meta-analyses of large groups of patients as well as these postmarketing surveys, provide no support for the concerns of emergent suicidality.

Anxiolytic Medications

Anxiety is a common symptom in many mental illnesses, including depression, bipolar disorder, and schizophrenia, and acute anxiety and agitation are associated with an increased risk of both suicide and suicide attempts. Additionally, anxiety is a prominent feature in suicidality that is related to psychosocial stressors. Benzodiazepines are the most commonly used medications to relieve anxiety in such cases. The data relating benzodiazepines to suicide are limited. There are, in fact, some reports (Melander et al., 1991; Neutel and Patten, 1997; Taiminen, 1993) that suggest that the use of benzodiazpines is associated with an *increased* risk of suicide. Causality is unknown and difficult to assess. The interpretation of this observation is confounded by the fact that benzodiazepines are often used as a means to complete suicide.

ELECTROCONVULSIVE THERAPY

Electroconvulsive therapy (ECT) is a safe and effective medical treatment for affective disorders (Avery and Winokur, 1977), particularly in severe refractory depression. It is most often used in the treatment of depression with or without psychotic features, acute mania, and schizophrenia (APA, 1990; Fink and Sackeim, 1996; Mukherjee et al., 1994), though rates of use are low, and in decline. Many texts and official recommendations indicate that when suicidal ideation and behavior is seen as a symptom of these mental disorders, ECT should be considered. It is clinically indicated in these cases of acute suicidality because of the rapid onset of its ameliorating effects (AHCPR, 1993; Goodwin and Jamison, 1990); the swift onset of action can provide time to decide on and implement appropriate long-term treatments such as anti-depressants and psychotherapy (APA, 1990). ECT is also recommended for people who have psychotic depression, for whom medications pose a medical risk, who have previously responded well to ECT, who have mixed manic episodes, and who are unresponsive to medications with catatonia, major depressive disorder, schizoaffective disorder, or melancholic symptoms.

Success rates for ECT have been found as high as 80–90 percent for unipolar and bipolar major depressive episodes and mania (Metzger, 1999), which is higher than most estimates of pharmacological treatment effectiveness, and is particularly notable given that ECT is often reserved for patients with medication resistant illnesses. In general, these studies did not differentiate by severity of illness and medication resistance status, and in studies that looked at this it was found that medication resistant patients show a 50–70 percent response rate (Prudic et al., 1990). Due to various methodological constraints, ECT has not been directly compared to drug therapy in terms of speed of onset. Thus, the commonly accepted belief that ECT is the fastest available treatment for depression (and thus indicated for acute suicidality) has not been subject to clinical studies (Roose and Nobler, 2001).

There is no evidence that ECT has a long-term effect on the suicide rate and suicidal behavior (Prudic and Sackeim, 1999). It is notable that the majority of studies have found a lower mortality rate for ECT treated psychiatric patients versus psychiatric patients with other treatment modalities, but these mortality risk studies are plagued by methodological problems. Interestingly, it has been found that the reduced mortality rate holds even after excluding suicides. Some of these studies have not noted the cause of death, so the conclusions to be drawn are limited. Even so, these studies may underestimate the positive effect of ECT on mortality since ECT is often used specifically for patients with suicidality, where a higher mortality rate would be expected. One naturalistic study of elderly patients with long-term follow-up found that the patients receiving ECT had lower mortality rates compared to patients receiving pharmacotherapy, but non-random assignment to treatment modality confounds these results; it appears that these patients may have been healthier at the outset (Philibert et al., 1995). Clinicians may be reluctant to recommend ECT in medically ill patients; however, medical illness, which may limit the tolerability of drug treatment, is a specific indication for the consideration of ECT.

There is evidence for a short-term effect of ECT on the reduction of suicidality. Given that suicidal ideation and behavior is a key symptom of the affective disorders, it would follow that an effective treatment for the disorder would also alleviate one of its symptoms. Additionally, Prudic and Sackeim (1999) found that both the ECT responders and the non-responders showed a large decrease in scores on the suicide item of the Hamilton Rating Scale for Depression, and this decrease was greater than the average improvement on the other items.

There has been much debate about the efficacy of ECT. Results have been fairly inconclusive due to methodological problems such as lack of controlled trials, and many variations in study protocol, which makes cross-study comparison extraordinarily difficult. Also the treated patients are often extremely diverse demographically, and in terms of their diagnoses. The case of suicide is particularly problematic because even when studies on ECT have been done, either they have not looked at suicide as an outcome, or the fact of suicide being such a low base rate behavior has thwarted any strong conclusions from being drawn. Knowledge about the effectiveness and mode of action of ECT has not grown as quickly as that for the psychotherapeutic drugs, which may in part be due to its controversial reputation among clinicians, the public, and mental health consumers.

PSYCHOTHERAPIES

Data show that medicine alone is not sufficient for treatment of mental disorders or suicidality. Individuals need to be supported while they pursue adequate care for the mental disorders that put them at increased risk for suicide. Psychiatric drugs can take over a month to take effect, and finding the right combination and doses to best treat an individual can take some months. During this time people experience often unpleasant side-effects, the stigma of mental disorders, and changes in life-circumstances secondary to the disorders in some cases. Furthermore, psychotherapeutic interventions target very different variables than do psychotropic drugs.

---

[2]Psychotherapy is one of several types of psychosocial treatments, which also includes social and vocational training, psychoeducation, and support groups. It is used in this text to refer broadly to non-pharmacological interventions.

There are several different types of psychotherapies,[2] including behavioral therapy, psychodynamic (or insight-oriented) therapy, and supportive therapy. Behavioral therapies include cognitive behavioral therapy (discussed further below) and focus on directly altering current behavior. Psychodynamic therapy, on the other hand, concentrates on increasing self-understanding (see also footnote 3). Supportive therapy provides patients with a non-judgmental environment in which to offer advice, attention, and sympathy. Psychotherapy often focuses on:

- changing long-term social-cognitive suicide risk factors such as hopelessness, low self-esteem and self-efficacy (see Chapter 3)
- interpersonal problem-solving deficits (see Chapter 3)
- socio-environmental risks such as family violence and parenting style (see Chapter 5)

Although certain psychotherapeutic interventions appear more effective in reducing suicide risk than others (see below), in the last 40 years mental health research has suggested that the most critical component of therapeutic treatment is the quality of the therapeutic relationship rather than the type of psychotherapy (e.g., Sexton and Whiston, 1991, see Chapter 6 for protective effects of social support).

The debt I owe my psychiatrist is beyond description. I remember sitting in his office a hundred times during those grim months and each time thinking, What on earth can he say that will make me feel better or keep me alive? Well, there never was anything he could say, that's the funny thing. It was all the stupid, desperately optimistic, condescending things he *didn't* say that kept me alive; all the compassion and warmth I felt from him that could not have been said; all the intelligence, competence, and time he put into it; and his granite belief that mine was a life worth living. He was terribly direct, which was terribly important, and he was willing to admit the limits of his understanding and treatments and when he was wrong. Most difficult to put into words, but in many ways the essence of everything: He taught me that the road from suicide to life is cold and colder and colder still, but—with steely effort, the grace of God, and an inevitable break in the weather—that I could make it. (Jamison, An Unquiet Mind: A Memoir of Moods and Madness, 1995: 118).

Given logistical constraints, evaluations of long-term therapeutic interventions are rare. Although numerous studies document the efficacy of therapeutic interventions, especially cognitive behavioral therapy (CBT),[3] in treating mental disorders such as depression and post-traumatic stress disorder that increase suicide risk (see Foa et al., 2000 and Chapter 3), far fewer studies document the direct effects of therapy on suicidal behavior and intent. As with pharmacotherapeutic interventions, many methodological problems currently plague studies of psychotherapeutic treatment efficacy for suicidality. Reviews of efficacy trials have noted a lack of operational definitions for the suicidal behavior studied (see Chapter 10) and paucity of standardized, reliable assessment tools to measure the suicidal outcome (see Chapter 7, above) (Hawton et al., 1998; Linehan, 1997). Many studies also fail to use blind assessment and true randomization procedures. These reviews further caution that therapist quality and adherence to treatment protocol are difficult to control and assess. Lastly, a critical limitation involves inadequate power as a risk in most of these studies, given that the infrequency of suicidal behavior makes most clinical trials too small to uncover treatment effects. Hawton and colleagues (1998), for example, estimated necessary sample sizes needed given expected effect sizes and concluded that even the pooled data from meta-analyses were probably of inadequate size (see also Chapter 10). This chapter reviews the relatively few studies utilizing adequate methodology and design.

Most studies on the efficacy of short-term treatment assessed the therapeutic potential of developing problem-solving skills, given suicidal individuals' serious skill deficits (see Chapter 3). In general, these studies have produced positive results for both adolescent and adult samples. Four studies of suicidal adolescents and young adults suggest that CBT with problem-solving components and general problem-solving therapy[4] reduces suicidal ideation and associated symptomatology such as depressive symptoms, hopelessness, and loneliness for at least 2 years (Harrington et al., 1998; Joiner et al., 2001; Lerner and Clum, 1990; Rudd et al., 1996). Three of these studies utilized group therapies; two used CBT

---

[3]The goals of CBT focus on restructuring current thoughts, perceptions, and beliefs of the client to facilitate behavioral and emotional change. During therapy, coping skills and abilities are also often assessed and further developed. Many short-term CBT interventions have been developed, and therapists use CBT for individual and group therapy. This contrasts with psychodynamic therapy that helps clients link current situations to past events, with the goal of better understanding how their emotional and cognitive states developed. This longer-term therapy usually remains unstructured and involves single individuals rather than groups.

[4]Problem-solving therapy generally involves the family unit and emphasizes the social context of the person's problems. Problem-solving therapy is usually a short-term, structured intervention that focuses on present circumstances and functioning.

with a problem-solving component (Joiner et al., 2001; Rudd et al., 1996) and the other used social problem-solving therapy (Lerner and Clum, 1990). Harrington et al. (1998) used a brief, home-based intervention targeting family-based problem solving. The positive effects of these interventions held even among high-risk, multiple-attempt patients and patients with comorbid mood and anxiety disorders (Joiner et al., 2001; Rudd et al., 1996). In addition, treatment adherence in such interventions appears to be greater for high-risk, multiple-attempt patients. However, these interventions do not appear to have a significant impact on the long-term rate of suicide attempts. Harrington and colleagues' (1998) study also found that their short-term family-based therapy specifically reduced suicidal ideation for those youth without major depression, pointing to a need for more research on the differential effects of interventions on suicidal subtypes.

Similar positive outcomes have been reported among adults receiving short-term, problem-solving and/or CBT treatments. In general, CBT and problem-solving treatment led to increased treatment adherence, reduced levels of suicidal ideation and attempts, and reductions in related symptomatology (Evans et al., 1999; Hawton et al., 1981; Hawton et al., 1987; Liberman and Eckman, 1981; McLeavey et al., 1994; Patsiokas and Clum, 1985; Salkovskis et al., 1990; van der Sande et al., 1997b). Reductions in suicide attempt rates, however, did not remain significant in long-term evaluations. Such short-term treatment approaches may prove cost effective, as indicated by Evans et al.'s (1999) pilot study.

These brief therapies in adults, as with youths, were effective even among high-risk, repeat suicide attempters, but with limitations. Liberman and Eckman (1981) compared brief (10-day) behavioral therapy including a problem-solving component versus insight-oriented therapy. The behavioral therapy group showed greater reductions in depression and suicidal ideation, but no between-group differences emerged with respect to suicide attempts over a 9-month follow-up. Patsiokas and Clum (1985) found similar results for cognitive therapy, problem-solving therapy, and supportive therapy over the course of 10 individual sessions, as all three groups showed reductions in hopelessness and suicide intent. Notably, patients who received problem-solving therapy demonstrated significantly greater reductions in hopelessness than patients who received supportive therapy. Other between-groups differences may have emerged if a larger sample had been used. Salkovskis et al. (1990) compared the relative efficacy of five sessions of CBT with a problem-solving component versus a referral to a general practitioner. Despite using a small sample (n=20), they found significantly reduced rates of suicidal ideation, depression, and hopelessness over a 12-month follow-up for the CBT group. The CBT group also showed a greater reduction in the rates of suicide attempt over a 6-month follow-up, but not over a 12-month follow-up. Finally, Evans et al. (1999) found that bibliotherapy[5] with cognitive therapy and aspects of dialectical behavior therapy (DBT)[6] led to decreased depressive symptoms, but no statistically significant decreases in suicide attempts, compared to treatment as usual.[7]

One of the only trials of long-term therapeutic interventions for suicidality involves DBT. In a randomized, controlled trial, Linehan and colleagues (1991) found that DBT consisting of weekly individual therapy, group skills training, and as-needed phone calls led to a greater reduction in the rate of suicide attempts and the number of hospitalized days for suicidal behaviors over a 12-month follow-up, as compared to a group who received a referral to other outpatient treatment. The DBT group also displayed greater treatment adherence. The groups did not differ with regard to depression, hopelessness, suicidal ideation, and reasons for living, however. A very small randomized, controlled trial recently found that a shortened version of DBT (all the components in half the dose) did reduce suicidal ideation, hopelessness, and depression compared to treatment as usual (Koons et al., 2001). Similarly, pilot results from a quasi-experimental trial of a 12-week DBT program for adolescents (DBT-A) suggest that DBT-A may be more effective than twice-weekly individual and family therapy at increasing treatment adherence and reducing suicide ideation, depression, impulsivity, and psychiatric hospitalizations (Miller et al., 1997).

Other forms of therapeutic intervention may also be effective. Guthrie (2001) investigated the efficacy of four weekly home-based sessions of brief psychodynamic interpersonal therapy. At a 6-month follow-up, the brief psychodynamic group showed a significantly greater reduction in the rate of suicide attempts and suicidal ideation. They also reported greater satisfaction with treatment than the control group in this study, which received treatment as usual (usually referral to their general practitioner).

Yet, some treatments are not definitively effective. Three months of task-centered casework with a social worker (Gibbons et al., 1978) was

---

[5]In this case, comprised of a manual of six short chapters covering problem solving, relapse prevention strategies, and basic cognitive techniques to manage emotions and negative thinking.

[6]A CBT-related therapy, DBT was developed specifically for the often treatment-refractive chronically suicidal population comprising mostly females with borderline personality disorder, though it is now being piloted with other samples. This therapy includes individual and group work, is quite structured, and is designed as a year-long intervention.

[7]Treatment as usual can vary from study to study. Often it is psychopharmacological treatment and intermittent supportive psychotherapy, but in some studies it can be simply referral to the care of a primary physician.

not more effective than referral to outpatient treatment in reducing suicide attempts or reducing depression and social problems. Inpatient crisis
intervention followed by either short-term outpatient psychotherapy with
the same clinician during and after hospitalization or a referral to outpatient suicide prevention services did not offer an advantage for rates of
suicide or suicide attempts (Möller, 1989). Both of these studies excluded
high-risk patients, however.

Certain psychotherapeutic interventions, therefore, hold promise to
reduce suicidality, even for (high-risk) individuals identified by at least
one prior attempt. Comparing across all CBT trials, two meta-analyses
reached different conclusions about behavioral interventions. Hawton and
colleagues (1998) included psychosocial crisis intervention and not DBT
in problem-solving therapy and did not find these interventions effective.
By contrast, van der Sande and colleagues (1997a) separated psychosocial
crisis interventions from CBT and included DBT and the CBT condition of
the Liberman and Eckman (1981) inpatient study in the CBT category.
Their meta-analysis found psychosocial crisis intervention ineffective, but
CBT effective. The studies reviewed in this section therefore indicate that
psychotherapy can more effectively reduce depression, hopelessness, suicidal ideation, and suicide attempts compared to treatment as usual.
Short-term psychotherapy with CBT and/or problem-solving training
components may also positively influence a wider range of suicide risk
factors than does solely supportive or insight-oriented therapy.

A critical finding from several studies of patients at higher risk involves the apparently separate treatment responses of depression and
suicidal behavior. Brent and colleagues (1997) compared CBT, systematic
behavior family therapy, and non-directive supportive treatment for 107
adolescents with major depressive disorder. They did not exclude participants based on suicide risk and at intake 36 percent reported current
suicidality and 24 percent had a history of at least one suicide attempt.
Results indicated comparable decreases in suicidality in all three treatment conditions, but significantly more rapid response in depression
symptoms with CBT. Lerner and Clum (1990) found comparable results
in comparison of problem-solving therapy and supportive therapy for
college students with suicidal ideation. All subjects showed reduced suicidal ideation following the treatment, but depressive symptoms were
significantly more reduced in the problem-solving condition. The opposite result was found by Linehan and colleagues (1991) in their comparison of DBT *versus* usual care for suicidal women with borderline personality disorder. In their study, there was a comparable decrease in
depression symptoms between treatment conditions, but significantly
fewer suicidal behaviors in the DBT condition. This highlights the gap in

the literature between what is known about general risk factors *versus* knowledge of specific etiological pathways to suicide. Several points should be noted that might explain the differing results in the efficacy literature. Linehan (1997) evaluated trials in her review based on the inclusion or exclusion of "high risk" patients (operationalized as needing immediate psychiatric treatment, at high risk of suicide or having characteristics known to increase suicide risk). Forty-five percent of the efficacy trials for treatment of suicidal behavior excluded high-risk individuals. (For comparison, this is fewer than the 88 percent exclusion for high-risk individuals in pharmacotherapy trials for depression [Beasley et al., 1991] but greater than one might think in studies on suicidal behavior.) Linehan then examined the 13 outpatient studies, of which six excluded high-risk individuals. None of the 6 studies excluding high-risk individuals showed beneficial effects, but six of the seven including high-risk did show significant effects. This effect may be one of power (i.e., the frequency of suicide attempts during follow-up is likely to be greater in high-risk individuals, thus creating a larger possible effect size), which suggests the need for larger trials. This also highlights, however, that high-risk individuals are able to benefit from outpatient interventions and, therefore, exclusion from such treatments is unwarranted (see Chapter 10 for further discussion of research issues).

INPATIENT AND FOLLOW-UP CARE FOR SUICIDALITY

Inpatient Care

Although suicidality is the most common precipitant for psychiatric inpatient admission (Friedman, 1989), no randomized clinical trials have been done to determine whether hospitalizing high-risk suicide attempters saves lives (AACAP, 2001). Between 60 and 75 percent of child, adolescent, and adult patients and 40 to 55 percent of geriatric patients are admitted to inpatient units with concerns of self-harm (Jacobson, 1999). Hospitalization may be voluntary or involuntary. Involuntary hospitalization is legally permitted when an individual meets criteria for mental illness and dangerousness to self or others, per each jurisdictions' laws.

Involuntary hospitalization is correlated with many of the common risk factors for suicide, including serious suicide attempts and completed suicide on the unit, a diagnosis of schizophrenia; history of prior attempts of high lethality; and history of living alone or living in a household without younger children (Roy and Draper, 1995).

The immediate priority upon hospitalization is to reduce the suicidal thoughts, anxiety, and other symptoms associated with the suicide attempt. Various pharmacological approaches are generally used. Patients are sometimes more responsive to medications during hospitalization than as outpatients (Kotin et al., 1973), perhaps because of increased adherence. ECT or sedation may be indicated (Möller, 2001). However, some patients may remain actively suicidal even if symptoms improve when life stresses are not resolved.

The effectiveness of brief hospitalizations is questionable, especially when they entail no psychiatric services or post-discharge services. One randomized controlled trial compared the efficacy of general hospital admission versus discharge in reducing the repetition of suicidal symptoms and suicide attempts over 4 months and found that short-term hospitalization (i.e., a mean of less than 24 hours) without psychiatric care produced no beneficial effect (Waterhouse and Platt, 1990). However, the follow-up period was short and only low-risk attempters could be included in the study, so this may have been a problem of insufficient power (see Hawton et al., 1998).

On the morning of August 7th, Tom, 23, visited a former middle school teacher and confided that he was contemplating suicide and had been very close to killing himself the day before. Tom also said that he had thought about hurting his former girlfriend, sold his car, bought a gun and ammunition, and planned to buy two more guns. The teacher and the school's principal called the police after obtaining Tom's consent. After speaking to the officer, Tom consented to being handcuffed and taken to the hospital.

The police emergency petition only required the hospital to evaluate him. Tom was kept overnight for psychiatric evaluation and released the next day. No medications were prescribed but a follow-up visit was scheduled. Tom shot himself two days later in an apartment next door to his girlfriend's home. His mother believes her son was released too soon (O'Hagan, 2001).

Name has been changed to maintain privacy.

Five to 6 percent of suicides in United States and Great Britain occurred during psychiatric hospitalization. Robins and coworkers (1959) reported that 7 percent of their patient population completed suicide while in a psychiatric hospital. Among different populations, the rate of suicides occurring during inpatient care is higher; for example, one study of manic-depressive patients found that of those who completed suicide, 27 percent did so while under hospital care (Weeke, 1979), although half of these had left the hospital either on a pass or unapproved absence. Most frequently, inpatient suicides occur early in the hospitalization. One study found that 43 percent of the suicides during hospitalization occurred during the first week (Crammer, 1984). However, longer stays do not prevent suicide in the hospital (Jacobson, 1999).

After Discharge Risk

The period directly following discharge from a psychiatric hospitalization is a period of significantly increased risk. There appear to be multiple reasons for this. Patients who are hospitalized are some of the most severely affected individuals. While in the hospital, they are under surveillance and do not have the opportunity or means to commit suicide. When these patients are released from the hospital, they frequently lose their support system and they again have the opportunity and the means to commit suicide. A study in Great Britain reported that within the first 28 days after discharge, suicide was more likely (7 times in men and 3 times in women) than during the remaining 48 weeks of the year (Goldacre et al., 1993). Another study similarly found that 24 percent of the suicides among discharged patients occurred within the first 3 months of discharge, primarily in the first week (see Figure 7-1) (Appleby et al., 1999b).

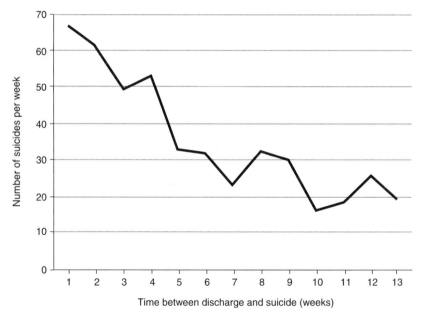

FIGURE 7-1. Number of suicides each week after discharge. SOURCE: Appleby et al., 1999b. Reprinted with permission from the BMJ Publishing Group.

Most of those who completed suicide were considered to be low risk. Discharged patients who completed suicide were 3.7 times more likely to have had their care reduced at their most recent outpatient appointment (Appleby et al., 1999a). A higher suicide rate was found to be associated with the loss of contact with the primary mental health professional (King et al., 2001). Other risk factors for suicide in recently discharged patients include living alone, hopelessness, relationship difficulties, loss of a job, a history of self harm, and a diagnosis of depression (King et al., 2001; McKenzie and Wurr, 2001). Patients who maintained care in the community (King et al., 2001) or maintained pharmacotherapy (Modestin et al., 1992) had lower suicide rates. These results suggest that discharged psychiatric patients are at higher risk of suicide for many reasons, but by maintaining some continuity of care and increasing adherence to treatment plans, some of the deaths may be prevented.

Although the risk of death by suicide appears low in medically hospitalized patients, estimated at 1.8 per 100,000 (Hung et al., 2000), the period immediately following hospitalization may be one of increased risk for these patients, as well. Dhossche and colleagues (2001) found that 73 percent (8 of 11) recently discharged medical patients who suicided were diagnosed with depression and/or substance abuse, whereas only 33 percent (11 of 33) of those who had not suicided had these diagnoses.

Angela, age 14, was treated in the emergency room after ingesting a "handful" of prescription pills in front of her mother and younger sister. This she did in retribution for being reprimanded and hit by her mother for staying out late. In the intake interview, she denied current suicidal ideation and stated that she was "glad" that her mother was worried. Once medically cleared, she was given an appointment with the outpatient psychiatry clinic for 9 days later, an appointment that was never kept. The nurse who attempted to contact the family by phone to follow up learned that the phone number given at intake had been disconnected for over 2 months (Berman & Jobes, Adolescent Suicide: Assessment and Intervention, 1991: 164).

Treatment Adherence

Individuals who do not adhere to their treatment regimens, including medication and therapy, are at greater risk for suicide. The period following hospitalization is a time of increased likelihood that individuals will stop taking their medications (Appleby, 2000). As described in a recent

IOM report (2001) and by Goodwin and Jamison (1990), the reasons for non-adherence can range from failure to understand the regimen or to appreciate the consequences of not following it, to adverse side effects. Lithium, for example, can cause cognitive impairment, weight gain, tremor, thirst, or lethargy (Goodwin and Jamison, 1990). It may also be that those who do not maintain their medication regimen had been reaping no benefit from it. This in turn is related to two possibilities. First, the individual may not have been on the medication for a long enough period of time to experience symptom relief; most psychiatric medications exert the desired beneficial effects only after taking them for multiple weeks. Meanwhile, unpleasant side-effects often occur during this initial period. Second, there are some people for whom the medications do *not* bring significant symptom relief; these "treatment resistant" individuals range upwards of 25 percent of those treated for some disorders. However, true non-response to medication is difficult to study because of the high incidence of non-adherence to dosing regimes for psychiatric drugs.

Non-adherence to treatment is a critical issue in suicide prevention since a large percentage of those taking psychiatric medications who complete suicide have been shown to have insufficient blood levels of the drugs to have reaped any benefits. Adherence to psychiatric treatment is lower than for treatment of somatic disorders, likely due to the societal stigma and unpleasant drug side effects, which typically start *before* the therapeutic benefit. In addition, for bipolar disorder and schizophrenia, suicide is most likely during the first years after diagnosis, often before consistent drug and therapy treatments have been established. These two disorders are most frequently diagnosed in early adulthood, a period when people may not yet have the maturity and/or financial resources to overcome the high stigma, tolerate the unpleasant side effects, and mount the barriers to accessing treatment and establishing a successful treatment regimen.

Follow-Up Care

Because of the high post-discharge suicide risk, many hospitals have implemented various forms of follow-up care for suicidal patients. Intensive follow-up, case management, telephone contacts, letters, or home visits sometimes improves treatment adherence (e.g., Termansen and Bywater, 1975; van Heeringen et al., 1995; Welu, 1977). Such interventions have produced mixed results with regard to suicidal behaviors: some have demonstrated decreased suicide attempts (Aoun, 1999; Termansen and Bywater, 1975; van Heeringen et al., 1995; Welu, 1977) and even completions (Motto and Bostrom, 2001), while others have found no effect on suicide attempts (Chowdhury et al., 1973; Litman and Wold, 1975).

Intervention efficacy may sometimes depend on the diagnosis of the suicidal individual (e.g., Byford et al., 1999).

Termansen and Bywater (1975) investigated the relative efficacies of no intervention, emergency room assessment alone, emergency room assessment plus as-needed follow-up care at a volunteer crisis center, and emergency room assessment plus a 3-month follow-up by the same mental health worker who conducted the assessment. Over the 3-month follow-up period, they found that the group who received follow-up by the same mental health worker demonstrated lower rates of suicide attempts and higher treatment adherence. Motto and Bostrum (2001) examined the impact of regular follow-up letters to suicidal individuals who refused ongoing treatment after discharge from a hospital. The study randomly assigned those refusing follow-up care or dropping out of follow-up care after hospitalization for severe depression or suicidality to either usual care or to receive regular letters from staff. Results of a survival analysis showed that for the first 2 years, the difference in the survival curves was significant, with the time to suicide longer in the contact vs. no contact group. When evaluated over the full five years the curves were not significantly different. It is important, however, that differences were greatest during the first 2 years, which is when suicides are most likely to occur. This was also when contact with the subjects was most frequent (in year 1). This is the only study to show a significant difference between experimental and usual care conditions for *completed* suicide.

In a comprehensive intervention, Aoun (1999) (1) instituted a standardized hospital protocol for dealing with cases of deliberate self-harm, (2) employed a suicide intervention counselor who worked with patients from within 48 hours of admission until 6 weeks post-discharge, and (3) provided professional and community education about intervention, risk assessment, and access to service. The experimental group received treatment from the suicide intervention counselor, and the control group received treatment as usual. Patients who received treatment from the suicide intervention counselor had significantly lower rates of hospital readmission for suicide attempts over a 22-month follow-up, as compared to readmission rates among patients who received treatment as usual and patients who were admitted prior to the start date of the intervention. Unfortunately, the findings of this study are limited by non-randomized groups and a variable length of follow-up depending on when the patient entered the study.

Rotheram-Borus, Piacentini, Cantwell, Belin, and Song (2000) provided specialized emergency room care to adolescent females with the goal of enhancing adherence to outpatient therapy. The intervention included a soap opera video regarding suicidality, a family therapy session, and staff training. The control group received standard emergency room care. At an 18-month follow-up, no significant between-group differences emerged in suicidal ideation or the rate of suicide attempts, although lack of power may have obscured treatment effects. Nevertheless, the experimental group showed significantly lower depressive symptoms and higher family cohesion, and these effects were greatest among those with higher suicidal symptomatology at admittance to the emergency department. This intervention also appears to improve treatment adherence among high-risk Latina adolescents (Rotheram-Borus et al., 1996; 1999).

CULTURAL CONSIDERATIONS AND FAITH-BASED INTERVENTIONS

When assessing risk and creating a treatment plan for suicidal individuals, as for any patient with mental illness (US DHHS, 2001), taking their cultural and spiritual views and needs into account emerges as a critical component of effective interventions. Language barriers prevent thousands of immigrants in the United States from receiving proper mental health care (US DHHS, 2001, see also Chapter 9 for discussion of barriers to treatment). Furthermore, racial and ethnic factors may affect how individuals respond metabolically to some common psychoactive medications (US DHHS, 2001). Individuals from ethnic and racial minority populations are far less likely to turn to professional mental health providers than are European Americans; some prefer traditional and/or spiritual methods of healing to mainstream medical and mental health strategies (see US DHHS, 2001, and Chapter 2, section on African Americans). Cultural and spiritual beliefs concerning self, psychobiological functioning (mind-body interactions), and disease causation influence the expression of mental disorders and response to treatment, including treatment adherence (Hsu, 1999; Marsella, 1988; Marsella and Yamada, 2000).

Clergy/spiritual ministers represent key gatekeepers for suicide prevention. In the United States, older adults, African Americans, and Hispanic Americans, in particular, more often turn to clergy than to professional mental health services when facing mental health issues, including suicide (Husaini and Moore, 1994; Starrett et al., 1992; Weaver and Koenig, 1996). Data from a large nationally representative study indicate that clergy see individuals with the same severity of mental disorders as do mental health professionals (Larson et al., 1988). Another study suggests that those who first go to clergy with mental health complaints are least likely to seek professional mental health services (Neighbors et al., 1998). A high percentage of clergy in Australia reported that they had been approached by suicidal adolescents (Leane and Shute, 1998). Studies in the United States document that older adults often seek help from clergy for suicidal crises, as well (Domino, 1985; Weaver and Koenig, 1996).

The few studies conducted on clergy knowledge and attitudes regarding suicide suggest that many clergy members need and desire training in assessing suicide risk (Domino, 1985; Leane and Shute, 1998). Although many congregations forge formal collaborations with professional mental health services (e.g., Thomas et al., 1994), Mannon and Crawford (1996) found that clergy from small congregations or from more conservative backgrounds are less likely to refer individuals to professional mental health services. They also reported that many clergy feel less confident about providing support and advice about severe mental disorders than about other matters. However, the African American ministers in their sample reported high levels of confidence even about handling serious mental disorders among their parishioners. Given the positive effects on mental health and suicidality of religious involvement and complementary faith-based treatment (e.g., Donahue, 1995; including seeking help from clergy, Koenig et al., 1998; Propst et al., 1992, see Chapter 6) and the widespread use of clergy, many comprehensive suicide prevention programs incorporate faith-based interventions into their strategies (see Chapter 8). Some researchers have also authored articles and handbooks delineating appropriate responses to suicidal and distressed elderly and youths for clergy (e.g., Koenig and Weaver, 1997; Weaver, 1993; Weaver et al., 1999).

To maximize treatment effectiveness and to reach under-served groups, collaborations of mental health professionals with culturally relevant providers, including spiritual ministers could be effective (Marsella and Yamada, 2000; Weaver, 1993). In recognition of the importance of cultural context, the Diagnostic and Statistical Manual of Mental Disorders (DSM-IV) (APA, 1994) provides guidelines for a culturological assessment of individuals presenting with mental disorders and includes mention of cultural variations in the expression of psychopathology. Nursing diagnoses have included spiritual distress and spiritual well-being for years (Johnson et al., 2001). The framework for culturally and spiritually sensitive approaches to treating and reducing mental disorders and suicidality is emerging.

FINDINGS

• Assessment tools are inadequate to determine acute suicide risk or to predict when a person will attempt or complete suicide. Assessment tools must be validated for various populations since they may not be generally applicable. Despite the limitations, tools for detection or risk assessment can be an important component of treatment when used appropriately.

The development of accurate measures for assessing acute suicide risk would likely enhance prevention efforts. Given the accuracy of certain measures in predicting lifetime risk for suicide, identified individuals should be referred for support and/or treatment.

• Large epidemiological studies demonstrate reductions in suicide rates with increased antidepressant use. Randomized, controlled trials of the effects of these anti-depressants on suicide have largely failed to reveal significant differences *versus* placebo, perhaps due to methodological limitations.

• Compelling evidence suggests that lithium maintenance treatment reduces suicide in certain populations. Evidence is mounting that clozapine treatment reduces suicide in specific populations, as well.

Important questions regarding lithium still remain. Controlled studies are needed to confirm the effectiveness of lithium and to define the factors (e.g., timing, dose, diagnosis) that influence it.

• Despite manifest anxiety and agitation often marking acute suicide risk, the effects of anti-anxiety drugs on suicidality remains largely unknown. Likewise, the literature contains virtually no new and only nonrandomized, uncontrolled studies regarding the potentially effective treatment modality of electroconvulsive therapy.

Carefully designed trials are necessary to understand the potential of pharmacotherapies to reduce suicidal behavior. Studies should include the antidepressants, lithium, clozapine, anti-anxiety drugs, as well as electroconvulsive therapy. The lack of long-term assessment of therapeutic strategies and the exclusion of high-risk patients from clinical trials represent critical gaps in the field.

• Medicine alone is not sufficient for treatment of suicidality, nor are treatments equally effective across individuals and diagnoses. Psychotherapy provides a necessary therapeutic relationship that reduces the risk of suicide. Cognitive-behavioral approaches that include problem-solving training seem to reduce suicidal ideation and attempts more effectively than treatment as usual or supportive therapy. As with drug therapy, research on the long-term effectiveness of these interventions is lacking.

Controlled clinical trials are necessary to determine the types and aspects of psychotherapy that are effective in reducing suicide for diverse individuals. Current evidence suggests that continued contact with a psychotherapist is critical. This needs to be rigorously evaluated.

• Suicide is far more likely to occur in the first month after discharge from a psychiatric hospital than subsequently; low treatment adherence poses a major risk for suicidal individuals. Long-term follow-up care of discharged suicidal individuals holds promise for reducing suicide. For example, a psychosocial intervention that effectively reduced completed suicides entailed regularly mailing letters to those patients who refused or dropped out of follow-up care.

Further research on the peri-hospital period to assess the risk and protective effects of hospitalization, the relationships between length of stay and outcomes, and the factors post-hospital that account for the increased risk for suicide would provide critical information for suicide reduction strategies. The efficacy of different approaches to follow-up care in reducing suicide across populations must also be established, and successful interventions should be replicated and widely disseminated.

• Efficacy studies of both psychopharmacological and psychosocial interventions demonstrate that suicidality often either fails to remit or returns even when symptoms of a mental disorder decrease due to treatment. The most effective psychopharmacological and psychosocial treatment strategies generally involve long-term and/or maintenance treatment. Maintenance treatment with lithium, clozapine, and electroconvulsive therapy, during which patients must regularly see health care professionals, appears more effective in reducing suicidality than only prophylactic treatments; regular contact with health care staff via mail and weeks or months of psychotherapy also appear to reduce suicide.

Longitudinal research is needed to assess outcomes of prophylactic/short-term versus maintenance/long-term treatment for suicidality. The course of suicidality across the life span suggests it may at times represent a life-long condition requiring sustained treatment; further life-course research is required to verify this.

REFERENCES

AACAP (American Academy of Child and Adolescent Psychiatry). 2001. Summary of the practice parameters for the assessment and treatment of children and adolescents with suicidal behavior. *Journal of the American Academy of Child and Adolescent Psychiatry*, 40(4): 495-499.

AHCPR (Agency for Health Care Policy and Research). 1993. *Clinical Practice Guideline 5. Depression in Primary Care: Volume 2. Treatment of Major Depression.* AHCPR publication 93-0551. Rockville, MD: United States Department of Health and Human Services, Agency for Health Care Policy and Research.

Aoun S. 1999. Deliberate self-harm in rural Western Australia: Results of an intervention study. *Australian and New Zealand Journal of Mental Health Nursing*, 8(2): 65-73.

APA (American Psychiatric Association Task Force on ECT). 1990. *The Practice of ECT: Recommendations for Treatment, Training and Privileging.* Washington, DC: American Psychiatric Association.

APA (American Psychiatric Association). 1994. *The Diagnostic and Statistical Manual of Mental Disorders.* 4th ed. Washington, DC.

Appleby L. 2000. Prevention of suicide in psychiatric patients. In: Hawton K, van Heeringen K, Editors. *The International Handbook of Suicide and Attempted Suicide.* (pp. 617-630). Chichester, UK: John Wiley and Sons.

Appleby L, Dennehy JA, Thomas CS, Faragher EB, Lewis G. 1999a. Aftercare and clinical characteristics of people with mental illness who commit suicide: A case-control study. *Lancet*, 353(9162): 1397-1400.

Appleby L, Shaw J, Amos T, McDonnell R, Harris C, McCann K, Kiernan K, Davies S, Bickley H, Parsons R. 1999b. Suicide within 12 months of contact with mental health services: National clinical survey. *British Medical Journal*, 318(7193): 1235-1239.

Apter A, Horesh N, Gothelf D, Graffi H, Lepkifker E. 2001. Relationship between self-disclosure and serious suicidal behavior. *Comprehensive Psychiatry*, 42(1): 70-75.

Avery D, Winokur G. 1977. The efficacy of electroconvulsive therapy and antidepressants in depression. *Biological Psychiatry*, 12(4): 507-523.

Baldessarini RJ, Tondo L. 1999. Antisuicidal effect of lithium treatment in major mood disorders. In: Jacobs DG, Editor. *The Harvard Medical School Guide to Suicide Assessment and Intervention.* (pp. 355-371). San Francisco: Jossey-Bass Publishers.

Baldessarini RJ, Tondo L, Hennen J. 1999. Effects of lithium treatment and its discontinuation on suicidal behavior in bipolar manic-depressive disorders. *Journal of Clinical Psychiatry*, 60(Suppl 2): 77-84.

Barbui C, Campomori A, D'Avanzo B, Negri E, Garattini S. 1999. Antidepressant drug use in Italy since the introduction of SSRIs: National trends, regional differences and impact on suicide rates. *Social Psychiatry and Psychiatric Epidemiology*, 34(3): 152-156.

Beasley CM Jr, Dornseif BE, Bosomworth JC, Sayler ME, Rampey AH Jr, Heiligenstein JH, Thompson VL, Murphy DJ, Masica DN. 1991. Fluoxetine and suicide: A meta-analysis of controlled trials of treatment for depression. *British Medical Journal*, 303(6804): 685-692.

Bech P, Olsen LR, Niméus A. 2001. Psychometric scales in suicide assessment. In: Wasserman D, Editor. *Suicide: An Unnecessary Death.* (pp. 147-157). London: Martin Dunitz.

Beck AT, Kovacs M, Weissman A. 1979. Assessment of suicidal intention: The Scale for Suicide Ideation. *Journal of Consulting and Clinical Psychology*, 47(2): 343-352.

Berman AL, Jobes DA. 1991. *Adolescent Suicide: Assessment and Intervention.* Washington, DC: American Psychological Association.

Blazer DG, Hybels CF, Simonsick EM, Hanlon JT. 2000. Marked differences in antidepressant use by race in an elderly community sample: 1986-1996. *American Journal of Psychiatry*, 157(7): 1089-1094.

Bowden CL. 2000. Efficacy of lithium in mania and maintenance therapy of bipolar disorder. *Journal of Clinical Psychiatry*, 61: 35-40.

Bowden CL, Lecrubier Y, Bauer M, Goodwin G, Greil W, Sachs G, Von Knorring L. 2000. Maintenance therapies for classic and other forms of bipolar disorder. *Journal of Affective Disorders*, 59: S57-S67.

Brent DA, Holder D, Kolko D, Birmaher B, Baugher M, Roth C, Iyengar S, Johnson BA. 1997. A clinical psychotherapy trial for adolescent depression comparing cognitive, family, and supportive therapy. *Archives of General Psychiatry*, 54(9): 877-885.

Brodersen A, Licht RW, Vestergaard P, Olesen AV, Mortensen PB. 2000. Sixteen-year mortality in patients with affective disorder commenced on lithium. *British Journal of Psychiatry*, 176: 429-433.

Brown GK. 2000. *A Review of Suicide Assessment Measures for Intervention Research With Adults and Older Adults.* Technical report submitted to NIMH under Contract No. 263-MH914950. Bethesda, MD: National Institute of Mental Health.

Brown GK, Beck AT, Steer RA, Grisham JR. 2000. Risk factors for suicide in psychiatric outpatients: A 20-year prospective study. *Journal of Consulting and Clinical Psychology*, 68(3): 371-377.

Byford S, Harrington R, Torgerson D, Kerfoot M, Dyer E, Harrington V, Woodham A, Gill J, McNiven F. 1999. Cost-effectiveness analysis of a home-based social work intervention for children and adolescents who have deliberately poisoned themselves. Results of a randomised controlled trial. *British Journal of Psychiatry*, 174: 56-62.

Calabrese JR, Rapport DJ, Shelton MD, Kimmel SE. 2001a. Evolving methodologies in bipolar disorder maintenance research. *British Journal of Psychiatry. Supplement*, 41: S157-S163.

Calabrese JR, Shelton MD, Bowden CL, Rapport DJ, Suppes T, Shirley ER, Kimmel SE, Caban SJ. 2001b. Bipolar rapid cycling: Focus on depression as its hallmark. *Journal of Clinical Psychiatry*, 62 (Suppl 14): 34-41.

Chan DW. 1995. Reasons for living among Chinese adolescents in Hong Kong. *Suicide and Life-Threatening Behavior*, 25(3): 347-357.

Chowdhury N, Hicks RC, Kreitman N. 1973. Evaluation of an after-care service for parasuicide (attempted suicide) patients. *Social Psychiatry*, 8(2): 67-81.

Conwell Y, Duberstein PR, Cox C, Herrmann JH, Forbes NT, Caine ED. 1996. Relationships of age and axis I diagnoses in victims of completed suicide: A psychological autopsy study. *American Journal of Psychiatry*, 153(8): 1001-1008.

Crammer JL. 1984. The special characteristics of suicide in hospital in-patients. *British Journal of Psychiatry*, 145: 460-463.

Danish University Antidepressant Group. 1993. Moclobemide: A reversible MAO-A-inhibitor showing weaker antidepressant effect than clomipramine in a controlled multicenter study. *Journal of Affective Disorders*, 28(2): 105-116.

Dhossche DM, Ulusarac A, Syed W. 2001. A retrospective study of general hospital patients who commit suicide shortly after being discharged from the hospital. *Archives of Internal Medicine*, 161(7): 991-994.

Domino G. 1985. Clergy's attitudes toward suicide and recognition of suicide lethality. *Death Studies*, 9(3-4): 187-199.

Donahue MJ. 1995. Religion and the well-being of adolescents. *Journal of Social Issues*, 51(2): 145-160.

Eberhard G, von Knorring L, Nilsson HL, Sundequist U, Bjorling G, Linder H, Svard KO, Tysk L. 1988. A double-blind randomized study of clomipramine versus maprotiline in patients with idiopathic pain syndromes. *Neuropsychobiology*, 19(1): 25-34.

Evans K, Tyrer P, Catalan J, Schmidt U, Davidson K, Dent J, Tata P, Thornton S, Barber J, Thompson S. 1999. Manual-assisted cognitive-behavior therapy (MACT): A randomized controlled trial of a brief intervention with bibliotherapy in the treatment of recurrent deliberate self-harm. *Psychological Medicine*, 29: 19-25.

Fawcett J, Clark DC, Scheftner WA. 1991. The assessment and management of the suicidal patient. *Psychiatric Medicine*, 9(2): 299-311.

Fink M, Sackeim HA. 1996. Convulsive therapy in schizophrenia? *Schizophrenia Bulletin*, 22(1): 27-39.

Foa EB, Keane TM, Friedman MJ, Editors. 2000. *Effective Treatments for PTSD: Practice Guidelines From the International Society for Traumatic Stress Studies.* New York: The Guilford Press.

Friedman RS. 1989. Hospital treatment of the suicidal patient. In: Jacobs DG, Brown HP, Editors. *Suicide: Understanding and Responding.* (pp. 379-402). Madison, CT: International Universities Press.

Gibbons JS, Butler J, Urwin P, Gibbons JL. 1978. Evaluation of a social work service for self-poisoning patients. *British Journal of Psychiatry,* 133: 111-118.

Goldacre M, Seagroatt V, Hawton K. 1993. Suicide after discharge from psychiatric inpatient care. *Lancet,* 342(8866): 283-286.

Goldstein RB, Black DW, Nasrallah A, Winokur G. 1991. The prediction of suicide. Sensitivity, specificity, and predictive value of a multivariate model applied to suicide among 1906 patients with affective disorders. *Archives of General Psychiatry,* 48(5): 418-422.

Goldston DB. 2000. *Assessment of Suicidal Behaviors and Risk Among Children and Adolescents.* Technical report submitted to NIMH under Contract No. 263-MD-909995. Bethesda, MD: National Institute of Mental Health.

Goldston DB, Daniel SS, Reboussin BA, Reboussin DM, Frazier PH, Harris AE. 2001. Cognitive risk factors and suicide attempts among formerly hospitalized adolescents: A prospective naturalistic study. *Journal of the American Academy of Child and Adolescent Psychiatry,* 40(1): 91-99.

Gonella G, Baignoli G, Ecari U. 1990. Fluvoxamine and imipramine in the treatment of depressive patients: A double-blind controlled study. *Current Medical Research and Opinion,* 12(3): 177-184.

Goodwin FK, Ghaemi SN. 2000. The impact of mood stabilizers on suicide in bipolar disorder: A comparative study. *CNS Spectrum 5,* 2(Supplement 1): 12-18.

Goodwin FK, Jamison KR. 1990. *Manic-Depressive Illness.* New York: Oxford University Press.

Goodwin GM. 1999. Prophylaxis of bipolar disorder: How and who should we treat in the long term? *European Neuropsychopharmacology,* 9: S125-S129.

Greil W, Ludwig-Mayerhofer W, Erazo N, Engel RR, Czernik A, Giedke H, Muller-Oerlinghausen B, Osterheider M, Rudolf GA, Sauer H, Tegeler J, Wetterling T. 1996. Comparative efficacy of lithium and amitriptyline in the maintenance treatment of recurrent unipolar depression: A randomised study. *Journal of Affective Disorders,* 40(3): 179-190.

Greil W, Ludwig-Mayerhofer W, Erazo N, Engel RR, Czernik A, Giedke H, Muller-Oerlinghausen B, Osterheider M, Rudolf GA, Sauer H, Tegeler J, Wetterling T. 1997a. Lithium vs carbamazepine in the maintenance treatment of schizoaffective disorder: A randomised study. *European Archives of Psychiatry and Clinical Neuroscience,* 247(1): 42-50.

Greil W, Ludwig-Mayerhofer W, Erazo N, Schochlin C, Schmidt S, Engel RR, Czernik A, Giedke H, Muller-Oerlinghausen B, Osterheider M, Rudolf GA, Sauer H, Tegeler J, Wetterling T. 1997b. Lithium versus carbamazepine in the maintenance treatment of bipolar disorders—A randomised study. *Journal of Affective Disorders,* 43(2): 151-161.

Guthrie E, Kapur N, Mackway-Jones K, Chew-Graham C, Moorey J, Mendel E, Marino-Francis F, Sanderson S, Turpin C, Boddy G, Tomenson B. 2001. Randomised controlled trial of brief psychological intervention after deliberate self poisoning. *British Medical Journal,* 323(7305): 135-138.

Harrington R, Kerfoot M, Dyer E, McNiven F, Gill J, Harrington V, Woodham A, Byford S. 1998. Randomized trial of a home-based family intervention for children who have deliberately poisoned themselves. *Journal of the American Academy of Child and Adolescent Psychiatry,* 37(5): 512-518.

Harris EC, Barraclough B. 1997. Suicide as an outcome for mental disorders. A meta-analysis. *British Journal of Psychiatry*, 170: 205-228.

Hawton K, Arensman E, Townsend E, Bremner S, Feldman E, Goldney R, Gunnell D, Hazell P, van Heeringen K, House A, Owens D, Sakinofsky I, Träskman-Bendz L. 1998. Deliberate self harm: Systematic review of efficacy of psychosocial and pharmacological treatments in preventing repetition. *British Medical Journal*, 317(7156): 441-447.

Hawton K, Bancroft J, Catalan J, Kingston B, Stedeford A, Welch N. 1981. Domiciliary and out-patient treatment of self-poisoning patients by medical and non-medical staff. *Psychological Medicine*, 11(1): 169-177.

Hawton K, McKeown S, Day A, Martin P, O'Connor M, Yule J. 1987. Evaluation of out-patient counselling compared with general practitioner care following overdoses. *Psychological Medicine*, 17(3): 751-761.

Healy D, Langmaak C, Savage M. 1999. Suicide in the course of the treatment of depression. *Journal of Psychopharmacology*, 13(1): 94-99.

Henriksson S, Boethius G, Isacsson G. 2001. Suicides are seldom prescribed antidepressants: Findings from a prospective prescription database in Jamtland county, Sweden, 1985-95. *Acta Psychiatrica Scandinavica*, 103(4): 301-306.

Hirschfeld RM. 2000. Suicide and antidepressant treatment. *Archives of General Psychiatry*, 57(4): 325-326.

Hsu SI. 1999. Somatisation among Asian refugees and immigrants as a culturally-shaped illness behaviour. *Annals of the Academy of Medicine, Singapore*, 28(6): 841-845.

Hung CI, Liu CY, Liao MN, Chang YH, Yang YY, Yeh EK. 2000. Self-destructive acts occurring during medical general hospitalization. *General Hospital Psychiatry*, 22(2): 115-121.

Husaini BA, Moore ST. 1994. Psychiatric symptoms and help-seeking behavior among the elderly: An analysis of racial and gender differences. *Journal of Gerontological Social Work*, 21(3): 177-195.

Inman W, Kubota K, Pearce G, Wilton L. 1993. PEM report number 6: Paroxetine. *Pharmacoepidemiology and Drug Safety*, 2: 393-422.

IOM (Institute of Medicine). 2001. *Health and Behavior: The Interplay of Biological, Behavioral, and Societal Influences.* Washington, DC: National Academy Press.

Isacsson G. 2000. Suicide prevention—a medical breakthrough? *Acta Psychiatrica Scandinavica*, 102(2): 113-117.

Isacsson G, Bergman U, Rich CL. 1994. Antidepressants, depression and suicide: An analysis of the San Diego study. *Journal of Affective Disorders*, 32(4): 277-286.

Isacsson G, Bergman U, Rich CL. 1996. Epidemiological data suggest antidepressants reduce suicide risk among depressives. *Journal of Affective Disorders*, 41: 1-8.

Isacsson G, Boethius G, Bergman U. 1992. Low level of antidepressant prescription for people who later commit suicide: 15 years of experience from a population-based drug database in Sweden. *Acta Psychiatrica Scandinavica*, 85(6): 444-448.

Isacsson G, Holmgren P, Druid H, Bergman U. 1997. The utilization of antidepressants—a key issue in the prevention of suicide: An analysis of 5281 suicides in Sweden during the period 1992-1994. *Acta Psychiatrica Scandinavica*, 96(2): 94-100.

Isacsson G, Holmgren P, Druid H, Bergman U. 1999. Psychotropics and suicide prevention. Implications from toxicological screening of 5281 suicides in Sweden 1992-1994. *British Journal of Psychiatry*, 174: 259-265.

Isacsson G, Holmgren P, Wasserman D, Bergman U. 1994. Use of antidepressants among people committing suicide in Sweden. *British Medical Journal*, 308(6927): 506-509.

Isometsa ET, Henriksson MM, Aro HM, Heikkinen ME, Kuoppasalmi KI, Lönnqvist JK. 1994. Suicide in major depression. *American Journal of Psychiatry*, 151(4): 530-536.

Jacobson G. 1999. The inpatient management of suicidality. In: Jacobs DG, Editor. *The Harvard Medical School Guide to Suicide Assessment and Intervention.* (pp. 383-405). San Francisco, CA: Jossey-Bass Publishers.

Jamison KR. 1995. *An Unquiet Mind: A Memoir of Moods and Madness.* New York: A.A. Knopf.

Jamison KR, Akiskal HS. 1983. Medication compliance in patients with bipolar disorder. *Psychiatric Clinics of North America,* 6(1): 175-192.

Jamison KR, Gerner RH, Goodwin FK. 1979. Patient and physician attitudes toward lithium: Relationship to compliance. *Archives of General Psychiatry,* 36: 866-869.

Johnson M, Bulecheck G, McCloskey Dochterman J, Maas M, Moorhead S, Editors. 2001. *Nursing Diagnoses, Outcomes, and Interventions: NANDA, NOC, and NIC Linkages.* St. Louis, MO: Mosby.

Joiner TEJr, Voelz ZR, Rudd MD. 2001. For suicidal young adults with comorbid depressive and anxiety disorders, probem-solving treatment may be better than treatment as usual. *Professional Psychology—Research & Practice,* 32(3): 278-282.

Judd FK, Moore K, Norman TR, Burrows GD, Gupta RK, Parker G. 1993. A multicentre double blind trial of fluoxetine versus amitriptyline in the treatment of depressive illness. *Australian and New Zealand Journal of Psychiatry,* 27(1): 49-55.

Kasper S, Moller HJ, Montgomery SA, Zondag E. 1995. Antidepressant efficacy in relation to item analysis and severity of depression: A placebo-controlled trial of fluvoxamine versus imipramine. *International Clinical Psychopharmacology,* 9 (Suppl 4): 3-12.

Keller MB, Lavori PW, Klerman GL, Andreasen NC, Endicott J, Coryell W, Fawcett J, Rice JP, Hirschfeld RM. 1986. Low levels and lack of predictors of somatotherapy and psychotherapy received by depressed patients. *Archives of General Psychiatry,* 43(5): 458-466.

Khan A, Khan SR, Leventhal RM, Brown WA. 2001. Symptom reduction and suicide risk in patients treated with placebo in antidepressant clinical trials: A replication analysis of the Food and Drug Administration Database. *International Journal of Neuropsychopharmacology,* 4(2): 113-118.

Khan A, Warner HA, Brown WA. 2000. Symptom reduction and suicide risk in patients treated with placebo in antidepressant clinical trials: An analysis of the Food and Drug Administration database. *Archives of General Psychiatry,* 57(4): 311-317.

King EA, Baldwin DS, Sinclair JM, Baker NG, Campbell MJ, Thompson C. 2001. The Wessex Recent In-Patient Suicide Study, 1. Case-control study of 234 recently discharged psychiatric patient suicides. *British Journal of Psychiatry,* 178: 531-536.

Koenig HG, Pargament KI, Nielsen J. 1998. Religious coping and health status in medically ill hospitalized older adults. *Journal of Nervous and Mental Disease,* 186(9): 513-521.

Koenig HG, Weaver AJ. 1997. *Counseling Troubled Older Adults: A Handbook for Pastors and Religious Caregivers.* Nashville, TN: Abingdon Press.

Koivumaa-Honkanen H, Honkanen R, Viinamaki H, Heikkila K, Kaprio J, Koskenvuo M. 2001. Life satisfaction and suicide: A 20-year follow-up study. *American Journal of Psychiatry,* 158(3): 433-439.

Koons CR, Robins CJ, Tweed JL, Lynch TR, Gonzalez AM, Morse JQ, Bishop GK, Butterfield MI, Bastian LA. 2001. Efficacy of dialectical behavior therapy in women veterans with borderline personality disorder. *Behavior Therapy,* 32(2): 371-390.

Kotin J, Post RM, Goodwin FK. 1973. Drug treatment of depressed patients referred for hospitalization. *American Journal of Psychiatry,* 130(10): 1139-1141.

Lapierre YD. 1991. Controlling acute episodes of depression. *International Clinical Psychopharmacology,* 6 (Suppl 2): 23-35.

Larson DB, Hohmann AA, Kessler LG, Meador KG, Boyd JH, McSherry E. 1988. The couch and the cloth: The need for linkage. *Hospital and Community Psychiatry,* 39(10): 1064-1069.

Lawrenson RA, Tyrer F, Newson RB, Farmer RD. 2000. The treatment of depression in UK general practice: Selective serotonin reuptake inhibitors and tricyclic antidepressants compared. *Journal of Affective Disorders*, 59(2): 149-157.

Leane W, Shute R. 1998. Youth suicide: The knowledge and attitudes of Australian teachers and clergy. *Suicide and Life-Threatening Behavior*, 28(2): 165-173.

Leon AC, Keller MB, Warshaw MG, Mueller TI, Solomon DA, Coryell W, Endicott J. 1999. Prospective study of fluoxetine treatment and suicidal behavior in affectively ill subjects. *American Journal of Psychiatry*, 156(2): 195-201.

Lerner MS, Clum GA. 1990. Treatment of suicide ideators: A problem-solving approach. *Behavior Therapy*, 21(4): 403-411.

Letizia C, Kapik B, Flanders WD. 1996. Suicidal risk during controlled clinical investigations of fluvoxamine. *Journal of Clinical Psychiatry*, 57(9): 415-421.

Liberman RP, Eckman T. 1981. Behavior therapy vs insight-oriented therapy for repeated suicide attempters. *Archives of General Psychiatry*, 38(10): 1126-1130.

Linehan MM. 1997. Behavioral treatments of suicidal behaviors. Definitional obfuscation and treatment outcomes. *Annals of the New York Academy of Sciences*, 836: 302-328.

Linehan MM, Armstrong HE, Suarez A, Allmon D, Heard HL. 1991. Cognitive-behavioral treatment of chronically parasuicidal borderline patients. *Archives of General Psychiatry*, 48(12): 1060-1064.

Linehan MM, Goodstein JL, Nielsen SL, Chiles JA. 1983. Reasons for staying alive when you are thinking of killing yourself: The reasons for living inventory. *Journal of Consulting and Clinical Psychology*, 51(2): 276-286.

Litman RE, Wold C. 1975. Beyond crisis intervention. In: Shneidman E, Editor. *Suicidology: Contemporary Developments*. (pp. 528-546). New York: Grune & Stratton.

MacKinnon DR, Farberow NL. 1976. An assessment of the utility of suicide prediction. *Suicide and Life-Threatening Behavior*, 6(2): 86-91.

Macqueen GM, Young LT. 2001. Bipolar II disorder: Symptoms, course, and response to treatment. *Psychiatric Services*, 52(3): 358-361.

Mahapatra SN, Hackett D. 1997. A randomised, double-blind, parallel-group comparison of venlafaxine and dothiepin in geriatric patients with major depression. *International Journal of Clinical Practice*, 51(4): 209-213.

Mann JJ, Goodwin FK, O'Brien CP, Robinson DS. 1993. Suicidal behavior and psychotropic medication. Accepted as a consensus statement by the ACNP Council, March 2, 1992. *Neuropsychopharmacology*, 8(2): 177-183.

Mann JJ, Kapur S. 1991. The emergence of suicidal ideation and behavior during antidepressant pharmacotherapy. *Archives of General Psychiatry*, 48(11): 1027-1033.

Mannon JD, Crawford RL. 1996. Clergy confidence to counsel and their willingness to refer to mental health professionals. *Family Therapy*, 23(3): 213-231.

Marchesi C, Ceccherininelli A, Rossi A, Maggini C. 1998. Is anxious-agitated major depression responsive to fluoxetine? A double-blind comparison with amitriptyline. *Pharmacopsychiatry*, 31(6): 216-221.

Markowitz JC. 2001. Antidepressants and suicide risk. *British Journal of Psychiatry*, 178: 477.

Marsella AJ. 1988. Cross-cultural research on severe mental disorders: Issues and findings. *Acta Psychiatrica Scandinavica. Supplement*, 344: 7-22.

Marsella AJ, Sanborn KO, Kameoka V, Shizuru L, Brennan J. 1975. Cross-validation of self-report measures of depression among normal populations of Japanese, Chinese, and Caucasian ancestry. *Journal of Clinical Psychology*, 31(2): 281-287.

Marsella AJ, Yamada A. 2000. Culture and mental health: An introduction and overview of foundations, concepts, and issues. In: Cuellar I, Paniagua FA, Editors. *Handbook of Multicultural Mental Health: Assessment and Treatment of Diverse Populations*. (pp. 3-24). San Diego, CA: Academic Press.

Marzuk PM, Tardiff K, Leon AC, Hirsch CS, Stajic M, Hartwell N, Portera L. 1995. Use of prescription psychotropic drugs among suicide victims in New York City. *American Journal of Psychiatry*, 152(10): 1520-1522.

McKenzie W, Wurr C. 2001. Early suicide following discharge from a psychiatric hospital. *Suicide and Life-Threatening Behavior*, 31(3): 358-363.

McLeavey BC, Daly RJ, Ludgate JW, Murray CM. 1994. Interpersonal problem-solving skills training in the treatment of self-poisoning patients. *Suicide and Life-Threatening Behavior*, 24(4): 382-394.

Meehl PE, Rosen A. 1955. Antecedent probability and the efficiency of psychometric signs, patterns, or cutting scores. *Psychological Bulletin*, 52: 194-216.

Melander A, Henricson K, Stenberg P, Lowenhielm P, Malmvik J, Sternebring B, Kaij L, Bergdahl U. 1991. Anxiolytic-hypnotic drugs: Relationships between prescribing, abuse and suicide. *European Journal of Clinical Pharmacology*, 41(6): 525-529.

Meltzer HY. 1999. Suicide and schizophrenia: Clozapine and the InterSePT study. International Clozaril/Leponex Suicide Prevention Trial. *Journal of Clinical Psychiatry*, 60 (Suppl 12): 47-50.

Meltzer HY, Alphs L, Altamura C, Kerwin R, Chouinard G, Green A, Lindenmayer JP, Potkin S, Islam Z, Kane J, Krishnan R, Anand R. 2001. *Effect of Clozapine on the Reduction of Suicidality in Schizophrenia and Schizoaffetive Disorder.* Abstract # 175 at the annual meeting of the American College of Neuropsychopharmacology in Kona, Hawaii, December 2001.

Meltzer HY, Okayli G. 1995. Reduction of suicidality during clozapine treatment of neuroleptic-resistant schizophrenia: Impact on risk-benefit assessment. *American Journal of Psychiatry*, 152(2): 183-190.

Metzger ED. 1999. ECT and suicide. In: Jacobs DG, Editor. *The Harvard Medical School Guide to Suicide Assessment and Intervention.* (pp. 406-413). San Francisco, CA: Jossey-Bass Publishers.

Miller AL, Rathus JH, Linehan MM, Wetzler S, Leigh E. 1997. Dialectical behavior therapy adapted for suicidal adolescents. *Journal of Practical Psychiatry and Behavioral Health*, 3(2): 78-86.

Modestin J, Schwarzenbach FA, Wurmle O. 1992. Therapy factors in treating severely ill psychiatric patients. *British Journal of Medical Psychology*, 65 (Pt 2): 147-156.

Möller HJ. 1989. Efficacy of different strategies of aftercare for patients who have attempted suicide. *Journal of the Royal Society of Medicine* 82: 643-647.

Möller HJ. 2001. Pharmacological treatment of underlying psychiatric disorders in suicidal patients. In: Wasserman D, Editor. *Suicide: An Unnecessary Death.* (pp. 173-178). London: Martin Dunitz.

Möller HJ, Steinmeyer EM. 1994. Are serotonergic reuptake inhibitors more potent in reducing suicidality? An empirical study on paroxetine. *European Neuropsychopharmacology*, 4(1): 55-59.

Montgomery DB, Roberts A, Green M, Bullock T, Baldwin D, Montgomery SA. 1994. Lack of efficacy of fluoxetine in recurrent brief depression and suicidal attempts. *European Archives of Psychiatry and Clinical Neuroscience*, 244(4): 211-215.

Montgomery S, Cronholm B, Asberg M, Montgomery DB. 1978. Differential effects on suicidal ideation of mianserin, maprotiline and amitriptyline. *British Journal of Clinical Pharmacology*, 5 (Suppl 1): S77-S80.

Montgomery SA, Dunner DL, Dunbar GC. 1995. Reduction of suicidal thoughts with paroxetine in comparison with reference antidepressants and placebo. *European Neuropsychopharmacology*, 5(1): 5-13.

Montgomery SA, Schatzberg AF, Guelfi JD, Kasper S, Nemeroff C, Swann A, Zajecka J. 2000. Pharmacotherapy of depression and mixed states in bipolar disorder. *Journal of Affective Disorders*, 59: S39-S56.

Morrison LL, Downey DL. 2000. Racial differences in self-disclosure of suicidal ideation and reasons for living: Implications for training. *Cultural Diversity and Ethnic Minority Psychology*, 6(4): 374-386.

Motto JA, Bostrom AG. 2001. A randomized controlled trial of postcrisis suicide prevention. *Psychiatric Services*, 52(6): 828-833.

Mukherjee S, Sackeim HA, Schnur DB. 1994. Electroconvulsive therapy of acute manic episodes: A review of 50 years' experience. *American Journal of Psychiatry*, 151(2): 169-176.

Müller-Oerlinghausen B, Berghofer A. 1999. Antidepressants and suicidal risk. *Journal of Clinical Psychiatry*, 60(Suppl 2): 94-99.

Negron R, Piacentini J, Graae F, Davies M, Shaffer D. 1997. Microanalysis of adolescent suicide attempters and ideators during the acute suicidal episode. *Journal of the American Academy of Child and Adolescent Psychiatry*, 36(11): 1512-1519.

Neighbors HW, Musick MA, Williams DR. 1998. The African American minister as a source of help for serious personal crises: Bridge or barrier to mental health care? *Health Education and Behavior*, 25(6): 759-777.

Neutel CI, Patten SB. 1997. Risk of suicide attempts after benzodiazepine and/or antidepressant use. *Annals of Epidemiology*, 7(8): 568-574.

O'Hagan M. 2001, August 23. Man sought help, then killed self. *The Washington Post*. H3

Ohberg A, Vuori E, Klaukka T, Lonnqvist J. 1998. Antidepressants and suicide mortality. *Journal of Affective Disorders*, 50(2-3): 225-233.

Ohberg A, Vuori E, Ojanpera I, Lonnqvist J. 1996. Alcohol and drugs in suicides. *British Journal of Psychiatry*, 169(1): 75-80.

Oquendo MA, Malone KM, Ellis SP, Sackeim HA, Mann JJ. 1999. Inadequacy of antidepressant treatment for patients with major depression who are at risk for suicidal behavior. *American Journal of Psychiatry*, 156(2): 190-194.

Osman A, Downs WR, Kopper BA, Barrios FX, Baker MT, Osman JR, Besett TM, Linehan MM. 1998. The Reasons for Living Inventory for Adolescents (RFL-A): Development and psychometric properties. *Journal of Clinical Psychology*, 54(8): 1063-1078.

Patsiokas AT, Clum GA. 1985. Effects of psychotherapeutic strategies in the treatment of suicide attempters. *Psychotherapy*, 22(2): 281-290.

Philibert RA, Richards L, Lynch CF, Winokur G. 1995. Effect of ECT on mortality and clinical outcome in geriatric unipolar depression. *Journal of Clinical Psychiatry*, 56(9): 390-394.

Pokorny AD. 1983. Prediction of suicide in psychiatric patients. Report of a prospective study. *Archives of General Psychiatry*, 40(3): 249-257.

Propst LR, Ostrom R, Watkins P, Dean T, Mashburn D. 1992. Comparative efficacy of religious and nonreligious cognitive-behavioral therapy for the treatment of clinical depression in religious individuals. *Journal of Consulting and Clinical Psychology*, 60(1): 94-103.

Prudic J, Sackeim HA. 1999. Electroconvulsive therapy and suicide risk. *Journal of Clinical Psychiatry*, 60(Suppl 2): 104-110.

Prudic J, Sackeim HA, Devanand DP. 1990. Medication resistance and clinical response to electroconvulsive therapy. *Psychiatry Research*, 31(3): 287-296.

Reid WH, Mason M, Hogan T. 1998. Suicide prevention effects associated with clozapine therapy in schizophrenia and schizoaffective disorder. *Psychiatric Services*, 49(8): 1029-1033.

Rich CL. 1999. Relationship between antidepressant treatment and suicide. *Journal of Clinical Psychiatry*, 60(5): 340.

Rich CL, Isacsson G. 1997. Suicide and antidepressants in south Alabama: Evidence for improved treatment of depression. *Journal of Affective Disorders*, 45(3): 135-142.

Rihmer Z, Belso N, Kalmar S. 2001. Antidepressants and suicide prevention in Hungary. *Acta Psychiatrica Scandinavica*, 103(3): 238-239.

Rihmer Z, Rutz W, Pihlgren. 1995. Depression and suicide on Gotland: An intensive study of all suicides before and after a depression-training programme for general practitioners. *Journal of Affective Disorders*, 35: 147-152.

Rihmer Z, Rutz W, Pihlgren H, Pestality P. 1998. Decreasing tendency of seasonality in suicide may indicate lowering rate of depressive suicides in the population. *Psychiatry Research*, 81(2): 233-240.

Robins E, Murphy GE, Wilkinson RHJr, Gassner S, Kayes J. 1959. Some clinical considerations in the prevention of suicide based on a study of 134 successful suicides. *American Journal of Public Health*, 49: 888-899.

Roose SP, Nobler M. 2001. ECT and onset of action. *Journal of Clinical Psychiatry*, 62 (Suppl 4): 24-26; discussion 37-40.

Rotheram-Borus MJ, Piacentini J, Cantwell C, Belin TR, Song J. 2000. The 18-month impact of an emergency room intervention for adolescent female suicide attempters. *Journal of Consulting and Clinical Psychology*, 68(6): 1081-1093.

Rotheram-Borus MJ, Piacentini J, Van Rossem R, Graae F, Cantwell C, Castro-Blanco D, Feldman J. 1999. Treatment adherence among Latina female adolescent suicide attempters. *Suicide and Life-Threatening Behavior*, 29(4): 319-331.

Rotheram-Borus MJ, Piacentini J, Van Rossem R, Graae F, Cantwell C, Castro-Blanco D, Miller S, Feldman J. 1996. Enhancing treatment adherence with a specialized emergency room program for adolescent suicide attempters. *Journal of the American Academy of Child and Adolescent Psychiatry*, 35(5): 654-663.

Rothschild AJ, Locke CA. 1991. Reexposure to fluoxetine after serious suicide attempts by three patients: The role of akathisia. *Journal of Clinical Psychiatry*, 52(12): 491-493.

Rouillon F, Phillips R, Serrurier D, Ansart E, Gerard MJ. 1989. Recurrence of unipolar depression and efficacy of maprotiline. *L'Encephale*, 15(6): 527-534.

Roy A, Draper R. 1995. Suicide among psychiatric hospital in-patients. *Psychological Medicine*, 25(1): 199-202.

Rudd MD, Rajab MH, Orman DT, Joiner T, Stulman DA, Dixon W. 1996. Effectiveness of an outpatient problem-solving intervention targeting suicidal young adults: Preliminary results. *Journal of Consulting and Clinical Psychology*, 64(1): 179-190.

Rutz W. 2001. Preventing suicide and premature death by education and treatment. *Journal of Affective Disorders*, 62(1-2): 123-129.

Rutz W, von Knorring L, Walinder J. 1989a. Frequency of suicide on Gotland after systematic postgraduate education of general practitioners. *Acta Psychiatrica Scandinavica*, 80(2): 151-154.

Rutz W, Walinder J, Eberhard G, Holmberg G, von Knorring AL, von Knorring L, Wistedt B, Aberg-Wistedt A. 1989b. An educational program on depressive disorders for general practitioners on Gotland: Background and evaluation. *Acta Psychiatrica Scandinavica*, 79(1): 19-26.

Salkovskis PM, Atha C, Storer D. 1990. Cognitive-behavioural problem solving in the treatment of patients who repeatedly attempt suicide. A controlled trial. *British Journal of Psychiatry*, 157: 871-876.

Sclar DA, Robinson LM, Skaer TL, Galin RS. 1998. Trends in the prescribing of antidepressant pharmacotherapy: Office-based visits, 1990–1995. *Clinical Therapeutics*, 20(4): 871-884; 870.

Sexton TL, Whiston SC. 1991. A review of the empirical basis for counseling: Implications for practice and training. *Counselor Education and Supervision*, 30(4): 330-354.

Sheehan D, Dunbar GC, Fuell DL. 1992. The effect of paroxetine on anxiety and agitation associated with depression. *Psychopharmacology Bulletin*, 28(2): 139-143.

Soloff PH, George A, Nathan RS, Schulz PM, Perel JM. 1986. Paradoxical effects of amitriptyline on borderline patients. *American Journal of Psychiatry*, 143(12): 1603-1605.

Starrett RA, Rogers D, Decker JT. 1992. The self-reliance behavior of the Hispanic elderly in comparison to their use of formal mental health helping networks. *Clinical Gerontologist*, 11(3-4): 157-169.

Taiminen TJ. 1993. Effect of psychopharmacotherapy on suicide risk in psychiatric inpatients. *Acta Psychiatrica Scandinavica*, 87(1): 45-47.

Teicher MH, Glod C, Cole JO. 1990. Emergence of intense suicidal preoccupation during fluoxetine treatment. *American Journal of Psychiatry*, 147(2): 207-210.

Termansen PE, Bywater C. 1975. S.A.F.E.R.: A follow-up service for attempted suicide in Vancouver. *Canadian Psychiatric Association Journal*, 20(1): 29-34.

Thies-Flechtner K, Muller-Oerlinghausen B, Seibert W, Walther A, Greil W. 1996. Effect of prophylactic treatment on suicide risk in patients with major affective disorders. Data from a randomized prospective trial. *Pharmacopsychiatry*, 29(3): 103-107.

Thomas SB, Quinn SC, Billingsley A, Caldwell C. 1994. The characteristics of northern black churches with community health outreach programs. *American Journal of Public Health*, 84(4): 575-579.

Tollefson GD, Fawcett J, Winokur G, Beasley CM, Potvin JH, Faries DE, Rampey AH, Sayler ME. 1993. Evaluation of suicidality during pharmacologic treatment of mood and nonmood disorders. *Annals of Clinical Psychiatry*, 5(4): 209-224.

Tondo L, Baldessarini RJ. 2000. Reduced suicide risk during lithium maintenance treatment. *Journal of Clinical Psychiatry*, 61 (Suppl 9): 97-104.

Tondo L, Baldessarini RJ, Hennen J, Floris G, Silvetti F, Tohen M. 1998. Lithium treatment and risk of suicidal behavior in bipolar disorder patients. *Journal of Clinical Psychiatry*, 59(8): 405-414.

Tondo L, Hennen J, Baldessarini RJ. 2001. Lower suicide risk with long-term lithium treatment in major affective illness: A meta-analysis. *Acta Psychiatrica Scandinavica*, 104(3): 163-172.

Tondo L, Jamison KR, Baldessarini RJ. 1997. Effect of lithium maintenance on suicidal behavior in major mood disorders. *Annals of the New York Academy of Sciences*, 836: 339-351.

US DHHS (U.S. Department of Health and Human Services). 2001. *Mental Health: Culture, Race and Ethnicity—A Supplement to Mental Health: A Report of the Surgeon General.* Rockville, MD: U.S. Department of Health and Human Services, Substance Abuse and Mental Health Services Administration, Center for Mental Health Services, National Institutes of Health, National Institute of Mental Health.

van der Sande R, Buskens E, Allart E, van der Graaf Y, van Engeland H. 1997a. Psychosocial intervention following suicide attempt: A systematic review of treatment interventions. *Acta Psychiatrica Scandinavica*, 96(1): 43-50.

van der Sande R, van Rooijen L, Buskens E, Allart E, Hawton K, van der Graaf Y, van Engeland H. 1997b. Intensive in-patient and community intervention versus routine care after attempted suicide. A randomised controlled intervention study. *British Journal of Psychiatry*, 171: 35-41.

van Heeringen C, Jannes S, Buylaert W, Henderick H, De Bacquer D, Van Remoortel J. 1995. The management of non-compliance with referral to out-patient after-care among attempted suicide patient: A controlled intervention study. *Psychological Medicine*, 25(5): 963-970.

Verkes RJ, Van der Mast RC, Hengeveld MW, Tuyl JP, Zwinderman AH, Van Kempen GM. 1998. Reduction by paroxetine of suicidal behavior in patients with repeated suicide attempts but not major depression. *American Journal of Psychiatry*, 155(4): 543-547.

Vestergaard P, Licht RW, Brodersen A, Rasmussen N-A, Christensen H, Arngrim T, Gronvall B, Kristensen E, Poulstrup I. 1998. Outcome of lithium prophylaxis: A prospective follow-up of affective disorder patients assigned to high and low serum lithium levels. *Acta Psychiatrica Scandinavica*, 98(4): 310-315.

Walker AM, Lanza LL, Arellano F, Rothman KJ. 1997. Mortality in current and former users of clozapine. *Epidemiology*, 8(6): 671-677.

Waterhouse J, Platt S. 1990. General hospital admission in the management of parasuicide. A randomised controlled trial. *British Journal of Psychiatry*, 156: 236-242.

Weaver AJ. 1993. Suicide prevention: What clergy need to know. *Journal of Psychology and Christianity*, 12(1): 70-79.

Weaver AJ, Koenig HG. 1996. Elderly suicide, mental health professionals, and the clergy: A need for clinical collaboration, training, and research. *Death Studies*, 20(5): 495-508.

Weaver AJ, Preston JD, Jerome LW. 1999. *Counseling Troubled Teens and Their Familes: A Handbook for Pastors and Youth Workers.* Nashville, TN: Abingdon Press.

Weeke A. 1979. Causes of death in manic-depressives. In: Schou M, Strömgren E, Editors. *Origin, Prevention and Treatment of Affective Disorders.* (pp. 289-299). London: Academic Press.

Welu TC. 1977. A follow-up program for suicide attempters: Evaluation of effectiveness. *Suicide and Life-Threatening Behavior*, 7(1): 17-20.

Wheadon DE, Rampey AH Jr, Thompson VL, Potvin JH, Masica DN, Beasley CM Jr. 1992. Lack of association between fluoxetine and suicidality in bulimia nervosa. *Journal of Clinical Psychiatry*, 53(7): 235-241.

Zaninelli R, Meister W. 1999. The treatment of depression with paroxetine in psychiatric practice in Germany: The possibilities and current limitations of drug monitoring. *Pharmacopsychiatry*, 30: 9-20.

And Levin, a happy father and a man in perfect health, was several times so near suicide that he hid the cord, lest he be tempted to hang himself, and was afraid to go out with his gun, for fear of shooting himself. But Levin did not shoot himself, and did not hang himself; he went on living.

—LEO TOLSTOY
Anna Karenina

8

Programs for Suicide Prevention

Over the last 15–20 years, the first two generations of suicide prevention efforts have yielded valuable information on risk and protective factors, empirically based methods for preventing suicidal behavior, and improved research methods (Berman and Jobes, 1995; PHS, 2001). During this time, the following developments have been observed in the area of suicide prevention (1) a proliferation of curriculum-based suicide prevention programs in schools (cf., Garland et al., 1989) accompanied by increased attention and concerns voiced over format, goals, theoretic orientation, and safety issues (Hazell and King, 1996) that led to improved methods and prevention program designs (cf., Breton et al., 1998; Kalafat and Ryerson, 1999; Orbach and Bar-Joseph, 1993); (2) increased efforts to undertake empirical research on suicide prevention, prompted by a 1990 US Congressional mandate, and accompanied by the rapid development of suicidology as a multidisciplinary subspecialty with national and international professional organizations, new journals, and the establishment of centers for the study and prevention of suicide (PHS, 1999; 2001); (3) a new precisely defined prevention framework that places prevention programs on a continuum of universal, selective, and indicated interventions (Gordon, 1987; IOM, 1994); (4) the emergence of research on suicide prevention programs designed to target higher risk populations (e.g., Eggert et al., 1995b; Thompson et al., 2001); (5) improved screening tools and measures of suicide and suicidal behaviors (e.g., Eggert et al., 1994; Pfeffer et al., 2000; Reynolds, 1991; Reynolds, 1998; Shaffer and Craft, 1999; Thompson and Eggert, 1999), and (6) key advances in research methods, including improved analytic tools and sophisticated models for measuring change over time in prevention trials (Brown and Liao, 1999).

In contrast to clinical approaches that explore the history and health conditions leading to suicide in the individual, the public health approach to suicide prevention focuses on identifying broader patterns of suicide and suicidal behavior throughout a group or population. The public health approach to suicide prevention is also reflected in an organized five-step process that has been developed for ensuring the effectiveness of preventive efforts (PHS, 2001: 11). This chapter will describe the current public health preventive framework and then review some of the interventions for preventing suicide at each level. The focus will be primarily on school-based programs. As with all other behavioral interventions, the best effects are most likely to be achieved with multidimensional interventions (IOM, 2001), given the overlapping nature of risk and protective factors across domains of influence. The chapter then explores examples of programs targeting specific populations and concludes with an analysis of an integrated approach for reducing the incidence of suicide in the broad population.

FRAMEWORK FOR PREVENTION

The prevailing prevention model in the interdisciplinary field of prevention science is the Universal, Selective, and Indicated (USI) prevention model. This USI model focuses attention on defined populations—from everyone in the population, to specific at-risk groups, to specific high-risk individuals—i.e., three population groups for whom the designed interventions are deemed optimal for achieving the unique goals of each prevention type.

Universal strategies or initiatives address an entire population (the nation, state, local county or community, school or neighborhood). These prevention programs are designed to influence everyone, reducing suicide risk though removing barriers to care, enhancing knowledge of what to do and say to help suicidal individuals, increasing access to help, and strengthening protective processes like social support and coping skills. Universal interventions include programs such as public education campaigns, school-based "suicide awareness" programs, means restriction, education programs for the media on reporting practices related to suicide, and school-based crisis response plans and teams.

Selective strategies address subsets of the total population, focusing on at-risk groups that have a greater probability of becoming suicidal. Selective prevention strategies aim to prevent the onset of suicidal behaviors among specific subpopulations. This level of prevention includes screening programs, gatekeeper training for "frontline" adult caregivers and peer "natural helpers," support and skill building groups for at-risk groups in the population, and enhanced accessible crisis services and referral sources.

Indicated strategies address specific high-risk individuals within the population—those evidencing early signs of suicide potential. Programs are designed and delivered in groups or individually to reduce risk factors and increase protective factors. At this level, programs include skill-building support groups in high schools and colleges, parent support training programs, case management for individual high-risk youth at school, and referral sources for crisis intervention and treatment.

UNIVERSAL PREVENTIONS

Using health promotion strategies to combat symptoms of mental illness, including suicidality, represents a primary aspect of many universal suicide prevention programs. Although the field has traditionally separated health promotion from prevention (IOM, 1994), preventionists in the United States and abroad have increasingly turned to mental health promotion as a means of universal prevention (Beautrais, 1998; Cowen, 1994; Durlak, 2000; Waring et al., 2000). Reviews (Cowen, 1994; NRC, 2002) and at least one meta-analysis (Durlak, 2000) demonstrate that school-based programs employing such a health promotion approach can effectively prevent and/or reduce suicide risk factors and correlates like adolescent pregnancy, externalizing disorders (such as delinquency and substance abuse), and depression. These programs also promote protective factors against suicide including: self-efficacy, interpersonal problem solving, self esteem, and social support (see Chapters 3 and 6). Furthermore, throughout the 1990s, the World Health Organization developed evidence-based policies and recommendations for how schools can effectively engage in health promotion using a four-level model (see, WHO, 2002). The WHO model promotes universal prevention, targeting environmental conditions and mental health education for all students, as well as selective and indicated prevention, providing psychosocial interventions and professional treatment for those with mental illness or at significant risk (see also Waring et al., 2000; WHO, 1999; 2000a). As mentioned in Chapter 3, the U.S. Surgeon General (PHS, 2001), the United Nations (1996), and the World Health Organization (1999) have endorsed promoting mental health/resiliency as part of universal suicide reduction strategies.

Population-based prevention programs with a school or community focus have an important advantage over those aimed at individuals. There is usually a high participation rate in such programs because all students are exposed, for instance, to a teacher's classroom management practices and control of aggressive behavior (Kellam et al., 1998) or to a middle school drug prevention program (Botvin et al., 1995). These programs also have the advantage, because of inoculation, of having potential impact on not only those who are currently at risk, but also those whose risk status changes after the intervention takes place. Finally, many of these broad prevention programs target multiple outcomes, so overall risk for suicide may be reduced by diminishing developmental risk through multiple pathways.

Policy changes represent another universal strategy for reducing suicide. For example, Birckmayer and Hemenway (1999) conclude in their review of minimum drinking age policies in each state from 1970 to 1990 that increases in the legal drinking age reduce not only motor vehicle deaths but also suicides.

Media Campaigns

A traditional universal public health approach to behavior-related problems has been widespread education through mass-media campaigns. This technique has been used with varying levels of success for smoking, AIDS, and coronary heart disease (see IOM, 2002). A few countries, including the United Kingdom and Norway, have implemented such mass-media campaigns for suicide prevention as part of overall mental health promotion; evaluations of results are not yet available. Extensive media campaigns for suicide prevention are not common, largely due to fear of engendering suicide imitation. Media initiatives more often have focussed on modifying portrayals of suicide to reduce the likelihood of imitation. Since data are limited on use of media for education, this section discusses what is known about suicide imitation through the media, followed by a description of efforts to address this problem and the evidence for their effectiveness.

The Evidence for Imitation

Throughout history, people have expressed concern about suicide imitation, and have seen the opportunity for intervention in such matters, as evidenced by various anecdotal accounts in the literature of suicide imitation and clustering. For example, Goethe's 1774 novel *The Sorrows of Young Werther*, in which the title character shoots himself after a failed love affair, was banned in Denmark, Saxony, and Milan in order to prevent further suicides that were thought to be a result of young men imitating the behavior of Werther (Phillips, 1974, 1985). These events led to the term the "Werther Effect" being used to describe imitation of this sort.

Today this effect is referred to as either suicide contagion or suicide imitation/modeling. Although they are often used interchangeably, each is based on a different theoretical framework. Each theoretical framework is useful, but Schmidtke and Schaller (2000) propose that the language of imitation and modeling is preferable to the language of a contagious process because it relies on active learning processes that do not imply the exclusion of individual volitional factors.

Imitation and modeling, which play a role in other harmful behaviors such as drug use and bullying, occur with suicide in several circumstances, such as in the case of temporal clusters of suicides in a particular community or culture (see Chapter 2), suicide among family members (see Chapter 5), and suicide following exposure to a media[1] presentation of a real or fictional suicide.

Research shows that suicide contagion through the media is real (for review, see Gould, 2001a; 2001b). Recent meta-analyses report that studies conducted by clinically oriented investigators yield the strongest support for suicide imitation (cited in Schmidtke and Schaller, 2000). However, many of the studies of suicide imitation are beset with methodological problems; for example, many are based on aggregate-level data, which preclude the possibility of ruling out the influence of other factors.

Imitation can be linked to newspaper accounts of suicide (for review, see Gould, 2001b; Hassan, 1995; Phillips, 1974; Stack, 1996). Newspaper coverage of suicide is related to an increase in the rate of suicide, and the magnitude of the increase is proportional to the duration, prominence and amount of media coverage (Gould, 2001a). There has been less conclusive research on the consequences of television news programs on suicide imitation. Kessler et al. (1988; 1989) found no association over an 11 year period in the United States, but recent studies suggest imitation in specific groups (e.g., in the elderly, see Stack, 1990).

The influence of fictional presentations of suicide on imitation is less clear. Research into fictional portrayals has examined attempts or other suicidal behavior (such as ideation) rather than just rates of completed suicides, which allows for actual measurement of exposure. Some studies indicate that imitation occurs (e.g., Gould et al., 1988; Hawton et al., 1999); others do not (e.g., Phillips and Paight, 1987); still others are inconclusive (Berman, 1988).

Aspects of both the media presentation and the individual interact to produce imitation. The person who is likely to imitate a suicidal behavior

---

[1]Media refers to literature, the press, music, broadcasting, films, TV, theater, and the Internet.

has underlying vulnerabilities. A healthy person is not likely to kill him-
or herself as a result of seeing an example of suicide. Different media (e.g.,
book vs. television) are likely to exert differential effects on different populations. Both the form (headline, placement) and content (celebrity, mental illness, murder-suicide) of suicide coverage clearly impact the likelihood of imitation. Attractive models are more likely to cause imitation.
    Similarities between a vulnerable person and the reported suicide
victim increase the likelihood of contagion. This has been shown with age
effects in both the young (Phillips and Carstensen, 1988) and the elderly
(Stack, 1999, cited in Schmidtke and Schaller, 2000). Similarly, ethnicity is
an important factor; Stack (1996) found that suicides of foreigners did not
cause imitation among native populations.

Encouraging Responsible Coverage of Suicide

Many elements of media presentations influence the likelihood of
imitation, and these all provide opportunities for prevention. In efforts to
prevent contagion, several countries (including Australia, Austria,
Canada, Germany, Japan, New Zealand, and Switzerland) and organizations, including the World Health Organization (United Nations, 1996;
WHO, 2000b) have formulated guidelines for media coverage of suicide.
    The National Strategy for Suicide Prevention in the United States
includes as one of its major goals improving "the reporting and portrayals of suicidal behavior, mental illness, and substance abuse in the enter-
tainment and news media" (PHS, 2001). To advance that goal, guidelines
for media coverage of suicide were formulated by the Annenberg Public
Policy Center of the University of Pennsylvania, the American Association of Suicidology (AAS) and the American Foundation for Suicide Prevention (AFSP) in collaboration with several government agencies (CDC,
NIMH, Office of the Surgeon General, Substance Abuse and Mental
Health Services Administration [SAMSHA]), the WHO, and other international suicide prevention groups. They were released in August 2001,
and the full text of these guidelines can be found on the sites of the
partner organizations that developed them, including www.appcpenn.org
and www.afsp.org. These guidelines, "Reporting on Suicide: Recommendations for the Media" update those developed in 1989 at a national consensus conference on the topic.
    The media guidelines include the stipulation that media accounts of
suicide should neither romanticize nor normalize suicide; that is, individuals who kill themselves should not inadvertently be idealized as he-
roic or romantic. They also urge the inclusion of factual information on
suicide contagion and mental illness, provide suggestions for questions to
ask of relatives and friends of the victim, and suggest that information on

treatment resources be included. The guidelines also address issues of language such as the use of terms like "a successful suicide," and speak to special situations that may arise such as a celebrity death by suicide. Finally, they suggest that media professionals address suicide as an issue in its own right, reporting on stigma, treatments, and trends in suicide rates, rather than only in response to a tragedy (AFSP, 2001). With shifts in focus and inclusion of educational material, the same articles that report on an unfortunate event can become part of universal preventive measures. This echoes other areas in the injury prevention field (Hemenway, 2001). The media now indicate the status of smoke detectors when a fire is reported, for example. Likewise, helmet use is indicated when reporting a bicycle accident.

Currently, many comprehensive suicide prevention programs include components to improve media response to suicide, including the Finland National Program, Maryland (see later in this chapter) and the Washington State Youth Suicide Prevention Program (Eggert et al., 1997), with the state programs often utilizing the nationally formulated guidelines. The Washington program included a media education component that was designed to impact reporting practices by (1) educating media personnel in ways to report youth suicide stories that prevent potential contagion effects and (2) educating select personnel such as crisis line workers, gatekeepers, and school personnel in how to respond to media requests for information and stories related to youth suicide and suicide prevention. It also focused on ensuring that the youth suicide prevention message was "in the news" by providing information to the media and encouraging ongoing and responsible coverage of suicide and suicide prevention.

Despite such efforts to shape discussion of suicide in the media, very little evidence exists to show that initiatives to promote responsible reporting in the media have a direct, significant effect on suicide rates. In Switzerland, implementation of media guidelines did increase responsible reporting of suicides; less sensational and higher quality stories resulted (Michel et al., 2000). But this has not yet been related to changes in suicide rates. An evaluation of media guidelines in Austria showed significant success in reducing suicides. The guidelines in that country were specifically formulated to address concerns that the increase in the number of suicides and suicide attempts on the subway in Vienna was related to the highly publicized and dramatic accounts of the deaths. Subsequent to the release of the guidelines, newspaper reporting of subway suicides decreased greatly and what was reported was much less prominent. The number of subway suicides significantly decreased in the second half of the year after release. In the 4 years following, the overall suicide rate decreased by 20 percent and the rate of subway suicides decreased by 75 percent with no substitution of method (Etzersdorfer and Sonneck, 1998; Etzersdorfer et al., 1992; Sonneck et al., 1994).

Reducing Access to Means

Universal measures can be used to reduce the availability of common tools for suicide. More restrictive legislation regarding firearms, barriers on bridges, or blister packs for medications are interventions that may be effective in reducing suicide or suicide attempts. This section focuses on the role of availability of methods of suicide, including the role that method availability and barrier restrictions may play in suicide by firearms, acetaminophen overdose, prescription drugs, jumping from buildings or bridges, domestic gas, automobile carbon monoxide, and railway suicides. Much of the research discussed has been done in Western societies, but suicide in rural Asian societies has been largely linked with availability of insecticides (Van der Hoek et al., 1998; Yip et al., 2000). Research is limited, but this underscores the need for implementing safe storage of agricultural poisons and using safety caps to reduce impulsive swallowing.

Firearms[2]

Epidemiological studies have consistently shown that firearms are most common method of suicide for all demographic groups in the United States (CDC, 1994). The association between suicide and firearms in the home is strong across all age groups, but is particularly high in the 24 and younger group (Odds Ratios[3] [ORs] of 10.4 vs. 4.0–7.2 for those 25 and older) (Kellermann et al., 1992). The dramatic increase in the American youth suicide rate since 1960 is primarily attributable to an increase in suicide by firearms (see Figure 8-1a,b; Boyd, 1983; Boyd and Moscicki, 1986). In one study of youth suicide in Allegheny County from 1960–1983, the rate of suicide by firearms increased 330 percent, but the rate of suicide by other means increased only 150 percent (Brent et al., 1987b). The more recent increase in the suicide rate by African American males is also attributable primarily to an increase in suicide by firearms.

---

[2]This section was abstracted from Brent DA. 2001. Firearms and suicide. *Annals of the New York Academy of Sciences*, 932: 225240. Reprinted by permission of the New York Academy of Sciences.
[3]The Odds Ratio is the ratio of the odds of an outcome (suicide) for the experimental group relative to the odds of the outcome in the control group.

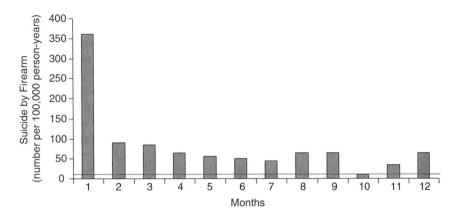

FIGURE 8-1a Rates of suicide by firearm in the **first year** after purchase among persons who purchased handguns in California in 1991. The horizontal line indicates the age- and sex-adjusted average annual rate of suicide by firearm in California in 1991 and 1992 (11.3 per 100,000 persons per year). SOURCE: Wintemute et al. 1999. Copyright © 1999 Massachusetts Medical Society. All rights reserved.

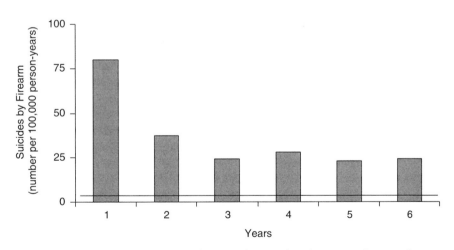

FIGURE 8-1b Rates of suicide by firearm during the **six years** after purchase among persons who purchased handguns in California in 1991. The horizontal line indicates the age- and sex-adjusted average annual rate of suicide by firearm in California in 1991 through 1996 (10.7 per 100,000 persons per year). SOURCE: Wintemute et al. 1999. Copyright © 1999 Massachusetts Medical Society. All rights reserved.

Ray, age 14, had made three suicide attempts prior to completing his suicide. Each time there had been someone there to stop him. He communicated often about his intent, remarking that "Life's a bitch" and asking others about which way they thought it would be better to kill oneself. The day before his death, he asked his mother whether it would be better to stick a gun "in your mouth or in your temple?" He chose the latter, using a .357 Magnum that had been kept fully loaded, in his mother's nightstand (Berman & Jobes, Adolescent Suicide: Assessment and Intervention, 1991: 189).

Alcohol and illicit drug abuse in the home greatly increase the risk of violent death, including suicide (Rivara et al., 1997). Youth who were drinking at the time of their suicide were much more likely to use a gun than were youth who were not drinking (Brent et al., 1987b; Brent et al., 1993; Hlady and Middaugh, 1988). The increase in youth alcohol abuse and in firearms availability over the past 3 decades may be related to the increase in youth suicide in general, and in youth firearms suicide in specific. However, it is important to note that youth suicide has also dramatically increased in geographic regions where firearms ownership and firearms suicides are relatively rare (e.g., New Zealand; Beautrais et al., 1996). Therefore, it would be an oversimplification to say that the increase in youth suicide, in the United States, or anywhere else in the world, is *solely* a function of increased firearms availability.

Several studies (Beautrais et al., 1996; Brent et al., 1991; Brent et al., 1988; Kellermann et al., 1992) have demonstrated that the presence of a gun in the home is highly predictive of its use for completed suicide (see Table 8-1). Firearms were between 31.1 and 107.9 times more likely to be used for the suicide if a gun was already in the home. This was even true in New Zealand, where firearms is a much less common method choice

TABLE 8-1 Case-Control Studies: Guns in the Home and the Method of Suicide

	Brent 1993	Kellerman 1992	Beautrais 1996
Use of gun if kept in home	87.8%	88%	33%
Use of gun if not kept in home	18.8%	6%	0.5%
Guns in home and firearms as method (Odds Ratio [OR])	31.1	69.5	107.9
Firearms and alcohol use (OR [95%CI])	7.3	—	—
Bought gun within two weeks of suicide	—	3%	—

for suicide than in the United States (14 percent vs. 55–60 percent, Beautrais et al., 1996). Conversely, if a gun was not in the home, it was used as a method of suicide quite infrequently. Furthermore, in a study by Kellermann et al. (1992), only 3 percent of those who completed suicide had bought a gun within 2 weeks of the suicide. Wintemute et al. (1999) examined the standardized mortality rates (SMRs) of purchasers of handguns in California, who are registered by state law, and found an extremely high rate of suicide right after purchase. However, the rates remained elevated for the 6 years of analysis. This suggests that firearms are purchased for the purpose of completing suicide even though most of the suicides occurred some time after the purchase. Together, these data strongly suggest that it is the immediate gun availability that conveys the risk for firearms suicide, and supports method restriction as one means to prevent firearms suicide.

Method of storage and the type and number of guns modify suicide risk substantially. Higher risk is associated with handguns than with long guns, loaded guns than unloaded guns, and unlocked than locked guns (see Table 8-2, Brent et al., 1993; Kellermann et al., 1992). Long guns convey an increased risk to males, but not females, and handguns convey a particularly increased risk for females (Brent et al., 1993). Furthermore, in adolescents, long guns, but not handguns, convey an increased risk in rural areas (OR's 4.5 vs. 1.0), while in urban areas, this situation is re-

TABLE 8-2 Risk of Suicide in the Home in Relation to Various Patterns of Gun Ownership

Variable	Adjusted Odds Ratio[a]	95% Confidence Interval
Type of guns in the home		
One or more handguns	5.8	3.1–4.7
Long guns only	3.0	1.4–6.5
No guns in the home	1.0	—
Loaded guns		
Any gun kept loaded	9.2	4.1–20.1
All guns kept unloaded	3.3	1.7–6.1
No guns in the home	1.0	—
Locked guns		
Any guns kept unlocked	5.6	3.1–10.4
All guns kept locked up	2.4	1.0–5.7
No guns in the home	1.0	—

SOURCE: Kellermann et al., 1992. Copyright © 1992 Massachusetts Medical Society. All rights reserved.

versed, with handguns conveying a much higher risk than long guns (OR's 5.6 vs. 1.3) (Brent et al., 1993).

While firearms counseling has gained acceptance as an important component of health supervision, in reality this often fails to occur (Grossman et al., 1995). Depressed adolescent patients and their parents are often non-compliant with physician recommendations to secure or remove firearms (Weil and Hemenway, 1992). Only two studies have examined the impact of firearms counseling on the removal of firearms with the parents of youth at risk for suicide. In one study, eight parents of suicide attempters with firearms in the home were counseled about the danger conveyed by firearms in the home, and five either removed the gun, or stored the gun in a more secure manner (Kruesi et al., 1999). In a study of depressed adolescents who entered a randomized psychotherapy clinical trial, only 27 percent of parents who reported having guns in the home at intake removed the guns on follow-up after being urged by the clinician to do so (Brent et al., 2000). Therefore, it is unwise to assume that providing recommendations on removal of firearms from the home will automatically result in compliance. An alternative recommendation to improve the security of gun storage is often more favorably received (Webster et al., 1992).

The firearms suicide rate and the overall suicide rate are related to the strictness of gun control laws and the prevalence of gun ownership (Boor and Bair, 1990; Killias, 1993; Lester, 1988; Lester and Murrell, 1986). Quasi-experimental studies suggest that greater restrictiveness in gun control laws is associated with declines in firearms suicide, sometimes without compensatory method substitution (Loftin et al., 1991). In a particularly elegant cross-country comparison, the suicide rates were compared in two similar cities, Seattle and Vancouver. Because gun control is more restrictive in Canada, it was assumed suicide rates in Vancouver would be lower (Sloan et al., 1990). Instead, the overall suicide rates were similar in the two cities, albeit with a 10-fold higher rate of firearms suicides in Seattle. This was almost entirely reflected in 40 percent higher rate of suicide among 15–24 year olds in Seattle. These results suggest that the greater availability of firearms is particularly deleterious for younger people.

In a well-designed quasi-experimental study, Loftin et al. (1991) examined the relationship between legislation enacted in 1976 in the District of Columbia and subsequent time trends in suicide and homicide during the years 1968 through 1987. This legislation mandated the registration of all firearms, required that new purchasers meet "fitness" and knowledge of safety standards, and necessitated that owners store guns unloaded and disassembled, with certain occupational exceptions, such as law enforcement. The unusual aspect of this study was that changes in the rates of suicide and homicide in the District of Columbia were compared to changes in rates of suicide and homicide in neighboring Maryland and Virginia counties, where no such change in firearms legislation had taken place. In the District of Columbia, subsequent to the enactment of this legislation, a 23 percent decline in firearms suicide and a 9 percent decline in non-firearms suicide were noted. Over the same period of time, in the adjoining Maryland and Virginia counties, a 12 percent increase in firearms suicide and a 2 percent decline in non-firearms suicide were observed. One weakness of all ecological studies is that it is impossible to monitor the extent to which these regulations were enforced or circumvented. However, one might have expected diffusion of unlawful firearms from neighboring counties into the District of Columbia, which would have diluted the potentially salutary impact of the legislation. The inference of a causal relationship between the change in legislation and the decline in suicide is bolstered by the greater effect on firearms vs. non-firearms suicide and the geographic specificity of this effect. Method substitution did not occur to any substantial degree, and an overall decline in the suicide rate prevailed. The impact of the Brady Act has been controversial. Although Ludwig and Cook (2000) found a significant reduction in suicide rates following enactment, their breakdown by age and their choice of duration of analysis may be problematic (Kleck and Marvell, 2000; Lott, 2000). Given the complexity of gun availability and fluctuations of these relatively infrequent events over time, a final judgement on the effectiveness of this legislation in reducing suicide is unlikely to happen soon.

The impact of firearms legislation on suicide was examined in Queensland, Australia (Cantor and Slater, 1995). The law required both current and prospective owners of long guns to obtain a license. A 28-day waiting period ("cooling off period") was instituted prior to a new purchase, and owners were required to pass a safety test. The suicide rate by firearms declined among men in metropolitan areas and in provincial cities, but not in rural areas. This effect was most notable among individuals under the age of 30. However, method substitution occurred in all regions but the provincial cities, where overall suicide rates did decline. Two limitations of the study are the absence of a "control" community where no change in legislation had occurred and the brevity of the observation (only 1 year pre- and post-legislation).

Acetaminophen Overdose

The rate of acetaminophen (or paracetamol) self-poisoning from emergency room registries has been estimated 21.4/100,000 in one American emergency room, and as high as 70–90/100,0000 in one study based in

Scotland (Bond and Hite, 1999; McLoone and Crombie, 1996). In the Scottish study, the rates among male and female adolescents aged 15–19 were approximate 150 and 350/100,000, respectively (McLoone and Crombie, 1996). Hospitalizations due to acetaminophen rose rapidly from the 1970s through the early 1900s, especially in adolescents and young adults (McLoone and Crombie, 1996). This increase is explained in part by the increased availability of acetaminophen. High correlations have been noted between sales of acetaminophen and overdose rates in Oxford, England (r=.86) and in France (r=.99), with similar correlations between sales and completed suicide (Gunnell et al., 1997). In addition to availability, adolescents' general ignorance about the risk for hepatotoxicity appears to contribute to the use of acetaminophen. Almost half of adolescents underestimate the potential lethality and toxicity of acetaminophen (Harris and Myers, 1997; Myers et al., 1992). Awareness is also limited that ingestion of acetaminophen in combination with alcohol greatly increases the likelihood of both hospitalization and of hepatotoxicity (Schiodt et al., 1997).

Restriction of drug content per purchase and the use of blister packs (requiring individual pill removal from a card with each pill in its own "bubble") may reduce the morbidity and mortality due to acetaminophen overdose (Chan, 1996; Hawton et al., 1996). Restriction in the amount of drug available in a purchase resulted in a 4-fold lower fatality from overdose in France, compared to England (Gunnell et al., 1997). The introduction of blister packs as a method for dispensing acetaminophen was associated with a 21 percent reduction in overdoses and a 64 percent reduction in severe overdoses, whereas overdoses due to benzodiazepines, which were not subject to these restrictions, remained stable (Turvill et al., 2000).

Some have considered the benefit of labels warning of hepatotoxicity, but it is unclear if warnings would alter the behavior of impulsive adolescents (Harris and Myers, 1997). In one survey, only 25 percent thought that a warning would deter them (Hawton et al., 1996). The addition of methionine to prevent the hepatotoxic effects has been suggested but not yet evaluated.

Prescription Drugs

The rate of self-poisoning by prescription drugs in New York City is highest in Manhattan, which has the higher per-capita density of physicians of any of the boroughs of New York (Marzuk et al., 1992). The greater number of prescribed psychotropic agents is correlated with an increased risk of overdose, at an estimated rate of 3.8/1000 prescriptions (Forster and Frost, 1985). However, Moens and van Voorde (1989) found no relationship between availability of prescription drugs and completed suicide. The prescription of a psychotropic agent is itself a marker for suicidal risk and it is important to consider its lethality in prescribing for patients with mental disorders. Furthermore, there is a marked gradient in toxicity among antidepressants (Cassidy and Henry, 1987; Kapur et al., 1992). In a study conducted in the United Kingdom, desipramine was reported to have over twice the death rate by overdose per 1,000,000 prescriptions compared to amitriptyline, imipramine, or nortriptyline, and 9 times the death rate by overdose of mianserin (Cassidy and Henry, 1987). In data from the United States, the toxicity of different antidepressants was examined using two different databases—the Association of Poison Control Centers (APCC) and the Drug Abuse and Early Warning Network (DAWN) (Kapur et al., 1992). In the APCC database the rate of overdose was adjusted for prescription volume based on the National Prescription Audit. Both APCC and DAWN databases revealed that desipramine had a higher risk for suicide attempt and greater fatality given an overdose than either amitriptyline or imipramine. The DAWN analysis also demonstrated that the three tricyclic antidepressants had between a 2.5 and 8.5 greater risk of death due to overdose than fluoxetine. Therefore, alteration in prescription practices to favor SSRIs over TCAs might result in a decline in deaths by overdose of antidepressants.

Suicide and suicide attempt are markedly increased in patients with epilepsy (Brent, 1986; Hawton et al., 1980; Mackay, 1979; Matthews and Barabas, 1981; Sillanpaa, 1973). While interictal psychopathology related to epilepsy seems to be an important risk factor for suicidal behavior (Mendez et al., 1989), phenobarbital may be an iatrogenic cause of depression and suicidal behavior in epilepsy (Brent, 1986; Brent et al., 1990; Brent et al., 1987a; Ferrari et al., 1983). One naturalistic study suggested that exposure to phenobarbital caused about a 4-fold risk for depression, which was most likely to occur if there was a family history of depression and very unlikely to occur in the absence of a family history of depression (Brent et al., 1987a). Phenobarbital is no longer a first-line anticonvulsant in the United States, but because of its overall safety and cost, it still is used quite commonly in developing countries. Screening for a family history of depression may help to avoid the iatrogenic difficulties associated with this medication.

Jumping from Buildings or Bridges

Availability of high buildings or bridges provides another means for suicide. In New York City, suicide by jumping was highest in Manhattan, and lowest in Staten Island, the two extremes for access to buildings of 7 stories or higher (Marzuk et al., 1992). In another study in New York, 81 percent of all suicides jumped from their own residences (Fischer et al.,

1993). One report suggested the efficacy of a crisis telephone line on a bridge. Its use in 30 cases resulted in only one completed suicide. Nine people jumped from the bridge and did not use the phone; 5 of the 9 completed the suicide. The availability of the phone line, staffed by mental health experts and with an automatic police alert, may have deterred some suicides (Glatt, 1987). As with injury control approaches, the creation of mechanical barriers on bridges could make jumping more difficult or impossible. Mechanical barriers in private residences would be more difficult to develop and enforce.

Domestic Gas Poisoning

Domestic gas poisoning was one of the leading causes of suicide in Great Britain; due to its high carbon monoxide (CO) content, domestic gas could be highly lethal. A decrease in CO content of domestic gas associated with decline in mortality in Great Britain, Austria, and Japan (Kreitman, 1976; Lester and Abe, 1989), but not in the Netherlands (Sainsbury, 1986). Method substitution eventually offset this decline in suicide by the mid 1980s in Great Britain (McClure, 1984), but not Japan (Lester and Abe, 1989). Therefore, in some locales, the detoxification of domestic gas has had a lasting effect, and even in Great Britain, where method substitution did eventually take place, this occurred after a reduction in the suicide rate which lasted for a 15-year period.

Suicide by Auto Exhaust

The rate of suicide by auto exhaust is, not surprisingly, related to the availability of automobiles (Marzuk et al., 1992; Ohberg et al., 1995; Ostrom et al., 1996). Suicide by auto exhaust is much more common in Queens and Staten Island (.46 and .40 per 100,000) than in Manhattan or the Bronx (0 and .08 per 100,000, Marzuk et al., 1992). A relationship between per-capita automobile ownership and suicide by carbon monoxide poisoning was also found in Finland (Ohberg et al., 1995).

Suicide by auto exhaust is often relatively impulsive and frequently occurs under influence of alcohol (Skopek and Perkins, 1998). Several suggestions for reducing the lethality of this method have been raised: a brief computer administered screen for sobriety as a condition for starting the car; decreasing the amount of CO in exhaust through a catalytic converter; having the engine cutoff if idling for too long; and modification of the end of the exhaust tail pipe to make it impossible to put a hose on the end (Ostrom et al., 1996). In the United States detoxification of car exhaust began in 1968 (8.5 percent CO content) and continued through 1980 (0.05 percent CO content). An examination of the suicide rate by this means between 1950 and 1984 failed to show a straightforward relationship between detoxification and suicide rates. Suicide among men by this method began to decline along with detoxification until 1979, at which point it began to rise again. A decline in female suicides by this method began in 1975 (Clarke and Lester, 1986).

Railway Suicides

The rate of railway suicide (e.g., jumping in front of a train) also is related to access. In New York, the rate of railway or subway suicide is proportional to the amount of track in a given borough (Marzuk et al., 1992). However, among cities internationally, there are marked variations in the suicide rate per passenger. Rates are extremely low in Singapore, Tokyo, Budapest, and Hong Kong but much higher in London, Barcelona, Rio de Janeiro, and Paris (O'Donnell et al., 1994).

Because the case fatality rate is high (estimated at 55 percent) and prediction is difficult, injury control methods have been suggested to reduce fatality. Suggestions include physical separation of passengers from the train bed, improved surveillance of passengers by station staff, liaison to hospital staff in stations with a high density of chronic mental patients, availability of emergency hotline telephones, redesign of bumper of train (including the addition of an airbag), increasing the distance between the train and the train bed, and a slower speed of approach to the station (Beskow et al., 1994; Clarke and Poyner, 1994). In addition to design issues, curbing media publicity about railway suicides may diminish the likelihood of imitation (Schmidtke and Hafner, 1988; Sonneck et al., 1994, see earlier section).

Hotlines and Crisis Centers

Research on the effectiveness of hotlines and crisis centers in reducing suicide is scarce, and what does exist is inconsistent. Yet the high prevalence of such services and their high usage warrants research so that the most effective services can be provided. There are over 350 Befrienders International Centers, associated with The Samaritans, in over 40 countries (see Scott, 2000), and there are over 1000 teen suicide hotlines alone in the United States as of 1992 (CDC, 1992). Hotlines and crisis intervention services include a broad scope of services including anonymous or non-anonymous phone counseling for suicidal individuals and/or their family and friends, face-to-face counseling, and referrals by professionals, paraprofessionals, and/or volunteers with various training. These services can intervene during an acute suicidal crisis and connect individuals to additional mental health services that they might not otherwise seek. Certification is available through the American Association of Suicidology for North American phone help lines, and from the Samaritans for membership in Befrienders International, based in London, England. Yet accreditation or membership does not require formal evaluation of services, nor is monitoring of services provided (Mishara and Daigle, 2001).

Research on the effectiveness of hotlines and crisis intervention is hampered by at least two methodological problems. First, suicide is a low-base rate behavior and studies typically include those who both did and did not have contact with the services in the community. Second, suicide prevention accounts for only 5–20 percent of the services provided by many such organizations (Eastwood et al., 1976; France, 1982; Knickerbocker and McGee, 1973; Lester, 1972). Hence, the noted changes in mental health status of the community may be attributable to other aspects of the organizations' work.

The research on hotline and crisis center effectiveness in reducing suicide shows three over-arching findings. First, the available data show either reductions (Bagley, 1968) or no change (Barraclough and Jennings, 1977; Lester, 1990) in suicide rates; *no* increased rates have been documented. Second, until recently young white females most frequently utilized these services (CDC, 1992; Stengel, 1964). Some studies examining suicide rates in white women 25 years and younger found significant decreases in counties with suicide prevention centers (Miller et al., 1984), but *only* for this demographic. Third, users of these services report high satisfaction with them and often use the services again. Numerous studies have found that about 80 percent of individuals report positive experiences with the hotlines (e.g., King, 1977; Motto, 1971; Stein and Lambert, 1984; Tekavcic-Grad and Zavasnik, 1987). These findings may be inflated due to reporting bias, since response rates to these inquiries range from 40–80 percent and may disproportionally include those who found the intervention helpful. Two researchers found that callers to hotlines may be more likely to attempt than complete suicide (Bagley, 1968), which may limit the potential usefulness of hotlines in reducing suicide rates.

Demographics of hotline use may be changing with an increase in usage by middle aged individuals (Scott, 2000). Baby-boomers are more likely than previous generations to use mental health services including hotlines, so that the demographics of highest usage may follow this cohort. Analogously, the majority of current teenagers look up health information on the Internet as their first resource (Borzekowski and Rickert, 2001a; Flowers-Coulson et al., 2000). Planning for interventions for this demographic will need to address the credibility of Internet health information (Borzekowski and Rickert, 2001).

No-Suicide Contracts

Suicide prevention contracts are widely used in all mental health settings as risk management tools, but they remain poorly evidenced. Also known as contracts for safety or no-suicide contracts, suicide prevention contracts ask the patient to make a commitment either verbally or in writing to avoid self-destructive behavior and to keep the clinician informed of any such suicidal impulses. However, there is no standardization in the form or content of the contract, nor in indications for use. Generally, no-suicide contracts are used in cases of acute suicidal thoughts, impulses, and behaviors, although chronic self-destructive behavior may also prompt the clinician to propose a contract.

There is scant evidence to support the efficacy of this widely used intervention, simply because so little evaluation has been done. One retrospective medical record study found that suicide prevention contracts did not prevent self-harm behaviors (Drew, 2001). Still, surveys of clinicians have found that suicide prevention contracts are commonly used, and that there is a general perception that they are helpful (Davidson et al., 1995; Green and Grindel, 1996).

A reason for the large variability in suicide prevention contracts as seen in practice is that they are not part of the formal, written tradition of suicide assessment. More often their use is perpetuated by word of mouth. A survey of psychiatrists and psychologists at Harvard Medical School points to the lack of formal training in the use of no-suicide contracts. Whereas 86 percent of the psychiatrists surveyed and 71 percent of the psychologists surveyed worked in places where contracts were regularly used, only 30–40 percent had received formal training or education during internship or residency concerning their use (Miller et al., 1998). This is just one element of the larger-scale problem in clinician training for treating suicidal patients, as discussed in Chapter 9. These data and other anecdotal accounts indicate that no-suicide contracts are a widely used intervention, but the precise prevalence rates of use are not known.

No-suicide contracts should never be used in place of appropriate suicide risk assessment and treatment (Miller, 1999; Simon, 1999). Refusal to sign a no-suicide contract does not necessarily indicate that the patient is in imminent danger of suicide, just as agreement to a contract does not mean that the risk of suicide and self-destructive behavior is lessened. The mental state of a patient is not static, and patients may have inconsistent and complex motivations for agreeing to or refusing a contract (Simon, 1999). A risk of using no-suicide contracts is that they may provide a false sense of security to the clinician and cause lessened diligence about the danger of suicide (Simon, 1999).

The usefulness of the suicide prevention contract may be dependent upon the strength of therapeutic relationship between the clinician and patient. In an emergency setting, for example, the patient has no investment in or commitment to the clinician, and thus, signing a contact would mean very little. In the context of a long-term therapeutic alliance, however, the commitment by the patient may carry more weight.

Additionally, the process of creating a contract can be either helpful or hurtful to the clinician–patient relationship. It may be beneficial if the process demonstrates to the patient a measure of caring and concern on the part of the clinician (Egan et al., 1997; Kroll, 2000) and may be harmful if the patient perceives that the clinician is attempting to reduce his or her own responsibility and involvement in the treatment (Miller et al., 1998). Other possible benefits of contracts include the opportunity to assess the nature of the therapeutic alliance, identify clear goals for treatment, and support coping mechanisms in some patients (Miller, 1999). Stanford and colleagues (1994) recommend that suicide prevention contracts be used as an assessment tool that can provide useful diagnostic information.

The legal implications of a no-suicide contract have been extensively explored by Simon (1999). He has concluded that the suicide prevention contract is not a legal contract and does not provide protection to the clinician in the event of a lawsuit. Alternate terminology is suggested, such as agreement, pact, or understanding (Simon, 1992). It should be recognized that suicide prevention contracts do not provide protection from lawsuits (and may have the opposite effect if it is determined that the contract took the place of a thorough assessment; Miller, 1999). As discussed in Chapter 10, suicide can be considered an expected outcome of some mental illnesses, and is very difficult to predict. Although the fear of lawsuits is understandable, the societal atmosphere that blames the clinician when a patient kills himself should not dictate clinical decisions.

In conclusion, suicide prevention contracts are likely overvalued and should never be used as the sole treatment for a patient with suicidal behavior. There is no convincing evidence to support the practice, and some evidence that points to its potential for harm with certain patients. The informed consent model proposed by Miller (1999) uses an agreement as one part of the collaboration between clinician and patient to create an ongoing treatment plan. This informed consent process involves exploring and fully explaining different treatment options and their various risks and benefits, including the risk of suicide, to the patient, and outlines the mutual commitment of the two parties to follow through with the plan. Of course, the patients' ability to provide informed consent must be assessed (see Chapter 10).

Awareness and Skills Training

A number of studies have explored the impact on suicidality of universal prevention interventions at the middle and high school level. Suicide awareness training is the dominant strategy of these universal programs in the United States, although more schools are turning to broad-based competence-promoting programs as evidence mounts for their effectiveness in reducing the burden of behavioral and mental disorders (see introduction to universal approaches). As would be expected with a universal program assessed shortly after its completion, the changes in suicidal behaviors and related risk factors have generally been promising yet modest. Universal programming assumes a healthy population and is not necessarily designed to impact acute risk factors directly, but rather targets contextual variables, protective processes, and predisposing factors, including reducing barriers to care. It is delivered at a dose and in a format that is not generally appropriate for changing risk factors or suicidal behaviors in the short term, but rather long-term. The greatest and most sustainable changes in behavior appear to follow interventions employing the multi-dimensional approach typical of health-promoting prevention strategies, especially with skills training components embedded in an environment with trained, supportive adults.

Eleven universal suicide prevention strategies at the high school level were reviewed for this analysis of programming typical for the United States; 15 published papers were found that examine the efficacy of these programs (Ashworth et al., 1986; Ciffone, 1993; Eggert et al., 1999; Kalafat, 2000; Kalafat and Elias, 1994; Kalafat and Ryerson, 1999; Klingman and Hochdorf, 1993; Nelson, 1987; Orbach and Bar-Joseph, 1993; Overholser et al., 1989; Shaffer et al., 1991; Shaffer et al., 1990; Spirito et al., 1988; Vieland et al., 1991; Zenere and Lazarus, 1997). Typically, one individual delivered the majority of the programs to a classroom of students. The 11 programs reviewed varied from 1-to-12 sessions, and ranged in duration from 55 minutes to more than 16 hours. These programs primarily used didactic presentations that cover warning signs, provide information to dispel myths and promote healthy attitudes, and review strategies for accessing resources. Several of the programs showed gains in knowledge (Ciffone, 1993; Eggert et al., 1999; Kalafat and Elias, 1994; Klingman and Hochdorf, 1993; Nelson, 1987; Shaffer et al., 1991; Spirito et al., 1988) that seem to be enhanced when youth use this knowledge to teach others (Eggert et al., 1999).

In addition, programs that included the importance of telling adults and seeking help for self or friends (Ciffone, 1993; Eggert et al., 1999; Kalafat and Elias, 1994; Shaffer et al., 1991) did produce positive changes in attitudes toward helping and behavioral intentions to help. Specifically, changes occurred in willingness to tell a friend or an adult, and in recommending resources, thus generally increasing the helping capacity among youth networks. A mixed response to seeking out a mental health professional was found that deserves attention. The finding at 18-months follow-up of various short-term curriculum-based programs that actual helping was not significantly different between participants and controls (Vieland et al., 1991) speaks to the importance of program length and need for skills training or practice, as differential effects were noted among youth who had participated in a more intensive, skill-based program (Eggert et al., 1999). Changes in helping behavior probably will not occur simply by fostering helping attitudes and increasing intentions to help; youth need skills training to act on these new attitudes and intentions. Behavioral intentions also improved for adults in the one skills-based program that reported on adult behaviors (Eggert et al., 1999). Although the program was delivered to youth, adults in the communities where the campaigns were delivered also showed benefits as opposed to comparison communities. For example, adults who had had contact with a youth showing signs of suicide risk were more likely to ask about suicide thoughts and give advice on where to get help.

Universal programs including skills-training components yield additional gains. Skills training as described was quite variable: a single session on active listening and other social skills for supporting a peer (Overholser et al., 1989); positive self-talk, situational analysis, empathy training, role playing, biblioguidance, interrupting automatic thoughts, rehearsal and skills strengthening (Klingman and Hochdorf, 1993); role-play with a suicidal peer emphasizing help-seeking (Kalafat and Elias, 1994); suicide-specific content included in the context of a 10th grade semester-long mental health course entitled "Life Management Skills" (Zenere and Lazarus, 1997); and a suicide intervention workshop, media training, and script writing and role-playing steps to helping a suicidal peer (Eggert et al., 1999).

Such programs increased adaptive coping skills (Klingman and Hochdorf, 1993; Overholser et al., 1989) and evidenced slight decreases in hopelessness (Ashworth et al., 1986; Orbach and Bar-Joseph, 1993; Overholser et al., 1989; Spirito et al., 1988). Furthermore, some studies have observed decreases in suicidal ideation (Klingman and Hochdorf, 1993; Orbach and Bar-Joseph, 1993) and suicide attempts (Zenere and Lazarus, 1997). Some evaluations have even noted decreases in rates of suicide completions among youth after program implementation (Kalafat, 2000; Kalafat and Ryerson, 1999; Zenere and Lazarus, 1997). For example, evaluation of the short behaviorally-oriented awareness program described by Kalafat and Elias (1994) has demonstrated long-term reductions in completed suicides compared to state and national rates (Kalafat and Ryerson, 1999). Evaluation of a comprehensive, skills-based, required mental health curriculum (Zenere and Lazarus, 1997) reported a decline in annual suicide rate from an average of 12.9 to 4.6 during the implementation of the district-wide pre-K–12 program as part of a suicide prevention strategy. Although this study employed no control data from comparable districts and the program was implemented following a year in which the district had experienced 19 suicides, Kalafat (2000) analyzed the county data in comparison to state and national suicide rates from 9 years before to 7 years after the initial program implementation and found a consistently lower post-program rate of completed suicide.

The current data support the importance of longer-term and skills-training prevention programs for schools that include accessible services. A broad review (Garland et al., 1989) of 115 school-based programs in the United States found that generally short-term interventions were not effective among past suicide attempters, specifically, and suggested that they might actually be harmful because they provided inadequate time to deal with the issues raised. Single-presentation interventions show limited effectiveness, and some studies found increased reporting of distress after the program (e.g., 2 of 14 youth suicide in Shaffer et al., 1990). Brief programs have also shown limited changes in attitude toward suicide (Ciffone, 1993; Nelson, 1987; Overholser et al., 1989; Shaffer et al., 1991). This may be due to the tendency to give socially desirable responses to attitude items, and the limited effectiveness of brief programs (Kalafat and Elias, 1994; Shaffer et al., 1991).

As with other issue-specific programs, the type of approach holds particular importance for outcomes. For example, film-based suicide awareness programs that depict suicidal acts may have negative effects because of potential imitation by suicidal adolescents (see earlier section, Gould and Shaffer, 1986; Shaffer et al., 1988). Given that prevention programs can exert differential effects on sub-groups, evaluation should examine how specific programs affect various sub-populations. Further, researchers have voiced concern about programs that do not use a solid scientific base, especially a tendency among some to ignore or even contradict research implicating mental illness in suicide (Shaffer et al., 1988).

In response to these issues about format of school-based suicide prevention programs, some United States researchers argue that universal interventions are inappropriate and recommend, instead, screening for those at risk (e.g., Shaffer and Craft, 1999). Others, such as the U.S. Task Force on Youth Suicide Prevention, have decided that suicide prevention should be integrated into "broader health promotion programs . . . directed at preventing other self-destructive behaviors, such as alcohol and substance abuse" (ADAMHA, 1989). The Surgeon General's conference report on children's mental health (PHS, 2000) reiterates the necessity and efficacy of school-based universal mental health promotion programs to invest in children's social and emotional development and thereby reduce numerous harmful outcomes. The World Health Organization has also endorsed school-based universal mental health promotion as a component of effective suicide prevention (WHO, 1999). In response to the mixed results of didactic suicide awareness programming in the United States and the World Health Organization's school health promotion model (e.g., WHO, 2000a; WHO, 2002), New Zealand, Australia, and Sweden have developed mental health promotion curricula as components of their comprehensive suicide prevention strategies (Beautrais, 1998; Ramberg, 2000; Waring et al., 2000). Following WHO philosophy, their approach focuses on influencing health-related behaviors via knowledge, skills, attitudes, and support; creating conditions in the school and community that are conducive to health; and preventing leading causes of death, illness, and disability, including suicide.

Although these countries have only recently established their programs and results therefore represent only preliminary analyses, outcomes suggest important differences relative to typical short-term United States efforts. Sweden, for example, uses a film to depict teenagers who wrestled with suicidal thoughts and crises and emerged feeling that they had learned and grown from their adverse experiences (Ramberg, 2000). Teachers who want to show this film must first complete a 2-day training. The film's objective involves helping students know about sources of help and understand that, when facing suicidal ideation, they are not alone. Unlike with many of the United States programs, high-risk students seem positive and interested in the film and indicate it helped them. Sweden's full mental health curriculum includes suicidality and teaches about the medical aspects of mental illness and then the socio-environmental aspects of mental illness. Evaluation necessarily comprises a quasi-experimental design that limits outcome validity, but preliminary results indicate an as-yet nonsignificant trend in the intervention group toward fewer suicide attempts but no decrease in reports of suicidal ideation (Ramberg, 2000). This echoes results of the similar United States program reviewed by Zenere and Lazarus (1997), as described above. Current international suicide prevention strategies (described in a subsequent section) require evaluation of program elements, and will therefore provide much-needed information about which programs most effectively reduce suicide for various populations. Australia, for example, has started piloting its school programs and is publishing reports on common barriers to effective, sustained program implementation (e.g., Wyn et al., 2000).

Given that many schools in the United States employ short-term school-based suicide awareness interventions that may be ineffective and even potentially harmful, evaluation of various models and dissemination of those found safe and effective emerges as a priority. The most effective United States and international programs integrate suicide prevention into a competence-promotion and stress-protection framework, suggesting closer examination of health promotion as a prevention strategy. The evidence reviewed here supports carefully designed, science-based programs, particularly longer-term approaches couched in a broader context of teaching skills and establishing appropriate follow-through and services, as part of an effective armamentarium against suicide. Brief, didactic suicide prevention programs with no connection to services should be avoided.

SELECTIVE PREVENTION

Prevention initiatives at the selective level include: (1) screening programs to identify and assess at-risk groups; (2) gatekeeper training, consultation, and education services; (3) support/skills training; and (4) crisis response and referral resources. This review focuses on the available empirical evidence regarding school-based suicide prevention efforts. For selective prevention, screening is a critical first step. Systematic identification can be accomplished when screening is routine. Tools such as the *Suicide Ideations Questionnaire* (Pinto et al., 1997; Reynolds, 1998) are available, and studies have suggested that screening combined with supportive intervention can work to decrease suicidal behaviors (Eggert et al., 1995b; Randell et al., 2001; Thompson et al., 2001). (The limitations of suicide assessment tools, however, are discussed in Chapter 7.) Because an adolescent's suicidal feelings are often short-term in duration and episodic in nature, repeated screening of high-risk populations is required to identify youth at risk for suicide in order to intervene to prevent impulsive behavior. The use of screening to identify at-risk and high-risk youth creates a demand for trained gatekeepers and programs designed to increase personal competencies. Gatekeepers need to consider multiple risk factors that suggest greater risk of suicide in addition to suicide ideation, such as substance abuse, history of physical or sexual abuse, conduct disorder, aggression/impulsivity, and family discord. Systematic identification of these youth should not be undertaken until social network resources are in place to respond to the needs identified by these screening procedures.

Gatekeeper Training

School-based Programs

Two gatekeeper-training activities were identified that were part of an integrated school-based program: LivingWorks Suicide Intervention

Workshop (SIW) and Suicide, Options, Awareness and Relief (Project SOAR).

SIW delivered five modules over 2 full days (Ramsey et al., 1994). Upon completion of the 2-day SIW training participants acquired basic knowledge about how to assess and intervene with youth at risk of suicide. The program was evaluated by comparisons between the gatekeepers' knowledge and helping intentions immediately post-training, and that of the general public who had been exposed to a public media campaign (Eggert et al., 1997). Trained gatekeepers were significantly more likely to know the suicide warning signs (Eggert et al., 1997).

Project SOAR was a mandatory 8-hour training course for school counselors in Dallas, Texas. School counselors who had completed SOAR as part of their district-wide training (48 percent in the last 3 years) were very knowledgeable about warning signs correctly identifying depression, previous attempts, low self-esteem and recent relationship breakups 87 percent of the time or better. They also were very knowledgeable about suicide intervention steps correctly responding (90 percent of the time or better) that they would call a parent, listen to the student, notify the principal, and ask for assistance from school resources. In the SOAR project, competencies were sustained for up to 3 years post-training and enhanced by actual assessment of suicidal youth. Knowledge of intervention steps was also significantly greater when counselors had 6 or more years of experience (King and Smith, 2000). Information provided by program participants suggested that participants in SOAR performed at a level above the national average based on a national survey (King and Smith, 2000).

The two programs demonstrated that motivated adult helpers/professionals have little difficulty learning critical facts regarding suicide and the associated warning signs/risk factors when delivered as part of a gatekeeper-training curriculum. Adults participating in skill-based, action-oriented programs endorse appropriate helper attitudes, have high behavioral intentions to help, demonstrate appropriate helping competencies in simulations, and report being comfortable when helping. Participation in gatekeeper training programs appears to produce significantly greater gains when compared to informational messages alone. "Booster" training every 2 to 3 years and mock assessment/intervention role-plays may be useful to maintain competence.

Primary Care Physicians: The Gotland Program

On the Swedish island of Gotland, Rutz and colleagues (Rutz et al., 1989) implemented a program of physician education. This effort included a structured educational program for general medicine physicians on recognition and treatment of depressive disorders. Training included interactive seminars. A primary goal of the program was to increase general practitioners' responsibility for treating depressive disorders. Several variables were monitored, including psychiatric referrals, sick leave for depression, psychiatric inpatient hospitalization, suicides, and prescriptions for antidepressant and anti-anxiety (anxiolytic) medications. When compared to suicide rates of the preceding 4 years, Rutz and colleagues (Rutz et al., 1989) found a significant decrease after the physician training. Referrals to psychiatry for depression decreased by over 50 percent and inpatient care for depression decreased by approximately 75 percent. The number of prescriptions for antidepressants increased, whereas the number of prescriptions for anxiolytics *decreased*. It should be mentioned that the analysis of the results was subsequently debated (Macdonald, 1995; e.g., Williams and Goldney, 1994), and the suicide rate increased again over time, coinciding with about half of the trained physicians leaving their positions (Rutz et al., 1992; see also discussion in Chapter 7).

Primary care provides a critical opportunity for suicide reduction in the United States as well (Chapter 9). However, significant barriers need to be addressed before primary care can serve as an effective conduit to mental health treatment including the treatment of suicidality. These include fractionation of services, lack of motivation of consumers and providers for mental health services, as well as economic barriers (DHHS 2002; see Chapter 9).

Support/Skills Training

The personal competency training program for youth in five urban high schools, Reconnecting Youth (RY) (Eggert et al., 1995a), serves as a model program for this review. Because approximately 35–40 percent of youth at risk for school failure are also at risk for suicide (Thompson and Eggert, 1999), potential high school dropouts are the targeted audience. This program is delivered in high school classrooms to small groups of 10 youths per teacher/ facilitator. The class was offered as an elective as part of the student's school schedule. It was offered usually on a daily basis for 55 minutes over a full semester (90 sessions), or following the schedule used for other classes in the school's time table.

All students participated in a comprehensive suicide-risk assessment (using the Measure of Adolescent Potential for Suicide [MAPS], Eggert et al., 1994) and social connections intervention, called Counselors-CARE (C-CARE). They were sorted into three groups: Group I youth participated in one semester of RY; Group II youth completed two semesters of RY; and Group III, the "usual care" comparison group, had the comprehensive assessment only. When at-risk youth participated in support/

skills training activities, they experienced clinically significant declines in suicide-risk behaviors; significant decreasing trends in depression, hopelessness, anger, and stress; significant gains in self-esteem and personal control; and increases in social support (Eggert et al., 1995).

The C-CARE assessment and social connection protocol appeared to be essentially as effective as the RY class (either the 1-semester or the 2-semester version) in reducing suicide-risk behaviors and related risk factors (Eggert et al., 1994). Similarly, it worked equally well to increase self-esteem and support resources. Importantly, youth participating in RY, both the 1-semester as well as the 2-semester versions, demonstrated significant gains in personal control (self-efficacy) not evidenced by the usual care/C-CARE group. The observation that a brief assessment protocol reduced suicidal behaviors and emotional distress that are sustained over a 10-month period is noteworthy, as well. Gains in personal control are more likely to be associated with lasting changes and sustained reductions in risk factors over time; longitudinal follow-up is necessary to answer this critical question. Results also point to the critical nature of leader support in building a positive peer culture and creating a context in which effective skills training occurs.

INDICATED PREVENTION

Programs for Youth

Youth identified as being at risk, evidencing early warning signs of suicide risk, need indicated suicide prevention. Among the initiatives designated as indicated are: (1) family support training; (2) skill-building support groups for high-risk individuals; (3) case management/alternative programming; and (4) referral resources for crisis intervention/treatment. This section focuses on two school-based suicide prevention efforts (Counselors CARE [C-CARE] and Project CAST [Coping and Support Training]) primarily addressing skills training support groups and case management/alternative programming for high-risk youth.

Included in both interventions were strategies designed to enhance a youth's sense of personal control. C-CARE is described as an in-depth motivational interview for assessing a comprehensive list of direct suicide-risk factors, related-risk factors, and protective factors. The interventions were designed for potential high school dropouts, all of whom had evidenced specific, early warning signs of suicide- and related-risk factors on the Suicide Risk Screen (Thompson and Eggert, 1999).

The two programs were tested with 150 youth in C-CARE, 155 youth in CAST, relative to 155 similar youth in a "usual care" control group. These "usual care" high-risk youth received a very brief assessment interview (15–30 min), and standardized social connections procedures (as in C-CARE) with parents and designated school personnel.

Both CAST and C-CARE involved school support personnel, resources, and policies related to student suicidal behaviors. Delivery occurred with youth in grades 9–12 and at the students' schools. C-CARE starts with a one-to-one, 2-hour assessment interview. An additional 1.5 to 2 hours counseling session and social "connections" intervention with parents and school personnel follows. A brief assessment/counseling "booster" session is held 6–8 weeks later. Project CAST adds a 12-session (12 hours) small-group skills training program combined with the C-CARE individual approach. It includes the initial and booster sessions of C-CARE. These 12 sessions focus on enhancing personal resources (self-esteem, personal control of moods, school performance, drug use, positive coping strategies, and monitoring/setting goals and staying on track) and support resources (giving and receiving group support; identifying support needs to ask for from school personnel, family, and friends). Key prevention strategies common to both interventions were assessment and feedback for empathy and motivation, access to help and support from school personnel and parents, control of lethal means as indicated, and school crisis-team support. Changes were assessed at four time points, including a 9-month follow-up (Thompson et al., 2001).

CAST was most effective in enhancing and sustaining increases in problem-solving coping and personal control (self-efficacy) (Thompson et al., 2001). Both CAST and C-CARE were effective in enhancing self-esteem over the short term to increase self-esteem. The greatest differences between youth in CAST vs. C-CARE and usual-care were in problem-solving coping at follow-up (Randell et al., 2001). C-CARE and CAST effectively reduced depression and hopelessness compared to "usual care." Both programs reduced anxiety and anger control problems in females. All youth showed significant decreases in hard drug use (Eggert et al., in press) but CAST was better at reducing alcohol and marijuana use (Eggert et al., in press). Growth curve analyses showed significant rates of decline in suicidal behaviors including suicidal ideation in both programs. Rates of suicide communications and attempts were unaffected; however, their low base-rate limited their outcome measures.

Programs for Aging Populations

As discussed in Chapter 9, late-life suicide victims typically see their primary care physicians in the month prior to death and face many obstacles to receiving appropriate care. A recent study on treatment outcome in suicidal versus non-suicidal depressed elderly patients showed that the two groups had identical remission rates (77 percent versus 78 percent) when treated with combined pharmacotherapy and interpersonal psychotherapy, but that the relapse rate was higher among suicidal elderly (26% versus 13%, Szanto et al., 2001). These data suggest that elderly suicidal depressed patients have an overall favorable treatment outcome, but that treatment response may be more brittle and may require the continuing use of adjunctive medication to prevent early relapse.

A recent "indicated" preventive intervention in the elderly looks promising. An NIMH-supported study on Prevention of Suicide in Primary Care Elderly: Collaborative Trial (PROSPECT; Bruce and Pearson, 1999) is testing the effectiveness of placing depression care managers in primary care practices in preventing and reducing suicidal ideation and behavior, hopelessness, and depressive symptomatology. The study is obtaining a sample representative of practice populations and is over-sampling patients with depression and the very old, i.e., those aged 75 and above. The essential tasks of the depression care manager are to convey clinical information to the primary care physician, to monitor the patient's treatment compliance with treatment that is informed by Agency for Health Care Policy and Research guidelines, to assess the patient's clinical status, to provide psychotherapy when requested, and to arrange specialist referrals. Preliminary data suggest that PROSPECT's intervention is more effective than treatment as usual. Although both patient populations had similar base rates, after 12 months, 10 percent of the patients in the intervention group had suicidal ideation compared to 17 percent of those in usual care; and only 5 percent expressed hopelessness compared to 17 percent in usual care (Reynolds et al., 2001). These data suggest that a depression care manager can be an effective intervention.

INTEGRATED APPROACHES TO PREVENTION

The World Health Organization (WHO) began espousing national responses to the problem of suicide by 1989, and in 1996 the United Nations formulated official guidelines for national suicide prevention strategies that urged governments to adopt comprehensive approaches to reducing suicidality and increasing personal resilience and community connectedness (United Nations, 1996). Currently, Asian countries generally experience significant lack of basic mental health services, and often only have either the volunteer "Befrienders" services (see hotlines section) for those contemplating suicide or a few crisis centers staffed by volunteers. Furthermore, some countries still consider suicide a crime, thus limiting health care services available to attempters (for review, see Murthy, 2000).

A number of European national and United States state governments, however, have responded to the complex nature of suicide by developing comprehensive suicide prevention strategies that incorporate all levels of prevention methods. In accordance with UN/WHO recommendations, such programs typically target both the reduction of mental illness and the promotion of mental health, employing everything from macro-level changes in social policy and the media to gatekeeper training and coordinated services for high-risk individuals. Many of these programs also establish improved data-gathering and surveillance systems. Although some comprehensive suicide prevention programs appear to reduce rates of suicide, evaluation of such programs remains challenging given the multitude of variables on the individual and aggregate level that interact to affect suicide rates. Omission of data collection from non-medical paradigms and lack of adequate planning and funding for evaluation have seriously hampered prevention efforts. Recent prevention strategies in Norway and Australia, for example, have therefore designated evaluation of all aspects of their programs as requirements for funding. As evaluation of comprehensive prevention models continues, nations and states will have more concrete information about what specific strategies effectively reduce suicide, how much funding such efforts require, and how best to coordinate efforts within and between levels of intervention.

Maryland Youth Suicide Prevention Strategy

The State of Maryland implemented a comprehensive suicide prevention model in the mid-1980s, but decided to focus on reducing youth, not general, suicide. According to a study by the Big Horn Center for Public Policy using data from the Centers for Disease Control and Prevention, Maryland has seen a reduction in suicide rates across age groups after program implementation. The greatest reduction has occurred in the 15–24 year old range targeted by the prevention strategy, with a drop of 21.4 percent in Maryland, while youth suicide increased 11 percent nationally over the same decade (Westray, 2001a). This evaluation has not, however, ruled out other causal explanations for this lower suicide rate in Maryland. Nonetheless encouraged by the apparent success of the Maryland strategy, the program's coordinators have trained 20 other United States states in how to implement its model and accepted an invitation from Australia to provide consultation to its national youth suicide prevention team.

As a means of organizing and administering the various components of the prevention strategy, Maryland created the "Governor's Inter-Agency Workgroup on Suicide Prevention." The Workgroup builds on existing agencies already targeting suicide risk factors such as substance abuse, child abuse, and mental disorders, and includes the involvement of the Maryland Department of Juvenile Justice, Education, and the Office of Chief Medical Examiners, as well. Various subcommittees then focus on particular levels of intervention, such as media education, the Maryland youth crisis hotline, and gun control efforts.

Maryland represents the first state to institute a statewide, toll-free youth crisis telephone hotline. Six centers comprise the hotline network, with several of them offering walk-in counseling, emergency shelter, and community education. Trained local crisis intervention counselors staff the hotline, and, in addition to making general mental health referrals, counselors make appointments at local mental health centers for those adolescents willing to disclose their identity. In the 10 years since its inception, Maryland has seen a 47 percent increase in calls to the hotline, with the modal age group increasing from 12–17 to 18–24 (Westray, 2001b).

A significant aspect of Maryland's youth suicide prevention plan involves funds for schools to develop prevention programs. Every district chooses a particular focus: some have implemented general mental health curriculum, others have established school gatekeeper training and crisis response teams, and others employ peer helper programs, suicide awareness education, and mental health referral systems. If properly evaluated, such program diversity could perhaps give insight into which approaches most effectively reduce youth suicide.

The Maryland youth suicide prevention plan, in contrast to Finland's program, for example, targets reduction of access to means by working to change policy regarding gun use and by educating the public on the relationship between handguns and suicide. The program also initiated an AIDS hotline in English and Spanish to reach traditionally underserved populations at risk for suicide. The Maryland model also includes educating the media on appropriate reporting practices concerning suicide, and uses public service announcements to influence community awareness of youth suicide and available services. Finally, the program collaborates with the University of Maryland to obtain research expertise for evaluation of program elements and for data surveillance.

Air Force Suicide Prevention Strategy

In response to an increased awareness of suicide as the second leading cause of death among active duty United States Air Force personnel (CDC, 1999), the Air Force formed a committee of civilian and military multidisciplinary experts to design a service-wide comprehensive suicide prevention strategy in 1996–1997. Drawing from the experiences of previous models, the Air Force prevention approach, dubbed "LINK," emphasizes the social and community aspects of suicide alongside individual, psychiatric elements. The Air Force suicide prevention program therefore targets both suicide risk reduction and mental and behavioral health promotion, goals that concur with those of the United Nations and the World Health Organization recommendations (United Nations, 1996). Primary aspects of the LINK strategy include encouraging early mental health intervention and offering coordinated services among agencies, normalizing help-seeking behavior, and increasing protective factors such as social connectedness, support, and effective coping skills (USAFMS, 2000). Further, the Air Force has implemented suicide awareness training for staff, changed certain Air Force policies in response to epidemiological research, and developed a database for collecting a broad array of information regarding suicide attempts and completions throughout Air Force personnel and their families.

The Air Force has aggressively pursued increasing community awareness of suicide risks and available services and decreasing the stigma surrounding accessing mental health services. Senior Air Force staff reinforce the perspective that suicide prevention is a community effort and regularly distribute notices to personnel regarding the problem of suicide within the Air Force (USAFMS, 2000). Regular staff development courses have also now incorporated suicide prevention education for all officers. Such training describes the risk and protective factors for suicide, including contexts and symptoms of acute suicide risk, and when and to whom to refer individuals at risk of suicide. Further, LINK espouses establishing "buddy care," in which everyone is encouraged to look out for others within the community. Enhancing the mental well-being of the entire unit is therefore conveyed as *each* staff member's responsibility. Supervisors and unit members alike are encouraged to persuade those facing mental health issues (including substance abuse and domestic violence) to self-refer to services. The Air Force presents such actions as a means of increasing unit productivity and helping the individual reach his or her fullest potential, and explicitly states these goals as motivation for commander-directed mental health evaluations when individuals do not self-refer (USAFMS, 2000). After reviewing personnel surveys regarding behavioral health concerns, the Air Force has recently expanded its education program to include violence and homicide risk (Staal, 2001).

Given the research on overlapping risk factors for suicidality, the Air Force recognized a need to coordinate its mental health and social services. The suicide prevention program established a collaboration among six agencies: chaplains, child and youth programs, family advocacy, family support, health promotion/health and wellness centers, and mental health clinics. This Integrated Delivery System oversees and organizes overlapping suicide prevention efforts while maintaining individual agencies' unique missions. The Delivery System therefore offers its services at schools, work sites, and community facilities in addition to usual care at the member agency facilities. Representatives from member agencies and senior military installation commanders form the Community Action Information Boards that manage collaborative efforts among Delivery System agencies and between the Delivery System and their respective communities (USAFMS, 2000).

After epidemiological research regarding suicide among Air Force personnel demonstrated that situations such as legal investigations increased suicide risk, the Air Force suicide prevention program spearheaded policy changes to encourage help-seeking in these contexts. Specifically, the Air Force initiated a "hand-off" policy requiring that anyone facing legal issues be released to a supervisor or, minimally, only after notification of the supervisor, to ensure that an authority figure would be ready to refer the individual to helping agencies if deemed necessary (USAFMS, 2000). The Air Force implemented an additional measure that departs from military tradition by extending limited patient privilege to those under legal investigation. Thus, Air Force personnel receiving mental health treatment know that what they share with their mental health provider will not be used against them in military court or to characterize their service at the time of their separation from the military.

After implementing its comprehensive suicide prevention program, the Air Force saw a significant decrease in suicide rates among its active-duty personal, from 16.4 per 100,000 to 9.4 per 100,000 ($p< 0.002$) between 1994 and 1998 (Litts et al., 2000). By 1999, the rate dropped to 5.6 per 100,000. These rates represent a 78 percent decline in the suicide rate among active duty Air Force personnel over the last 5 years (Staal, 2001). In contrast, over the same period, suicide rates in other branches of the United States military (Navy, Army, and Marines) have not shown the same sustained decline (Litts et al., 2000). As with the other programs reviewed here, despite apparent success, the Air Force has not established that this reduction in suicide follows directly from LINK's implementation (Litts et al., 2000; USAFMS, 2000).

An external evaluation of the program is currently under way at the University of Rochester School of Medicine's Center for the Study and Prevention of Suicide. The Air Force also plans to continue analyzing its data to determine the effects of its suicide prevention efforts (Staal, 2001; USAFMS, 2000), and has established an epidemiological database and surveillance system. This system collects psychological, social, behavioral, economic, and relationship factors surrounding suicide attempts and completions among active and non-active duty cases. This database operates independently from other Air Force databases to enhance the confidentiality of mental health provider reports and to include data from Reservists, National Guard, and Department of Defense members. If analysis of the Air Force LINK model finds it effective in reducing suicide, exporting it to other communities could prove valuable. However, difficulties are anticipated. For example, the Air Force is a controlled environment in which commanding officers can forcibly refer individuals deemed at high risk for suicide to mental health services. Moreover, given personnel assignments to units, military service membership creates a salient community. Program elements establishing social support, sense of belonging, and social responsibility therefore take root much more easily in such a setting than in the broader society. Furthermore, the Air Force can routinely include suicide/mental health education into staff development and can form system-wide policies aimed at specific suicide-reduction efforts more quickly and with greater power to enforce such policies than the United States government as a whole. The Centers for Disease Control thus recommends first using the Air Force's LINK model in occupation-related communities such as law enforcement and investigative agencies (CDC, 1999). The Department of Defense is currently implementing the LINK model, which should yield more information about its effectiveness in reducing suicide.

Suicide Prevention Programs for Rural American Indian Communities

Integrated approaches to suicide prevention have been used effectively in several American Indian reservation communities in the United States and Canada for at least three decades. These efforts were in response to either high suicide rates or apparent suicide clusters. They utilized universal, selected, and indicated intervention/prevention methods through community and public service agencies.

In the 1960s, the Shoshone-Bannock Tribal Council worked to reduce the high rate of suicide of 98 per 100,000 (mostly involving adolescents and young adults) in their community (Dizmang, 1969; Dizmang et al., 1974; Shore et al., 1972), but the rate continued to rise into the early 1970s. A partnership was formed among the tribe, NIMH, and the Indian Health Service (IHS) in 1968 in response to this crisis. Epidemiological research during the early part of this program identified acute alcohol intoxication, arrest for minor infraction, and high family disruption as risk factors for suicide, and services were designed to reduce these risks (Dizmang et al., 1974; Levy, 1988; May, 1987; Shore et al., 1972). This program included social and economic improvements, traditional Indian cultural enhancement programs, and increasing mental health services (Dizmang, 1969).

One of the hallmarks of this program was the active and enthusiastic participation of the local tribal members. Community awareness and organizing was used, and a tribal holding facility was established for youths "at risk" for suicide, or who had made low lethality suicide attempts. Here they received informal counseling, help, and support from volunteers from the Shoshone-Bannock tribal members who were on call around the clock. These volunteers had been trained by local mental health professionals and had ongoing support from health, mental health, and law enforcement officials. The suicide rate fell from a high of 173.1 per 100,000 in 1972–1976 to 21.5 in 1977–1980, but then rose again to 45.4 in 1981–1984 (May, 1987).

The suicide rate had also been very high in another Native American community, the Jicarilla Apache Tribe of northern New Mexico; 41 to 61 per 100,000 for a 10 year period (1969–1979) (VanWinkle and May, 1986; 1993). The rate was extraordinarily high among adolescents and young adults, exceeding 160 per 100,000 among those aged 15–24 during this same time-span (VanWinkle and May, 1986; 1993). Again, as with the Shoshone-Bannock, a partnership was formed between the Jicarilla Apache Tribal Council and Tribal Health Programs, with the Indian Health Service, and later the CDC. The program utilizes multiple agencies in the community including the IHS clinic, tribal mental health and substance abuse programs, the high school, and law enforcement. As a result of this partnership, this Jicarilla Apache community has had a comprehensive youth suicide prevention program since 1989 targeting 15–18 year olds in school and in the community with a variety of measures including public education, risk assessment, counseling, and alcohol abuse prevention initiatives (Serna et al., 1998).

Like the Shoshone-Bannock community program, the Jicarilla Apache program emphasized the use of "Natural Helpers" (local, indigenous persons trained to recognize symptoms of self-destruction and perform lay counseling) as key vehicles for prevention. The Natural Helpers work with the support and utilization of mental health professionals who serve as therapists for the highest risk and most serious cases. Professionals also provide training, advice, and support to community and staff alike. The program has drastically lowered the rate of suicide gestures, attempts, and completions combined (Serna et al., 1998). One of the consistent effects is not only a significant lowering of the rate of attempted and completed suicide in the targeted ages of 15–18, but a gradual lowering of the rates in older age brackets (e.g., 19–24), as the target population ages (P. May, University of New Mexico, personal communication, December 2001; VanWinkle and Williams, 2001).

Since the majority of suicides among American Indians occur among the young, schools have been a primary focus of some American Indian suicide prevention programs. An effective school-based suicide prevention program was developed and implemented among the people of the Zuni Pueblo Tribe in western New Mexico (LaFramboise, 1996). This approach arose from the concern of the indigenous administrators of the Zuni Tribal School District over a 20-year pattern of 2 suicides per year in their high school. American Indian psychology and counseling researchers were brought into the community from Stanford University, the University of Oklahoma, and the University of Wisconsin to examine and define the situation among the youth and to develop strategies for the prevention of suicide. A number of risk factors and possible solutions were identified from survey research among the students, teachers, tribal leaders, and others within the community. The research at Zuni pinpointed correlates of suicide specific to this community that identified high risk youths as having experience similar to that of other populations (e.g., suicide ideation, depression, poor social support, and hopelessness, among others), but also identified variables of help-seeking behavior, communication, and cultural resources that were specific to this particular tribal community and clearly differentiated those Zuni youths that were high risk and those that were not (Bee-Gates et al., 1996; Howard-Pitney et al., 1992). The research and the school collaboration led to the development of a comprehensive school curriculum that covered everything from building self-esteem, dealing with emotions and stress, and communication, to recognizing self-destructive behavior and helping those who may be suicidal (LaFramboise, 1996). The program was integrated into the language arts classes of the school rather than presented as a stand-alone course. Detailed research analysis indicated that students who were exposed to the program scored better than a no-intervention group at post test in hopelessness, problem-solving ability, and suicide intervention skills, with nonsignificant yet encouraging declines in suicide probability, as well (LaFramboise and Howard-Pitney, 1995). Though no formal evaluation of post-program suicide completions has been conducted, the school has experienced a reversal of its 20-year suicide rate, with zero completions noted since the program was taught in the late 1980s (P. May, University of New Mexico, and H. Lewis, past superintendent of the Zuni Public School District, personal communication, February 2002).

The fourth and final program discussed in this section on rural American Indian communities was implemented in Canada. After a suicide cluster of eight young adults in 1974–1975 on an Ottawa reserve in northern Canada, risk factors were identified by case control research within the community (Ward and Fox, 1977). Social isolation, family disruption, and poor coping skills were identified, in addition to acute and chronic misuse of alcohol (Ward and Fox, 1977). Because of the link of suicide with alcohol problems, suicide awareness, prevention strategies, and a counseling program were all placed into service in the community via the counselors of the alcohol treatment program and with support from other mental health professionals and educators. Five years later the suicide rate in this community had fallen 10-fold, from 267 per 100,000 to 26.7. In addition, the overall violent death rate dropped from 253 per 100,000 to 109 (Fox et al., 1984; Ward, 1984). For a critical review of these and other suicide prevention programs among American Indians and Alaska Native communities, see Middlebrook et al., 2001.

International Programs

Lessons from Finland

Finland countered its unusually high rate of suicide (see La Vecchia et al., 1994) by establishing the world's first nationally implemented, research-based comprehensive suicide prevention program. Organized into a research (1986–1991), implementation (1992–1996), and evaluation (1997–1998) phase, Finland's National Suicide Prevention Project has offered itself as a learning opportunity for the world's suicidologists. Both internal and external international teams have evaluated the project, and the United Nations/World Health Organization guidelines (1996) have included the model as a prime example for others to follow. Finland saw a peak in suicide rates in 1990 before project implementation, and then a 20 percent reduction between 1991 and 1996. The suicide rate has since stabilized at 9 percent below pre-project levels (Beskow et al., 1999).

The Suicide Prevention Project seeks to combine reducing suicide and promoting mental health, and therefore includes selective and indicated strategies, such as improving responsibility and cooperation between health services agencies, and universal measures such as enhancing individuals' inner resources and living conditions. A foundational strategy involved building a national network of contact persons, primarily in health care, but also in the social services, churches, and police and rescue departments. Many prevention components arose from this network as schools and churches developed prevention projects specific to their settings, for example. National policy created better care for suicide attempters, increased knowledge among members of the media about suicide and mental illness, and promulgated media guidelines for reporting on suicide. Furthermore, the national players created an organizational frame for increased mental health research. An acclaimed national depression program targeting the general population that features coordinated basic and specialized services for all ages has also arisen from the Suicide Prevention Project.

Noted shortcomings of Finland's project include, however, no selected or indicated focus on the elderly. The project also fails to include policies on reducing access to means. From a research perspective, Finland's prevention project falls short in planning for sound evaluation; program developers did not collect data that could enable researchers to control for possible confounding variables. An international evaluation team further noted a lack of data collected from social psychological, sociological, and cultural perspectives that could enhance the science of suicide prevention (Beskow et al., 1999).

Finland did not implement its prevention program in a traditional fact-oriented, didactic fashion, but rather in a collaborative manner of guiding and supporting practitioners and service providers through joint reflections on prevention methods based on their expertise and existing activities. Evaluators note that participants found this approach and its attendant emphasis on "learning by doing" rewarding and psychologically effective, with key players/gatekeepers embracing the model. However, a general lack of studies on effective program implementation processes currently hampers prevention efforts. The Finland project, for example, still experiences tensions between the public and private sectors regarding hierarchy and organization (Beskow et al., 1999).

In summarizing the primary lessons from Finland's experience with comprehensive suicide prevention programming, Beskow and colleagues (1999) mention the need for prevention strategies to carefully plan economic resources and evaluation. They also stress that a strong anchoring of the prevention strategy with city administrators and politicians and within professional organizations ensures its continuation.

Of paramount importance stands the need to understand and bridge differences between medical and other paradigms. Beskow's evaluation team laments the presence of such conflicts in Finland that remain even after 11 years. The prestige of medical research can lend authority to a prevention strategy based on psychiatric-epidemiological research. Published results of a national psychological autopsy study alone brought suicide to the national consciousness in Finland and evoked willingness among professionals to tackle the problem. Ignoring other research paradigms, however, hampered evaluation efforts, for example, and made determining whether the prevention program accounts for the reduction in suicide rates virtually impossible. The program evaluators cite the encouraging trend within biopsychosocial research to use cross-disciplinary approaches as reason to believe that divisions between paradigms will be diminishing.

Other Recent International Programs

Certain other countries have designed comprehensive suicide prevention programs that will be evaluated continuously, yielding invaluable information about best practices for other governments. Australia, for example, used UN/WHO guidelines, the Finland experience, and consultation with the State of Maryland to design a national youth suicide prevention strategy that has now expanded to the general population. The Australia program uses evidenced-based practices to deliver and enhance cross-sectoral services; has developed and started implementing national university suicide prevention curriculum for doctors, nurses, teachers, and journalists; is re-orienting health services to focus on mental health promotion; and has started piloting a mental health curriculum for schools. The program also includes social change strategies such as media education, reducing access to lethal means, and investing in parenting programs (Commonwealth Department of Health and Family Services, 1997; Waring et al., 2000; Wyn et al., 2000). New Zealand's youth suicide prevention program incorporates virtually the same elements, including the parenting interventions (Beautrais, 1998). Sweden's program is very similar (Ramberg, 2000; The National Council for Suicide Prevention, 1996).

Norway, however, departs from these models by considering universal prevention and promotion factors as valuable social resources, but not part of a national strategy. Norway's program therefore focuses on selected and indicated prevention, particularly increasing services to attempters after hospital release, though it does also support training for health providers and media education to reduce the stigma surrounding suicide (Norwegian Board of Health, 1995).

Finally, England represents a different approach by couching mental health issues within a truly comprehensive health strategy (Great Britain Department of Health, 1999). England's prevention and health promotion efforts encompass physical and mental health, with suicide reduction a key element of their mental health program (see also Thornicroft, 1999). Concerning suicide, England engages in very similar cross-cutting activities as the previously mentioned programs, with policies to reduce access to lethal means, public education campaigns, improved mental health services, and mental health promotion components for youth and adults.

Summary of Integrated Approaches

Suicidologists and preventionists have monitored a number of comprehensive suicide prevention models implemented in sundry settings and cultures. These programs demonstrate that government workgroups can, through cooperative efforts, mobilize health professionals and change service delivery, access to means, and public awareness regarding suicide. The Maryland and Air Force models, in particular, offer insight into how to establish effective inter-agency cooperation of services, and Finland has produced suicide prevention guidebooks for many specific settings (e.g., churches, police force). The programs of various American Indian communities provide models of culture-specific approaches to suicide reduction, especially for marginalized/ minority populations. Research from Finland and Australia provides valuable information regarding barriers to program implementation and the importance of pilot projects.

Currently evaluated comprehensive programs offer the striking lesson that lack of evaluation planning has seriously handicapped the field of suicide prevention. Although each of these programs based their strategy on the scientific literature regarding suicide, they lack the means to determine accurately whether their methods have specifically affected suicide rates. Suicide prevention researchers therefore have voiced concern about how funders and scientists have poured the bulk of their resources into more well-developed fields while communities continue to establish prevention efforts whose true effects remain largely unknown. Recently launched programs have responded to this by requiring evaluation, and will therefore fill much of the gap in knowledge concerning implementation and effectiveness of comprehensive national approaches to suicide prevention.

ASSESSING THE EFFECTIVENESS OF PREVENTION APPROACHES

To effectively reduce the incidence of suicide in the population, both the relative risk associated with a particular risk factor and its rate of occurrence within the population must be taken into consideration. It is very difficult to have broad population impact by focusing on a risk factor (as predictive of suicide as it might be) if it is itself a rare event. An analysis by Brown (2001) demonstrates that high-risk, and therefore also low-prevalence conditions, are always linked with low population-atttributable risk[4] (PAR) and population preventive effects[5] (PPE) (see Table 8-3a,b). Those who are hospitalized for unipolar depression, for example, have an extremely high relative risk, but the low prevalence of

---

[4]Population-attributable risk expresses the proportion of an outcome that could be eliminated if the risk factor were removed.

[5]Population preventive effect measures the relative reduction in an outcome within a population if an intervention is applied to the full population.

TABLE 8-3 High-Risk Strategies for Reducing Attempted and Completed Suicide

High-Risk Group	p(X)[a]	RR[b]	PAR[c]	IE(X)[d]	IE(X^c)	PPE[e]
a. Reducing Completed Suicide						
Serious Suicide Attempt	0.30%	25.9	7%	50%	0%	4%
Psychiatric Hospitalization 1st Month	0.09%	129	10%	50%	0%	6%
Psychiatric Hospitalization 1st Year	0.09%	34	3%	50%	0%	2%
Unipolar Depression Hospitalization	0.03%	100	3%	50%	0%	2%
Unemployed	6.00%	2.5	8%	50%	0%	8%
Psychotic Like Symptoms	0.50%	15	7%	50%	0%	4%
b. Reducing Attempted Suicide						
Teen Suicide Attempt	3.00%	10	21%	50%	0%	15%
Psychiatric Diagnoses	10.00%	4	23%	50%	0%	20%
Major Depressive Disorder	9.00%	4	21%	50%	0%	18%
3 or More Symptoms	12.00%	3.5	23%	50%	0%	21%
2 or More Symptoms	23.00%	3.6	37%	50%	0%	41%
1 or More Symptoms	38.00%	2.7	39%	50%	0%	51%

[a]P(x) is the percentage of population with the trait or risk factor X.

[b]Relative risk (RR) is defined as the proportion of people with a disorder among those exposed to a particular risk factor divided by the proportion of people with the disorder among those not exposed to the risk factor.

[c]The population attributable risk, PAR, is the relative decrease in the disorder that we would expect if we were able to reduce the risk associated with X in a population at risk to that of the rest of the population not at risk.

[d]Intervention effectiveness, IE, is the relative reduction in disorder that would occur if the intervention were implemented for the full population. IE(X) and IE(X^c) represent the intervention's effectiveness on the subgroup sharing risk factor X and the subgroup without risk factor X. IE takes into account factors such as level of program implementation and participation. Thus IE can be no larger than the participation rate.

[e]Population preventive effect, PPE, is the relative reduction in the disorder within a population, if the intervention were applied to the full population.

SOURCE: Brown, 2001.

this population implies that targetting this group alone will not make a large impact on suicide in the general population. Note also that the last three rows, indicating number of psychiatric symptoms, have a decreasing relationship with both PAR and PPE. This indicates that broadening the target group can lead to a higher population effect than a strategy relying on a very high risk group.

When population-based strategies are considered, a larger impact can be effected. This can be illustrated with an example for early risk interventions such as prevention of aggression and conduct disorder, and substance abuse. In this illustration, it is estimated that the early risk factor (whichever example might be chosen) has 15 percent prevalence in the population (similar to early aggressive behavior). Because the risk factor has relatively high prevalence, its relative risk is rather modest (a value of 2 is selected for analysis). Two situations are considered for early risk interventions (see Table 8-4). The first is based on the highly optimistic assumption that a broad-based prevention program has completely successful impact on the high-risk group but produces only a 5 percent decrease in risk among the low-risk group. In this case, the overall reduction in risk is 34 percent. A second alternative is to assume 50 percent impact in the high-risk group and no impact in the low-risk group. This still produces a respectable 15 percent reduction in overall risk for suicide.

These strategies compare quite favorably with the impact of strategies involving crisis telephone lines. Crisis lines are now being used by about 2 percent of the population. Various technologies currently exist to improve participation in prevention programs and through higher utilization increase hotline effectiveness; the analysis here uses 5 percent. Even with the assumption of a very liberal relative risk of 2.5–10 for

TABLE 8-4 PAR and PPE for Alternative Population-Based Prevention Programs

	p(X)	RR	PAR	IE(X)	IE(X^c)	PPE
Early Risk	15.00%	2	13%	100%	5%	34%
	15.00%	2	13%	50%	0%	15%
Crisis Line	2.00%	2.5	3%	10%	0%	1%
	5.00%	2.5	7%	10%	0%	1%
	2.00%	10	15%	10%	0%	2%
	5.00%	10	31%	10%	0%	5%
Gatekeeper	10.00%	2.5	13%	10%	0%	3%
	20.00%	2.5	23%	20%	0%	10%

SOURCE: Brown, 2001.

suicide among would-be crisis line callers, the PAR and PPE are still quite small (Table 8-4). Their value in making a dramatic reduction in suicide is limited because of two factors—they are not used by a high percentage of those at risk, and successful treatment referral is also modest (Gould and Kramer, 2001).

For gatekeeper training, there is some opportunity for significant benefit, provided sufficient numbers of gatekeepers can reach out to those at risk. Two situations are compared to give a range of potential benefit (Table 8-4). In the first situation, the assumption is that gatekeepers are effective in reaching the upper 10 percent who are at risk, and they are only 10 percent effective in reducing their risk. Under these conditions, PAR and PPE are quite modest. On the other hand, if gatekeepers can work more effectively with the top 20 percent at risk, this could lead to sizable reductions in suicide.

In summary, high-risk strategies alone cannot suffice to significantly reduce the incidence of suicide. Our current knowledge forces us to examine universal and selective strategies that can reach individuals early on, when developmental patterns leading to youth problem behavior and psychiatric symptoms can potentially be changed.

FINDINGS

• Imitation of suicides depicted in the media occurs. Education of media professionals can change reporting practices and such changes seem to reduce suicide in certain contexts but the data are limited.

Long-term public education campaigns and media training should be evaluated for their effectiveness both to change the public's knowledge and attitudes and to reduce suicide and suicidal behaviors.

• Reduction in access to a means of suicide can result in a decline in the use of that method. This decline sometimes occurs without substitution of means, thereby reducing suicide. Access to firearms is a particular risk factor for youth. Families often do not comply with counseling about the removal of guns from the home or securing the firearms. Evidence suggests that legislation can be effective.

Measures should be taken to reduce the fatality of all methods. Access to guns should be reduced, especially for those at high risk of suicide. Health care providers should involve families in working to reduce access to means. Education of health care providers about these issues would increase their knowledge regarding concerns and options and should be implemented.

• Universal, selective, and indicated prevention programs that provide skills training show promise in increasing coping skills and to reducing hopelessness. School-based programs have been shown to enhance social support, self-efficacy, and self-esteem and may reduce depression, substance abuse, and suicidality. Training gatekeepers including responsible school staff or primary care physicians may be effective for identifying individuals at risk and obtaining assistance. Placing depression care managers in primary care practices may prove to be of benefit in reducing suicidal behaviors. The value of intervention programs, however, is frequently difficult to assess because of their short duration, often inadequate control populations, and limited long-term follow-up.

School-based intervention programs at the universal, selective, and indicated levels can help to limit suicide among youths and should be pursued. Efforts should provide skills training, gatekeeper training, a crisis response plan, and screening for youth at risk. Evidence-based programs, especially longer-term approaches couched in a broader context of teaching skills and establishing appropriate follow-through and services appear the most effective against suicide. Brief, didactic suicide prevention programs with no connection to services should be avoided.

• Some suicide prevention programs targeting special populations have shown promise. Such models can inform national efforts regarding specific strategies for implementing effective programs in high-risk or special populations, such as policemen, indigenous peoples, and the elderly.

• Comprehensive, integrated state and national suicide prevention strategies that target suicide risk and barriers to treatment across levels and domains appear to reduce suicide. Evaluation of such programs remains challenging given the multitude of variables on the individual and aggregate level that interact to affect suicide rates. Lack of adequate planning and funding for evaluation have seriously hampered prevention efforts.

Prevention and intervention trials must be carefully designed with appropriate controls and rigorously evaluated with long-term follow-up in order to know what works. Furthermore, it is critical that these interventions be assessed to determine if they can be applied to populations other than those in the original test and to define the characteristics that make a program generally effective.

REFERENCES

ADAMHA (Alcohol, Drug Abuse, and Mental Health Administration). 1989. *Report of the Secretary's Task Force on Youth Suicide.* Washington, DC: U.S. Government Printing Office.

AFSP (American Foundation for Suicide Prevention). 2001. *Reporting on Suicide: Recommendations for the Media.* [Online]. Available: http://www.afsp.org/index-1.htm [accessed December 5, 2001].

Ashworth S, Spirito A, Colella A, Drew CB. 1986. A pilot suicidal awareness, identification, and prevention program. *Rhode Island Medical Journal,* 69(10): 457-461.

Bagley C. 1968. The evaluation of a suicide prevention scheme by an ecological method. *Social Science and Medicine,* 2(1): 1-14.

Barraclough BM, Jennings C. 1977. Suicide prevention by the Samaritans. A controlled study of effectiveness. *Lancet,* 2(8031): 237-239.

Beautrais A. 1998. *A Review of Evidence: In Our Hands—The New Zealand Youth Suicide Prevention Strategy.* Wellington, New Zealand: Ministry of Health, New Zealand.

Beautrais AL, Joyce PR, Mulder RT. 1996. Access to firearms and the risk of suicide: A case control study. *Australian and New Zealand Journal of Psychiatry,* 30(6): 741-748.

Bee-Gates D, Howard-Pitney B, LaFromboise T, Rowe W. 1996. Help-seeking behavior of Native American Indian high school students. *Professional Psychology—Research and Practice,* 27(5): 495-499.

Berman AL. 1988. Fictional depiction of suicide in television films and imitation effects. *American Journal of Psychiatry,* 145(8): 982-986.

Berman AL, Jobes DA. 1991. *Adolescent Suicide: Assessment and Intervention.* Washington, DC: American Psychological Association.

Berman AL, Jobes DA. 1995. Suicide prevention in adolescents (age 12-18). *Suicide and Life-Threatening Behavior,* 25(1): 143-154.

Beskow J, Kerkhof A, Kokkola A, Uutela A. 1999. *Suicide Prevention in Finland 1986–1996: External Evaluation by an International Peer Group.* Helsinki: Ministry of Social Affairs and Health.

Beskow J, Thorson J, Ostrom M. 1994. National suicide prevention programme and railway suicide. *Social Science and Medicine,* 38(3): 447-451.

Birckmayer J, Hemenway D. 1999. Minimum-age drinking laws and youth suicide, 1970–1990. *American Journal of Public Health,* 89(9): 1365-1368.

Bond GR, Hite LK. 1999. Population-based incidence and outcome of acetaminophen poisoning by type of ingestion. *Academic Emergency Medicine,* 6(11): 1115-1120.

Boor M, Bair JH. 1990. Suicide rates, handgun control laws, and sociodemographic variables. *Psychological Reports,* 66: 923-930.

Borzekowski DL, Rickert VI. 2001a. Adolescent cybersurfing for health information: A new resource that crosses barriers. *Archives of Pediatrics and Adolescent Medicine,* 155(7): 813-817.

Borzekowski DL, Rickert VI. 2001b. Adolescents, the internet, and health: Issues of access and content. *Journal of Applied Developmental Psychology,* 22(1): 49-59.

Botvin GJ, Baker E, Dusenbury L, Botvin EM, Diaz T. 1995. Long-term follow-up results of a randomized drug abuse prevention trial in a white middle-class population. *Journal of the American Medical Association,* 273(14): 1106-1112.

Boyd JH. 1983. The increasing rate of suicide by firearms. *New England Journal of Medicine,* 308(15): 872-874.

Boyd JH, Moscicki EK. 1986. Firearms and youth suicide. *American Journal of Public Health,* 76(10): 1240-1242.

Brent DA. 1986. Overrepresentation of epileptics in a consecutive series of suicide attempters seen at a children's hospital, 1978–1983. *Journal of the American Academy of Child Psychiatry,* 25(2): 242-246.

Brent DA, Baugher M, Birmaher B, Kolko DJ, Bridge J. 2000. Compliance with recommendations to remove firearms in families participating in a clinical trial for adolescent depression. *Journal of the American Academy of Child and Adolescent Psychiatry*, 39(10): 1220-1226.

Brent DA, Crumrine PK, Varma R, Brown RV, Allan MJ. 1990. Phenobarbital treatment and major depressive disorder in children with epilepsy: A naturalistic follow-up. *Pediatrics*, 85(6): 1086-1091.

Brent DA, Crumrine PK, Varma RR, Allan M, Allman C. 1987a. Phenobarbital treatment and major depressive disorder in children with epilepsy. *Pediatrics*, 80(6): 909-917.

Brent DA, Perper JA, Allman CJ. 1987b. Alcohol, firearms, and suicide among youth: Temporal trends in Allegheny County, Pennsylvania, 1960 to 1983. *Journal of the American Medical Association*, 257(24): 3369-3372.

Brent DA, Perper JA, Allman CJ, Moritz GM, Wartella ME, Zelenak JP. 1991. The presence and accessibility of firearms in the homes of adolescent suicides: A case-control study. *Journal of the American Medical Association*, 266(21): 2989-2995.

Brent DA, Perper JA, Goldstein CE, Kolko DJ, Allan MJ, Allman CJ, Zelenak JP. 1988. Risk factors for adolescent suicide. A comparison of adolescent suicide victims with suicidal inpatients. *Archives of General Psychiatry*, 45(6): 581-588.

Brent DA, Perper JA, Moritz G, Baugher M, Schweers J, Roth C. 1993. Firearms and adolescent suicide. A community case-control study. *American Journal of Diseases of Children*, 147(10): 1066-1071.

Breton JJ, Boyer R, Bilodeau H, Raymond S, Joubert N, Nantel MA. 1998. *Review of Evaluative Research on Suicide Intervention and Prevention Programs for Young People in Canada: Theoretical Context and Results.* Montreal, Quebec, Canada: Université de Montréal.

Brown CH. 2001. *Designs to Evaluate High-Risk and Population-Based Suicide Prevention Programs: Maximizing Our Potential for Reducing Completed Suicide:* Paper commissioned for the Institute of Medicine.

Brown CH, Liao J. 1999. Principles for designing randomized preventive trials in mental health: An emerging developmental epidemiology paradigm. *American Journal of Community Psychology*, 27(5): 673-710.

Bruce ML, Pearson JL. 1999. Designing and intervention to prevent suicide: PROSPECT (Prevention of Suicide in Primary Care Elderly: Collaborative Trial). *Dialogues in Clinical Neuroscience*, 1(2): 100-112.

Cantor CH, Slater PJ. 1995. The impact of firearm control legislation on suicide in Queensland: Preliminary findings. *Medical Journal of Australia*, 162(11): 583-585.

Cassidy S, Henry J. 1987. Fatal toxicity of antidepressant drugs in overdose. *British Medical Journal (Clinical Research Edition)*, 295(6605): 1021-1024.

CDC (Centers for Disease Control and Prevention). 1992. *Youth Suicide Prevention Programs: A Resource Guide.* Atlanta: Centers for Disease Control.

CDC (Centers for Disease Control and Prevention). 1994. Deaths resulting from firearm- and motor-vehicle-related injuries—United States, 1968–1991. *Journal of the American Medical Association*, 271(7): 495-496.

CDC (Centers for Disease Control and Prevention). 1999. Suicide prevention among active duty Air Force personnel—United States, 1990–1999. *Morbidity and Mortality Weekly Report*, 48(46): 1053-1057.

Chan TY. 1996. Safety packaging of acetaminophen combination preparations and severity of adult poisoning. *Journal of Toxicology. Clinical Toxicology*, 34(6): 747-749.

Ciffone J. 1993. Suicide prevention: A classroom presentation to adolescents. *Social Work*, 38(2): 197-203.

Clarke RV, Lester D. 1986. Detoxification of motor vehicle exhaust and suicide. *Psychological Reports*, 59(3): 1034.

Clarke RV, Poyner B. 1994. Preventing suicide on the London Underground. *Social Science and Medicine*, 38(3): 443-446.

Commonwealth Department of Health and Family Services, Mental Health Branch. 1997. *Youth Suicide in Australia: the National Youth Suicide Prevention Strategy*. Canberra, Australia: Australian Government Publishing Service.

Cowen EL. 1994. The enhancement of psychological wellness: Challenges and opportunities. *American Journal of Community Psychology*, 22(2): 149-179.

Davidson MW, Wagner WG, Range LM. 1995. Clinicians' attitudes toward no-suicide agreements. *Suicide and Life-Threatening Behavior*, 25(3): 410-414.

Dizmang LH. 1969. Observations on suicidal behavior among the Shoshone-Bannock Indians. *U.S. Senate Committee on Labor and Public Welfare, Part 5. Special Subcommittee on Indian Education*. (pp. 2351-2355). Washington, DC: U.S. Governement Printing Office.

Dizmang LH, Watson J, May PA, Bopp J. 1974. Adolescent suicide at an Indian reservation. *American Journal of Orthopsychiatry*, 44(1): 43-49.

Drew BL. 2001. Self-harm behavior and no-suicide contracting in psychiatric inpatient settings. *Archives of Psychiatric Nursing*, 15(3): 99-106.

Durlak JA. 2000. Health promotion as a strategy in primary prevention. In: Cicchetti D, Rappaport J, Sandler I, Weissberg RP, Editors. *The Promotion of Wellness in Children and Adolescents*. (pp. 221-241). Washington, DC: CWLA Press.

Eastwood MR, Brill L, Brown JH. 1976. Suicide and prevention centres. *Canadian Psychiatric Association Journal*, 21(8): 571-575.

Egan MP, Rivera SG, Robillard RR, Hanson A. 1997. The 'no suicide contract': Helpful or harmful? *Journal of Psychosocial Nursing and Mental Health Services*, 35(3): 31-33.

Eggert LL, Karovsky PP, Pike KC. 1999. *School-Based Public Education Campaign. Washington State Youth Suicide Prevention Program: Pathways to Enhancing Community Capacity in Preventing Youth Suicidal Behaviors. Final Report*. Seattle: University of Washington.

Eggert LL, Nicholas LJ, Owen LM. 1995a. *Reconnecting Youth: A Peer Group Approach to Building Life Skills*. Bloomington, IN: National Educational Service.

Eggert LL, Randell BR, Thompson EA, Johnson CL. 1997. *Washington State Youth Suicide Prevention Program: Report of Activities*. Seattle, WA: University of Washington.

Eggert LL, Thompson EA, Herting JR. 1994. A measure of adolescent potential for suicide (MAPS): Development and preliminary findings. *Suicide and Life-Threatening Behavior*, 24(4): 359-381.

Eggert LL, Thompson EA, Herting JR, Nicholas LJ. 1995b. Reducing suicide potential among high-risk youth: Tests of a school-based prevention program. *Suicide and Life-Threatening Behavior*, 25(2): 276-296.

Eggert L, Thompson E, Pike K, Randell B. in press. Preliminary effects of two brief school-based approaches for reducing youth suicide-risk behaviors, depression and drug involvement. *Journal of Child and Adolescent Psychiatric Nursing*.

Etzersdorfer E, Sonneck G. 1998. Preventing suicide by influencing mass-media reporting: The Viennese experience 1980–1996. *Archives of Suicide Research*, 4: 67-74.

Etzersdorfer E, Sonneck G, Nagel-Kuess S. 1992. Newspaper reports and suicide. *New England Journal of Medicine*, 327(7): 502-503.

Ferrari M, Barabas G, Matthews WS. 1983. Psychologic and behavioral disturbance among epileptic children treated with barbiturate anticonvulsants. *American Journal of Psychiatry*, 140(1): 112-113.

Fischer EP, Comstock GW, Monk MA, Sencer DJ. 1993. Characteristics of completed suicides: Implications of differences among methods. *Suicide and Life-Threatening Behavior*, 23(2): 91-100.

Flowers-Coulson PA, Kushner MA, Bankowski S. 2000. The information is out there, but is anyone getting it? Adolescent misconceptions about sexuality education and reproductive health and the use of the Internet to get answers. *Journal of Sex Education and Therapy*, 25(2-3): 178-188.

Forster DP, Frost CE. 1985. Medicinal self-poisoning and prescription frequency. *Acta Psychiatrica Scandinavica*, 71(6): 567-574.

Fox J, Manitowabi D, Ward JA. 1984. An Indian community with a high suicide rate—5 years after. *Canadian Journal of Psychiatry*, 29(5): 425-427.

France MH. 1982. Seniors helping seniors: A model of peer counseling for the aged. *Canada's Mental Health*, 30(3): 13-15.

Garland A, Shaffer D, Whittle B. 1989. A national survey of school-based, adolescent suicide prevention programs. *Journal of the American Academy of Child and Adolescent Psychiatry*, 28(6): 931-934.

Glatt KM. 1987. Helpline: Suicide prevention at a suicide site. *Suicide and Life-Threatening Behavior*, 17(4): 299-309.

Gordon R. 1987. An operational classification of disease prevention. In: Steinberg JA, Silverman MM, Editors. *Preventing Mental Disorders*. (pp. 20-26). Rockville, MD: Department of Health and Human Services.

Gould MS. 2001a. Suicide contagion. Workshop presentation at the Institute of Medicine's Workshop on Suicide Prevention and Intervention, May 14, 2001. Summary available in: Institute of Medicine. *Suicide Prevention and Intervention: Summary of a Workshop*. (pp. 8-10). Washington, DC: National Academy Press.

Gould MS. 2001b. Suicide and the media. *Annals of the New York Academy of Sciences*, 932: 200-221; discussion 221-224.

Gould MS, Kramer RA. 2001. Youth suicide prevention. *Suicide and Life-Threatening Behavior*, 31 (Suppl): 6-31.

Gould MS, Shaffer D. 1986. The impact of suicide in television movies. Evidence of imitation. *New England Journal of Medicine*, 315(11): 690-694.

Gould MS, Shaffer D, Kleinman M. 1988. The impact of suicide in television movies: Replication and commentary. *Suicide and Life-Threatening Behavior*, 18(1): 90-99.

Great Britain Department of Health. 1999. *Saving Lives: Our Healthier Nation*. London: The Stationery Office. [Online]. Available: http://www.archive.official-documents.co.uk/document/cm43/4386/4386.htm [accessed April 8, 2002].

Green JS, Grindel CG. 1996. Supervision of suicidal patients in adult inpatient psychiatric units in general hospitals. *Psychiatric Services*, 47(8): 859-863.

Grossman DC, Mang K, Rivara FP. 1995. Firearm injury prevention counseling by pediatricians and family physicians. Practices and beliefs. *Archives of Pediatrics and Adolescent Medicine*, 149(9): 973-977.

Gunnell D, Hawton K, Murray V, Garnier R, Bismuth C, Fagg J, Simkin S. 1997. Use of paracetamol for suicide and non-fatal poisoning in the UK and France: Are restrictions on availability justified? *Journal of Epidemiology and Community Health*, 51(2): 175-179.

Harris HE, Myers WC. 1997. Adolescents' misperceptions of the dangerousness of acetaminophen in overdose. *Suicide and Life-Threatening Behavior*, 27(3): 274-277.

Hassan R. 1995. Effects of newspaper stories on the incidence of suicide in Australia: A research note. *Australian and New Zealand Journal of Psychiatry*, 29(3): 480-483.

Hawton K, Fagg J, Marsack P. 1980. Association between epilepsy and attempted suicide. *Journal of Neurology, Neurosurgery, and Psychiatry*, 43(2): 168-170.

Hawton K, Simkin S, Deeks JJ, O'Connor S, Keen A, Altman DG, Philo G, Bulstrode C. 1999. Effects of a drug overdose in a television drama on presentations to hospital for self poisoning: Time series and questionnaire study. *British Medical Journal*, 318(7189): 972-977.

Hawton K, Ware C, Mistry H, Hewitt J, Kingsbury S, Roberts D, Weitzel H. 1996. Paracetamol self-poisoning. Characteristics, prevention and harm reduction. *British Journal of Psychiatry*, 168(1): 43-48.

Hazell P, King R. 1996. Arguments for and against teaching suicide prevention in schools. *Australian and New Zealand Journal of Psychiatry*, 30(5): 633-642.

Hemenway D. 2001. Firearm availability and suicide. Workshop presentation at the Institute of Medicine's Workshop on Suicide Prevention and Intervention, May 14, 2001. Summary available in: Institute of Medicine. *Suicide Prevention and Intervention: Summary of a Workshop.* (pp. 17-20). Washington, DC: National Academy Press.

Hlady WG, Middaugh JP. 1988. Suicides in Alaska: Firearms and alcohol. *American Journal of Public Health*, 78(2): 179-180.

Howard-Pitney B, LaFromboise TD, Basil M, September B, Johnson M. 1992. Psychological and social indicators of suicide ideation and suicide attempts in Zuni adolescents. *Journal of Consulting and Clinical Psychology*, 60(3): 473-476.

IOM (Institute of Medicine). 1994. Mrazek PJ, Haggerty RJ, Editors. *Reducing Risks for Mental Disorders: Frontiers for Preventive Intervention Research.* Washington, DC: National Academy Press.

IOM (Institute of Medicine). 2001. *Health and Behavior: The Interplay of Biological, Behavioral, and Societal Influences.* Washington, DC: National Academy Press.

IOM (Institute of Medicine). 2002. *Speaking of Health: Assessing Health Communication Strategies for Diverse Populations.* Washington, DC: National Academy Press.

Kalafat J. 2000. Issues in the evaluation of youth suicide prevention initiatives. In: Joiner T, Rudd MD, Editors. *Suicide Science: Expanding the Boundaries.* (pp. 241-249). Boston: Kluwer Academic Publishers.

Kalafat J, Elias M. 1994. An evaluation of a school-based suicide awareness intervention. *Suicide and Life-Threatening Behavior*, 24(3): 224-233.

Kalafat J, Ryerson DM. 1999. The implementation and institutionalization of a school-based youth suicide prevention program. *Journal of Primary Prevention*, 19: 157-175.

Kapur S, Mieczkowski T, Mann JJ. 1992. Antidepressant medications and the relative risk of suicide attempt and suicide. *Journal of the American Medical Association*, 268(24): 3441-3445.

Kellam SG, Ling X, Merisca R, Brown CH, Ialongo N. 1998. The effect of the level of aggression in the first grade classroom on the course and malleability of aggressive behavior into middle school. *Development and Psychopathology*, 10(2): 165-185.

Kellermann AL, Rivara FP, Somes G, Reay DT, Francisco J, Banton JG, Prodzinski J, Fligner C, Hackman BB. 1992. Suicide in the home in relation to gun ownership. *New England Journal of Medicine*, 327(7): 467-472.

Kessler RC, Downey G, Milavsky JR, Stipp H. 1988. Clustering of teenage suicides after television news stories about suicides: A reconsideration. *American Journal of Psychiatry*, 145(11): 1379-1383.

Kessler RC, Downey G, Stipp H, Milavsky JR. 1989. Network television news stories about suicide and short-term changes in total U.S. suicides. *Journal of Nervous and Mental Disease*, 177(9): 551-555.

Killias M. 1993. International correlations between gun ownership and rates of homicide and suicide. *Canadian Medical Association Journal*, 148(10): 1721-1725.

King GD. 1977. An evaluation of the effectiveness of a telephone counseling center. *American Journal of Community Psychology*, 5(1): 75-83.

King KA, Smith J. 2000. Project SOAR: A training program to increase school counselors' knowledge and confidence regarding suicide prevention and intervention. *Journal of School Health*, 70(10): 402-407.

Kleck G, Marvell T. 2000. Impact of the Brady Act on homicide and suicide rates. *Journal of the American Medical Association*, 284(21): 2718-2719; discussion 2720-2721.

Klingman A, Hochdorf Z. 1993. Coping with distress and self harm: The impact of a primary prevention program among adolescents. *Journal of Adolescence*, 16(2): 121-140.

Knickerbocker DA, McGee RK. 1973. Clinical effectiveness of nonprofessional and professional telephone workers in a crisis intervention center. In: Lester D, Brockopp GW, Editors. *Crisis Intervention and Counseling by Telephone*. (pp. 298-309). Springfield, IL: Charles C. Thomas.

Kreitman N. 1976. The coal gas story. United Kingdom suicide rates, 1960–71. *British Journal of Preventive and Social Medicine*, 30(2): 86-93.

Kroll J. 2000. Use of no-suicide contracts by psychiatrists in Minnesota. *American Journal of Psychiatry*, 157(10): 1684-1686.

Kruesi MJ, Grossman J, Pennington JM, Woodward PJ, Duda D, Hirsch JG. 1999. Suicide and violence prevention: Parent education in the emergency department. *Journal of the American Academy of Child and Adolescent Psychiatry*, 38(3): 250-255.

La Vecchia C, Lucchini F, Levi F. 1994. Worldwide trends in suicide mortality, 1955–1989. *Acta Psychiatrica Scandinavica*, 90(1): 53-64.

LaFramboise TD. 1996. *American Indian Life Skills Development Curriculum*. Madison, WI: University of Wisconisn Press.

LaFramboise TD, Howard-Pitney B. 1995. The Zuni Life Skills Development Program: Description and evaluation of a suicide prevention program. *Journal of Counseling Psychology*, 42: 479-486.

Lester D. 1972. The myth of suicide prevention. *Comprehensive Psychiatry*, 13(6): 555-560.

Lester D. 1988. Gun control, gun ownership, and suicide prevention. *Suicide and Life-Threatening Behavior*, 18(2): 176-180.

Lester D. 1990. Was gas detoxification or establishment of suicide prevention centers responsible for the decline in the British suicide rate? *Psychological Reports*, 66(1): 286.

Lester D, Abe K. 1989. The effect of restricting access to lethal methods for suicide: A study of suicide by domestic gas in Japan. *Acta Psychiatrica Scandinavica*, 80(2): 180-182.

Lester D, Murrell ME. 1986. The influence of gun control laws on personal violence. *Journal of Community Psychology*, 14: 315-318.

Levy JE. 1988. The effects of labeling on health behavior and treatment programs among North American Indians. *American Indian and Alaska Native Mental Health Research*, 1 (Mono 1): 211-231; discussion 232-243.

Litts DA, Moe K, Roadman CH, Janke R, Miller J. 2000. From the Centers for Disease Control and Prevention. Suicide prevention among active duty Air Force personnel— United States, 1990–1999. *Journal of the American Medical Association*, 283(2): 193-194.

Loftin C, McDowall D, Wiersema B, Cottey TJ. 1991. Effects of restrictive licensing of handguns on homicide and suicide in the District of Columbia. *New England Journal of Medicine*, 325(23): 1615-1620.

Lott JR Jr. 2000. Impact of the Brady Act on homicide and suicide rates. *Journal of the American Medical Association*, 284(21): 2718; discussion 2720-2721.

Ludwig J, Cook PJ. 2000. Homicide and suicide rates associated with implementation of the Brady Handgun Violence Prevention Act. *Journal of the American Medical Association*, 284(5): 585-591.

Macdonald AJ. 1995. Suicide prevention in Gotland. *British Journal of Psychiatry*, 166(3): 402.

Mackay A. 1979. Self-poisoning—a complication of epilepsy. *British Journal of Psychiatry*, 134: 277-282.

Marzuk PM, Leon AC, Tardiff K, Morgan EB, Stajic M, Mann JJ. 1992. The effect of access to lethal methods of injury on suicide rates. *Archives of General Psychiatry*, 49(6): 451-458.

Matthews WS, Barabas G. 1981. Suicide and epilepsy: A review of the literature. *Psychosomatics*, 22(6): 515-524.

May PA. 1987. Suicide and self-destruction among American Indian youths. *American Indian and Alaska Native Mental Health Research*, 1(1): 52-69.

McClure GM. 1984. Recent trends in suicide amongst the young. *British Journal of Psychiatry*, 144: 134-138.

McLoone P, Crombie IK. 1996. Hospitalisation for deliberate self-poisoning in Scotland from 1981 to 1993: Trends in rates and types of drugs used. *British Journal of Psychiatry*, 169(1): 81-85.

Mendez MF, Lanska DJ, Manon-Espaillat R, Burnstine TH. 1989. Causative factors for suicide attempts by overdose in epileptics. *Archives of Neurology*, 46(10): 1065-1068.

Michel K, Frey C, Wyss K, Valach L. 2000. An exercise in improving suicide reporting in print media. *Crisis*, 21(2): 71-79.

Middlebrook DL, LeMaster PL, Beals J, Novins DK, Manson SM. 2001. Suicide prevention in American Indian and Alaska Native communities: A critical review of programs. *Suicide and Life-Threatening Behavior*, 31 (Suppl): 132-149.

Miller HL, Coombs DW, Leeper JD, Barton SN. 1984. An analysis of the effects of suicide prevention facilities on suicide rates in the United States. *American Journal of Public Health*, 74(4): 340-343.

Miller MC. 1999. Suicide-prevention contracts: Advantages, disadvantages, and an alternative approach. In: Jacobs DG, Editor. *The Harvard Medical School Guide to Suicide Assessment and Intervention.* (pp. 463-481). San Francisco: Jossey-Bass Publishers.

Miller MC, Jacobs DG, Gutheil TG. 1998. Talisman or taboo: The controversy of the suicide-prevention contract. *Harvard Review of Psychiatry*, 6(2): 78-87.

Mishara B, Daigle M. 2001. Helplines and crisis intervention services: Challenges for the future. In: Lester D, Editor. *Suicide Prevention: Resources for the Millennium.* (pp. 153-171). Philadelphia, PA: Brunner-Routledge.

Moens GF, van de Voorde H. 1989. Availability of psychotropic drugs and suicidal self-poisoning mortality in Belgium from 1971–1984. *Acta Psychiatrica Scandinavica*, 79(5): 444-449.

Motto JA. 1971. Evaluation of a suicide prevention center by sampling the population at risk. *Suicide and Life-Threatening Behavior*, 1(1): 18-22.

Murthy RS. 2000. Approaches to suicide prevention in Asia and the Far East. In: Hawton K, van Heeringen K, Editors. *The International Handbook of Suicide and Attempted Suicide.* Chichester, UK: John Wiley and Sons.

Myers WC, Otto TA, Harris E, Diaco D, Moreno A. 1992. Acetaminophen overdose as a suicidal gesture: A survey of adolescents' knowledge of its potential for toxicity. *Journal of the American Academy of Child and Adolescent Psychiatry*, 31(4): 686-690.

Nelson FL. 1987. Evaluation of a youth suicide prevention school program. *Adolescence*, 22(88): 813-825.

Norwegian Board of Health. 1995. *The National Plan for Suicide Prevention 1994–1998.* [Online]. Available: http://www.helsetilsynet.no/english.htm [accessed December 22, 2001].

NRC (National Research Council). 2002. Eccles J, Gootman JA, Editors. *Community Programs to Promote Youth Development.* Washington, DC: National Academy Press.

O'Donnell I, Arthur AJ, Farmer RD. 1994. A follow-up study of attempted railway suicides. *Social Science and Medicine*, 38(3): 437-442.

Ohberg A, Lonnqvist J, Sarna S, Vuori E, Penttila A. 1995. Trends and availability of suicide methods in Finland. Proposals for restrictive measures. *British Journal of Psychiatry*, 166(1): 35-43.

Orbach I, Bar-Joseph H. 1993. The impact of a suicide prevention program for adolescents on suicidal tendencies, hopelessness, ego identity, and coping. *Suicide and Life-Threatening Behavior*, 23(2): 120-129.

Ostrom M, Thorson J, Eriksson A. 1996. Carbon monoxide suicide from car exhausts. *Social Science and Medicine*, 42(3): 447-451.

Overholser JC, Hemstreet AH, Spirito A, Vyse S. 1989. Suicide awareness programs in the schools: Effects of gender and personal experience. *Journal of the American Academy of Child and Adolescent Psychiatry*, 28(6): 925-930.

Pfeffer CR, Jiang H, Kakuma T. 2000. Child-Adolescent Suicidal Potential Index (CASPI): A screen for risk for early onset suicidal behavior. *Psychological Assessment*, 12(3): 304-318.

Phillips DP. 1974. The influence of suggestion on suicide: Substantive and theroretical implications of the Werther effect. *American Sociological Review*, 39(3): 340-354.

Phillips DP. 1985. The Werther effect. Suicide, and other forms of violence, are contagious. *Sciences*, 25: 32-39.

Phillips DP, Carstensen LL. 1988. The effect of suicide stories on various demographic groups, 1968–1985. *Suicide and Life-Threatening Behavior*, 18(1): 100-114.

Phillips DP, Paight DJ. 1987. The impact of televised movies about suicide. A replicative study. *New England Journal of Medicine*, 317(13): 809-811.

PHS (Public Health Service). 1999. *The Surgeon General's Call to Action to Prevent Suicide.* Rockville, MD: U.S. Department of Health and Human Services.

PHS (Public Health Service). 2000. *Report of the Surgeon General's Conference on Children's Mental Health: A National Action Agenda.* Rockville, MD: U.S. Department of Health and Human Services.

PHS (Public Health Service). 2001. *National Strategy for Suicide Prevention: Goals and Objectives for Action.* Rockville, MD: U.S. Department of Health and Human Services.

Pinto A, Whisman MA, McCoy KJM. 1997. Suicidal ideation in adolescents: Psychometric properties of the Suicideal Ideation Questionnaire in a clinical sample. *Psychological Assessment*, 9(1): 63-66.

Ramberg IL. 2000. *Presentation of a Youth Suicide Prevention Programme.* Presentation at Youth Suicide Prevention: European Conference, September 19-20, 2000 in Nantes, France.

Ramsey RF, Tanney BL, Tierney RJ, Lang WA. 1994. *Suicide Intervention Handbook.* Calgary, Alberta, Canada: Living Works Education.

Randell BP, Eggert LL, Pike KC. 2001. Immediate post intervention effects of two brief youth suicide prevention interventions. *Suicide and Life-Threatening Behavior*, 31(1): 41-61.

Reynolds CF, Schulberg HC, Bruce M, Alexopoulos GS, Katz IR, Mulsant BH. 2001. *Depression Treatment in Primary Care Elderly: Preliminary Outcomes of the NIMH PROSPECT Collaborative.* Abstract presented at the annual meeting of the American College of Neuropsychopharmacology in Kona, Hawaii, December 10, 2001.

Reynolds WM. 1991. A school-based procedure for the identification of adolescents at risk for suicidal behaviors. *Family and Community Health*, 14: 64-75.

Reynolds WM. 1998. *Suicide Ideation Questionnaire: A Professional Manual.* Odessa, FL: Psychological Assessment Resources.

Rivara FP, Mueller BA, Somes G, Mendoza CT, Rushforth NB, Kellermann AL. 1997. Alcohol and illicit drug abuse and the risk of violent death in the home. *Journal of the American Medical Association*, 278(7): 569-575.

Rutz W, von Knorring L, Walinder J. 1989. Frequency of suicide on Gotland after systematic postgraduate education of general practitioners. *Acta Psychiatrica Scandinavica*, 80(2): 151-154.

Rutz W, von Knorring L, Walinder J. 1992. Long-term effects of an educational program for general practitioners given by the Swedish Committee for the Prevention and Treatment of Depression. *Acta Psychiatrica Scandinavica*, 85(1): 83-88.

Sainsbury P. 1986. The epidemiology of suicide. In: Roy A, Editor. *Suicide*. (pp. 17-40). Baltimore: Williams and Wilkins.

Schiodt FV, Rochling FA, Casey DL, Lee WM. 1997. Acetaminophen toxicity in an urban county hospital. *New England Journal of Medicine*, 337(16): 1112-1117.

Schmidtke A, Hafner H. 1988. The Werther effect after television films: New evidence for an old hypothesis. *Psychological Medicine*, 18(3): 665-676.

Schmidtke A, Schaller S. 2000. The role of mass media in suicide prevention. In: Hawton K, Van Heeringen K, Editors. *The International Handbook of Suicide and Attempted Suicide*. (pp. 675-697). Chichester, UK: John Wiley and Sons.

Scott V. 2000. Crisis services: Befrienders International: Volunteer action in preventing suicide. In: Lester D, Editor. *Suicide Prevention: Resources for the Millenium*. (pp. 265-273). Ann Arbor, MI: Sheridan Books.

Serna P, May P, Sitaker M. 1998. Suicide prevention evaluation in a Western Athabaskan American Indian Tribe—New Mexico, 1988–1997. *Morbidity and Mortality Weekly Report*, 47(13): 257-261.

Shaffer D, Craft L. 1999. Methods of adolescent suicide prevention. *Journal of Clinical Psychiatry*, 60(Suppl 2): 70-74.

Shaffer D, Garland A, Gould M, Fisher P, Trautman P. 1988. Preventing teenage suicide: A critical review. *Journal of American Academy of Child and Adolescent Psychiatry*, 27(6): 675-687.

Shaffer D, Garland A, Vieland V, Underwood M, Busner C. 1991. The impact of curriculum-based suicide prevention programs for teenagers. *Journal of the American Academy of Child and Adolescent Psychiatry*, 30(4): 588-596.

Shaffer D, Vieland V, Garland A, Rojas M, Underwood M, Busner C. 1990. Adolescent suicide attempters: Response to suicide-prevention programs. *Journal of the American Medical Association*, 264(24): 3151-3155.

Shore JH, Bopp JF, Waller TR, Dawes JW. 1972. A suicide prevention center on an Indian reservation. *American Journal of Psychiatry*, 128(9): 1086-1091.

Sillanpaa M. 1973. Medico-social prognosis of children with epilepsy. Epidemiological study and analysis of 245 patients. *Acta Paediatrica Scandinavica. Supplement*, 237: 3-104.

Simon RI. 1992. Clinical risk management of suicidal patients: Assessing the unpredictable. In: Simon RI, Editor. *Review of Clinical Psychiatry and the Law, Volume 3*. (pp. 3-63). Washington, DC: American Psychiatric Press.

Simon RI. 1999. The suicide prevention contract: Clinical, legal, and risk management issues. *Journal of the American Academy of Psychiatry and Law*, 27(3): 445-450.

Skopek MA, Perkins R. 1998. Deliberate exposure to motor vehicle exhaust gas: The psychosocial profile of attempted suicide. *Australian and New Zealand Journal of Psychiatry*, 32(6): 830-838.

Sloan JH, Rivara FP, Reay DT, Ferris JAJ, Path MRC, Kellermann AL. 1990. Firearms regulations and rates of suicide: A comparison of two metropolitan areas. *New England Journal of Medicine*, 322(6): 369-373.

Sonneck G, Etzersdorfer E, Nagel-Kuess S. 1994. Imitative suicide on the Viennese subway. *Social Science and Medicine*, 38(3): 453-457.

Spirito A, Overholser J, Ashworth S, Morgan J, Benedict-Drew C. 1988. Evaluation of a suicide awareness curriculum for high school students. *Journal of the American Academy of Child and Adolescent Psychiatry*, 27(6): 705-711.

Staal MA. 2001. The assessment and prevention of suicide for the 21st century: The Air Force's community awareness training model. *Military Medicine*, 166(3): 195-198.

Stack S. 1990. Audience receptiveness, the media, and aged suicide. *Journal of Aging Studies*, 4: 195-209.

Stack S. 1996. The effect of the media on suicide: Evidence from Japan, 1955–1985. *Suicide and Life-Threatening Behavior*, 26(2): 132-142.

Stanford EJ, Goetz RR, Bloom JD. 1994. The no-harm contract in the emergency assessment of suicidal risk. *Journal of Clinical Psychiatry*, 55(8): 344-348.

Stein DM, Lambert MJ. 1984. Telephone counseling and crisis intervention: A review. *American Journal of Community Psychology*, 12(1): 101-126.

Stengel E. 1964. *Suicide and Attempted Suicide*. Harmondsworth, England: Penguin Books.

Szanto K, Mulsant BH, Houck PR, Miller MD, Mazumdar S, Reynolds CF 3rd. 2001. Treatment outcome in suicidal vs. non-suicidal elderly patients. *American Journal of Geriatric Psychiatry*, 9(3): 261-268.

Tekavcic-Grad O, Zavasnik A. 1987. Comparison between counselor's and caller's expectations and their realization on the telephone crisis line. *Crisis*, 8(2): 162-177.

The National Council for Suicide Prevention. 1996. *Support in Suicidal Crises*. Stockholm, Sweden: The National Council for Suicide Prevention.

Thompson EA, Eggert LL. 1999. Using the Suicide Risk Screen to identify suicidal adolescents among potential high school dropouts. *Journal of the American Academy of Child and Adolescent Psychiatry*, 38(12): 1506-1514.

Thompson EA, Eggert LL, Randell BP, Pike KC. 2001. Evaluation of indicated suicide risk prevention approaches for potential high school dropouts. *American Journal of Public Health*, 91(5): 742-752.

Thornicroft G, Chairman, Expert Reference Group. 1999. *National Service Framework for Mental Health*. London: Great Britain Department of Health.

Turvill JL, Burroughs AK, Moore KP. 2000. Change in occurrence of paracetamol overdose in UK after introduction of blister packs. *Lancet*, 355(9220): 2048-2049.

United Nations. 1996. *Prevention of Suicide: Guidelines for the Formulation and Implementation of National Strategies*. New York: United Nations.

USAFMS (U.S. Air Force Medical Service). 2000. *The Air Force Suicide Prevention Program: A Description on Program Intiatives and Outcomes*. AFPAM 44-160. Washington, DC: United States Air Force.

Van der Hoek W, Konradsen F, Athukorala K, Wanigadewa T. 1998. Pesticide poisoning: A major health problem in Sri Lanka. *Social Science and Med*, 46(4-5): 495-504.

VanWinkle NW, May PA. 1986. Native American suicide in New Mexico, 1957–1979: A comparative study. *Human Organization*, 45(4): 296-309.

VanWinkle NW, May PA. 1993. An update on American Indian suicide in New Mexico, 1980–1987. *Human Organization*, 52(3): 304-315.

VanWinkle NW, Williams M. 2001. *Evaluation of the National Model Adolescent Suicide Prevention Project: A Comparison of Suicide Rates Among New Mexico American Indian Tribes, 1980–1998*. Tulsa, Oklahoma: Oklahoma State University, College of Osteopathic Medicine.

Vieland V, Whittle B, Garland A, Hicks R, Shaffer D. 1991. The impact of curriculum-based suicide prevention programs for teenagers: An 18-month follow-up. *Journal of the American Academy of Child and Adolescent Psychiatry*, 30(5): 811-815.

Ward JA. 1984. Preventive implications of a Native Indian mental health program: Focus on suicide and violent death. *Journal of Preventive Psychiatry*, 2(4): 371-385.

Ward JA, Fox J. 1977. A suicide epidemic on an Indian reserve. *Canadian Psychiatric Association Journal*, 22(8): 423-426.

Waring T, Hazell T, Hazell P, Adams J. 2000. Youth mental health promotion in the Hunter region. *Australian and New Zealand Journal of Psychiatry*, 34(4): 579-585.

Webster DW, Wilson ME, Duggan AK, Pakula LC. 1992. Parents' beliefs about preventing gun injuries to children. *Pediatrics*, 89(5 (Pt 1)): 908-914.

Weil DS, Hemenway D. 1992. Loaded guns in the home. Analysis of a national random survey of gun owners. *Journal of the American Medical Association*, 267(22): 3033-3037.

Westray H Jr. 2001a. *The Maryland Suicide Prevention Model: A Caring Community Saves Lives.* Baltimore, MD: Presented at the 13th Annual Maryland Youth Suicide Prevention Conference, October 11, 2001.

Westray H Jr. 2001b. *Maryland Youth Crisis Hotline.* Baltimore, MD: Presented at the 13th Annual Maryland Youth Suicide Prevention Conference, October 11, 2001.

WHO (World Health Organization). 1999. *Violence Prevention: An Important Element of a Health-Promoting School.* WHO/SCHOOLS/98.3, WHO/HPR/HEP/98.2. Geneva: World Health Organization WHO Information Series on School Health.

WHO (World Health Organization). 2000a. *Local Action: Creating Health Promoting Schools.* WHO/NMH/HPS/00.3, WHO/SCHOOL/00.2. Geneva: World Health Organization WHO Information Series on School Health.

WHO (World Health Organization). 2000b. *Preventing Suicide: A Resource for Media Professionals.* Geneva.

WHO (World Health Organization). 2002. *Global School Health Initiative.* [Online]. Available: http://www.who.int/hpr/archive/gshi/index.html [accessed January 9, 2002].

Williams JM, Goldney RD. 1994. Suicide prevention in Gotland. *British Journal of Psychiatry*, 165(5): 692.

Wintemute GJ, Parham CA, Beaumont JJ, Wright M, Drake C. 1999. Mortality among recent purchasers of handguns. *New England Journal of Medicine*, 341(21): 1583-1589.

Wyn J, Cahill H, Holdsworth R, Rowling L, Carson S. 2000. MindMatters, a whole-school approach promoting mental health and wellbeing. *Australian and New Zealand Journal of Psychiatry*, 34(4): 594-601.

Yip PS, Callana C, Yuen HP. 2000. Urban/rural and gender differentials in suicide rates: East and west. *Journal of Affective Disorders*, 57(1-3): 99-106.

Zenere FJ 3rd, Lazarus PJ. 1997. The decline of youth suicidal behavior in an urban, multicultural public school system following the introduction of a suicide prevention and intervention program. *Suicide and Life-Threatening Behavior*, 27(4): 387-402.

Encompass'd with a thousand dangers,
Weary, faint, trembling with a thousand terrors . . .
I . . . in a fleshy tomb, am
      Buried above ground.

—William Cowper (1731-1800)
From the poem "Lines Written During a Period of Insanity".

Cowper on several occasions tried to hang, poison, or stab himself. The lines above were composed after one of his suicide attempts.

9

Barriers to Effective Treatment and Intervention

The barriers to receiving effective mental health treatment are nothing short of daunting (US DHHS, 1999). This chapter describes the constellation of barriers deterring use of mental health treatment by people who are either suicidal or who have major risk factors for suicidality: a mental disorder[1] or a past suicide attempt (Chapters 2, 3).

A close examination of barriers to treatment is warranted by several striking findings: (1) the vast majority (90–95 percent) of people in the United States who complete suicide have a diagnosable mental disorder, yet only about half of them are diagnosed and treated appropriately (Conwell et al., 1996; Fawcett et al., 1991; Harris and Barraclough, 1997; Isometsa et al., 1994b; Robins et al., 1959); (2) many are symptomatic for several years before suicide (Fawcett et al., 1991; Shaffer and Craft, 1999); (3) many have made a past suicide attempt (Harris and Barraclough, 1997); and (4) most who complete suicide make contact with health services in the days to months before their death. Nearly 20 percent make contact with primary care providers in the *week* before suicide, nearly 40 percent make contact within the month before suicide (Pirkis and Burgess, 1998), and nearly 75 percent see a medical professional within their last year (Miller and Druss, 2001). Among older people, the rates are higher, with about 70 percent making contact within the month before

---

[1]Includes alcohol and substance use disorders.

331

suicide (Barraclough, 1971; Miller, 1976). However, suicide victims are three times more likely to have difficulties accessing health care than people who died from other causes (Miller and Druss, 2001).

These findings underscore the importance of sifting through reasons why people escape detection or fail to receive adequate diagnosis and treatment for risk factors and suicidality. They also underscore the importance of taking a broad view of barriers—focusing on suicidality, as well as on risk factors—because their treatment is so intertwined.

The barriers discussed in this chapter collectively weigh against treatment. Each barrier is unlikely to act in isolation, but likely interacts with and reinforces the others. The complex relationship of various precipitative, exacerbative, and maintenance effects of barriers is unique in each clinical case. Deeper and more nuanced understanding of the multiple barriers to treatment is essential for design, development, and implementation of preventive interventions. Prospective longitudinal studies can help to elucidate relationships among barriers as they change across the life-span and across the development of suicidality.

The chapter works its way from general to more specific barriers. It first looks broadly at barriers to treatment—such as stigma, cost, and the fragmented organization of mental health services. It then covers barriers raised *within* a range of therapeutic settings—by *both* clinician and patient. Finally, the chapter focuses on barriers for groups at greatest risk for suicide: older people, adolescents, certain ethnic populations, and incarcerated persons.

GENERAL BARRIERS TO TREATMENT

Stigma and Discrimination

The stigma of mental illness is one of the foremost barriers deterring people who need treatment from seeking it (US DHHS, 1999). About two-thirds of people with diagnosable mental disorders do not receive treatment (Kessler et al., 1996; Regier et al., 1993; US DHHS, 1999). Stigma toward mental illness is pervasive in the United States and many other nations (Bhugra, 1989; Brockington et al., 1993; Corrigan and Penn, 1998).

Stigma refers to stereotypes and prejudicial attitudes held by the public. These pejorative attitudes induce them to fear, reject, and distance themselves from people with mental illness (Corrigan and Penn, 1998; Hinshaw and Cicchetti, 2000; Penn and Martin, 1998). The stigma of mental illness is distinct from the stigma surrounding the act of suicide itself. The stigma of mental illness deters people from seeking treatment for mental illness, and thereby creates greater risk for suicide. The stigma surrounding suicide is thought to act in the opposite direction—to deter people from completing suicide.[2] A prominent nationally representative survey conducted in the early 1990s found that 44 percent of Americans are opposed to suicide under any circumstances; most of the remainder are opposed to suicide except in the case of terminal illness (Agnew, 1998). In some situations, however, the stigma of suicide acts to increase suicide risk because it may prevent people from disclosing to clinicians their suicidal thoughts or plans. Studies cited later in this chapter clearly indicate that patients often do not discuss their suicidal plans with their clinician. This, in turn, leads to their under-treatment and thus increases their likelihood of suicide.

The existence of stigma surrounding mental illness is best supported by nationally representative studies of public attitudes. Studies find that about 45–60 percent of Americans want to distance themselves from people with depression and schizophrenia. The figures are even greater for substance use disorders (Link et al., 1999). Stigma leads the public to discriminate against people with mental illness in housing and employment (Corrigan and Penn, 1998). It also discourages the public from paying for treatment through health insurance premiums (Hanson, 1998). Public attitudes toward mental health treatment are somewhat contradictory: while nationally representative surveys find that Americans generally support mental health treatment for people with disorders, the public is less willing to use formal services if they anticipate a mental health problem for themselves (Pescosolido et al., 2000; Swindle et al., 2000).

For people with mental illness, the consequences of societal stigma can be severe: diminished opportunities, lowered self-esteem, shame and concealment of symptoms, and lower help-seeking behavior (Hornblow et al., 1990; Link et al., 1997; Sussman et al., 1987; Wahl, 1999). The National Comorbidity Survey, one of the only nationally representative studies to investigate why individuals with mental illnesses do not seek treatment, found that almost 1 in 4 males and 1 in 5 females with Posttraumatic Stress Disorder cite stigma as their reason (Kessler, 2000). While the majority with mental illness do not seek treatment, there is wide demographic variability: women and younger adults (ages 18-44) are more likely to reach some kind of care, whereas ethnic minorities and older people are less likely (Bland et al., 1997; Gallo et al., 1995; Narrow et al., 2000; US DHHS, 1999; US DHHS, 2001). If they make contact with primary care providers, stigma inhibits them from bringing up their mental health concern. Patients may instead report more somatic symptoms of

---

[2]Both stigmas can feed into the emotional burden in the wake of a suicide attempt by someone with mental illness. They may experience the stigma of mental illness, as well as the stigma of having tried to die by suicide.

mental illness, such as dizziness and stomach disturbances, because these are more culturally acceptable (US DHHS, 2001). Even if patients begin treatment for mental illness, stigma can deter them from staying in treatment. These problems are especially relevant for older people (Sirey et al., 2001), adolescents, and certain ethnic populations. These groups are discussed later in the chapter because they are at high risk for suicide.

Stigma also extends to family members. Family members of people with mental illness have lowered self-esteem and more troubled relationships with the affected family member (Wahl and Harman, 1989). Families of suicidal people tend to conceal the suicidal behavior to avoid the shame or embarrassment, or to avoid the societal perception that they are to blame (especially with a child or adolescent suicide). After suicide, family members suffer grief as well as pain and isolation from the community (PHS, 2001).

Financial Barriers

The cost of care is among the most frequently cited barriers to mental health treatment. About 60–70 percent of respondents in large, community-based surveys say they are worried about cost (Sturm and Sherbourne, 2001; Sussman et al., 1987). Economic analyses of patterns of use of mental health services clearly indicate that use is sensitive to price: use falls as costs rise, while use increases with better insurance coverage (Manning et al., 1986; Taube et al., 1986). Rises in co-payments of mental health services are associated with lower access (Simon et al., 1996a). The demand for mental health services is more responsive to price than is demand for other types of health services (Taube et al., 1986).

Having health insurance, through the private or public sector, is a major determinant of access to health services (Newhouse, 1993). People without health coverage experience greater barriers to care, delay seeking care, and have greater unmet needs (Ayanian et al., 2000). Overall, about 16 percent of Americans are uninsured, but rates are higher in racial and ethnic minorities (Brown et al., 2000). Having health insurance, however, does not guarantee receipt of mental health services because insurance typically carries greater restrictions for mental illness than for other health conditions (US DHHS, 1999).

Over the past decade, during the growth of managed care, disparities in coverage have led to a 50 percent decrease in the mental health portion of total health care costs paid by employer-based insurance (Hay Group, 1998). Not surprisingly, insured people with mental disorders in a large United States household survey in 1994 were twice as likely as those without disorders to have reported delays in seeking care and to have reported being unable to obtain needed care (Druss and Rosenheck, 1998).

A more recent household survey in 1998 found that people with a probable mental disorder are more likely than those without a disorder to have lost their health insurance and to report lower access to care (Sturm and Wells, 2000). The consequences of the disparities in insurance coverage for mental illness have led to legislative proposals at the state and federal level for parity—coverage for mental illness *equivalent to* that for other health conditions (US DHHS, 1999). While there do not appear to be any studies directly examining cost as a barrier to treatment for suicidal people, most researchers believe that cost does play a role.

Mental Health System Barriers

The fragmented organization of mental health services has been repeatedly recognized as a serious barrier to obtaining treatment (US DHHS, 1999). The vision, beginning in 1975, of the community support reform movement—an integrated, seamless service system that brings mental health services directly to the community—has not fully materialized. Mental health services continue to be so fragmented that they have been termed the "de facto" service system (Regier et al., 1993). People with mental illness frequently report their frustrations and waiting times as they navigate through a maze of disorganized services (Sturm and Sherbourne, 2001; Sussman et al., 1987). The disorganization is a product of historical reform movements, separate funding streams, varying eligibility rules, and disparate administrative sources—all of which have created artificial boundaries between treatment settings and sectors (Ridgely et al., 1990). Among the hardest hit are people with co-occurring substance abuse and mental health problems, a group at higher risk of suicidality. Co-occurring disorders are the rule rather than the exception in mental health and substance abuse treatment (US DHHS, 1999).

Linkages between different settings are critical for detection and treatment of mental disorders and suicidality (Mechanic, 1997). They include linkages between primary care and specialty mental health care; emergency department care and mental health care; substance abuse and mental health care; and, for adolescents, school-based programs with mental health or substance abuse care. The transition from inpatient care to community-based care is an especially critical period for suicidality in light of studies finding that a large proportion of completed suicides come after recent inpatient discharge, often before the first outpatient appointment (Appleby et al., 1999; Morgan and Stanton, 1997). In addition to improved linkages between different settings, many new programs strive to integrate mental health and primary care, through a variety of service configurations (e.g., a psychiatric nurse practicing with the primary care setting who treats some patients and is a referral source for others). Several approaches to integrating care have been found successful in the treatment of depression (Katon et al., 1996; Katon et al., 1999; Smith et al., 2000). Its utility for suicidality is being studied through ongoing trials (Mulsant et al., 2001; Reynolds et al., 2001).

Services research has focused for the past decades in developing better models of care that bridge these different sectors of care to deliver more integrated mental health care. Several successful models have been developed, most notably wraparound services including multisystemic treatment, for children and adolescents with serious emotional problems and assertive community treatment, a form of intensive case management for people with serious mental illness, combined services for people with mental and substance abuse disorders, and management programs for late life depression in primary care settings (US DHHS, 1999). One major problem, however, is lack of availability to these state-of-the-art services. Many communities simply do not provide them, and, when they do, there are often waiting times for treatment (US DHHS, 1999). Low availability of mental health services (of any kind) is a major problem in rural areas (Beeson et al., 1998; Fortney et al., 1999) and communities with large minority populations (US DHHS, 1999; US DHHS, 2001). People in rural areas report significantly more suicide attempts than their urban counterparts, partly as a result of lower access to mental health services (Rost et al., 1998).

Another major problem is adapting model services to the unique needs of different communities or populations. Programs found successful for some populations may not translate into other settings. For example, a new primary care program for veterans designed to expand access to specialty mental health failed to do so (Rosenheck, 2000), despite the success of similarly designed gateway programs for other populations. Tailoring programs to the needs of distinct populations, including minority groups, is essential, given that they are less likely to access mental health treatment than are whites (US DHHS, 2001).

Managed Care

In the past two decades, managed care has grown from relative obscurity to cover almost 72 percent of Americans with health insurance in 1999 (OPEN MINDS, 1999). Driven by the goal of cost-containment, managed care refers to a variety of strategies for organizing, delivering, and/ or paying for health services. Its promise has been to improve access to health care by lowering its cost, reducing inappropriate utilization, relying on clinical practice guidelines to standardize care, promoting organizational linkages, and by emphasizing prevention and primary care. Managed care's emphasis on treatment of mental health problems in primary care is potentially advantageous for certain populations, such as older people and minorities, which are less inclined toward use of specialty mental health care (US DHHS, 1999). Managed care's potential pitfalls are poorer quality of care, denial of needed care, under-treatment, and disruption in the continuity of clinician–patient relationships (IOM, 1997; Mechanic, 1997).

The impact of managed care on mental health services has been profound in terms of costs: there is strong evidence that managed care has lowered the cost of mental health services (US DHHS, 1999). The study cited above by the Hay Group (1998) indicated that during the growth of managed care, there was a 50 percent reduction in the mental health portion of total health care costs paid by employer-based insurance. Whether these cost reductions have lowered access to, and quality of, mental health services for people who need them is a critical topic for research, but one for which answers have been elusive. Research has been stymied by the dramatic pace of change in the health care marketplace, the difficulty of obtaining proprietary claims data, and the lack of information systems tracking mental health quality or outcome measures (Fraser, 1997; US DHHS, 1999). Most concerns center on potentially poorer quality and outcomes of care from limited access to mental health specialists, reduced length of inpatient care, and reductions in intensity of outpatient mental health services (Mechanic, 1997; Mechanic, 1998). There are also concerns that more impaired populations and children will be adversely affected (US DHHS, 1999). The 1999 *Surgeon General's Report on Mental Health* concluded that, while research is sparse, existing incentives in managed care did not encourage an emphasis on quality of mental health care (US DHHS, 1999).

The impact of managed care expressly on detection or treatment of suicide has been largely unstudied. The limited body of relevant research has focused on depression treatment, spotlighting problems in quality of care and outcomes. The first major studies of prepaid managed care versus traditional fee-for-service care found generally no overall differences in outcome, but poorer outcomes for patients with the most severe mental illness (Lurie et al., 1992; Rogers et al., 1993). Later studies, focusing exclusively on primary care, found that less than 50 percent of depressed patients in staff-model health maintenance organizations received antidepressant medication that met practice guidelines (Katon et al., 1995; Simon et al., 1996b). One of few managed care studies to have addressed suicide, at least tangentially, was of 1204 outpatients with depression receiving care from seven managed care organizations of varying organizational structures (Wells et al., 1999). Using patient questionnaires, the study found that about 48–60 percent of patients with depressive disorder received some sort of mental health care. Only 35–42 percent of depressed patients used medication at appropriate doses, leading the authors to conclude that overall quality of care was moderate to low. Two findings of the study are particularly relevant to suicide prevention: (1) patients with suicidal ideation did *not* receive higher rates of treatment than did patients without suicidal ideation (using measures of process and quality); (2) patients with both depression and alcohol abuse—which places them at higher risk of suicide—were not given more specialty referrals, as recommended by treatment guidelines (see later section on *Substance Abuse*). While the study did not assess outcomes of care, it did conclude that patients with suicidal ideation and other "silent," yet serious, symptoms are at particular risk for not receiving appropriate treatment by managed care organizations. Another study, of serious suicide attempters in Florida, found that managed care's criteria for approving admission to hospitals were not predictive of features seen in patients who made such attempts (Hall et al., 1999).

A largely unstudied question is whether reductions in intensity of outpatient services, or in length of stay in inpatient care, contribute to suicide risk. A case-control study of completed suicides in the UK found that "reduction in care" at the final service contact was associated with almost a *4-fold increase* in risk of suicide (Appleby et al., 1999). Reduction in care was defined by the study as one or more of the following: reduced appointment frequency, lowered doses of medication, less supervised location (e.g., transfer from day hospital or outpatient), or discharge from follow-up. While this study was not of managed care *per se*, it raises questions about cost containment strategies used by managed care to reduce intensity or frequency of services for people at risk of suicide. In related findings, initial results from a study of all hospital discharges in Pennsylvania found a 25 percent reduction in length of stay during a 3-year period for inpatient treatment of depression. Preliminary results suggest that the reduction in length of stay was accompanied by an increase in readmission rates, a finding that the study investigators interpreted as suggesting that caution should be used when implementing practice guidelines for length of stay (personal communication, J. Harman, University of Pittsburgh School of Medicine, December 18, 2001).

Given the concerns about quality of care and lack of monitoring by managed care, the Surgeon General's *National Strategy for Suicide Prevention* (PHS, 2001) explicitly recommends implementation of quality care/utilization management guidelines by managed care organizations and health insurance plans for effective response to, and treatment of, individuals at risk for suicide. Quality improvement guidelines have been demonstrated to be successful at improving productivity and outcomes of depression in managed care, according to a randomized controlled trial (Wells et al., 2000).

CLINICIAN BARRIERS TO TREATMENT

The overwhelming majority of suicide victims have a diagnosable mental disorder—most commonly a mood or substance use disorder (Chapter 3). Yet, as indicated earlier, most suicide victims do not have their disorder diagnosed or adequately treated at the time of suicide. This section explores the multiple barriers to treatment posed by clinicians in primary care, emergency care, and specialty care.

Barriers in Primary Care

Primary care has become a critical setting for detection of depression and alcohol use disorders (US Preventive Services Task Force, 1996) because of their high prevalence (Murphy, 2000). Primary care refers to family physicians, obstetrician-gynecologists, nurse practitioners, general internists, or pediatricians.

Depression

The detection and treatment of depression by primary care physicians is of great relevance to suicidology. Depression evaluation presents the first opportunity for primary care physicians to ask about suicidal ideation, which is one of several symptoms of major depressive disorder (APA, 1994), and a major risk factor for completed suicide (Harris and Barraclough, 1997). Treatment of depression in primary care is associated with reduced rates of completed suicide, according to an uncontrolled ecological study on the Swedish island of Gotland (see discussion in Chapters 7 and 8, Rutz et al., 1989; 1992). The effects of depression treatment in primary care on suicidal behavior are being studied in a controlled clinical trial in the United States. Preliminary results indicate reduced rates of hopelessness, suicidal ideation, and related symptoms of depression in older primary care patients (personal communication, C. Reynolds, G. Alexopoulos, and I. Katz, University of Pittsburgh School of Medicine, 2001).

In primary care, routine screening for depression is not currently recommended for all asymptomatic adults; however, routine screening for depression is recommended if the physician *suspects* depression or if the patient carries depression risk factors (Beck et al., 1979; Preboth, 2000; U.S. Preventive Services Task Force, 1996).[3] According the American

---

[3]New recommendations from the U.S. Preventive Task Force (2002, *Annals of Internal Medicine* 136: 760-764) now call for screening for depression in the primary care setting.

Medical Association council, considerable evidence indicates that a diagnostic interview for depression is comparable in sensitivity and specificity to many radiologic and laboratory tests commonly used in medicine (Preboth, 2000). During depression screening, guidelines explicitly recommend asking patients about suicidal intent and past suicide attempts. When a suicidal patient is identified, primary care physicians should refer them to specialty care and consider hospitalization (Beck et al., 1979; US Preventive Services Task Force, 1996). The role of primary care is likely to expand, however, as a result of recent health care trends and high level public health concern about suicide prevention. The Surgeon General's *National Strategy* (PHS, 2001) sets as national objectives screening for depression in federally-supported primary care settings (e.g., Medicare and Medicaid) and the use of such screening as a performance measure for evaluating the quality of managed health care plans.

The expanding role of primary care in detection and treatment of depression stems from at least four major factors. The first is awareness of how frequently depression is encountered in primary care. Depression is one of the most common of all mental and somatic diagnoses (Von Korff et al., 1987). About 6–10 percent of people attending primary care settings have major depression (Katon and Schulberg, 1992). The second is that many people with depression *prefer* to be treated in primary care or resist referral to specialty care (Cooper-Patrick et al., 1999; Orleans et al., 1985; Williams et al., 1999). Seventy-five percent of those seeking help for depression do so through their primary care physician rather than through a mental health professional (Goldman et al., 1999). One reason may be that they perceive primary care as less stigmatizing than specialty mental health care. The third factor is the advent of new classes of antidepressant medications that are less toxic when taken in overdose, thus making medication management less complex for non-specialists (Hirschfeld and Russell, 1997; US DHHS, 1999). The fourth factor is the trend in cost containment. Managed care generally encourages the receipt of mental health services in primary, rather than specialty, care because of lower costs (Mechanic, 1998). It is thus not surprising that about half of all people with depression and other mental disorders—either by preference or by financing—receive their mental health treatment in primary care (US DHHS, 1999). Primary care physicians handle nearly half of all antidepressant-related office visits (Pincus et al., 1998).

Only about 30–50 percent of adults with diagnosable depression are accurately diagnosed by primary care physicians (Higgins, 1994; Katon et al., 1992; Wells et al., 1994). Even more startling to suicide prevention are findings about the infrequency of suicide questioning during routine depression evaluation. Only 58 percent of a random sample of 3375 primary care clinicians directly questioned patients about suicide (Williams et al., 1999), despite the fact that such questions are supposed to be asked during a depression evaluation (Beck et al., 1979; US Preventive Services Task Force, 1996). When broken down by specialty, the study found 65 percent of family physicians, 52 percent of general internists, and 48 percent of obstetrician-gynecologists assessed suicide by direct questions. Through regression analyses, the study found that family physicians and general internists were significantly more likely to make direct assessments for suicide than were obstetrician-gynecologists (Williams et al., 1999). Reasons for physician reticence in asking about suicide are discussed in a later section.

Even when patients' depression is accurately diagnosed, only a *minority* of patients receive adequate treatment for depression (US DHHS, 1999; Young et al., 2001). Since the vast majority of primary care physicians prefer to treat depression with medication (Williams et al., 1999), studies often measure inadequate treatment by inadequate dosage or duration of medication, infrequent follow-up, lack of medication adjustment, and/or inadequate conformance to treatment guidelines. Although detection and treatment in primary care are improving, major professional efforts have been undertaken to highlight and respond to the problem (Beck et al., 1979; Hirschfeld et al., 1997).

What are the reasons for inadequate detection and treatment of depression by primary care physicians? The most frequently cited barriers relate to lack of knowledge and time. One recent survey of randomly selected primary care physicians found them to report widespread lack of knowledge about diagnostic criteria and treatment of depression. Overall, about one-third reported knowledge of formal diagnostic criteria and treatment, yet there was great variation between primary care specialties. Obstetrician–gynecologists reported the least knowledge, whereas family physicians reported the most knowledge (Williams et al., 1999). Inadequate time and competing demands created by other health problems—under the cost pressures of managed care—have been identified as barriers in several studies (Borowsky et al., 2000; Rost et al., 2000; Williams et al., 1999). The mean duration of a visit to a primary care physician is 16.3 minutes (Blumenthal et al., 1999), to which patients bring an average of six problems (cited in Williams et al., 1999). The time constraints on the primary care physician become immediately apparent, sparking concerns that primary care clinicians are ill-equipped for their enhanced role in detection of depression (Kane, 1996; Katon et al., 2001). Under-detection and under-treatment of depression are clearly associated with patient distress and disability (Hirschfeld et al., 1997).

Substance Abuse

Substance use disorders are second to mood disorders as the most common risk factor for suicide (Chapter 3). Substance abuse is an especially important risk factor for suicide in young adults (Chapter 3). Furthermore, substance abuse and mood disorders frequently co-occur, with 51 percent of suicide attempters having both (Suominen et al., 1996). Treatment of co-morbid alcoholism and depression with selective serotonin reuptake inhibitors (SSRI) reduces suicidality (Cornelius et al., 2000; Cornelius et al., 2001). Thus, detection and treatment of substance abuse and depression in primary care is important for suicide prevention (Murphy, 2000; PHS, 2001).

For the primary care setting, numerous professional groups recommend routine detection of problem drinking in all patients, as well as brief counseling for non-dependent problem drinkers (summarized in US Preventive Services Task Force, 1996). Nevertheless, problem drinking often goes undetected in primary care. In recent surveys, about 40 percent of primary care physicians do not perform routine screening for substance abuse (Bradley et al., 1995; Williams et al., 1999). The most commonly cited reasons are lack of time and fear of spoiling the relationship with the patient (Arborelius and Damstrom-Thakker, 1995).

For detection of drug abuse in primary care, professional guidelines diverge from those for problem drinking: they generally do not recommend screening all primary care patients for drug abuse. However, clinicians are recommended to be alert to signs and symptoms and to refer drug-abusing patients to specialized treatment (US Preventive Services Task Force, 1996). Standardized screening questionnaires are thought to be too insensitive to identify potential drug abusing patients. In a recent shift, arising from concern about suicide, the Surgeon General's *National Strategy* (PHS, 2001) sets as national objectives screening for substance abuse, depression, and suicide risk in federally-supported primary care settings (e.g., via Medicare and Medicaid) and the use of such screening as performance measures for managed health care plans. A later section deals with the treatment of substance abuse, with or without a co-occurring mental disorder, because it is reserved for specialty care (US Preventive Services Task Force, 1996).

Primary Care Barriers to Detection of Suicidality

It is well established that a large proportion of suicide victims are not detected in primary care in the days before suicide. A systematic review of published studies found that, in the week before death, contact with primary care was made for 16–20 percent of completed suicides. Within one month of death, the rate is 34–38 percent of completed suicides (Pirkis and Burgess, 1998). The frequency of contacts with primary care also increases in the month before death of *young* suicide victims (<35 years old) (Appleby et al., 1996). These findings are widely interpreted as suggesting that patients are motivated to seek help but are reluctant to bring up suicide as the reason during an office visit (Hirschfeld and Russell, 1997; Michel, 2000). Yet people with suicidal thoughts usually tell their physicians *if they are asked* (Delong and Robins, 1961).

Communication of suicidal intent is an interactive process. It depends on the patient's willingness to communicate, as well as the clinician's ability to listen, recognize, and ask questions about intentions. During the final contact with primary care, there is a striking breakdown in communication: physicians often do not ask about suicidal intent or ideation, and patients often do not spontaneously report it. A review of medical records of 61 completed suicides (<35 years) in Manchester, United Kingdom, found almost total absence of documentation of suicide risk by the general practitioner (Appleby et al., 1996). Suicide risk was commented upon in the medical record in only one case. Yet the physicians deemed that 64 percent of the patients had psychological concerns as the principal reason for the visit. A similar study of suicide deaths in Scottish adults (>16 years) found that only 3.3 percent of records indicated that patients expressed suicide ideation or communications at the time of the final consultation[4] (Matthews et al., 1994). The figures are somewhat higher in a study from Finland in which 19 percent of suicide completers with depression communicated their intent to medical providers (Isometsa et al., 1994c). Despite limitations of using case notes to infer what occurred during the final visit, these studies—as well as clinical experience—point to a major barrier in communication: patients are reluctant to communicate their suicidal intent, and primary care physicians are reluctant to ask (Hirschfeld and Russell, 1997).

The failure of physicians to detect suicidality was described in a now classic paper as an "error of omission" (Murphy, 1975). Numerous interrelated reasons are proffered to explain physicians' reticence to ask patients about suicide, yet there has been little systematic research.

One of the most common explanations for physicians' reticence stems from their concern that asking patients about suicide will trigger suicidal behavior (Michel, 2000). Clinical experience, however, suggests this concern to be unwarranted: *"There is universal agreement that asking questions about suicidal ideation does not trigger suicidal behavior . . ."* (Michel, 2000: 665). There is also indirect research support for this statement. The suicide

---

[4]The study did not indicate whether the general practitioner asked patients about suicide.

rate actually *decreased* on the Swedish island of Gotland after the introduction of a primary care educational program to improve depression identification and treatment. This reduction came in spite of investigators' initial concerns that the suicide rate might increase (Rutz et al., 1989). Furthermore, the vast majority of patients in primary care—both suicidal and nonsuicidal—hold the view that physicians *should* inquire about emotional health issues on a regular basis or at yearly checkups (Zimmerman et al., 1995).

Another reason for physician reticence comes from the lack of acute predictors for suicide assessment. Most studies have found low sensitivity and specificity of suicide prediction (Goldney, 2000; see Chapter 7; Pokorny, 1993). In a prospective study, long-term risk factors for suicide were unable to provide the means for acute prediction of suicide (Fawcett et al., 1987). Considering the rarity of suicide in primary care—one suicide every 3–5 years—physicians have little incentive to take active steps to become skilled in suicide assessment or treatment (Michel, 2000). Nor do professional guidelines recommend routine screening of asymptomatic patients. Many professional organizations do not have guidelines on suicide assessment. After expressly evaluating the evidence, the US Preventive Services Task Force in 1996 found "insufficient evidence" to recommend routine suicide screening of asymptomatic adults. The Canadian Task Force on Periodic Health Examination came to a similar conclusion in 1994 (Feightner, 1994). But a change in policy may occur with the release in 2001 of the Surgeon General's *National Strategy for Suicide Prevention*. This plan encourages development of guidelines for primary care settings. It also sets specific national objectives of screening for suicide risk in federally supported primary care settings (e.g., Medicare and Medicaid) and the use of such screening as a performance measure for managed health care plans.

A final reason cited for physician reticence is lack of clinical training (Bernstein and Feldberg, 1991; Ellis et al., 1998). A majority of primary care physicians are surprised by their patients' attempted suicide and desire more training (cited in Michel, 2000). More generally, they report insufficient training in dealing with mental health problems (Kane, 1996; Williams et al., 1999). In short, it is generally believed that primary care physicians do not ask about suicide because they feel ill-equipped—in terms of training and skills in suicide assessment and treatment—to handle an affirmative answer.

The United States Surgeon General has been consistent in urging better training of primary care providers to deal with mental health problems (PHS, 2001). More to the point, the Surgeon General sets as a national objective that physicians and physician assistants "should be skilled in talking with patients about the risk for suicide, in providing crisis intervention for those at imminent risk for the expression of suicidal behaviors . . . and in referring their patients for expert assessment and treatment" (PHS, 2001).

Barriers in Emergency Care

Suicidal patients are frequently encountered in the emergency department (ED). These patients present for care in four situations: (1) patients who mask their suicidal intent by complaining of other health problems; (2) overtly suicidal patients coming in on their own, or with the help of others; (3) patients who have already attempted suicide; and (4) patients pronounced dead in the ED from a suicide attempt and whose bereaved family must be consulted (Buzan and Weissberg, 1992).

Several barriers to care occur in the ED, all of which have been highlighted previously in the context of primary care. The first barrier is that patients with covert symptoms are not recognized. Another barrier is the lack of guidelines for suicide assessment by professional organizations. This prompted the Surgeon General to set as a national objective the development of guidelines expressly for the ED (PHS, 2001). Yet another barrier is the lack of training for ED staff. Seventy percent of emergency physician training programs in a 1990 survey reported not offering any training in the management of psychiatric emergencies (Weissberg, 1990).

Once diagnosed in the ED, suicide attempts are important to treat promptly, to admit to a psychiatric unit, and/or to arrange for effective care after discharge (Buzan and Weissberg, 1992). Suicide attempters are at risk of re-attempt or completed suicide (Chapter 3). However, they often do not receive follow-up care. For instance, up to *half* of all suicide attempts among adolescents did not receive subsequent care after an ED visit (Spirito et al., 1989). The need for effective linkages with follow-up care was set as a national objective by the Surgeon General (PHS, 2001). Yet barriers persist even with good linkage to care because many—more than 40 percent of adolescent attempters (Piacentini et al., 1995)—are nonadherent with treatment.

Barriers in Specialty Mental Health Care

A significant percentage of suicide completers make recent contact with specialty mental health care, either in the community or in the hospital. A review of the published literature found that about 41 percent of those who die by suicide have contact with inpatient care in the year before death. Up to 9 percent of them complete suicide within a day of discharge from inpatient care. The figures are slightly lower for community-based psychiatric care, with 11 percent making contact in the year before death and 4 percent within a day of contact (Pirkis and Burgess, 1998). About 5 percent of suicides occur during hospitalization (Crammer, 1984; Robins et al., 1959).

These figures imply the existence of lost opportunities and numerous barriers to effective treatment in the specialty setting. Barriers extend throughout the process—from the very beginning of diagnosis to after discharge. The problems are similar to those discussed in other clinical settings: the failure to assess suicidal risk and to treat patients who are suicidal or at risk for suicide.

There is an additional barrier to mental health treatment for individuals of racial, ethnic or cultural minorities. There is substantial underrepresentation of minorities among mental health providers, and cultural differences between provider and consumer can greatly interfere with both diagnosis and treatment (US DHHS, 2001).

Barriers to Detection of Suicidality

One overarching barrier to detection of suicidality is the lack of professional guidelines for both *assessment* and *treatment* of the suicidal patient in the specialty mental health care setting. The Surgeon General's National Strategy (PHS, 2001) calls for the development and implementation of professional guidelines for suicide assessment—as well as individualized policies, procedures, and evaluation programs for treatment in a full range of specialty mental health and substance abuse treatment centers. The lack of professional guidelines partly accounts for clinicians' reporting that they do not receive adequate training in suicide detection and treatment, as discussed above.

One early barrier to detection of suicidality, and thus treatment, comes in the form of *exclusion* of suicidal patients by certain types of providers. While research is sparse, one study found that 59 percent of training clinics affiliated with clinical and professional psychology doctoral programs had a policy of excluding patients with suicidal risk (Bernstein and Feldberg, 1991). There are likely many reasons governing the policy, but one salient reason is fear of malpractice. Though suicide-related malpractice claims are still relatively rare, they have increased in the last decades (Jobes and Berman, 1993). The payouts in settlement or verdict are disproportionately high relative to the percentage of claims. For example, among lawsuits for malpractice filed against psychiatrists, 21 percent involve a patient's suicide, yet 42 percent of the dollars paid out are in connection to these cases (Bongar et al., 1992). Clinicians' fear of being sued in the wake of a patient's suicide is considered widespread, even though court decisions usually do not hold clinicians liable if they have practiced according to a loosely defined standard of care (Bongar et al., 1992; Bongar et al., 1998).

Clinicians who accept suicidal patients are legally and ethically obligated to assess suicidal risk through a clinical interview, mental status examination, direct and indirect questioning about suicide, and history taking (see Chapter 7). From a legal perspective, the assessment of suicide risk does not mean *prediction* of risk, because the latter is not yet possible. Rather, it means that the clinician used reasonable prudence that other professionals would exercise in similar circumstances (Maris et al., 2000). In one of the few surveys, researchers asked practicing psychologists, psychiatrists, and clinical social workers about their methods of suicide assessment. Respondents reported infrequent use of assessment instruments (e.g., Hopelessness Scale and Suicide Intent Scale) and reported that they did not find them to be very useful. Psychologists frequently use various psychological tests (e.g., MMPI, Rorschach Ink Blot). The overwhelming majority (>80 percent of clinicians) use clinical observations about patient affect and appearance, as well as direct interview questions about suicide plans, suicide thoughts, method availability, history of drug/alcohol use, and previous attempt, among others (Jobes and Eyman, 1995). Although these findings are not nationally representative and are limited by low response rate, they indicate the need for better assessment instruments.

Another barrier related to the assessment of suicide concerns appropriate diagnosis of the associated mental disorder. If a mental disorder is not properly diagnosed in specialty care, then patients receive either no treatment or inappropriate treatment, placing them at risk for suicide. One misdiagnosis that enhances suicide risk relates to bipolar disorder. Patient surveys (N=600) indicate that 69 percent are misdiagnosed, and they frequently consult four physicians before a correct diagnosis is made (Lewis, 2001). Through review of patient charts at first clinical contact, bipolar disorder is misdiagnosed as unipolar depression in more than one-third of patients with affective disorder (Ghaemi et al., 2000). When treated with antidepressants, but not with mood stabilizers, these patients are risk for rapid cycling (Ghaemi et al., 2000; Kilzieh and Akiskal, 1999), which carries a poorer prognosis and higher risk of suicide (Goodwin, 1999; Schweizer et al., 1988). Bipolar depression carries markedly higher rates of suicidality than do other phases of bipolar disorder (Dilsaver et al., 1997; Isometsa et al., 1994c). Many patients also do not receive adequate treatment even when bipolar disorder is accurately diagnosed, as discussed in later sections.

Communication of Suicidal Intent

In a large number of completed suicides, clinicians are caught unaware of patients' suicidal intent. Across all treatment settings, about 22 percent of suicide victims communicate their intent to clinicians (Isometsa et al., 1995). The problem is worse in primary care, as discussed earlier, where the rate is lower. The situation is somewhat better in specialty care. A psychological autopsy study was conducted in Finland of *all* suicide victims over a 12-month period whose last appointment occurred 28 days before suicide (N=571). By interviewing health care professionals, investigators found that, during the last appointment, 39 percent and 30 percent of patients communicated their intent to outpatient and inpatient psychiatric care providers, respectively (Isometsa et al., 1995). In a related study, the same investigators found that 59 percent of suicide victims with depression communicated their intent to psychiatrists, as opposed to 19 percent to medical providers (Isometsa et al., 1994a). The communication of intent was determined by explicit notes in the medical records or from interviews of clinicians. The study confirmed an early psychological autopsy study that found an even greater disparity (87 percent of psychiatrists versus 17 percent of other physicians) in awareness of suicide communication or attempt (Murphy, 1975). None of these studies, however, indicated whether patients were explicitly asked about suicide by their clinician or whether they spontaneously reported their intent. While specialty care is associated with greater communication of intent, the fact remains that suicidal intent is not communicated in a sizable portion of all patients, regardless of treatment setting.

Barriers to Effective Treatment

The goal of suicide treatment in specialty care is to develop and implement a treatment plan, which includes monitoring of medication efficacy and safety, as well as discharge planning (Maris et al., 2000). The details of treatment, however, are not spelled out in clinical guidelines. Organizations of mental health specialists have developed no clinical guidelines for treatment of suicidality. Clinical guidelines for other areas of mental health treatment are typically developed on the basis of a strong body of evidence for efficacy (PHS, 2001; US DHHS, 2001). The clearest evidence to date suggests the efficacy of lithium, cognitive behavioral interventions, and the minimal contact-letter intervention (see Chapter 7). For suicide treatment, however the larger body of evidence for efficacy is beset by insufficient power and insufficient rigor in research design. It is thus difficult to conduct studies of suicide treatment effectiveness in the absence of clear guidelines for what constitutes effi-cacious treatment. Consequently, the few available studies of suicidal patients focus on whether clinicians in the practice setting ("usual care") administer appropriate treatment for the associated mental disorder, for which treatment guidelines are available (or for which there is more evidence of treatment efficacy). Studies also focus on process issues such as frequency of treatment.

Most of the available research on barriers to effective treatment per-tains to treatment of the mental disorder(s) associated with suicide. The following section covers the relationship between suicide and under-treat-ment of depression and substance abuse.

Under-Treatment

Depression. Psychological autopsy studies have found that a large per-centage of suicide victims with major depression were not receiving treat-ment or were receiving inadequate treatment. The majority of patients receiving antidepressants were prescribed inadequate doses (Isacsson et al., 1994; Isacsson et al., 1992; Isometsa et al., 1994b; Modestin and Schwarzenbach, 1992). Victims receiving psychotherapy rarely had visits as often as once a week (Isometsa et al., 1994b). These findings also apply to suicide attempters both *before* as well as *after* a suicide attempt (Suominen et al., 1998). Patients with depression and a history of past suicide attempts—a group at high risk for suicide—received inadequate pharmacological treatment in the 3 months before hospitalization (Oquendo et al., 1999).

Substance Abuse. Substance abuse is often under-treated in suicidal patients. Although not as well investigated as under-treatment for de-pression, studies indicate that alcohol dependence is under-treated in the vast majority of patients both before and after a suicide attempt (Suominen et al., 1999). As noted earlier, substance use and mental disorders fre-quently co-occur in completed (Henriksson et al., 1993) and attempted suicide (Suominen et al., 1996). Co-occurring disorders are best treated by programs that integrate mental health and substance abuse treatment (US DHHS, 1999). A major barrier to integrated treatment is the lack of such specialized programs (US DHHS, 1999).

PATIENT BARRIERS TO TREATMENT

The preceding sections have described the barriers deterring the ma-jority of people with symptoms from seeking mental health care: stigma, cost, and fragmentation of services. Additional patient barriers to care are fear of being hospitalized and thinking that they can handle their problems without formal treatment (Kessler, 2000; Sussman et al., 1987). If patients succeed in overcoming these general barriers to treatment, there are additional barriers confronting them within treatment itself.

Medication adherence is one key barrier. The term "adherence" is defined as the extent to which an individual's use of medication adheres to medical advice. About 24–28 percent of suicide victims are non-adherent with medication treatment in the month before death (Appleby et al., 1999). More generally, about one-third of patients with mood disorders or psychosis (regardless of whether they are suicidal) are non-adherent (Cramer and Rosenheck, 1998), thereby placing them at risk for suicide. The reasons for non-adherence are complex. Certainly the barriers operating against *reaching* care—cost, fragmentation of services, and stigma— also apply for patients who are *receiving* care. Patients may be non-adherent to avoid the stigma attached to having a mental disorder, considering that most psychiatric medications need to be taken on a chronic basis (Kihlstrom, 1998). Medication side effects represent another major reason for less than optimal adherence (Fenton et al., 1997). Other reasons for patient non-adherence include: impaired cognition from the underlying disorder or co-occurring substance use; lack of social support; attitudes against medication or treatment; and dissatisfaction with treatment or poor therapeutic alliance, including lack of information from clinicians about dose and side effects (Fawcett, 1995; Fenton et al., 1997; Schou, 1997).

Another major barrier operating in the treatment setting is that the vast majority of patients who are suicidal often do not spontaneously report their suicidal intent to their clinician. A study, cited earlier, found that only 22 percent of suicide victims communicate their intent to their clinicians (Isometsa et al., 1995). The reasons for patient underreporting of suicidal intent are complex and difficult to discern upon psychological autopsy. The most commonly asserted reasons are the hopelessness of suicidality or the underlying symptoms of mental illness. Patients perceive their condition as hopeless and their clinician as unhelpful or unable to meet their needs for counseling, medication, and information (Hintikka et al., 1998; Michel, 2000; Pirkis et al., 2001). Fifty percent of adults who previously attempted suicide retrospectively reported that they could not have accepted help at the time of their attempt (Michel et al., 1994). Their cognition, judgment, or memory may be impaired, thus undermining their ability to appreciate the therapeutic value of treatment (Fawcett, 1995)

BARRIERS TO TREATMENT FOR HIGH-RISK GROUPS

Older People

Older men have the highest rates of suicide in the United States; the overall rate of suicide among men over 65 is about 30 per 100,000 population (Chapter 2). These figures underscore the urgency of examining the barriers to treatment for older people, especially men. The barriers range from general ones—cost of services and stigma—to more specific barriers posed by clinicians and patients.

For older people, the major financier of health services is Medicare. In comparison with private insurance, Medicare carries fewer benefits for mental health services via lower coverage of office visits and limits on hospitalization (US DHHS, 1999).[5] Prescription drugs are not covered at all, although this may change under new policy initiatives. One-quarter of older people report that, because of Medicare restrictions, they would not seek mental health services if they needed them (Mickus et al., 2000). Other general barriers to treatment include limited transportation and stigma (Unutzer et al., 1999; US DHHS, 1999). Older people are less likely to accept a diagnosis of a mental disorder and they are less receptive to treatment than are other adults (Gallo et al., 1999; Leaf et al., 1988). They also perceive greater situational barriers to care (Leaf et al., 1988). If they enter treatment, they are more likely to discontinue prematurely because of stigma (Sirey et al., 2001). The significance of these barriers is borne out in overall patterns of utilization. Older persons are less likely to use mental health services than are other adults, and older males are less likely than older females (Burns et al., 2001; Leaf et al., 1987; Olfson and Pincus, 1996; Swartz et al., 1998). Thus, the demographic group most likely to complete suicide—older men—is the least likely to use services.

Several additional barriers, discussed below, relate specifically to suicidality: "ageism" in social attitudes; problems with detection and treatment of depression, the foremost risk factor for suicide in older people (Conwell et al., 1996); and problems in detection of suicidality.

Ageism refers to societal attitudes that devalue life as people age. It is manifest in stereotypes held by the public, older people, and clinicians. Members of the public, for example, perceive suicide in older people as less tragic than suicide in youth (Marks, 1988-1989). Clinicians, family members, and older adults report that suicidal ideation and depression

---

[5]Medicare requires a 50 percent copayment for most outpatient mental health services, as compared to 20 percent copayment for general medical services. It also carries a 190-day lifetime limit on hospitalization.

are part of the aging process (Duberstein et al., 1995; Seidlitz et al., 1995). The vast majority of surveyed primary care physicians think that, because of losses in late life, depression is understandable (Gallo et al., 1999). They are less alert to the complications of widowhood, which include depression, traumatic grief, and suicidality (Rosenzweig et al., 1997; Szanto et al., 1997; US DHHS, 1999). Depression and grief, in particular, are often misattributed to normal aging (Unutzer et al., 1999). Thus, stereotypes about aging thwart efforts to identify and diagnose depression and traumatic grief on the part of patients, families, and providers (US DHHS, 1999).

Under-detection and under-treatment of depression in older people is considered a major public health problem (Lebowitz et al., 1997; US DHHS, 1999). Most research focuses on primary care because this is where older patients present for, and prefer to receive, mental health care (Mickus et al., 2000; Unutzer et al., 1999). Most older people with depression in primary care remain undiagnosed (US DHHS, 1999). Detection of depression is worse in older than in younger patients, a well-recognized problem that does not appear to be improving (Harman et al., 2001c). Even with detection, up to 50 percent are given inadequate treatment (Katon et al., 1992; Unutzer et al., 2000; US DHHS, 1999), although a more recent study shows some improvement in treatment rates for depression (Harman et al., 2001b). More specifically, depressed older women are about two times more likely than depressed older men to receive antidepressants (Brown et al., 1995). Untreated or inadequately treated depression in primary care plays a role in suicide of older people (Lebowitz et al., 1997).

The reasons for lack of detection and treatment are a complex combination of clinician and patient factors (Pearson et al., 1997; Unutzer et al., 1999; US DHHS, 1999). Family physicians attribute their difficulty in detection to the atypical nature of depression's symptoms in older people (Gallo et al., 1999).[6] Further complicating the diagnosis is that older people commonly report somatic symptoms, as opposed to mental symptoms. Older men, in particular, are less likely than older women to be detected because they report fewer mood symptoms and crying spells (Unutzer et al., 1999). Greater reporting of somatic symptoms by older people might be an attempt to avoid the stigma of mental illness. It also might be that symptoms of physical disorders are amplified by depression (US DHHS, 1999), or that the depressive symptoms are relatively mild (Hotopf et al., 2001). Older persons are more likely to attribute their depression symp-

---

[6]Depression symptoms have somewhat different manifestations in older people. Many have "minor depression," a subsyndromal form of depression with fewer symptoms and less impairment (US DHHS, 1999).

toms to a physical illness (Heithoff, 1995; Knauper and Wittchen, 1994). Further, older patients are often non-adherent with depression medications (NIH Consensus Development Panel on Depression in Late Life, 1992), taking only 50–70 percent of prescribed doses. Their low adherence to depression medications results partly from cost, from polypharmacy (i.e., reluctance to add another medication to the substantial number they have to take for other disorders), and from sensory and cognitive impairment (US DHHS, 1999).

One unexplored reason for lower treatment adherence or dropout may also be a mismatch between clinicians and patients in treatment preferences. Primary care physicians treating older people overwhelming prefer to prescribe medications rather than psychotherapy (Kaplan et al., 1999). Yet people with depression who attend primary care prefer counseling over medication—a finding based on a mixed age population (Dwight-Johnson et al., 2000). There are no studies that directly assess older people's preferences for treatment and analyze findings by gender.

The detection of suicidality in older persons is a major opportunity considering that older people frequently make contact with their primary care physician before suicide. Some studies suggest that up to 70 percent of older people visit their clinician within 30 days of death (Barraclough, 1971; Caine et al., 1996; Conwell et al., 1991). Primary care clinicians are strongly in favor of suicidal assessment in depressed older patients (Harman et al., 2001a). Yet suicidality is complex to recognize in older persons for two main reasons: co-morbidities and infrequency of contacts with mental health specialists (Caine and Conwell, 2001). Co-morbid chronic illnesses are common in older people, they increase risk for depression and suicide, and they make symptom presentation more complicated to disentangle (US DHHS, 1999). To make accurate diagnoses, clinicians have to sort through symptoms of physical illness, depressive symptoms, and side effects of medications. When assessing for suicidality, only 44 percent of primary care providers ask about firearms access, despite the fact that firearms are the method of choice in older suicides (Kaplan et al., 1999). In this survey, general internal medicine physicians were the least likely primary care specialty to ask about firearms and reported the least confidence in assessing and treating suicidality. There is more recent evidence of improvement in physician attitudes about asking older patients about firearms access (Harman et al., 2001a).

There are no professional guidelines for screening older people for depression, substance abuse, or suicidality; however, the Surgeon General's National Plan calls for screening as a minimum standard of care for hospice and nursing homes supported by Medicaid and Medicare.

Adolescents

Barriers to treatment for suicidal adolescents are generally the same as those discussed throughout this chapter: low access to care, low help seeking behavior, low utilization, problems with clinician detection of suicidality, and problems with referral or adherence to care. The empirical basis of these findings is primarily from studies of adolescent suicide attempters. Extrapolating from studies of suicide attempters to completers is problematic for adolescents because attempters are more likely to be female, whereas completed suicides are more likely to be male. Female adolescents are more likely than males to identify a need for mental health help (Saunders et al., 1994).

Access to mental health care is one of the foremost problems. Adolescents at the highest risk for suicide completion have dropped out of school and are unemployed. Their odds for suicide compared to controls are increased 44-fold (Gould et al., 1996). These adolescents, by definition, would not have access to school-based mental health services or employer supportive services.

Adolescent suicide attempters typically first access care in emergency departments, but up to half receive no formal treatment after their emergency department visit (Spirito et al., 1989). Of those receiving care after a visit, non-adherence is exceedingly common. In an inner city hospital where they had received emergency care, 77 percent of adolescent suicide attempters dropped out of treatment in the outpatient psychiatry clinic. Attempters kept significantly fewer appointments than did non-attempters (Trautman et al., 1993). In a separate study at the same clinic, age was inversely related to treatment adherence in male adolescents: younger males (ages 11–15) were more likely to keep appointments after emergency care than were older male suicide attempters (ages 16–19; Piacentini et al., 1995). The reasons for failure of adolescents to attend treatment are likely to include parent resistance to treatment, repetitive evaluations, long waiting periods, and poor communication in the emergency department (Rotheram-Borus et al., 2000; Rotheram-Borus et al., 1994).

Medication adherence is also low among adolescents, although there appear to be no direct data in suicide attempters or completers. In a study of adolescents discharged from inpatient psychiatric care, only 38 percent were adherent. Substance abuse was a major predictor of non-adherence (Lloyd et al., 1998).

Detection of suicidality is another barrier to treatment. Only 9 percent of teachers and only one-third of high school counselors thought that they could recognize a student at risk (King et al., 1999a; King et al., 1999b). Despite the fact that previous suicide attempt is the strongest predictor of suicide, less than 20 percent of adolescent suicide attempters were actually asked about suicidal behavior by physicians at a medical clinic (Slap et al., 1992). A survey of pediatricians and family physicians in Maryland found that only 23 percent either frequently or always screened adolescents for suicide risk factors such as alcohol use or abuse, depression, physical or sexual abuse, or prior attempts (Frankenfield et al., 2000). The American Academy of Pediatrics recommends that pediatricians ask all adolescents about depression, suicidal thoughts, and other suicide risk factors during routine medical history (AAP, 2000). The American Medical Association also recommends annual screening of adolescents to identify those at risk for suicide (US Preventive Services Task Force, 1996).

Ethnic Groups

The general barriers to mental health care for racial and ethnic minorities are similar to those operating for whites—cost, fragmentation and availability of services, and stigma. Added to these barriers are several that are more unique to the minority experience in the US: fear and mistrust of treatment, which stems from the legacy of racism and discrimination, as well as miscommunication for non-English speakers. All of these barriers can act alone or together to deter minorities from accessing and utilizing mental health care. Their access is also lower than whites because of lower socioeconomic status and lower rates of health insurance (Brown et al., 2000). When they utilize care, minorities are more likely than whites to be misdiagnosed or receive inferior quality of care. These disparities between minorities and whites—lower access, lower utilization, and poorer quality of care—are documented in recent reports of the US Surgeon General and the Institute of Medicine (IOM, 2002; US DHHS, 2001). The Surgeon General's report also documents the similar overall prevalence of mental illness across distinct ethnic groups, including whites. Similar overall prevalence, combined with lower access, utilization, and quality, led to the conclusion that minorities suffer a greater burden of unmet mental health needs (US DHHS, 2001). Whether or not these general barriers expressly apply to detection and treatment of suicide in minority groups in community settings has not been empirically documented but can be assumed by extension.

Barriers to the detection and treatment of suicidality in American Indians and Alaska Natives require special focus because rates of suicide are 72 percent higher than those of the general United States population (see Chapter 2). The risk is greatest among young males under 40 years of age. The vast majority of suicides (69 percent) involve alcohol, although the rate varies depending on cultural group.

Of all ethnic groups in the United States, prevalence information is most limited with respect to Native populations. Although evidence is sparse, there are indications that Native youth and adults have somewhat higher prevalence of mental illness compared to the United States population and different distributions of disorders (US DHHS, 2001). The availability of mental health services is a major problem because of the rural, isolated location of many Native communities and the paucity of providers with Native backgrounds. Native populations living on reservations have access to services of the Indian Health Service (IHS), yet its resources for mental health services—especially for secondary and tertiary care—are limited. Furthermore, the majority of American Indians and Alaska Natives live in urban areas and thus do not have access to IHS facilities, which are mainly located on or near reservations. About 23 percent of American Indians and Alaska Natives who report not having IHS coverage lack any other health insurance, compared with 14 percent of whites (Brown et al., 2000).

For suicide victims, however, access to service does not necessarily translate into utilization. A major problem, from a case control study conducted on a Plains Indian reservation, is that victims are less likely to seek health care than are matched controls drawn from the same reservation health facility (Mock et al., 1996). This is in marked contrast to studies of the general United States population, where victims are more likely than controls to seek health care. During health visits within 6 months of suicide, cases on the reservation reported fewer psychological and interpersonal problems than did controls, and almost all had no record of use of mental health services during this period. Given the low rates of health care utilization, the investigators concluded that the clinic shows little promise for detection of those at risk for suicide and recommended stronger community outreach especially to those at greatest risk (i.e., males under age 40).

Incarcerated Persons

There are multiple barriers to providing adequate mental health care in correctional facilities. These barriers emanate from society and correctional facility environments, leadership, officers, health care staff, and inmates themselves. Some of the barriers are similar to those of other populations, but the context is unique in prisons and jails.

Societal Barriers

Before the early 1970s, the courts and society allowed correctional facilities to have broad discretionary powers in the way they treated inmates (Anno, 1991). This changed with a series of court cases in the 1970s and 1980s (*Newman v. Alabama* 1972[7]; *O'Connor v. Donaldson* 1975[8]; 1980 *Ruiz v. Estelle* 1980[9]; 1989 *Langley v. Coughlin* 1989[10]) that held that inmates deserved professional treatment and evaluation of psychiatric problems in appropriate settings. From the Estelle decision, inmates were assured of three basic rights applicable to mental health services: the right to access to care, the right to care that is ordered, and the right to a professional medical judgment.

In 1995 *Madrid v. Gomez*[11] added several factors that determine the constitutionality of a correctional mental health system: (1) an inmate must have a means of making his or her needs known to the medical staff; (2) sufficient staffing must allow individualized treatment of each inmate with serious mental illness; (3) an inmate must have speedy access to services; (4) there must be a system of quality assurance, and staff must be competent and well trained; and (5) there must be a system of responding to emergencies and preventing suicides. Despite the protections afforded by these court cases, in 1996, Congress passed the Prison Litigation Reform Act (PLRA), which curtails the authority of the federal courts to intervene in class actions suits concerning prison conditions, including the delivery of medical care.

Correctional Facility Barriers

The environment in correction facilities is itself a deterrent to mental health. Inmates are often unsafe from random violence, rape, and exploitation (Kupers, 1999). To the extent that these factors increase the hopelessness of some inmates, they increase risk factors related to suicide and are hard for health professionals to mediate.

The growth in the number of individuals confined in prisons and jails has doubled in the past decade and tripled in the past 20 years (Bell, In press). This growth in population frequently outpaces correctional facility health care infrastructure preventing adequate mental health services delivery. Escalating costs of caring for individuals infected with HIV has eroded some progress in quality of care achieved with correctional health care reform that began in the 1970s. (Bell, In press).

---

[7]Newman v. Alabama, 349 F. Supp. 285 (M.D. Ala. 1972); aff'd, 503 F, 2d 1320 (5th Cir. 1974); cert. Denied, 421 U.S. 948 (1975).

[8]O'Connor v. Donaldson, 422 U.S. 563 (1975).

[9]Ruiz v. Estelle, 503 F. Supp. 1265 (S.D. Tx. 1980).

[10]Langley v. Coughlin, 888 F2d 252 (2d Cir. 1989).

[11]Madrid v. Gomez, 889 F. Supp. 1146 (N.D. Cal. 1995).

The logistics of movement within corrections makes health care encounters much more difficult than in the free world. Thus, inmate access to mental health services becomes difficult (Schiff and Shansky, 1998). The mission of corrections is to house inmates in secure facilities that separate them from the rest of society. In correctional facilities, psychiatric needs may take a back seat to issues of security, order, and control (Wilmont, 1997). Accordingly, the roles and relationships among doctors, their inmate patients, and the correctional staff and authorities responsible for managing correctional facilities are often at odds.

Because of the high turnover of inmates in jails, it is difficult to provide complete health assessments that might uncover an inmate who is at high risk for suicide. Many facilities have addressed this problem by providing suicide-screening programs when the inmate first enters the institution. Screening is helped by directing attention to those inmates with a higher risk for suicide, such as young, white males. Other factors predisposing inmates to suicide include: legal complications such as denial of parole, bad news about "loved ones" at home, and victimization in sexual assault or other trauma. While 73 percent of jails report they have suicide prevention programs (Steadman and Veysey, 1997), the content of these programs remains unverified.

Health Care Staff

Even the most dedicated physicians find that jail and prison settings strain their ability to be compassionate (King, 1998) Thus, the attitudes and belief structures of the correctional staff and physicians also complicate the physician/inmate relationship. Within a correctional environment. medical staffs are often pressured to choose sides between correctional philosophy and attitudes and the ethical practice of medicine. "The prison medical community must resist the efforts that are made to tailor the quality and quantity of medical treatment to the exaggerated demands of institutional security, productivity, discipline, and administrative convenience. Every invitation or temptation to define the quality of professional care by the substandard criteria that may govern other facets of the prison's operation must be eschewed" (Nathan, 1984 as cited in King, 1998).

Complicating things is the reality that the typical mental health care professional's world is vastly different from the world from which the inmate comes. Class prejudices combined with ignorance about inmates' background, culture, and environment creates barriers to high-quality interactions and communication (Adebimpe, 1981; Dehoyos and Dehoyos, 1965; Gross et al., 1969). In addition, most service providers are members of the white population while the majority of inmates are nonwhite. This difference in origin and experiences frequently causes problems in inter-actions (US DHHS, 2001). Prejudices and imbalances of power and oppor-tunity produce a climate of mutual fear and distrust that is antithetical to the trust needed for health care (Schiff and Shansky, 1998).

Ethical dilemmas unique to correctional facilities also create barriers to mental health treatment in correctional facilities. The issues of the doc-tor/patient relationship; the quality, extent and power of patient author-ity; the process of informed consent and refusal; physician beneficence; the use, misuse, and control and possible abuse of medical technology; and research on human participants, with particular emphasis on espe-cially vulnerable populations including prisoners, are all issues of medi-cal ethics strained in correctional environments (Bell, In press; Dubler and Anno, 1991), and which interfere with the provision of correctional men-tal health care.

A doctor is ethically required to provide a patient with enough infor-mation to make informed consent decisions regarding their treatment. Patients outside of prison are free to choose a medical approach or to deny treatment even if it results in death. In prison settings, inmates can consent to care but may not, in all circumstances, refuse care.

One example is that of an inmate who was denied the right to refuse dialysis (Commissioner of Correction v. Meyer, 1992[12]) because the re-fusal was considered to be an attempt to manipulate the system to obtain a transfer.

Confidentiality is central to the doctor/patient relationship, but can be breached to protect injury to the patient or to others. In prison, confi-dentiality may not hold if the patient presents risks of escape or internal discord or riot. Patient concerns about confidentiality in a prison setting can seriously hinder appropriate care.

Inmates

Some inmates visit a health care facility as a route to escape from boredom, a place to meet friends in more relaxed and less supervised setting, or as a way of escaping from the monotony of work and programs that continue unrelentingly and are unresponsive to individual daily choice. Some inmates only get out of their cell when they seek health care. Thus, there is some overuse of the system for purposes other than seeking health care. This knowledge develops a sense of cynicism from guards about reasons inmates want to be seen (King, 1998).

Some inmates may be extraordinarily demanding and manipulative.

---

[12]Commisioner of Corrections v Meyer, 399 N.E.2d 452 (Mass. 1979).

Inmates may press health professionals for services or medications that they do not require. It is a rare prison physician (especially one new to corrections) who has not received repeated requests from inmates for medication for "nerves" or "sleeplessness" or "pain." Health providers must ensure that their patients receive the care they need. Simultaneously, they must recognize that succumbing to inmate demands for unnecessary care can do harm.

GLOBAL BARRIERS

Interventions in developing countries face many of the same barriers that are discussed above yet the obstacles are even greater. In developing countries, access to health care in general can be limited. Many countries have few primary care physicians, let alone specialists such as psychiatrists. For example, India has only 3 psychiatrists per million people (Murthy, 1998) and China has 10 per million (de Jong, 1996). In rural areas, the availability can be even less; there can be a physician patient ratio of 1:20,000—and worse for specialists (IOM, 2001).

In developing countries, medical care is often provided by community health centers and caregivers may have minimal education (IOM, 2001). Basic training for these providers—in interviewing and information recording, consultation, use of medication, and even increased awareness and management skills—may effectively improve mental health care (IOM, 2001). Limitations in the diagnostic and treatment capabilities of primary care physicians also have been noted (e.g., Al-Jaddou and Malkawi, 1997; Wright et al., 1989). Among physicians in Jordan, one study found that only 24 percent of the patients with mental disorders were identified (Al-Jaddou and Malkawi, 1997). In order for physicians to recognize the risk factors associated with suicide, they also require additional education. Yet in developing countries the financing of such training is a significant obstacle. A recent IOM report (2001) recommended that existing systems of primary care be extended and strengthened to deliver services for brain disorders, including mental illnesses. It suggested that the training be linked with secondary and tertiary care facilities and be integrated through national policies. Implementation of these recommendations would be likely to reduce the burden of suicides in these countries.

The stigma of mental illness is a major obstacle to treatment and increases the risk of suicide. In some countries, traditional beliefs increase the stigmatization of mental disorders (IOM, 2001). As in developed countries, stigma reduces the likelihood that an individual suffering with a mental disorder might seek out help. Without broad educational programs to reduce the discrimination faced by those with mental illness, many will forego potentially life-saving treatment.

Evaluating the problem of suicide globally is especially difficult because of the variability in the reporting of suicide and inadequate databases in developing countries. As described in Chapter 6, rates may be under-reported in countries where the predominant religion prohibits suicide, such as Catholicism in Ireland, because of the greater stigma (Kelleher et al., 1998; Myers and Farquhar, 1998). Furthermore, the reporting process can differ significantly and introduce additional artifacts. In developing countries, no registries may exist. The lack of accurate accounting for deaths by suicide makes assessment of risk factors and of effectiveness of interventions difficult if not impossible. Under-reporting and consequently underestimating the magnitude of the problem can reduce the effort and resources applied to finding solutions.

FINDINGS

• Stigma represents a major barrier to reducing suicide. The stigma against mental illness results in diminished opportunities and lower self-esteem. Stigma prevents people from seeking treatment for symptoms of mental illness. Untreated mental illness increases suicide risk.

Approaches to reduce the stigma associated with mental illnesses and their treatment must be sought.

• Most people who complete suicide had contact with a health professional within a year of their death, 40 percent within a month of their death. Screening for depression or substance abuse is not routine in primary care. Even when depression is accurately diagnosed, only a minority of patients receives adequate treatment. Primary care physicians lack training and evidence-based screening, assessment, and referral practices for suicidality.

Professional evidence-based guidelines for suicide risk screening, assessment, and referral need to be developed and implemented into primary health care settings. Screening, treatment, and referral for the major suicide risk factors depression and alcohol abuse disorders should be conducted in primary health care settings.

• Many individuals cannot access proper care for mental illness because of the fragmentation of services. This particularly affects those with co-occurring substance use.

Mental health services, including treatment for substance use disorders, should be delivered in an integrated fashion.

• Certain populations face additional barriers to treatment that increase their vulnerability to suicide. For minors and aged adults, transportation and/or permission of family members present challenges to obtaining treatment. Barriers for incarcerated populations include lack of mental health care staff and, at times, either outright denial of care or forced treatment. Minority populations face discrimination and may refuse seeking professional care because of mistrust. Developing countries suffer severe lack of specialist care.

Efforts should be made to bridge the barriers to proper treatment in under-served, at-risk populations. Culturally appropriate strategies to increase access and utilization of mental health services should be employed.

• Lack of adequate insurance coverage for mental health services represents a critical barrier to treatment for mental disorders, including substance use disorders, that increase suicide risk.

Insurance coverage equal to that of general health services should be extended to mental health services. Such action is projected to reduce suicide via increasing access to care for those at risk. Laws and policies mandating insurance coverage parity for mental health services are likely necessary before third-party payers will cover clinically adequate mental health services. Uninsured adults and children must be provided with effective treatment. Novel approaches to funding need to be explored, since current funding mechanisms are not adequate.

REFERENCES

AAP (American Academy of Pediatrics, Committee on Adolescence). 2000. Suicide and suicide attempts in adolescents. *Pediatrics*, 105(4 (Pt 1)): 871-874.

Adebimpe VR. 1981. Overview: White norms and psychiatric diagnosis of black patients. *American Journal of Psychiatry*, 138(3): 279-285.

Agnew R. 1998. The approval of suicide: A social-psychological model. *Suicide and Life-Threatening Behavior*, 28(2): 205-225.

Al-Jaddou H, Malkawi A. 1997. Prevalence, recognition and management of mental disorders in primary health care in Northern Jordan. *Acta Psychiatrica Scandinavica*, 96(1): 31-35.

Anno BJ. 1991. *Prison Health Care: Guidelines for the Management of an Adequate Delivery System.* Washington, DC: U.S. Department of Justice, Department of Corrections.

APA (American Psychiatric Association). 1994. *The Diagnostic and Statistical Manual of Mental Disorders.* 4th ed. Washington, DC.

Appleby L, Amos T, Doyle U, Tomenson B, Woodman M. 1996. General practitioners and young suicides: A preventive role for primary care. *British Journal of Psychiatry*, 168(3): 330-333.

Appleby L, Dennehy JA, Thomas CS, Faragher EB, Lewis G. 1999. Aftercare and clinical characteristics of people with mental illness who commit suicide: A case-control study. *Lancet*, 353(9162): 1397-1400.

Arborelius E, Damstrom-Thakker K. 1995. Why is it so difficult for general practitioners to discuss alcohol with patients? *Family Practice*, 12(4): 419-422.

Ayanian JZ, Weissman JS, Schneider EC, Ginsburg JA, Zaslavsky AM. 2000. Unmet health needs of uninsured adults in the United States. *Journal of the American Medical Association*, 284(16): 2061-2069.

Barraclough BM. 1971. Suicide in the elderly: Recent developments in psychogeriatrics. *British Journal of Psychiatry*, Suppl 6: 87-97.

Beck AT, Kovacs M, Weissman A. 1979. Assessment of suicidal intention: The Scale for Suicide Ideation. *Journal of Consulting and Clinical Psychology*, 47(2): 343-352.

Beeson PG, Britian C, Howell ML, Kirwan D, Sawyer DA. 1998. Rural mental health at the millenium. In: Manderscheid RW, Henderson MJ, Editors. *Mental Health United States, 1998*. (pp. 82-98). Rockville, MD: Center for Mental Health Services. (DHHS Pub. No. [SMA] 99-328).

Bell C. In press. Correctional Psychiatry. In: Sadock BJ, Sadock VA, Editors. *Comprehensive Textbook of Psychiatry*. 8th ed. Baltimore: Williams and Wilkins.

Bernstein RM, Feldberg C. 1991. After-hours coverage in psychology training clinics. *Professional Psychology: Research and Practice*, 22(3): 204-208.

Bhugra D. 1989. Attitudes towards mental illness. A review of the literature. *Acta Psychiatrica Scandinavica*, 80(1): 1-12.

Bland RC, Newman SC, Orn H. 1997. Help-seeking for psychiatric disorders. *Canadian Journal of Psychiatry*, 42(9): 935-942.

Blumenthal D, Causino N, Chang YC, Culpepper L, Marder W, Saglam D, Stafford R, Starfield B. 1999. The duration of ambulatory visits to physicians. *Journal of Family Practice*, 48(4): 264-271.

Bongar B, Maris RW, Berman AL, Litman RE. 1992. Outpatient standards of care and the suicidal patient. *Suicide and Life-Threatening Behavior*, 22(4): 453-478.

Bongar B, Maris RW, Berman AL, Litman RE. 1998. Outpatient standards of care and the suicidal patient. In: Bongar B, Berman AL, Maris RW, Silverman M, Harris EA, Packman WL, Editors. *Risk Management With Suicidal Patients*. New York: the Guilford Press.

Borowsky SJ, Rubenstein LV, Meredith LS, Camp P, Jackson-Triche M, Wells KB. 2000. Who is at risk of nondetection of mental health problems in primary care? *Journal of General Internal Medicine*, 15(6): 381-388.

Bradley KA, Curry SJ, Koepsell TD, Larson EB. 1995. Primary and secondary prevention of alcohol problems: U.S. internist attitudes and practices. *Journal of General Internal Medicine*, 10(2): 67-72.

Brockington IF, Hall P, Levings J, Murphy C. 1993. The community's tolerance of the mentally ill. *British Journal of Psychiatry*, 162: 93-99.

Brown ER, Ojeda VD, Wyn R, Levan R. 2000. *Racial and Ethnic Disparities in Access to Health Insurance and Health Care*. Los Angeles, CA: UCLA Center for Health Policy Research and the Henry J. Kaiser Family Foundation.

Brown SL, Salive ME, Guralnik JM, Pahor M, Chapman DP, Blazer D. 1995. Antidepressant use in the elderly: Association with demographic characteristics, health-related factors, and health care utilization. *Journal of Clinical Epidemiology*, 48(3): 445-453.

Burns MJ, Cain VA, Husaini BA. 2001. Depression, service utilization, and treatment costs among Medicare elderly: Gender differences. *Home Health Care Services Quarterly*, 19(3): 35-44.

Buzan RD, Weissberg MP. 1992. Suicide: Risk factors and therapeutic considerations in the emergency department. *Journal of Emergency Medicine,* 10(3): 335-343.

Caine ED, Conwell Y. 2001. Suicide in the elderly. *International Clinical Psychopharmacology,* 16 (Suppl 2): S25-S30.

Caine ED, Lyness JM, Conwell Y. 1996. Diagnosis of late-life depression: Preliminary studies in primary care settings. *American Journal of Geriatric Psychiatry,* 4(Suppl 1): S25-S30.

Conwell Y, Duberstein PR, Cox C, Herrmann JH, Forbes NT, Caine ED. 1996. Relationships of age and axis I diagnoses in victims of completed suicide: A psychological autopsy study. *American Journal of Psychiatry,* 153(8): 1001-1008.

Conwell Y, Olsen K, Caine ED, Flannery C. 1991. Suicide in later life: Psychological autopsy findings. *International Psychogeriatrics,* 3(1): 59-66.

Cooper-Patrick L, Gallo JJ, Powe NR, Steinwachs DM, Eaton WW, Ford DE. 1999. Mental health service utilization by African Americans and Whites: The Baltimore Epidemiologic Catchment Area Follow-Up. *Medical Care,* 37(10): 1034-1045.

Cornelius JR, Salloum IM, Haskett RF, Daley DC, Cornelius MD, Thase ME, Perel JM. 2000. Fluoxetine versus placebo in depressed alcoholics: A 1-year follow-up study. *Addictive Behaviors,* 25(2): 307-310.

Cornelius JR, Salloum IM, Lynch K, Clark DB, Mann JJ. 2001. Treating the substance-abusing suicidal patient. *Annals of the New York Academy of Sciences,* 932: 78-90; discussion 91-93.

Corrigan PW, Penn DL. 1998. Lessons from social psychology on discrediting psychiatric stigma. *American Psychologist,* 54: 765-776.

Cramer JA, Rosenheck R. 1998. Compliance with medication regimens for mental and physical disorders. *Psychiatric Services,* 49(2): 196-201.

Crammer JL. 1984. The special characteristics of suicide in hospital in-patients. *British Journal of Psychiatry,* 145: 460-463.

de Jong JT. 1996. A comprehensive public mental health programme in Guinea-Bissau: A useful model for African, Asian and Latin-American countries. *Psychological Medicine,* 26(1): 97-108.

Dehoyos A, Dehoyos G. 1965. Symptomology differentials between Negro and white schizohrenics. *International Journal of Social Psychiatry,* 11: 245-255.

Delong W, Robins E. 1961. The communication of suicidal intent prior to psychiatric hospitalization: A study of 87 patients. *American Journal of Psychiatry,* 117: 695-705.

Dilsaver SC, Chen YW, Swann AC, Shoaib AM, Tsai-Dilsaver Y, Krajewski KJ. 1997. Suicidality, panic disorder and psychosis in bipolar depression, depressive-mania and pure-mania. *Psychiatry Research,* 73(1-2): 47-56.

Druss BG, Rosenheck RA. 1998. Mental disorders and access to medical care in the United States. *American Journal of Psychiatry,* 155(12): 1775-1777.

Duberstein PR, Conwell Y, Cox C, Podgorski CA, Glazer RS, Caine ED. 1995. Attitudes toward self-determined death: A survey of primary care physicians. *Journal of the American Geriatrics Society,* 43(4): 395-400.

Dubler NN, Anno BJ. 1991. Ethical considerations and the inteface with custody. In: Anno BJ, Editor. *Prison Health Care: Guidelines for the Management of an Adequate Delivery System.* (pp. 53-69). Chicago: U.S. Department of Justice, Department of Corrections.

Dwight-Johnson M, Sherbourne CD, Liao D, Wells KB. 2000. Treatment preferences among depressed primary care patients. *Journal of General Internal Medicine,* 15(8): 527-534.

Ellis TE, Dickey TOI, Jones EC. 1998. Patient suicide in psychiatry residency programs: A national survey of training and postvention practices. *Academic Psychiatry,* 22(3): 181-189.

Fawcett J. 1995. Compliance: Definitions and key issues. *Journal of Clinical Psychiatry,* 56 (Suppl 1): 4-8; discussion 9-10.

Fawcett J, Clark DC, Scheftner WA. 1991. The assessment and management of the suicidal patient. *Psychiatric Medicine*, 9(2): 299-311.

Fawcett J, Scheftner W, Clark D, Hedeker D, Gibbons R, Coryell W. 1987. Clinical predictors of suicide in patients with major affective disorders: A controlled prospective study. *American Journal of Psychiatry*, 144(1): 35-40.

Feightner JW. 1994. Early detection of depression. In: Canadian Task Force on Periodic Health Examination. *Canadian Guide to Clinical Preventive Health Care*. (pp. 450-454). Ottawa: Health Canada.

Fenton WS, Blyler CR, Heinssen RK. 1997. Determinants of medication compliance in schizophrenia: Empirical and clinical findings. *Schizophrenia Bulletin*, 23(4): 637-651.

Fortney J, Rost K, Zhang M, Warren J. 1999. The impact of geographic accessibility on the intensity and quality of depression treatment. *Medical Care*, 37(9): 884-893.

Frankenfield DL, Keyl PM, Gielen A, Wissow LS, Werthamer L, Baker SP. 2000. Adolescent patients—healthy or hurting? Missed opportunities to screen for suicide risk in the primary care setting. *Archives of Pediatrics and Adolescent Medicine*, 154(2): 162-168.

Fraser I. 1997. Introduction: Research on health care organizations and markets—the best and worst of times. *Health Services Research*, 32(5): 669-678.

Gallo JJ, Marino S, Ford D, Anthony JC. 1995. Filters on the pathway to mental health care, II. Sociodemographic factors. *Psychological Medicine*, 25(6): 1149-1160.

Gallo JJ, Ryan SD, Ford DE. 1999. Attitudes, knowledge, and behavior of family physicians regarding depression in late life. *Archives of Family Medicine*, 8(3): 249-256.

Ghaemi SN, Boiman EE, Goodwin FK. 2000. Diagnosing bipolar disorder and the effect of antidepressants: A naturalistic study. *Journal of Clinical Psychiatry*, 61(10): 804-808.

Goldman LS, Nielsen NH, Champion HC. 1999. Awareness, diagnosis, and treatment of depression. *Journal of General Internal Medicine*, 14(9): 569-580.

Goldney RD. 2000. Prediction of suicide and attempted suicide. In: Hawton K, van Heeringen K, Editors. *The International Handbook of Suicide and Attempted Suicide*. (pp. 585-595). Chichester, UK: John Wiley and Sons.

Goodwin FK. 1999. Anticonvulsant therapy and suicide risk in affective disorders. *Journal of Clinical Psychiatry*, 60(Suppl 2): 89-93.

Gould MS, Fisher P, Parides M, Flory M, Shaffer D. 1996. Psychosocial risk factors of child and adolescent completed suicide. *Archives of General Psychiatry*, 53(12): 1155-1162.

Gross HS, Herbert MR, Knatterud GL, Donner L. 1969. The effect of race and sex on the variation of diagnosis and disposition in a psychiatric emergency room. *Journal of Nervous and Mental Disease*, 148(6): 638-642.

Hall RC, Platt DE, Hall RC. 1999. Suicide risk assessment: A review of risk factors for suicide in 100 patients who made severe suicide attempts. Evaluation of suicide risk in a time of managed care. *Psychosomatics*, 40(1): 18-27.

Hanson KW. 1998. Public opinion and the mental health parity debate: Lessons from the survey literature. *Psychiatric Services*, 49(8): 1059-1066.

Harman JS, Brown G, Brown E, Laidlaw K, Ten Have T, Mulsant BH, Bruce M. 2001a. *Physician Attitudes Toward Suicide and Suicide Assessment of Elderly Patients in Primary Care Practices*: Abstract presented at the Gerontological Society of America Annual Meeting, November 2001.

Harman JS, Mulsant BH, Kelleher KJ, Schulberg HC, Kupfer DJ, Reynolds CF III. 2001b. Narrowing the gap in treatment of depression. *International Journal of Psychiatry in Medicine*, 31(3): 239-253.

Harman JS, Schulberg HC, Mulsant BH, Reynolds CF III. 2001c. Effect of patient and visit characteristics on diagnosis of depression in primary care. *Journal of Family Practice*, 50(12): 1068.

Harris EC, Barraclough B. 1997. Suicide as an outcome for mental disorders. A meta-analysis. *British Journal of Psychiatry*, 170: 205-228.

Hay Group. 1998. *Health Care Plan Design and Cost Trends: 1988 Through 1997*. Washington, DC: Hay Group.

Heithoff K. 1995. Does the ECA underestimate the prevalence of late-life depression? *Journal of the American Geriatrics Society*, 43(1): 2-6.

Henriksson MM, Aro HM, Marttunen MJ, Heikkinen ME, Isometsa ET, Kuoppasalmi KI, Lonnqvist JK. 1993. Mental disorders and comorbidity in suicide. *American Journal of Psychiatry*, 150(6): 935-940.

Higgins ES. 1994. A review of unrecognized mental illness in primary care. Prevalence, natural history, and efforts to change the course. *Archives of Family Medicine*, 3(10): 908-917.

Hinshaw SP, Cicchetti D. 2000. Stigma and mental disorder: Conceptions of illness, public attitudes, personal disclosure, and social policy. *Development and Psychopathology*, 12(4): 555-598.

Hintikka J, Viinamaki H, Koivumaa-Honkanen HT, Saarinen P, Tanskanen A, Lehtonen J. 1998. Risk factors for suicidal ideation in psychiatric patients. *Social Psychiatry and Psychiatric Epidemiology*, 33(5): 235-240.

Hirschfeld RM, Keller MB, Panico S, Arons BS, Barlow D, Davidoff F, Endicott J, Froom J, Goldstein M, Gorman JM, Marek RG, Maurer TA, Meyer R, Phillips K, Ross J, Schwenk TL, Sharfstein SS, Thase ME, Wyatt RJ. 1997. The National Depressive and Manic-Depressive Association consensus statement on the undertreatment of depression. *Journal of the American Medical Association*, 277(4): 333-340.

Hirschfeld RM, Russell JM. 1997. Assessment and treatment of suicidal patients. *New England Journal of Medicine*, 337(13): 910-915.

Hornblow AR, Bushnell JA, Wells JE, Joyce PR, Oakley-Browne MA. 1990. Christchurch psychiatric epidemiology study: Use of mental health services. *New Zealand Medical Journal*, 103(897): 415-417.

Hotopf M, Wadsworth M, Wessely S. 2001. Is "somatisation" a defense against the acknowledgment of psychiatric disorder? *Journal of Psychosomatic Research*, 50(3): 119-124.

IOM (Institute of Medicine). 1997. Edmunds M, Frank R, Hogan M, McCarty D, Robinson-Beale R, Weisner C, Editors. *Managing Managed Care: Quality Improvement in Behavioral Health*. Washington, DC: National Academy Press.

IOM (Institute of Medicine). 2001. *Neurological, Psychiatric, and Developmental Disorders: Meeting the Challenge in the Developing World*. Washington, DC: National Academy Press.

IOM (Institute of Medicine). 2002. B.D. Smedley, A.Y. Stith, A.R. Nelson, Editors. *Unequal Treatment: Confronting Racial and Ethnic Disparities in Healthcare*. Washington, DC: National Academy Press.

Isacsson G, Bergman U, Rich CL. 1994. Antidepressants, depression and suicide: An analysis of the San Diego study. *Journal of Affective Disorders*, 32(4): 277-286.

Isacsson G, Boethius G, Bergman U. 1992. Low level of antidepressant prescription for people who later commit suicide: 15 years of experience from a population-based drug database in Sweden. *Acta Psychiatrica Scandinavica*, 85(6): 444-448.

Isometsa ET, Aro HM, Henriksson MM, Heikkinen ME, Lönnqvist JK. 1994a. Suicide in major depression in different treatment settings. *Journal of Clinical Psychiatry*, 55(12): 523-527.

Isometsa ET, Heikkinen ME, Marttunen MJ, Henriksson MM, Aro HM, Lönnqvist JK. 1995. The last appointment before suicide: Is suicide intent communicated? *American Journal of Psychiatry*, 152(6): 919-922.

Isometsa ET, Henriksson MM, Aro HM, Heikkinen ME, Kuoppasalmi KI, Lönnqvist JK. 1994b. Suicide in major depression. *American Journal of Psychiatry*, 151(4): 530-536.

Isometsa ET, Henriksson MM, Aro HM, Lönnqvist JK. 1994c. Suicide in bipolar disorder in Finland. *American Journal of Psychiatry*, 151(7): 1020-1024.

Jobes DA, Berman AL. 1993. Suicide and malpractice liability: Assessing and revising policies, procedures, and practice in outpatient settings. *Professional Psychology: Research and Practice*, 24(1): 91-99.

Jobes DA, Eyman JRYRI. 1995. How clinicians assess suicide risk in adolescents and adults. *Crisis Intervention*, 2: 1-12.

Kane FJJr. 1996. Need for better psychiatric training for primary care providers. *Academic Medicine*, 71(6): 574-575.

Kaplan MS, Adamek ME, Calderon A. 1999. Managing depressed and suicidal geriatric patients: Differences among primary care physicians. *Gerontologist*, 39(4): 417-425.

Katon W, Robinson P, Von Korff M, Lin E, Bush T, Ludman E, Simon G, Walker E. 1996. A multifaceted intervention to improve treatment of depression in primary care. *Archives of General Psychiatry*, 53(10): 924-932.

Katon W, Schulberg H. 1992. Epidemiology of depression in primary care. *General Hospital Psychiatry*, 14(4): 237-247.

Katon W, von Korff M, Lin E, Bush T, Ormel J. 1992. Adequacy and duration of antidepressant treatment in primary care. *Medical Care*, 30(1): 67-76.

Katon W, Von Korff M, Lin E, Simon G. 2001. Rethinking practitioner roles in chronic illness: The specialist, primary care physician, and the practice nurse. *General Hospital Psychiatry*, 23(3): 138-144.

Katon W, Von Korff M, Lin E, Simon G, Walker E, Unutzer J, Bush T, Russo J, Ludman E. 1999. Stepped collaborative care for primary care patients with persistent symptoms of depression: A randomized trial. *Archives of General Psychiatry*, 56(12): 1109-1115.

Katon W, Von Korff M, Lin E, Walker E, Simon GE, Bush T, Robinson P, Russo J. 1995. Collaborative management to achieve treatment guidelines. Impact on depression in primary care. *Journal of the American Medical Association*, 273(13): 1026-1031.

Kelleher MJ, Chambers D, Corcoran P, Williamson E, Keeley HS. 1998. Religious sanctions and rates of suicide worldwide. *Crisis*, 19(2): 78-86.

Kessler RC. 2000. Posttraumatic stress disorder: The burden to the individual and to society. *Journal of Clinical Psychiatry*, 61 (Suppl 5): 4-12; discussion 13-14.

Kessler RC, Berglund PA, Zhao S, Leaf P.J., Kouzis AC, Bruce ML, Freidman RL, Grosser RC, Kennedy C, Narrow WE, Kuehnel TG, Laska EM, Manderscheid RW, Rosenheck RA, Santoni TW, Schneir M. 1996. The 12-month prevalence and correlates of serious mental illness (SMI). In: Manderscheid RW, Sonnenschein MA, Editors. *Mental Health, United States, 1996*. Rockville, MD: Center for Mental Health Services. (Pub. No. [SMA] 96-3098).

Kihlstrom LC. 1998. Managed care and medication compliance: Implications for chronic depression. *Journal of Behavioral Health Services and Research*, 25(4): 367-376.

Kilzieh N, Akiskal HS. 1999. Rapid-cycling bipolar disorder. An overview of research and clinical experience. *Psychiatric Clinics of North America*, 22(3): 585-607.

King KA, Price JH, Telljohann SK, Wahl J. 1999a. How confident do high school counselors feel in recognizing students at risk for suicide? *American Journal of Health and Behavior*, 23(6): 457-467.

King KA, Price JH, Telljohann SK, Wahl J. 1999b. High school health teachers' perceived self-efficacy in identifying students at risk for suicide. *Journal of School Health*, 69(5): 202-207.

King LN. 1998. Doctors, patients, and the history of correctional medicine. In: Puisis M, Editor. *Clinical Practice in Correctional Medicine.* St. Louis: Mosby.

Knauper B, Wittchen HU. 1994. Diagnosing major depression in the elderly: Evidence for response bias in standardized diagnostic interviews? *Journal of Psychiatric Research,* 28(2): 147-164.

Kupers TA. 1999. *Prison Madness: The Mental Health Crisis Behind Bars and What We Must Do About It.* San Francisco: Jossey-Bass, Inc.

Leaf PJ, Bruce ML, Tischler GL, Freeman DH Jr, Weissman MM, Myers JK. 1988. Factors affecting the utilization of specialty and general medical mental health services. *Medical Care,* 26(1): 9-26.

Leaf PJ, Bruce ML, Tischler GL, Holzer CE 3rd. 1987. The relationship between demographic factors and attitudes toward mental health services. *Journal of Community Psychology,* 15(2): 275-284.

Lebowitz BD, Pearson JL, Schneider LS, Reynolds CF 3rd, Alexopoulos GS, Bruce ML, Conwell Y, Katz IR, Meyers BS, Morrison MF, Mossey J, Niederehe G, Parmelee P. 1997. Diagnosis and treatment of depression in late life. Consensus statement update. *Journal of the American Medical Association,* 278(14): 1186-1190.

Lewis LJ. 2001. *The Face of Bipolar Illness: Results of a National DMDA Survey.* New Orleans, LA: Presented at the American Psychiatric Association Annual Meeting, May 6, 2001.

Link BG, Phelan JC, Bresnahan M, Stueve A, Pescosolido BA. 1999. Public conceptions of mental illness: Labels, causes, dangerousness, and social distance. *American Journal of Public Health,* 89(9): 1328-1333.

Link BG, Struening EL, Rahav M, Phelan JC, Nuttbrock L. 1997. On stigma and its consequences: Evidence from a longitudinal study of men with dual diagnoses of mental illness and substance abuse. *Journal of Health and Social Behavior,* 38(2): 177-190.

Lloyd A, Horan W, Borgaro SR, Stokes JM, Pogge DL, Harvey PD. 1998. Predictors of medication compliance after hospital discharge in adolescent psychiatric patients. *Journal of Child and Adolescent Psychopharmacology,* 8(2): 133-141.

Lurie N, Moscovice IS, Finch M, Christianson JB, Popkin MK. 1992. Does capitation affect the health of the chronically mentally ill? Results from a randomized trial. *Journal of the American Medical Association,* 267(24): 3300-3304.

Manning WG Jr, Wells KB, Duan N, Newhouse JP, Ware JE Jr. 1986. How cost sharing affects the use of ambulatory mental health services. *Journal of the American Medical Association,* 256(14): 1930-1934.

Maris RW, Berman AL, Silverman MM. 2000. *Comprehensive Textbook of Suicidology.* New York: the Guilford Press.

Marks A. 1988-1989. Structural parameters of sex, race, age and eduction and their influence on attitudes toward suicide. *Omega,* 19(4): 327-336.

Matthews K, Milne S, Ashcroft GW. 1994. Role of doctors in the prevention of suicide: The final consultation. *British Journal of General Practice,* 44(385): 345-348.

Mechanic D. 1997. Approaches for coordinating primary and specialty care for persons with mental illness. *General Hospital Psychiatry,* 19(6): 395-402.

Mechanic D. 1998. Emerging trends in mental health policy and practice. *Health Affairs (Project Hope),* 17(6): 82-98.

Michel K. 2000. Suicide prevention and primary care. In: Hawton K, van Heeringen K, Editors. *International Handbook of Suicide and Attempted Suicide.* (pp. 661-674). Chichester, UK: John Wiley and Sons.

Michel K, Valach L, Waeber V. 1994. Understanding deliberate self-harm: The patients' views. *Crisis,* 15(4): 172-178.

Mickus M, Colenda CC, Hogan AJ. 2000. Knowledge of mental health benefits and preferences for type of mental health providers among the general public. *Psychiatric Services,* 51(2): 199-202.

Miller CL, Druss B. 2001. Datapoints: Suicide and access to care. *Psychiatric Services*, 52(12): 1566.

Miller M. 1976. Geriatric suicide: The Arizona Study. *Gerontologist*, 18: 488-495.

Mock CN, Grossman DC, Mulder D, Stewart C, Koepsell TS. 1996. Health care utilization as a marker for suicidal behavior on an American Indian Reservation. *Journal of General Internal Medicine*, 11(9): 519-524.

Modestin J, Schwarzenbach F. 1992. Effect of psychopharmacotherapy on suicide risk in discharged psychiatric inpatients. *Acta Psychiatrica Scandinavica*, 85(2): 173-175.

Morgan HG, Stanton R. 1997. Suicide among psychiatric in-patients in a changing clinical scene. Suicidal ideation as a paramount index of short-term risk. *British Journal of Psychiatry*, 171: 561-563.

Mulsant BH, Alexopoulos GS, Reynolds CF 3rd, Katz IR, Abrams R, Oslin D, Schulberg HC. 2001. Pharmacological treatment of depression in older primary care patients: The PROSPECT algorithm. *International Journal of Geriatric Psychiatry*, 16(6): 585-592.

Murphy GE. 1975. The physician's responsibility for suicide. II. Errors of omission. *Annals of Internal Medicine*, 82(3): 305-309.

Murphy GE. 2000. Psychiatric aspects of suicidal behavior: Substance abuse. In: Hawton K., Van Heeringen K, Editors. *International Handbook of Suicide and Attempted Suicide.* (pp. 135-146). Chichester, UK: John Wiley and Sons.

Murthy RS. 1998. Rural psychiatry in developing countries. *Psychiatric Services*, 49: 967-969.

Myers KA, Farquhar DR. 1998. Improving the accuracy of death certification. *Canadian Medical Association Journal*, 158(10): 1317-1323.

Narrow WE, Regier DA, Norquist G, Rae DS, Kennedy C, Arons B. 2000. Mental health service use by Americans with severe mental illnesses. *Social Psychiatry and Psychiatric Epidemiology*, 35(4): 147-155.

Nathan VM. 1984. *Correctional Health Care: The Perspective of a Special Master:* Presented at the annual meeting of the National Commission on Correctional Health Care. Cited in King (1998).

Newhouse JP. 1993. *Free for All: Lessons From the RAND Health Insurance Experiment.* Cambridge, MA: Harvard University Press.

NIH Consensus Development Panel on Depression in Late Life. 1992. NIH consensus conference. Diagnosis and treatment of depression in late life. *Journal of the American Medical Association*, 268(8): 1018-1024.

Olfson M, Pincus HA. 1996. Outpatient mental health care in nonhospital settings: Distribution of patients across provider groups. *American Journal of Psychiatry*, 153(10): 1353-1356.

OPEN MINDS. 1999. Over 72% of insured Americans are enrolled in MBHOs: Magellan Behavioral Health continues to dominate the market. *OPEN MINDS Behavioral Health and Social Service Industry Analyst*, 11: 9.

Oquendo MA, Malone KM, Ellis SP, Sackeim HA, Mann JJ. 1999. Inadequacy of antidepressant treatment for patients with major depression who are at risk for suicidal behavior. *American Journal of Psychiatry*, 156(2): 190-194.

Orleans CT, George LK, Houpt JL, Brodie HK. 1985. How primary care physicians treat psychiatric disorders: A national survey of family practitioners. *American Journal of Psychiatry*, 142(1): 52-57.

Pearson JL, Conwell Y, Lyness JM. 1997. Late-life suicide and depression in the primary care setting. *New Directions for Mental Health Services*, (76): 13-38.

Penn DL, Martin J. 1998. The stigma of severe mental illness: Some potential solutions for a recalcitrant problem. *Psychiatric Quarterly*, 69(3): 235-247.

Pescosolido BA, Martin JK, Link BG, Kikuzawa S, Burgos G, Swindle R, Phelan J. 2000. Americans' views of mental health and illness and century's end: Continuity and change. *Public Report on the MacArthur Mental Health Module, 1996 General Social Survey.* Bloomington, IN: Indiana Consortium of Mental Health Services Research, Indiana University and the Joseph P. Mailman School of Public Health, Columbia University.

PHS (Public Health Service). 2001. *National Strategy for Suicide Prevention: Goals and Objectives for Action.* Rockville, MD: U.S. Department of Health and Human Services.

Piacentini J, Rotheram-Borus MJ, Gillis JR, Graae F, Trautman P, Cantwell C, Garcia-Leeds C, Shaffer D. 1995. Demographic predictors of treatment attendance among adolescent suicide attempters. *Journal of Consulting and Clinical Psychology*, 63(3): 469-473.

Pincus HA, Tanielian TL, Marcus SC, Olfson M, Zarin DA, Thompson J, Magno Zito J. 1998. Prescribing trends in psychotropic medications: Primary care, psychiatry, and other medical specialties. *Journal of the American Medical Association*, 279(7): 526-531.

Pirkis J, Burgess P. 1998. Suicide and recency of health care contacts. A systematic review. *British Journal of Psychiatry*, 173: 462-474.

Pirkis J, Burgess P, Meadows G, Dunt D. 2001. Self-reported needs for care among persons who have suicidal ideation or who have attempted suicide. *Psychiatric Services*, 52(3): 381-383.

Pokorny AD. 1993. Suicide prediction revisited. *Suicide and Life-Threatening Behavior*, 23(1): 1-10.

Preboth M. 2000. Clinical review of recent findings on the awareness, diagnosis and treatment of depression. *American Family Physician*, 61(10): 3158, 3160, 3167-3168.

Regier DA, Narrow WE, Rae DS, Manderscheid RW, Locke BZ, Goodwin FK. 1993. The de facto US mental and addictive disorders service system. Epidemiologic catchment area prospective 1-year prevalence rates of disorders and services. *Archives of General Psychiatry*, 50(2): 85-94.

Reynolds CF 3rd, Degenholtz H, Parker LS, Schulberg HC, Mulsant BH, Post E, Rollman B. 2001. Treatment as usual (TAU) control practices in the PROSPECT Study: Managing the interaction and tension between research design and ethics. *International Journal of Geriatric Psychiatry*, 16(6): 602-608.

Ridgely MS, Goldman HH, Willenbring M. 1990. Barriers to the care of persons with dual diagnoses: Organizational and financing issues. *Schizophrenia Bulletin*, 16(1): 123-132.

Robins E, Murphy GE, Wilkinson RHJr, Gassner S, Kayes J. 1959. Some clinical considerations in the prevention of suicide based on a study of 134 successful suicides. *American Journal of Public Health*, 49: 888-899.

Rogers WH, Wells KB, Meredith LS, Sturm R, Burnam MA. 1993. Outcomes for adult outpatients with depression under prepaid or fee-for-service financing. *Archives of General Psychiatry*, 50(7): 517-525.

Rosenheck R. 2000. Primary care satellite clinics and improved access to general and mental health services. *Health Services Research*, 35(4): 777-790.

Rosenzweig A, Prigerson H, Miller MD, ReynoldsIII, CF. 1997. Bereavement and late-life depression: Grief and its complications in the elderly. *Annual Review of Medicine*, 48: 421-428.

Rost K, Nutting P, Smith J, Coyne JC, Cooper-Patrick L, Rubenstein L. 2000. The role of competing demands in the treatment provided primary care patients with major depression. *Archives of Family Medicine*, 9(2): 150-154.

Rost K, Zhang M, Fortney J, Smith J, Smith GR Jr. 1998. Rural-urban differences in depression treatment and suicidality. *Medical Care*, 36(7): 1098-1107.

Rotheram-Borus MJ, Piacentini J, Cantwell C, Belin TR, Song J. 2000. The 18-month impact of an emergency room intervention for adolescent female suicide attempters. *Journal of Consulting and Clinical Psychology*, 68(6): 1081-1093.

Rotheram-Borus MJ, Piacentini J, Miller S, Graae F, Castro-Blanco D. 1994. Brief cognitive-behavioral treatment for adolescent suicide attempters and their families. *Journal of the American Academy of Child and Adolescent Psychiatry*, 33(4): 508-517.

Rutz W, von Knorring L, Walinder J. 1989. Frequency of suicide on Gotland after systematic postgraduate education of general practitioners. *Acta Psychiatrica Scandinavica*, 80(2): 151-154.

Rutz W, von Knorring L, Walinder J. 1992. Long-term effects of an educational program for general practitioners given by the Swedish Committee for the Prevention and Treatment of Depression. *Acta Psychiatrica Scandinavica*, 85(1): 83-88.

Saunders SM, Resnick MD, Hoberman HM, Blum RW. 1994. Formal help-seeking behavior of adolescents identifying themselves as having mental health problems. *Journal of the American Academy of Child and Adolescent Psychiatry*, 33(5): 718-728.

Schiff G, Shansky R. 1998. Challenges to improving quality in the correctional setting. In: Puisis M, Editor. *Clinical Practice in Correctional Medicine*. (pp. 12-25). St. Louis: Mosby.

Schou M. 1997. The combat of non-compliance during prophylactic lithium treatment. *Acta Psychiatrica Scandinavica*, 95(5): 361-363.

Schweizer E, Dever A, Clary C. 1988. Suicide upon recovery from depression. A clinical note. *Journal of Nervous and Mental Disease*, 176(10): 633-636.

Seidlitz L, Duberstein PR, Cox C, Conwell Y. 1995. Attitudes of older people toward suicide and assisted suicide: An analysis of Gallup Poll findings. *Journal of the American Geriatrics Society*, 43(9): 993-998.

Shaffer D, Craft L. 1999. Methods of adolescent suicide prevention. *Journal of Clinical Psychiatry*, 60(Suppl 2): 70-74.

Simon GE, Grothaus L, Durham ML, VonKorff M, Pabiniak C. 1996a. Impact of visit copayments on outpatient mental health utilization by members of a health maintenance organization. *American Journal of Psychiatry*, 153(3): 331-338.

Simon GE, Von Korff M, Heiligenstein JH, Revicki DA, Grothaus L, Katon W, Wagner EH. 1996b. Initial antidepressant choice in primary care. Effectiveness and cost of fluoxetine vs tricyclic antidepressants. *Journal of the American Medical Association*, 275(24): 1897-1902.

Sirey JA, Bruce ML, Alexopoulos GS, Perlick DA, Raue P, Friedman SJ, Meyers BS. 2001. Perceived stigma as a predictor of treatment discontinuation in young and older outpatients with depression. *American Journal of Psychiatry*, 158(3): 479-481.

Slap GB, Vorters DF, Khalid N, Margulies SR, Forke CM. 1992. Adolescent suicide attempters: Do physicians recognize them? *Journal of Adolescent Health*, 13(4): 286-292.

Smith JL, Rost KM, Nutting PA, Elliott CE, Duan N. 2000. A primary care intervention for depression. *Journal of Rural Health*, 16(4): 313-323.

Spirito A, Brown L, Overholser J, Fritz G. 1989. Attempted suicide in adolescence: A review and critique of the literature. *Clinical Psychology Review*, 9(3): 335-363.

Steadman HJ, Veysey BM. 1997. Providing services for jail inmates with mental disorders. *Research in Brief*. Washington, DC: U.S. Department of Justice, National Institute of Justice.

Sturm R, Sherbourne CD. 2001. Are barriers to mental health and substance abuse care still rising? *Journal of Behavioral Health Services and Research*, 28(1): 81-88.

Sturm R, Wells K. 2000. Health insurance may be improving—but not for individuals with mental illness. *Health Services Research*, 35(1 (Pt 2)): 253-262.

Suominen K, Henriksson M, Suokas J, Isometsa E, Ostamo A, Lönnqvist J. 1996. Mental disorders and comorbidity in attempted suicide. *Acta Psychiatrica Scandinavica*, 94(4): 234-240.

Suominen KH, Isometsa ET, Henriksson MM, Ostamo AI, Lönnqvist JK. 1998. Inadequate treatment for major depression both before and after attempted suicide. *American Journal of Psychiatry*, 155(12): 1778-1780.

Suominen KH, Isometsa ET, Henriksson MM, Ostamo AI, Lonnqvist JK. 1999. Treatment received by alcohol-dependent suicide attempters. *Acta Psychiatr Scand*, 99(3): 214-9.

Sussman LK, Robins LN, Earls F. 1987. Treatment-seeking for depression by black and white Americans. *Social Science and Medicine*, 24(3): 187-196.

Swartz MS, Wagner HR, Swanson JW, Burns BJ, George LK, Padgett DK. 1998. Administrative update: Utilization of services. I. Comparing use of public and private mental health services: The enduring barriers of race and age. *Community Mental Health Journal*, 34(2): 133-144.

Swindle R Jr, Heller K, Pescosolido B, Kikuzawa S. 2000. Responses to nervous breakdowns in America over a 40-year period. Mental health policy implications. *American Psychologist*, 55(7): 740-749.

Szanto K, Prigerson H, Houck P, Ehrenpreis L, Reynolds CF 3rd. 1997. Suicidal ideation in elderly bereaved: The role of complicated grief. *Suicide and Life-Threatening Behavior*, 27(2): 194-207.

Taube CA, Kessler LG, Burns BJ. 1986. Estimating the probability and level of ambulatory mental health services use. *Health Services Research*, 21(2 (Pt 2)): 321-340.

Trautman PD, Stewart N, Morishima A. 1993. Are adolescent suicide attempters noncompliant with outpatient care? *Journal of the American Academy of Child and Adolescent Psychiatry*, 32(1): 89-94.

Unutzer J, Katon W, Sullivan M, Miranda J. 1999. Treating depressed older adults in primary care: Narrowing the gap between efficacy and effectiveness. *Milbank Quarterly*, 77(2): 225-256, 174.

Unutzer J, Simon G, Belin TR, Datt M, Katon W, Patrick D. 2000. Care for depression in HMO patients aged 65 and older. *Journal of the American Geriatrics Society*, 48(8): 871-878.

US DHHS (U.S. Department of Health and Human Services). 1999. *Mental Health: A Report of the Surgeon General*. Rockville, MD: U.S. Department of Health and Human Services, Substance Abuse and Mental Health Services Administration, Center for Mental Health Services, National Institutes of Health, National Institute of Mental Health.

US DHHS (U.S. Department of Health and Human Services). 2001. *Mental Health: Culture, Race and Ethnicity—A Supplement to Mental Health: A Report of the Surgeon General*. Rockville, MD: U.S. Department of Health and Human Services, Substance Abuse and Mental Health Services Administration, Center for Mental Health Services, National Institutes of Health, National Institute of Mental Health.

US Preventive Services Task Force. 1996. *Guide to Clinical Preventive Services. Second Edition*. Alexandria, VA: International Medical Publishing.

Von Korff M, Shapiro S, Burke JD, Teitlebaum M, Skinner EA, German P, Turner RW, Klein L, Burns B. 1987. Anxiety and depression in a primary care clinic. Comparison of Diagnostic Interview Schedule, General Health Questionnaire, and practitioner assessments. *Archives of General Psychiatry*, 44(2): 152-156.

Wahl OF. 1999. Mental health consumers' experience of stigma. *Schizophrenia Bulletin*, 25(3): 467-478.

Wahl OF, Harman CR. 1989. Family views of stigma. *Schizophrenia Bulletin*, 15(1): 131-139.

Weissberg M. 1990. The meagerness of physicians' training in emergency psychiatric intervention. *Academic Medicine*, 65(12): 747-750.

Wells KB, Katon W, Rogers B, Camp P. 1994. Use of minor tranquilizers and antidepressant medications by depressed outpatients: Results from the medical outcomes study. *American Journal of Psychiatry*, 151(5): 694-700.

Wells KB, Schoenbaum M, Unutzer J, Lagomasino IT, Rubenstein LV. 1999. Quality of care for primary care patients with depression in managed care. *Archives of Family Medicine*, 8(6): 529-536.

Wells KB, Sherbourne C, Schoenbaum M, Duan N, Meredith L, Unutzer J, Miranda J, Carney MF, Rubenstein LV. 2000. Impact of disseminating quality improvement programs for depression in managed primary care: A randomized controlled trial. *Journal of the American Medical Association*, 283(2): 212-220.

Williams JWJ, Rost K, Dietrich AJ, Ciotti MC, Zyzanski SJ, Cornell J. 1999. Primary care physicians' approach to depressive disorders. Effects of physician specialty and practice structure. *Archives of Family Medicine*, 8(1): 58-67.

Wilmont Y. 1997. Prison nursing: The tension between custody and care. *British Journal of Nursing*, 6: 333-336.

Wright C, Nepal MK, Bruce-Jones WD. 1989. Mental health patients in primary health care services in Nepal. *Asia-Pacific Journal of Public Health*, 3(3): 224-230.

Young AS, Klap R, Sherbourne CD, Wells KB. 2001. The quality of care for depressive and anxiety disorders in the United States. *Archives of General Psychiatry*, 58(1): 55-61.

Zimmerman M, Lish JD, Lush DT, Farber NJ, Plescia G, Kuzma MA. 1995. Suicidal ideation among urban medical outpatients. *Journal of General Internal Medicine*, 10(10): 573-576.

"Hope" is the thing with feathers—
That perches in the soul—
And sings the tune without the words—
And never stops—at all—

And sweetest—in the Gale—is heard—
And sore must be the storm—
That could abash the little Bird
That kept so many warm—

I've heard it in the chillest land—
And on the strangest Sea—
Yet, never, in Extremity,
It asked a crumb—of Me

—Emily Dickinson

Reprinted by permission of the publishers and the Trustees of Amherst College from *The Poems of Emily Dickinson*, Thomas H. Johnson, editor, Cambridge, Massachusetts: The Belknap Press of Harvard University Press, Copyright © 1951, 1955, 1979 by the President and Fellows of Harvard College.

10

Barriers to Research and Promising Approaches

Given its unique nature, research on suicide faces a series of obstacles that limit progress in the understanding, prevention, and treatment of the problem. Because the field is a conglomeration of several disciplines that grew up independently, issues of interdisciplinary research pose problems of communication, jargon, and disciplinary rivalries (see IOM, 2000). Furthermore, recruiting researchers to the field is difficult because of the many obstacles that the field faces, as discussed in this chapter. As indicated in Chapter 1, the terminology used among suicide researchers is inconsistent. Consequently, it is difficult to obtain reliable numbers about the incidence and prevalence of suicide and suicide attempts. Working with patients that present a risk of suicide presents ethical and safety concerns that can be difficult to resolve. Special measures must be taken to increase the statistical power of intervention and prevention studies, since suicide is a relatively infrequent event. These approaches range from using alternate endpoints such as suicidal ideation to finding ways to increase the size of the population under study. Each has limitations.

This chapter first explores the methodological issues that affect the collection of data. Next, it addresses the ethical and safety issues surrounding research protocols with suicidal participants. Statistical approaches to addressing some of these barriers are presented. Options for working with the limitation of suicide's low base-rate are presented at various points in the chapter. Finally, the chapter presents a center-based approach that can be used to advance the study of suicide.

METHODOLOGY

Research on suicide is plagued with many methodological problems that limit progress in the field. Definitions lack uniformity, proximal measures are not always predictive of suicide, reporting of suicide is inaccurate, and its low frequency exacerbates all of these problems.

Terminology

There is a need for researchers and clinicians in suicidology to use a common language or set of terms in describing suicidal phenomena. Thirty years ago, NIMH convened a conference on suicide prevention at which a committee was charged with recommending a system for defining and communicating about suicidal behaviors (Beck et al., 1973). As a result of this committee's work, operational definitions for basic terms such as suicidal ideation, suicide attempts, and completed suicide were proposed. Definitional issues were revisited in the mid-1990s at workshops held by the American Association of Suicidology, NIMH, and the Center for Mental Health Services, and through informal discussions among suicidologists (O'Carroll et al., 1996). Once again, the difficulties caused by lack of efficient communication and cross-talk were described, and a specific nomenclature with objective definitions of suicidal behaviors was proposed. Interestingly, many of the definitions proposed in this article were not appreciably different from those proposed for researchers more than a quarter of a century ago by the NIMH committee. Despite this seeming consensus, terminology continues to be an obstacle (see also Chapter 1). For example, "suicide attempt" does not uniformly include the intent to die. Since some who harm themselves do not actually intend to die (Linehan, 1986), assessing suicidal behavior is difficult. Not only are terms used differently across the field, they only infrequently are operationally defined in studies. Furthermore, often researchers do not reliably assess behavioral intent, since interviews can be unreliable (Linehan, 1997). Comparisons across studies also are complicated by differences in scales and instruments used to measure suicidality (see also Chapter 7). Many studies use only selected questions from questionnaires instead of the complete validated tool. Many of the studies do not report validity and reliability of instruments used.

Low Base-Rate Event

The base-rate of completed suicide is sufficiently low to preclude all but the largest of studies. When such studies are performed, resultant comparisons are between extremely small and large groups of individuals (suicide completers versus non-suicide completers, or suicide attempters versus non-suicide attempters). Use of suicidal ideation as an outcome can increase incidence and alleviate the problem to some extent; however, it is unclear whether suicidal ideation is a strong predictor of suicide completion. Using both attempts and completions can confound the analysis since attempters may account for some of the suicides completed within the study period. Because the duration of the prevention studies is frequently too brief to collect sufficient data on the low frequency endpoints of suicide or suicide attempt, proximal measures such as changes in knowledge or attitude are used. Yet the predictive value of these variables is unconfirmed. Statistical approaches (see Appendix A) and proximal endpoints may provide solutions, but a large population base is preferable.

Psychological Autopsy

A psychological autopsy is the reconstruction of the events leading up to the death; ascertainment of the circumstances of the death, including suicidal intent; and an in-depth exploration of other significant risk factors for suicide (Beskow et al., 1991; Brent et al., 1988; Brent et al., 1993; Cooper, 1999; Hawton et al., 1998; Kelly and Mann, 1996; Velting et al., 1998). The psychological autopsy is the standard approach to augmenting the information obtained from a death certificate. Information is gathered through a semi-structured interview with key informants, and discrepancies are resolved by re-interviewing informants and through a case conference using "best estimate" procedures (Mitchell, 1982). Among the key issues and risk factors addressed are:

- Circumstances and method of suicide
- Psychopathology
- Family history of psychopathology and suicidal behavior
- Social adjustments and functioning
- Personality characteristics, especially aggression/impulsivity
- Life stressors and supports, including religion
- Characteristics of treatment, especially in the 90 days prior to death.
- Physical health and medical history
- Socioeconomic background and family constellation
- Communication of suicidal intent
- Other record linkage (birth records, child welfare, school, criminal justice)

Most studies have found that the optimal time to conduct this kind of investigation is between 2 and 6 months after the death. Informants' emotions may be too raw to conduct an extensive interview prior to 2 months after the death. Longer than 6 months after the death, many informants want closure on the suicide and no longer are willing to open up and discuss emotionally difficult topics. The quality of information, measured by the number of diagnoses generated, did not vary as a function of the amount of time since the death (Brent et al., 1988). Caution should be used when interpreting information gathered from friends and relatives; one experimental study found that subjects' descriptions of psychological distress varied with characteristics of the deceased and aspects of the manner of death (Telcser, 1996). Use of a comparison group of individuals who died accidentally by similar means could strengthen validity of findings. In general, when case-control methods are used in psychological autopsy studies, the comparisons are made to individuals who died by natural causes matched on demographic variables or psychiatric diagnoses.

The psychological autopsy has many similarities to the Family History-Research Diagnostic Criteria or any other indirect interview. The interview is less informative than a direct interview (Andreasen et al., 1977; 1986) but improves with the number of informants. Certain informants may provide specific information that may not be available from others. For example, friends of adolescent suicide victims may be more aware of substance use and abuse than parents (Brent et al., 1988). Employers and co-workers may be able to describe the victim's functional ability on the job; for younger victims, interview of teachers and review of school records may play an analogous role.

Certain types of information are very difficult, or even impossible, to obtain with a psychological autopsy approach. For example, sexual orientation is information that the victim may have been subliminally aware of, or may not have confided to a friend or parent. Information processing style, or other laboratory-based measures obviously cannot be obtained without the victim's self-report. However, psychological autopsy studies can help to identify living individuals whose characteristics closely resemble suicide victims who can then be studied using more dynamic assessments.

Combining biological findings with information about psychopathology, personality, family history, treatment history, and history of family adversity may provide a much more complete picture about the neurobiology of suicidal behavior. For example, altered serotonin in the brain may be a consequence of adverse rearing environments (Kaufman et al., 1998; Kraemer et al., 1989; Pine et al., 1997), and may very well be a consistent finding across different mental disorders. Conversely, psychological autopsy data may allow for the selection of relatively homogeneous sub-samples that can be subjected to genetic analyses. Complementary concurrent methods with intense, highly focused ethnography can improve knowledge about setting, process, motivations, and outcome, and thereby increase validity of data.

SURVEILLANCE OF SUICIDE AND SUICIDE ATTEMPTS

To address suicide as a public health problem requires the sustained and systematic collection, analysis and dissemination of accurate information on the incidence, prevalence and characteristics of suicide and suicide attempts. Surveillance is a cornerstone of public health, allowing realistic priority setting, the design of effective prevention initiatives, and the ability to evaluate such programs (IOM, 1999). Official suicide rates have been used to chart trends in suicide; monitor the impact of change in legislation, treatment policies, and social change; and to compare suicides across regions, both within and across countries. In addition, suicide rates have offered a way to assess risk and protective factors for geographical areas (counties, states and countries). However, there exist serious inadequacies in the availability and quality of information. The sources of data that are currently available remain "fragmentary and unlinked" (Berman, 2001). The need for improved and expanded surveillance systems is highlighted as one of the central goals of the National Strategy for Suicide Prevention (PHS, 2001).

Completed Suicide: Sources of Variability in Suicide Statistics

The suicide rate information available on a national level is derived from state vital records systems that collect data from local death certificate registries. States forward the information to the National Center for Health Statistics of the CDC which maintains the National Vital Statistics System (Davies et al., 2001). The utility and accuracy of these data are constrained by the variability in suicides statistics. As described in Chapter 2, there are at least four sources of this variability (Jobes et al., 1987; O'Carroll, 1989), including:

- regional differences in the definition of suicide and how ambiguous cases are classified
- regional differences in the requirements and political arrangements for the office of coroner or medical examiner
- differences in terms of the extent to which cases are investigated
- variations that have to do with the quality of data management involved in preparing official statistics.

Ambiguous Cases

Classifications of deaths vary regionally (see also Chapter 6). Some jurisdictions, for example, require a suicide note in order to render a verdict of suicide, yet fewer than half of all suicide victims leave a note. Russian roulette deaths are called suicides in some jurisdictions but accidents in others (Keck et al., 1998). Religious traditions, life insurance policies, or actual legal sanctions may motivate underreports of suicide. Some jurisdictions tend to call any deaths with prominent intoxication an accident. All of these differences interfere in cross-site comparisons (Brent et al., 1987; McCarthy and Walsh, 1975).

The verdict of "undetermined" (also known as "open verdict" in the United Kingdom) harbors many unreported suicides, with estimates ranging from 50–100 percent of all undetermined cases being true suicides (Brent et al., 1987; Cavanagh et al., 1999; Holding and Barraclough, 1975; 1978; Ovenstone, 1973). Undetermined verdicts appear to be more likely if the victim is older, died by poisoning, and is female, perhaps because this profile may not fit the archetypal suicide completer (Ohberg and Lönnqvist, 1998; Ovenstone, 1973). Studies suggest that the official suicide rate underestimates the true rate by about 30 percent, but that time trends are unaffected by classification errors (Brent et al., 1987; Gist and Welch, 1989; Sainsbury and Jenkins, 1982).

There are other types of ambiguous cases that may be misclassified as accidents or homicides. For instance, some controversy exists about the degree to which vehicular deaths might be due to suicide (Jenkins and Sainsbury, 1980; Phillips and Ruth, 1993; Schmidt et al., 1977). "Victim precipitated suicides," often in the context of "suicide by cop," (Mohandie and Meloy, 2000; Wolfgang, 1958) are difficult to determine definitively, but may contribute to the underestimation of suicide. The availability of routine toxicology, physical evidence, autopsy, and psychological data can influence the classification of suicide. Larger jurisdictions may be able to investigate most comprehensively, making inter-jurisdiction comparisons unreliable (Nelson et al., 1978). Differential investigation by ethnic group and differences in willingness to share information with an investigator can also distort the picture of suicide.

Training and Background of Coroner/Medical Examiner

There are marked differences in the training and background of the persons who by law certify a death as a suicide among states within the United States (O'Carroll, 1989) and internationally (see also Chapter 6). In the United States, the qualifications range from simply having an interest in the job (e.g., Indiana) to specialized training in forensic pathology (e.g.,

Oklahoma). Medico-legal officials may be elected, appointed or serve ex-officio (e.g., elected county sheriffs). Investigations may be centralized within a state (e.g., Rhode Island) or organized by each county (e.g., Utah). Each of these factors affects the nature, extent, and quality of the investigation and the classification of deaths as suicide.

Danish and English coroners differ significantly by their threshold for certification of suicide (Atkinson et al., 1975). Yet, one British study showed that changes in coroners (within a country) did not result in significant changes in certification practices (Sainsbury and Jenkins, 1982). While some have reported that examiners with a medical background are more willing to certify a suicide as such, others found that more highly trained medical examiners were more likely to classify a death as "undetermined" (Murphy et al., 1986; Pescosolido and Mendelsohn, 1986). More recent studies have suggested substantial variability between different coroners' courts and even within courts (O'Donnell and Farmer, 1995). Furthermore, reported rates in countries that are predominantly Catholic, such as Ireland, may be artificially lower because of a greater stigma associated with suicide and consequent greater reluctance to certify a death as a suicide (Jobes et al., 1987; Myers and Farquhar, 1998). Similarly, the low rates of suicide reported by Muslim countries may reflect possible diagnosis or reporting bias due to stigma (Wasserman and Varnik, 1998). Ongoing concern exists about the lack of quality monitoring of the persistently idiosyncratic death certification process (Maudsley and Williams, 1996).

Local, State, and National Surveillance

National data provide perspective on the scale of the problem of suicide, and permit the evaluation of the impact of federal laws. Given the low-base rate of completed suicide, national level data are necessary to aggregate enough cases to identify patterns of suicide across populations. National data also allow for the analysis of variations in the suicide rate by regions of the country and by different environments (e.g., urban vs. rural). However, state and local data are essential in order to examine suicide as it occurs in specific communities. The map found later in this chapter (Figure 10.1) demonstrates how suicide rates can vary widely across relatively small geographical areas. Understanding which specific qualities of the areas and populations tend to influence the suicide rate is critical for designing programs to enhance protective factors and reduce risk factors. Since many suicide prevention programs are implemented in community and school settings, more precise data are needed at these levels to be able to evaluate their effectiveness, recognize what services

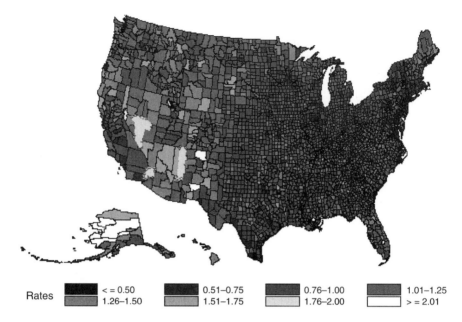

Rates
| | < = 0.50 | | 0.51–0.75 | | 0.76–1.00 | | 1.01–1.25 |
| | 1.26–1.50 | | 1.51–1.75 | | 1.76–2.00 | | > = 2.01 |

FIGURE 10-1. Bayes Estimates of County-Level Deviations from the National Annual Suicide Rates per 100,000 (1996–1998). Adjusted for Age, Sex, and Race.

may still be needed, and identify populations that have not been targeted. In addition, the evaluation of state and local policies and laws can only occur through state and local data collected over time.

There is no precedent for federal law to require the reporting of health conditions to the national government. However, state regulations frequently mandate that details of various diseases and conditions be reported to the Centers for Disease Control and Prevention (CDC). For example, confirmed diagnoses of tuberculosis and various sexually transmitted diseases including AIDS are required by law to be reported in all states (Bunk, 1997). In the case of AIDS reporting, the CDC encouraged the states to pass such statutes by requiring the existence of surveillance regulation in order to receive funding for state AIDS prevention and treatment programs (Gostin et al., 1997). Similarly, for suicide surveillance, data should be collected at the local and state levels in a standardized manner so that it can be aggregated for a national reporting system.

Fatality Analysis Reporting System (FARS)

The potential benefits of a state-based, national reporting system for suicides are great. Such systems have successfully been used to monitor the incidence and characteristics of public health concerns such as infectious diseases and motor-vehicle injuries. For example, the National Highway Traffic Safety Administration (NHTSA) maintains the longstanding Fatality Analysis Reporting System (FARS) to track the circumstances and incidence of motor-vehicle related deaths, which are similar to suicide in number (~40,000/year) (Barber et al., 2000; NHTSA, 2001). The system collects detailed information from the 50 states, the District of Columbia, and Puerto Rico within 30 days of the occurrence. A FARS report includes over 100 coded pieces of data on each crash and the vehicle and people involved (Davies et al., 2001). A state employed FARS analyst collects the required information from a variety of sources: police accident reports, state vehicle registration files, state driver licensing files, state highway department data, vital statistics death certificates, coroner/ medical examiner reports, hospital medical records and emergency medical service reports (NHTSA, 2001).

Since its inception in 1975, surveillance data from FARS has improved our understanding of motor-vehicle injuries and the state and federal laws that affect traffic safety. For example, FARS data and vital statistics data were used to assess the effects of establishing 21 (vs. 18) as the minimum age to purchase alcoholic beverages (Cook and Tauchen, 1984; GAO, 1987). Based on their results, a federal law was passed that made federal highway funding to states contingent upon the establishment of 21 as the minimum age for purchasing alcohol (Wagenaar, 1993), and this policy is estimated to have saved 16,513 lives between 1975 and 1996 (NHTSA, 1996).

National Violent Death Reporting System (NVDRS)

A National Violent Death Reporting System (NVDRS) has been designed by researchers at the Harvard Injury Control and Research Center to collect information on homicides and suicides as well as other firearm deaths. It is based on FARS and on a pilot called the National Violent Injury Statistics System (NVISS) (Azrael et al., 2001).

Currently 11 states and metropolitan areas are collaborating with NVISS to design and pilot test NVDRS. Ten sites have received grants from the project and collect data covering the states of Connecticut, Maine, Maryland, Michigan, Utah, and Wisconsin and in Allegheny County (PA), Miami-Dade County, metropolitan Atlanta, and San Francisco (HICRC, 2001). Legislation for Fiscal Year 2002 funding programs under the Departments of Labor, Health and Human Services, and Education (P.L. 107-116) included designated funding to the CDC's National Center for Injury Prevention and Control of $1.5 million for continued planning and preliminary implementation of the NVDRS in selected states (AAST, 2002). It is estimated that a fully implemented system covering every state would require approximately $20 million per year (AAST, 2002).

NVDRS collects information from four sources: death certificates, coroner/medical examiner reports, police Uniform Crime Reports (and, in some jurisdictions, police incident reports), and crime laboratories (HICRC, 2001). This diversity of sources is expected to allay some of the quality of data limitations that exist due to the irregular information available from the medical examiner/coroner system (see above, and IOM, 1999). NVDRS will collect detailed information on both victims and offenders, including basic demographics, substance use, relationship to one another, the circumstances leading to the injury, whether the event occurred at their home or work, specific of the incidents (e.g., date and location), and weapon type. For suicide deaths, this information will be supplemented by data on physical and mental health, treatment status, and possible precipitating life stresses. In the case of firearm involvement, the weapon's type, make, model, and caliber will also be collected, and for deaths involving under-age shooters, information regarding how the weapon was obtained will be sought (HICRC, 2001). The researchers and pilot sites have developed uniform data elements, reporting protocols, and software for the reporting system (NFFIRS Workgroup, 2001; NVISS Workgroup, 2002). These technical details are centrally important to the future success of implementing this system on a national level; other concerns that must be addressed include ongoing technical assistance and extensive training to ensure quality and consistency of data (Gallagher, 2001).

Surveillance of Attempted Suicides

The quality of the data on suicide attempts is even more tenuous than that of completed suicides. The concerns about nomenclature (Garrison et al., 1991; O'Carroll et al., 1996) and accurate reporting (PHS, 2001) apply here even more than with suicide deaths. There is neither systematic nor mandatory reporting of suicide attempts in the United States. The two major sources of data on suicide attempts comes from the National Comorbidity Survey conducted between 1990 and 1992 (Kessler et al., 1999) and the Epidemiological Catchment Area study conducted in the 1980s (Moscicki et al., 1988). Other epidemiological data on attempts are available from small surveys in localized areas. Risk factors for attempts, especially clinical factors, are surveyed, but often not through population-based surveys that would avoid the bias and lack of generalizability of clinical populations (Feinstein, 1977). Most information regarding suicide attempts must be collected from data systems designed for other purposes (PHS, 2001). This section describes a few of the potential models and sources of information on suicide attempts: the National Electronic Injury Surveillance System, the Youth Risk Behavior Survey, and the Oregon State Adolescent Suicide Attempt Data System.

National Electronic Injury Surveillance System (NEISS).

The NEISS has been operated by the U.S. Consumer Product Safety Commission (CPSC) for almost 30 years. In 2000, the system was expanded to collect data on all injuries, and since 1992 NEISS has collected information on all nonfatal firearm-related injuries seen in NEISS emergency rooms (Annest et al., 1995; Davis et al., 1996); some of these incidences may represent suicide attempts. NEISS is based on injury data gathered from the emergency departments of 100 representative hospitals selected as a probability sample of all 5,300+ U.S. hospitals with emergency departments (EDs) (grouped into 5 "strata," four representing EDs of differing sizes and one from children's hospitals) (CPSC, 2001).

Given its current sampling system, the utility of NEISS is limited; the data can only be used for national estimates and are invalid at regional, state and local levels (GAO, 1997). In addition, because it does not use the International Classification of Diseases (ICD) coding system both the detail of data collected and the ease with which the data can be shared with other systems are limited (AdvanceMed, 2001).

Youth Risk Behavior Survey (YRBS).

The YRBS is managed by the CDC and includes national, state, territorial, and local school-based surveys of representative samples of students in grades 9–12 in participating jurisdictions. Its intent is to monitor risk behaviors associated with the leading causes of injury and death among adolescents (Kann et al., 1998). In 1997, the YRBS was conducted by 38 states, 4 territories and 17 large cities, in addition to the national-level representative survey (STIPDA, 1999). Concerns regarding the validity of self-reports presents particular problems for collecting information on suicide attempts by the YRBS (Ivarsson et al., 2002). In addition, some jurisdictions, especially less populous ones, choose not to include the items about suicidality out of concerns for liability and imitation. This introduces bias into the results when comparing geographical areas. However, given that some suicide attempts may never come to medical attention or result in hospitalization, self-report measures like YRBS remain a valuable source of information.

Oregon State Adolescent Suicide Attempt Data System (ASADS)

In 1987, Oregon became the only state with a law requiring the reporting of suicide attempts by youth under 18 to the state health department (Hopkins et al., 1995). Failure to comply with this regulation is a Class A misdemeanor; however, it has been unnecessary to charge any hospital thus far (personal communication, D. Hopkins, Oregon Department of Human Services, April 19, 2002). Oregon law also specifies that the treating hospital must refer attempters to "in-patient or out-patient community resources, crisis intervention or other appropriate intervention by the patient's attending physician, hospital social work staff or other appropriate staff[1]".

ASADS contains information such as demographics, date, county, method, place of attempt, living arrangement, psychological history, drug/alcohol use, previous attempt(s), reason(s), and seriousness and intent of attempt. Data are collected from emergency department records for all youth treated for a suicide attempt. Under-reporting is thought to occur. Training of staff and consistency of information is also an issue since only the information included in the patient's medical chart can be collected. The system could be improved through better documentation by the health care provider (personal communication, L. Millet, Oregon Department of Human Services, April 22, 2002).

Limitations of the Model Systems

There exist many potential sources of information, but most often these are unlinked and in some cases represent redundant efforts. Most of what is available is based on hospitalization records or self-reports; however, studies have shown that injury surveillance based on hospitalization information alone may underestimate incidence by as much as 65 percent (Washington Department of Health, 1997). Currently, there is no systematic way of following repeat attempters over time. Elderly patients have among the highest rates of suicide completion, yet they are not included in some of the attempt surveillance systems that exist. Addi-

---

[1]Oregon Revised Statutes, 441.750. Suicide attempts by minors; referral; report; disclosure of information; limitation of liability.

tional sources of information that could be consulted include emergency medical services data, school health services records, community and private health care providers data, etc. However, there are serious technical and practical limitations to integrating these sources.

Coding

External Cause of Injury codes (E-codes) were developed by the World Health Organization (WHO) as a supplemental code for use with the International Classification of Diseases (ICD). These codes provide a systematic way to classify diagnostic information that health care providers have entered into the medical record. They are standardized internationally and thus permit comparisons of data among communities, states, and countries (Educational Development Center, 1999). Since 1999 mortality data in the United States has been coded using the 10th Revision of the ICD (ICD-10), while morbidity data is coded using a clinical modification of the 9th Revision of the ICD (ICD-9CM) (Annest et al., 1998). ICD-10CM is currently being developed, and is expected to improve the specificity and accuracy for descriptions of non-fatal injuries (Annest et al., 1998). Currently, 26 states either mandate or have rates over 90 percent for use of E-codes in their Hospital Discharge Data Systems (ICRIN, 2001), and 11 states require their use in Emergency Department Data Systems (Annest et al., 1998).

The usefulness of E-codes for a surveillance system rests on the consistency of their use, and technical concerns regarding the compatibility of the format and type of different systems (CDC, 1995). For example, the number of permitted fields on reporting forms would need to be standardized since more than one field allows much more detailed and informative coding. The CDC is currently pilot-testing its National Electronic Disease Surveillance System (NEDSS), an initiative that will standardize public health data systems for infectious disease to allow integrated and electronically compatible national, state, and local surveillance systems. NEDSS also will support surveillance of other public health concerns including causes of injury (CDC, 2001b). In the future, use of a NEDSS compatible system will be a requirement for CDC surveillance funding of infectious diseases (CDC, 2001a). An ongoing international effort seeks to develop a new multi-axial classification system for external causes of injury which is intended to be used in both mortality and morbidity databases (Annest and Pogostin, 2000). Such a system needs to be compatible with existing data coding systems in order to maintain consistency of monitoring and to increase the feasibility of large-scale implementation (IOM, 1999).

Issues of Confidentiality

Surveillance systems are usually organized either by the name of the individuals, by a unique identification number, or by a record identification number for each incident. Each of these approaches presents methodological and ethical concerns. With a name-based system concerns of privacy and the possibility of reluctance to report could limit effectiveness and compliance. To avoid this, the Oregon ASADS system (discussed above) assigns a record number to each attempt (personal communication, D. Hopkins, Oregon Department of Human Services, April 19, 2002). Surveillance for HIV/AIDS provides a valuable precedent for use of a name-based system. The organization of the HIV/AIDS reporting system was and remains a highly contentious issue. This debate echoes a larger ongoing discussion regarding the privacy of health information in the computerized age. Unique identification numbers presented particular problems in pilot programs for expanding from AIDS to HIV/AIDS reporting with the recounting of cases at diagnosis and again with onset of the syndrome, and with incomplete reporting due to technical and operational difficulties (for review, see CDC, 1999). Critics of name-based systems cite concerns about the stigma of HIV/AIDS and the ensuing discrimination. Anecdotal evidence is cited that providing names would discourage individuals from getting tested. However, the CDC and six state health departments determined that rates of testing did not decrease when name-based testing was instituted (Nakashima et al., 1998).

Many of the same issues exist with suicide attempts, particularly with regard to tracking individuals over time. Because a previous suicide attempts is one of the strongest predictors of completed suicide, and repeat attempters are at higher risk for completed suicide, it is important to be able to track individuals over time.

All of these factors contribute to the tension that exists between the need for quality surveillance to promote the public's health and an individual's right to privacy. In the surveillance of many other health conditions (e.g., HIV/AIDS), state health departments remove identifying information prior to sending the data to the CDC for national reporting (CDC, 1995). The CDC also maintains specific administrative policies and technical program procedures to protect the security of both paper-based and electronic records. Reports are reviewed before public dissemination to ensure that potential individual identifiers are not released (CDC, 1995). Oregon's ASADS does not collect identifying information such as the name or school of the attempter. In addition, data from ASADS are not released when there is a possibility of identification of a particular individual; more explicitly, data from a jurisdication are withheld if it reports fewer than 10 attempts or if the population at risk numbers less than 50. There is limited staff access to the database, and they have not experienced any inappropriate releases of information (personal communication, D. Hopkins, Oregon Department of Human Services, April 19, 2002).

ETHICS AND SAFETY

Since suicide, by definition, involves intent to die, including people at risk of suicide in research on prevention and intervention presents a number of unique and complex ethical dilemmas. Ethical arguments can be made for both inclusion and exclusion of those at risk for suicide in clinical trials. Excluding suicidal participants has been standard industry practice for trials of psychoactive medicines in an effort to reduce the risk of death. On the other hand, excluding those at risk for suicide can be considered unethical since it precludes evaluation of treatments for this population. Furthermore, such screening is impractical since it is not possible to totally screen out people at risk for suicide.

Intervention research with suicidal patients is a complex and risky undertaking. The elements required for ethical intervention research with suicidal patients are similar to those for other types of clinical research: social and scientific value, scientific rigor and validity, fair participant selection, favorable risk–benefit ratio, independent review by a data and safety monitoring board, informed consent, and respect for potential and enrolled participants (Emanuel et al., 2000).

This section reviews the issues of informed consent and safe conduct of clinical trials and presents a statistical approach that can facilitate clinical research with suicidal participants.

Informed Consent

As reviewed earlier (Chapter 3), most suicide is associated with a diagnosis of a major mental disorder. The National Bioethics Advisory Commission (1998) recently issued a report providing guidelines for research on persons with impaired decision making that focused on those with mental disorders. Depression, for example, was included because of the resultant impairment in information processing (Hartlage et al., 1993), reasoning (Baker and Channon, 1995) and possibly decision making (Elliot, 1997; Lee and Ganzini, 1992). Before a person can consent to be part of a clinical trial, they must understand the purpose, the risks, and the possible benefits of the research (National Bioethics Advisory Commission, 1998). To give informed consent requires the ability to express choice, to understand, to reason, and to appreciate the relevance to oneself of the research and any intervention it entails (Appelbaum and Grisso,

1995). It has been argued that a depressed person might understand the risks of a research protocol but may not care about, or may even welcome, the risks. (Elliot, 1997). On the other hand, one might argue that a desperately ill cancer patient or a patient with end-stage cardiac disease awaiting mechanical assistance may be equally unconcerned about the risks. We have no *direct* data regarding the decision-making capacity of suicidal patients. For some people, as seen with depressed patients, the hopelessness and despair may impair their reasoning about risks and benefits. There is a clear need for empirical research to test hypotheses on the capacity of suicidal patients to give informed consent.

Some mental disorders are accompanied by fluctuating decision-making ability (like bipolar disorder) or by progressive impairment (such as Alzheimer's dementia). It is important to note that suicidal ideation also fluctuates and that suicidal acts, especially in the young, are often impulsive (Brent et al., 1999; Hawton et al., 1982). There are alternatives to providing consent at the time of the clinical trial (National Bioethics Advisory Commission, 1998). These options include advance directives[2] or the consent of a legally authorized representative. Another option is assent/ objection, which means that a person who may be partially impaired but still functional can enroll in a low-risk study from which he/she could withdraw at any time. Such approaches would be useful in studies with suicidal participants. Here, it may be appropriate and reasonable to utilize advance research directives or to reevaluate the patient's understanding of the research at some point after the patient has entered the trial and is better able to understand, reason, and appreciate what is being asked of him/her.

In the absence of direct, empirical research on decision-making capacity in suicidal patients, additional safeguards to ensure safety and ethical conduct of research must entail involving family members or other surrogates. This is especially true in cases where there may be reduced capacity for consent such as with highly suicidal participants and/or members of special populations, including minors and elders, patients who are severely mentally ill or psychotic, and prisoners. Community consultation, the process of conferring with representatives who can adequately reflect the concerns of the prospective research participants, is also important under these circumstances. As risk rises, increased formality, objectivity, and documentation of capacity assessment and the informed consent process is wise.

---

[2]An advance directive is a document in which an individual provides specific information about their health care and related wishes in the event that they lose the capacity to express their preferences at some later date.

No Undue Risk

Conducting clinical trials with suicidal patients involves managing risk at many levels and in many ways. As with all clinical trials, investigators need to take appropriate precautions to protect their participants in order to prevent exposure to unnecessary risk. Risk should not be greater than under ordinary, usual, or standard care. Commonly used precautions in clinical trials include frequent and ongoing team-based clinical monitoring of participants, an explicit protocol to follow in the face of acutely increased risk, the specification of rules for participant withdrawal (either temporarily or permanently), and the use of Data and Safety Monitoring Boards to assess: (1) the risk to benefit ratio for participants, (2) investigator adherence to protocol, and (3) the need for and appropriateness of study continuation versus termination (National Bioethics Advisory Commission, 2001). Other standards of protocol safety should include a process of informed consent and avoidance of coercion (see above), documentation of discussions about the clinical and protocol management of participants, adherence to national and local standards of care as appropriate, provision of a safety net for participants and their care givers, avoidance of conflict of interest on the part of investigators, and clarity about who pays the costs of care and injury (e.g., sponsor, institution, insurer; National Bioethics Advisory Commission, 2001). Finally, other risk reduction strategies may include experimental procedures such as the use of adaptive randomization,[3] as well as early termination of a study when the null hypothesis has been disconfirmed. These practices are standard for all clinical trials and can apply to suicidal patients as well. To address some of these concerns, NIMH issued a report on "Issues to Consider in Intervention Research with Persons at High Risk for Suicidality" (Pearson et al., 2000).

One example of how safety and ethical concerns for patients at risk for suicide can be addressed in an intervention trial is the PROSPECT study (Reynolds et al., 2001). In this study, primary care practices are randomly assigned to either the intervention arm of the study (which utilizes depression care managers to improve the recognition and treatment of depression) or to the usual care arm of the practice (which provides screening and assessment services, but no treatment; treatment re-

---

[3]In adaptive randomization the probability of the next treatment assignment is altered on the basis of the responses of previous patients enrolled. As a consequence, more patients receive the best treatment. An example is the "play the winner rule," in which an observed success generates a future trial with the successful treatment on another patient, and a failure generates a future trial with the alternative treatment.

mains the prerogative of the primary care physician [PCP]). Treatment as usual in older primary care patients has been linked to under-recognition of depression and elevated rates of suicide completion. Although treatment as usual is a necessary and credible control condition, the ethical requirement not to expose participants to undue risk requires that patients and their PCP's be informed of the results of psychiatric assessments performed as part of the PROSPECT protocol. Thus, if a patient in a treatment as usual practice is found to have suicidal and/or homicidal ideation, the patient's PCP is promptly informed, as are the patient's caregivers. Although this type of information enhances what is actually and usually available in usual care, it is necessary to meet the ethical demand to do no harm by withholding such crucial information. At the same time, however, this ethically necessary practice potentially prejudices a fair test of the main study hypothesis (intervention practices will lower rates of suicidal ideation, hopelessness, and suicidal behavior to a greater extent than treatment as usual practices). Nonetheless, ethical issues inevitably attend the conduct of intervention studies addressing life and death issues like suicide and must be dealt with forthrightly.

Exclusion from Trials

Because of the concerns about death by suicide, however, people who exhibit suicidal behaviors are often excluded from clinical trials (Pearson et al., 2000). The practice of excluding these patients from trials limits the opportunity for this population to benefit from such research. The Food and Drug Administration's (FDA) requirement to prevent undue risk is frequently noted as the reason for the exclusion. However, suicidal behavior is not expressly excluded by the regulations (personal communication, P. David, FDA, November 15, 2001).

Institutional review boards (IRBs)[4] are charged with protecting participants in research trials to ensure that they are provided with all the information they need for informed consent, protected from unnecessary harm, provided with maximal benefit possible, and provided with appropriate (or usual) medical care if not part of the experimental arm of the protocol.[5] All research protocols using human participants are required to

---

[4]IRBs are comprised of at least five members who are primarily clinical and/or scientific professionals. The board must include at least one non-scientific member, often a legal professional or a clergy member. At least one person must be unaffiliated with the institution at which the work is being done.

[5]Protection of Human Subjects, Code of Federal Regulations, Title 45, Part 46 (1991). Available: http://ohrp.osophs.dhhs.gov/humansubjects/guidance/45cfr46.htm

have IRB approval. In carrying out this charge, IRBs often require patients at risk for suicide to be excluded from trials (Ethical considerations, 2001). The concerns are that the participants' risk exceeds their benefit and that the investigators and/or the treatment protocols are inadequate to monitor and address suicide (Pearson et al., 2000).

Excluding suicidal patients from clinical trials has serious repercussions. The number of studies that assess changes in suicidal behavior with new pharmacological treatments is extremely limited (Linehan, 1997). Treatments for suicidality have not been, for the most part, subject to controlled clinical trials. The evidence base for care is lacking. Linehan in 1997 could locate only 20 clinical trials that selected suicidal participants. Among the 13 outpatient studies in this list, 6 excluded those at high risk for suicide. These 6 studies showed no significant effects of experimental treatment. In contrast, 6 of the 7 remaining studies that included high-risk patients were able to demonstrate effectiveness of an intervention. This analysis clearly demonstrates how critical it is to include suicidal patients in a trial if we are to develop effective treatment protocols for those at risk.

As discussed in Chapter 3, suicide is, unfortunately, a medically expectable outcome of many mental illnesses. Death in a cancer clinical trial may be predictable, or even inevitable, but trials do not exclude terminally ill patients. Likewise, suicide attempts and completed suicide are also expectable, if unpredictable, events in severely mentally ill persons. One might logically reframe the perspective in this way: the outcome of suicide is a result of the mental illness, not the research or therapeutic intervention. Similarly, one might argue that a suicide attempt (or relapse) should *not* automatically exclude continuing participation, since it is necessary and desirable from a public health perspective to establish whether a particular intervention is effective in preventing further attempts or completed suicide in high-risk participants.

RESEARCH DESIGN AND ANALYSIS ISSUES

Statistical analysis and display of suicide data are complex problems, and there are many different approaches to their solution. This section considers several statistical issues in the design and analysis of studies of suicide. Many of the issues presented are well known in the suicide literature (e.g., estimating prevalence) whereas some are new to the study of suicide (e.g., use of empirical Bayes estimates in studying geographic variation in suicide rates). Throughout the chapter, a distinction is made between the analysis of suicide rates, where the unit of observation is typically a geographic area (e.g., a county) and the analysis of suicide as an outcome where the unit of analysis is an individual. The section discusses 1) the problem of computing lifetime risk of suicide and describes an appropriate methodology, 2) the problem of identifying suicide clusters, 3) statistical approaches that can inform suicide research, and 4) issues in the design of suicide studies. These issues include, case-control studies, risk-based allocation, and sample size and statistical power. Technical details of the statistical models are presented in Appendix A. The methods described here are by no means an exhaustive list of potentially useful approaches in the analysis of suicide data. It is hoped that these examples will provide a perspective on the power of appropriate statistical methodologies in suicide research.

Lifetime Risk of Suicide

Based on the work of Guze and Robins (1970), much of the psychiatric literature purports that 15 percent of depressed patients will die by suicide. To better understand the foundation of this estimate it is important to understand the various ways in which lifetime risk can be computed. In the case of Guze and Robins (1970), lifetime risk is defined as the proportion of the dead who died by suicide, often termed "proportionate mortality" (see also Goodwin and Jamison, 1990). As pointed out by Bostwick and Pankratz (2000), proportionate mortality is a reasonable estimator of lifetime risk only when the participants are followed until death. In general, however, the studies synthesized in the report by Guze and Robins, typically followed patients for no more than a few years. Furthermore, the participants were hospitalized psychiatric patients, often hospitalized as a precaution for suicide. Both this selection effect and the use of proportionate mortality as an estimator of lifetime risk, lead to an increase in the estimated lifetime prevalence. To obtain a more accurate assessment, Inskip, Harris, Barraclough (1998) calculated percent death by suicide to percent dead overall in a large number of studies. Analyses were stratified by diagnostic group (alcohol dependence, affective disorder, schizophrenia). Unfortunately, the majority of these studies had overall mortality rates of less than 50 percent, so the estimates of lifetime risk (i.e., 100 percent mortality) were extrapolated from the available data. Nevertheless, the lifetime suicide risk estimates were 7 percent for alcohol dependence, 6 percent for affective disorder, and 4 percent for schizophrenia.

In the most statistically rigorous approach to date, Bostwick and Pankratz (2000) compared proportionate mortality to "case fatality prevalence," which is the number of suicides divided by the total number of patients at risk. Based on a synthesis of 29 studies of hospitalized affective disorder inpatients (19,723 patients), the pooled estimate of proportionate mortality prevalence was 20.0 percent, but only 4.1 percent for case fatality prevalence. As one might expect, in outpatients the rate for case fatality prevalence decreased to 2.0 percent in the analysis of 7 studies of 7,444 affective disorder outpatients. In contrast, the rate actually increased slightly to 24.6 percent for proportionate mortality prevalence.

Bostwick and Pankratz (2000) computed lifetime risk of suicide, using Bayes theorem, as the probability of suicide given death times the probability of death. For example, the overall probability of death in the 29 studies of affective disorder inpatients was 20 percent and of those, 20 percent died by suicide. The product of these two probabilities (i.e., the conditional probability of suicide given death and the prior probability of death) is the Bayes estimate of lifetime risk, which in this case is 4 percent. The Bayes estimate is remarkably close to the case fatality prevalence of 4.1 percent. This finding was consistent for all of the groups examined in their study (affective disorder outpatients = 2.2 percent, affective disorder inpatients = 4.0 percent, Guze and Robins data = 4.8 percent, Goodwin and Jamison data = 3 percent, and the general population = 0.5 percent).

Suicide Clustering

Suicidal behavior in adolescents is a major public health problem (NCHS, 1988). Data suggest that teen suicides often occur in temporal and geographic proximity of one another. This phenomenon is not unlike the concept of an outbreak of a disease in a particular community. Naturally, some clustering of suicides occurs by chance alone even if suicides occur at random. In the study of suicide clusters, the goal is to determine whether or not the outbreaks are occurring to an extent greater than would be expected by chance variation. Past studies have used various populations, such as psychiatric in-patients, high school and college students, marine troops, prison inmates, religious sects etc. (Gould et al., 1990). However, county of residence may be a more sensitive space unit to define a cluster (Gould et al., 1990).

Several statistical methods have been used to detect and statistically assess the time-space clustering of disease (see Gould et al., 1990). The Ederer-Myers-Mantel method (Ederer et al., 1964) is found to be sensitive to temporal clustering as well as time-space clustering. A method proposed by Knox (1964) considers all possible pairs of cases and the time and space distances between them. It establishes clustering by demonstrating a positive relation between the time and space distances of a pair, but required specification of the critical values for time and space to define closeness. This approach was modified by Smith (1982) to define "close in space" as occurring within the same geographic area. Wallenstein and colleagues (1989) provided a formula to assess the practical significance of clusters as well as the statistical significance. Gibbons et al. (1990)

took this further to decompose the overall distribution of suicide rates into a mixture of two Poisson distributions, the first to characterize the normal rate and the second to characterize the elevated rate, possibly due to one or more "suicide epidemics." When they fit the model to 10 years (1977–1987) of monthly suicide rate data from Cook County (Chicago area), they found no evidence for a contribution of the second distribution. However, as described in Appendix A, using this analysis on the spatial distribution of suicide has identified qualitatively distinct geographic groupings of suicide rates across the United States. During the past decade, statistical research on finite mixture distributions has developed greatly (for review, see Böhning, 1999) and holds great promise for application to suicide. Appendix A describes the general statistical theory and developments.

Statistical Models for Assessment of Suicide Rates

Poisson Regression Models

In the analysis of suicide rate data, Poisson regression models are a natural choice. With this approach, the data are modeled as Poisson counts whose means are expressed as a function of covariates. For example, the data may consist of yearly county-level suicide rates, broken down by age, sex, and race for that year. For these type of rate estimates a fixed-effects model is usually used. When there is a mixture of fixed (e.g., age, sex, and race) and random effects (e.g., unobservable county-specific effects), the more general mixed-effects Poisson regression model is used. In the case of suicide, the rates are considered to be nested within geographic locations (e.g., counties) and can represent multiple rates obtained over time (e.g., yearly suicide rates for a given county) or rates for different strata within a given county (e.g., males and females) or both. The random effects would modify the rate for each county from the population average.

Often, it is of interest to estimate values of the random effects within a sample. In the present context, these estimates would represent the deviation of the suicide rate for a given county from the national mean suicide rate, conditional on model covariates such as age, race, and sex, which may be either fixed or random effects. This can be done by using an empirical Bayes estimator of *cluster*-specific effects.[6] Thomas et al. (1992)

---

[6]In this context, *cluster* does not refer to suicide clusters but rather to the group or category of an observation.

have used this kind of analysis to describe hospital mortality rates where *cluster*-specific (hospital-specific) effects represent how much the death rates for patients at a particular hospital differ from the national rates for patients with the same covariate values (i.e., matched patients). Longford (1994) provides extensive references to applications involving empirical Bayes estimates of random effects.

An alternative approach to the analysis of suicide rate data is based on Generalized Estimating Equations (GEEs) models, which were introduced by Liang and Zeger (1986) and Zeger and Liang (1986). The GEE method models the marginal expectation (i.e., average response for observations having the same covariates) of outcomes as a function of the explanatory variables. In this approach, the coefficients measure differences in the average response for a unit change in the predictor; in contrast the mixed-effect model produces predictions that are *cluster*-specific. An important property of the GEE method is that the parameter estimates are consistent even if the working correlation matrix is misspecified as long as the model for the mean is correct. A disadvantage of GEE is that it does not provide *cluster*-specific (e.g., county-level) suicide rate estimates adjusted for case mix (i.e., covariate effects). Appendix A outlines the statistical foundations of both fixed-effects and mixed-effects Poisson regression models, as well as the alternative approach based on GEE.

To illustrate how Poisson regression models can be used to estimate the effects of age, race, and sex on *clustered* (i.e., within counties) suicide rate data, this example considers the effects of age divided into five categories (5–14, 15–24, 25–44, 45–64, and 65 and older), sex, and race (African American versus Other) in the prediction of suicide rates across the United States for the period of 1996–1998. These categories were used so that there would be sufficient sample sizes available to compare observed and expected annual suicide rates for both GEE and mixed-effects Poisson regression models. In general, the GEE and mixed effect parameter estimates were remarkably similar.

Table 10-1 displays observed and expected annual suicide rates for both methods of estimation, broken down by age, sex, and race calculated from the parameter estimates. Inspection of Table 10-1 reveals several interesting results. In general, suicide increases with age, is higher in males, and is lower in African Americans. Black females have the lowest suicide rates across the age range. In non-Black males, the suicide rate increases with age whereas in all other groups, the suicide rate either is constant or decreases after age 65. Comparison of the expected frequencies for the GEE and mixed-effects models reveal that they are quite similar and the GEE does a slightly better job of predicting the observed rates.

A special feature of the mixed-effects model is the ability of estimating county-specific rates using empirical Bayes estimates of the random

TABLE 10-1 Observed and Expected Suicide Rates by Age, Race, and Sex

Age Group	Race	Sex	Number of Suicides	Population	Observed Rate	Expected Rate[a]	Expected Rate[b]
05–14	Black	Male	79	9,256,227	0.000009	0.000010	0.000009
05–14	Black	Female	28	8,978,221	0.000003	0.000003	0.000002
05–14	Other	Male	620	50,356,003	0.000012	0.000014	0.000012
05–14	Other	Female	206	47,847,778	0.000004	0.000005	0.000004
15–24	Black	Male	1,333	8,389,386	0.000159	0.000177	0.000160
15–24	Black	Female	191	8,352,196	0.000023	0.000024	0.000021
15–24	Other	Male	9,482	47,906,710	0.000198	0.000222	0.000198
15–24	Other	Female	1,673	45,396,608	0.000037	0.000042	0.000037
25–44	Black	Male	2,546	15,274,935	0.000167	0.000184	0.000164
25–44	Black	Female	474	17,191,095	0.000028	0.000033	0.000030
25–44	Other	Male	27,209	109,106,670	0.000249	0.000283	0.000250
25–44	Other	Female	6,977	108,864,081	0.000064	0.000072	0.000064
45–64	Black	Male	861	7,741,680	0.000111	0.000124	0.000111
45–64	Black	Female	224	9,633,227	0.000023	0.000026	0.000023
45–64	Other	Male	17,358	72,740,945	0.000239	0.000267	0.000239
45–64	Other	Female	5,307	76,289,629	0.000070	0.000078	0.000070
65+	Black	Male	415	3,295,133	0.000126	0.000142	0.000131
65+	Black	Female	83	5,140,632	0.000016	0.000014	0.000013
65+	Other	Male	14,074	38,889,596	0.000362	0.000398	0.000361
65+	Other	Female	2,814	55,229,051	0.000051	0.000057	0.000051

[a]Mixed-effect model
[b]GEE model

effects as described in the previous section. This allows an estimate of county-specific, expected suicide rates, which directly incorporate the effects race, sex, and age of that county. Table 10-2 provides a comparison of observed and expected numbers of suicides (1996-1998) for 100 randomly selected counties. Inspection of Table 10-2 reveals remarkably close agreement between observed and expected numbers of suicides.

This approach also allows the use of Bayes estimates directly to obtain county-level suicide rates adjusted for the effects of race, sex, and age. For example, a Bayes estimate of 1.0 represents an adjusted rate that is equal to the national rate, while a Bayes estimate of 2.0 represents a doubling of the national rate, and a Bayes estimate of 0.5 represents one-half of the national rate. Figure 10-1 (found on page 382) displays the Bayes estimates by county across the United States and reveals that even after accounting for these important demographic variables, considerable spatial variability remains. This map provides a useful tool for qualitative research into the etiology of suicide through an assessment of the spatial

TABLE 10-2 Observed and Expected Number of Suicides for 100 Randomly Selected Counties

State	County	Observed # of Deaths	Expected # of Deaths	State	County	Observed # of Deaths	Expected # of Deaths
56	7	16	10.3	51	75	5	5.9
53	63	169	170.4	20	159	6	4.5
5	91	14	13.6	21	103	14	8.7
47	111	13	9.4	40	45	1	1.6
54	93	1	2.8	31	61	1	1.5
28	5	9	5.5	31	91	0	0.3
27	141	22	21.7	40	73	9	6.3
38	47	0	1.0	20	203	1	1.0
21	59	25	27.5	1	5	8	8.2
48	451	54	50.2	38	51	0	1.4
48	87	3	1.4	38	39	2	1.3
18	97	391	385.3	21	95	11	12.0
35	7	8	6.2	48	73	32	25.8
48	383	2	1.5	23	11	38	39.6
31	41	3	4.3	55	101	58	59.5
18	7	2	3.4	17	107	9	10.8
45	61	6	5.9	47	127	1	1.9
19	1	4	3.4	55	55	28	28.1
8	119	13	9.9	21	223	5	3.4
36	3	22	20.9	30	97	1	1.4
19	93	2	2.9	19	51	2	3.0
12	95	303	314.1	47	129	4	6.4
49	49	89	91.1	48	9	2	3.0
28	45	30	24.1	19	5	9	6.7
18	107	19	16.9	28	69	3	3.0
5	1	6	6.8	46	19	6	4.1
17	167	64	64.8	27	171	31	30.8
39	89	43	44.7	28	53	1	2.4
28	1	9	9.5	20	31	2	3.1
53	23	0	0.9	51	47	18	15.0
48	213	30	28.8	46	123	3	2.7
55	107	9	7.1	12	81	135	129.6
31	177	6	6.7	2	122	22	20.4
17	49	12	12.2	21	61	0	3.4
55	75	18	17.5	21	25	7	6.3
8	55	3	2.7	26	13	6	4.0
29	121	4	5.4	18	157	42	44.1
40	125	34	30.2	21	165	2	2.2
20	73	3	3.2	48	447	2	0.8
21	109	7	5.5	13	265	3	0.6
29	197	2	1.8	2	100	2	1.0
51	133	7	5.0	55	11	4	5.2
29	105	8	10.0	48	81	0	1.3
47	181	14	9.7	21	229	6	4.6
51	103	9	5.5	55	35	32	32.3
16	15	3	2.2	39	151	112	113.5
38	55	2	3.5	28	89	17	18.4
39	17	91	93.6	19	167	4	8.2
55	51	3	2.8	23	27	17	15.7
19	119	3	4.2	38	1	0	1.1

distribution of Bayes estimates for outliers. For example, in the western continental United States and Alaska where suicide rates are typically high, a few counties have Bayes estimates consistent with the national average. Similarly, in the central United States where there is a high concentration of counties with the lowest suicide rates, a few counties exhibit the highest suicide rates. What are the risk and protective factors that have produced these spatial anomalies? Are these spatial anomalies simply due to reporting bias or some other unmeasured characteristic? Based on a review of the literature, it does not appear that this type of statistical approach to this problem has been previously considered. Examining these spatial anomalies in greater detail is a fruitful area for further research.

Mixed-effects Ordinal Regression Models

To study suicidal ideation, attempts, and completion in individual participants under various conditions, mixed-effects ordinal and nominal regression models can be used. The basic concept is to develop an ordinal scale of suicidal behavior, ranging from no suicidal ideation, low, medium, and high suicidal ideation, suicide attempt, and ending at suicide completion. Several authors have described models including both random and fixed effects (e.g., Agresti and Lang, 1993; Ezzet and Whitehead, 1991; Harville and Mee, 1984; Hedeker and Gibbons, 1994; Jansen, 1990; Ten Have, 1996). Statistical details are presented in Appendix A.

A reanalysis of the longitudinal data from Rudd et al. (1996) on suicidal ideation and attempts in a sample of 300 suicidal young adults (personal communication, Dr. M. David Rudd, Professor of Psychology, Baylor University) serves as an illustration of an application of the mixed-effects ordinal logistic regression model. In the original study, 180 participants were assigned to an outpatient intervention group therapy condition and 120 participants received treatment as usual. This re-analysis assigns the ordinal outcome measure of 0=low suicidal ideation, 1=clinically significant suicidal ideation, and 2=suicide attempt. Suicidal ideation was defined as a score of 11 or more on the Modified Scale for Suicide Ideation (MSSI, Miller et al., 1986). Model specification included main effects of month (0, 1, and 6) and treatment (0=control, 1=intervention), and the treatment by month interaction. Although data at 12, 18 and 24 months were also available, the dropout rates at these later months were too large for a meaningful analysis. In addition, to illustrate the flexibility of the model, depression as measured by the Beck Depression Inventory (BDI, Beck and Steer, 1987) and anxiety as measured by the Millon Clinical Multiaxial Inventory (MCMI-A, Millon, 1983) were treated as time-varying covariates in the model, to relate fluctuations in depressed mood and anxiety to shifts in suicidality. Details of the analysis are in Appendix A.

Briefly, the analysis reveals that both of the time-varying covariates, depression and anxiety, were significantly associated with suicidality. By contrast, the treatment by time interaction was not significant, indicating that the intervention did not significantly effect the rate of suicide ideation or attempts over time. Treatment was found to be ineffective even after excluding the effects of anxiety and depression, which could mask treatment and treatment by time interactions. The random month effect was significant, indicating appreciable inter-individual variability in the rates of change over time.

Interval Estimation

Three types of statistical intervals, confidence intervals, prediction intervals, and tolerance intervals, can provide information relevant to suicide. A confidence interval can be used to describe our uncertainty in the overall suicide rate. A prediction limit can estimate an upper bound on a future rate. A statistical tolerance limit can set an upper bound on a specified proportion of all future monthly or yearly suicides incidences, with a specified level of confidence. General discussion of Poisson confidence, prediction, and tolerance limits are presented in Hahn and Meeker (1991) and Gibbons (1994), and in Appendix A.

As an example, consider the case in which after 61 months of observation for a particular county, with a population of 100,000 people, 123 suicides are recorded. The 95 percent confidence interval for the true population suicide rate is between 1.659 and 2.373 suicides per month per 100,000 (details of this computation are provided in Appendix A). In contrast, a 95 percent upper prediction limit for the actual number of suicides in the next month is 4 suicides. Finally, to have 95 percent confidence that the limit will not be exceeded in 99 percent of all future months (not just the next single month), the 95 percent confidence 99 percent coverage tolerance limit is 7 suicides per month (see Appendix A for computational details). These calculations are useful to determine if an event (e.g., a television program about teen suicide) has an impact on suicide rates. If the number of suicides in the month following the event exceeds the calculated prediction (in the example, 4 suicides), then the television program may have been related to an increase in the suicide rate that is inconsistent with chance expectation based on the previous 61 months of data. If the tolerance limit is exceeded (in the example 7 suicides in the month), there is evidence that the rate is beyond chance expectations given the 61 months of historical data. The advantage of the tolerance limit over the prediction limit is that the tolerance limit preserves the confidence level over a large number of future comparisons, whereas the prediction limit applies to a single future time period. Complete computational details are provided in Appendix A.

Study Design Issues

The following sections touch on some experimental design issues that may be useful in future studies of suicide either at the level of the individual or at the population level.

Case-Control Studies

Retrospective case-control studies are often used to examine risk factors of completed suicide. Logistic regression is typically the standard method for analysis of these case-control studies where multiple risk factors are assessed. For low-base rate conditions such as suicide, risk factors such as previous suicide attempts are often not seen in matched controls. For example, in a study by Brent et al. (1999) that attempted to relate past suicide attempts to completed suicide in female adolescents, 13 of 21 completed suicides, but none of the 39 controls, had a previous suicide attempt. The problem has been termed "complete separation" by Hosmer and Lemeshow (1989). As a consequence, parameter estimation becomes difficult and often the logistic regression model fails to converge. Some investigators (e.g., Shaffer et al., 1996) have simply eliminated previous attempts as a predictor. Chen, Iyengar, and Brent (unpublished) developed a hybrid model to handle the case of zero cells caused by variables like previous suicide attempts. The model is essentially a mixture of a standard logistic regression model estimated from both cases and controls and a risk estimate for previous attempts (or some other low-rate risk factor), which is the conditional probability of suicide given a past attempt. Parameters are estimated by subtracting the risk attributable to previous attempts from the overall risk and then modeling the residual risk over the rest of the risk factors using a logistic regression model. Innovative statistical approaches such as this are needed to deal with some of the special problems associated with the modeling of low-rate events such as completed suicide.

Risk-Based Allocation

Risk-based allocation, a non-randomized design could be quite useful in the study of suicide. It allows participants at higher risk, or with greater disease severity, to benefit from the potentially superior experimental treatment, assuring that all of the sickest patients will receive the experimental treatment. Consequently, the design is sometimes called an "assured allocation" design (Finkelstein et al., 1996a; 1996b). Because the design is non-randomized, it should only be considered in those situations where a randomized trial would not be possible.

The design first requires a quantitative measure of risk, disease severity, or prognosis, which is observed at or before enrollment into the study, together with a pre-specified threshold for receiving the experimental therapy. All participants above the threshold receive the experimental treatment, while all participants below the threshold receive the standard treatment. The risk-based design also requires a prediction of what the outcomes would have been in the sicker patients if they had received the standard treatment. One example of such a model might be an appropriate regression model of the relationship between pre-treatment suicidal ideation on post-treatment suicidal ideation in a group of depressed patients treated with the standard antidepressant therapy. The validity of this model can then be tested by comparing the observed and predicted levels of the of suicidal ideation in the low-risk control participants that were given the standard treatment. This is the basis of another novel feature of the risk-based design: to estimate the difference in average outcome between the high-risk participants who received the experimental treatment, compared with what the same participants would have experienced on the standard treatment.

The model for the standard treatment (but only the standard treatment) needs to relate the average or expected outcome to specific values of the baseline measure of risk used for the allocation. Because the parameters of the model will be estimated from the concurrent control data and extrapolated to the high-risk patients, only the functional form of the model is required, not specific values of the model parameters. This offers a real advantage over historical estimates. All one needs to assume for the risk-based design is that the mathematical form of the model relating outcome to risk is correctly specified throughout the entire range of the risk measure. This is a strong assumption, to be sure, but with sufficient experience and prior data on the standard treatment, the form of the model can be validated.

The risk-based allocation clearly creates a "biased" allocation and, obviously, the statistical analysis appropriate to estimate the treatment effect is not the simple comparison of mean outcomes in the two groups, as it would be in a randomized trial. Instead, the theory of general empirical Bayes estimation can be applied (Robbins, 1993; Robbins and Zhang, 1988; Robbins and Zhang, 1989; Robbins and Zhang, 1991). There are several cautions to observe. The population of participants entering a trial with risk-based allocation should be the same as that for which the model was validated, so that the form of the assumed model is correct. Clinicians enrolling patients into the trial need to be comfortable with the allocation rule, because protocol violations raise difficulties just as they do in randomized trials. Finally, the standard error of estimates will reflect the effect of extrapolation of the model predictions for the higher-risk patients based on the data from the lower-risk patients. Because of this, a randomized design with balanced arms will have smaller standard errors than a risk-based design with the same number of patients.

Sample Size Considerations

When designing studies for low-base rate events, such as suicide incidence, attempts, and ideation, statistical power considerations can lead to studies with quite different sample size requirements. The lower the base-rate and the greater the need for precision, the larger the population size necessary to achieve significance. In addition, large samples are required to increase the confidence limits. Table 10-3 provides a summary of required sample sizes for computing incidence rates and corresponding levels of precision, with three levels of confidence. For a 90 percent confidence interval for a rate of 10 per 100,000 (plus or minus 5 per 100,000), approximately 100,000 participants are needed. By contrast, if the assessment is in a high-risk population where the mean incidence is 50 per

TABLE 10-3 Sample Size Estimates for Estimating the Population Proportion of Suicide or Suicide Attempts

Rate	Confidence		
	80%	90%	95%
0.0001 ± 0.00005	65,689	96,684[a]	>100,000
0.0005 ± 0.00025	13,133	21,634	30,717
0.001 ± 0.0005	6,563	10,812	15,351
0.005 ± 0.0025	1,308	2,154	3,058
0.01 ± 0.005	651	1,072	1,522
0.05 ± 0.01	781	1,286	1,825
0.05 ± 0.025	125	206	292
0.10 ± 0.01	1,479	2,435	3,458
0.10 ± 0.02	370	609	865
0.10 ± 0.03	165	271	385
0.10 ± 0.04	93	153	217
0.10 ± 0.05	60	98	139

[a]88% confidence

100,000 with a 95 percent confidence interval from 25 to 75 per 100,000, 30,717 participants are required. For measurement of risk of suicide attempts in a high-risk population (estimated at 10 percent, for instance), a sample size of 3458 is required for precision of 1 percent, but only 139 participants are needed for precision of 5 percent.

Study designs frequently compare suicide, or suicide attempts, or suicidal ideation as an outcome in two groups of individuals. Several factors affect the necessary sample size. Table 10-4 illustrates required sample sizes for a two-group comparison of suicide (completion, attempts, or ideation) rates based on a Type I error rate of 5 percent, power of 0.8, for one to ten repeated evaluations, assuming either intra-class (i.e., intra-subject) correlations (ICC) of 0.3, 0.5, or 0.7. The larger the ICC, the less independent information available, and the larger the required sample size for a given effects size. Furthermore, the larger the ICC, the less impact taking multiple repeated measurements has on the required number of participants. If there is only one repeated measurement, the sample

TABLE 10-4 Sample Size Estimates for Comparison of Two Groups

Difference	Number of Repeated Measurements									
	1	2	3	4	5	6	7	8	9	10
ICC = .3										
1% vs 2%	1826	1187	974	867	803	761	730	708	690	676
5% vs 10%	343	223	183	163	151	143	137	133	129	127
10% vs 20%	157	102	84	75	69	65	63	61	59	58
25% vs 50%	46	30	24	22	20	19	18	18	17	17
ICC = .5										
1% vs 2%	1826	1370	1217	1141	1096	1065	1043	1027	1014	1004
5% vs 10%	343	257	228	214	206	200	196	193	190	188
10% vs 20%	157	118	105	98	94	92	90	88	87	86
25% vs 50%	46	34	30	28	27	27	26	26	25	25
ICC = .7										
1% vs 2%	1826	1552	1461	1415	1388	1369	1356	1347	1339	1333
5% vs 10%	343	291	274	265	260	257	254	253	251	250
10% vs 20%	157	133	126	122	119	118	117	116	115	115
25% vs 50%	46	39	36	35	35	34	34	34	33	33

Suicide completion, suicide attempts, or suicide ideation for a one-tailed test, α =0.05, power of 0.8, 1 to 10 repeated measurements, and intra-class correlation (ICC) of 0.3, 0.5, or 7 (entries are n/group).

sizes are for a cross-sectional study. For more than one repeated measurement, the strength of the correlation of events over time must be considered and based on preliminary data. Obviously, for completed suicide, there would be only one repeated measurement and consequently the required sample size would be larger. Note that Table 10-4 provides an example of study sizes needed when the incidence of the outcome is at least 1 percent (i.e., 1000/100,000). As demonstrated in both Table 10-3 and Table 10-4, population sizes must be much larger when working with a low base-rate event. The estimates in Table 10-4 are based on the method of Hsieh (1988).

CENTERS

Because of its low base rate, the difficulties in assessment, and the long-term, interdisciplinary nature of the risk and protective factors, the optimal approach to learn about suicide is to use large populations with cultural and genetic diversity for long-duration, interdisciplinary studies. A centrally coordinated, population-based approach would provide the infrastructure necessary to estimate more reliably the incidence of suicidal behavior (including attempts and completions) in different racial and ethnic groups and in different groups of mentally ill persons. Such an approach would also facilitate longitudinal studies of risk and protective factors (biological and psychosocial) and of preventive interventions. Research centers have often been the mechanism used to address similar research objectives. Large research centers have the additional advantage of being able to provide training opportunities and thereby attract new researchers to a difficult field. Furthermore, centers provide the opportunities for tissue banks and registries that are necessary resources to advance the field. At large research centers, the collaboration of researchers from different but complementary disciplines can significantly enhance progress. For example, integration of ethnographic assessments with psychological and biological evaluations can considerably deepen and contextually validate psychological autopsies to provide a better understanding of the interplay between community and individual risk, and to more successfully develop interdisciplinary preventive interventions that can be rigorously assessed.

In the early 1960s, there was a drive to understand the reasons for and the consequences of the rapidly increasing world population. To address these issues, the Ford Foundation funded the creation of several population research centers around the world, including centers at Georgetown University (2001), the University of Michigan (2002), and the University of the Philippines (2002), which are still flourishing today. The scientific questions required a prospective approach with many years of follow up and a large population base to ensure statistical significance (Garenne et al., 1997). In these characteristics, the study of populations encountered some of the same challenges as the study of suicide. With the creation of the population research centers and ongoing support from the Ford Foundation, Rockefeller Foundation, and the Population Council, the field of demography blossomed. Research efforts created new links among biomedical research, economic analyses, and cultural context. It brought population issues to the attention of policy makers, especially in developing countries (Nagelberg, 1985).

More recently, research centers have been established to tackle difficult public health issues. Many different approaches have been used and some examples are described below.

To study the prevention and treatment of tobacco use, Transdisciplinary Tobacco Use Research Centers were created through a collaborative funding effort of the National Cancer Institute, NIDA and the Robert Woods Johnson Foundation. They created seven academic institutions with a commitment of $84 million over 5 years (NIDA, 1999). Each center is organized around a particular theme, such as Relapse, Tobacco Dependence, or Biobehavioral Basis of Use. Using cultural, genetic, behavioral, and other approaches, scientists at each center focus their research on their particular theme.

The Centers for Disease Control and Prevention (CDC) has established Injury Control Research Centers to explore the prevention, care and rehabilitation needs presented by various types of injury. In fiscal year 2001, the CDC had plans to fund ten centers (Injury prevention, 2001) at an estimated cost of $900,000 each (Grants for injury control, 2001) for up to 5 years each. The Centers are asked to conduct research in prevention, acute care, and rehabilitation and to serve as training centers and information centers for the public. Studies may be organized around a single theme but this is not a requirement. One such center at the University of North Carolina was funded during its first seven years (1987–1993) at an average of $3 million per year. The CDC provided the core funding, which was 20–25 percent of the total (University of North Carolina, 2001).

The National Institute on Aging (NIA) supports about 30 Alzheimer's Disease Research Centers to foster basic and clinical studies of Alzheimer's Disease and related disorders. According to NIA's request for proposals (NIA, 2000), the Centers are intended to "provide financial, intellectual, patient and tissue resources to support research projects that have been reviewed and supported on an individual basis . . . [and] to provide an environment that will strengthen research, increase productivity, and generate new ideas through formal interdisciplinary collaborative efforts." The centers are mandated to include an administrative core, a clinical core to recruit patients, a neuropathology core to archive specimens, and an educational core. The centers support short pilot projects as well as multi-year research efforts. NIA funds each center at a level up to $1.4 million each year for five years, with competitive renewals (NIA, 1998; NIA, 2000). In 1994, NIA was committing $35 million per year on 28 centers (Benowitz, 1996). By supporting both basic and clinical research, the centers enhance the translation of research advances into improved care and diagnosis. With the advent of the centers, progress in understanding neurodegenerative dementias has been remarkable (see IOM, 2000).

The National Cancer Institute (NCI) has established 60 cancer centers throughout the United States to provide a broad-based, interdisciplinary effort in cancer research (NCI, 2001a). NCI has found that the centers provide the opportunity to apply complex research strategies and to undertake novel multidisciplinary approaches to the critical questions facing prevention, assessment, and treatment of cancer (NCI, 2001b). Because of the long duration of funding and centralized support that centers provide, it is possible to follow through on studies of etiology and treatment that would be difficult to undertake in a different setting (NCI, 2001b). Many of the same issues facing researchers in suicide (assessment of risk factors, the necessity for large clinical studies, multidisciplinary issues, etc.) have been successfully addressed through these centers. The Cancer Centers vary greatly in their structure and scope. The centers might encompass basic science, clinical trials, population studies, and/or clinical care. They might be part of a university, freestanding institutes, or jointly run by multiple institutions (NCI, 2000a). In Fiscal Year 2000, $169 million was allocated for funding these 60 centers through NCI (NCI, 2000b). This averages to almost $2.8 million for each center that year. Because of the many sources from which cancer researchers can obtain funds, the general guideline of NCI is that NCI funding should be no more than 20 percent of the total funding of the center (NCI, 2001c). This means that if NCI provides $2.5 million per year to a center, it is expected that the total annual funding is about $12.5 million. Although the support from NCI is only a small part of the total, it is key to the support of the infrastructure, provides shared resources, and allows flexibility in the use of funds. Through these means, NCI funding of the centers helps to stimulate innovation and collaboration in cancer research (NCI, 2000a).

The Conte Center for the Neuroscience of Mental Disorders, funded by the National Institute of Mental Health, is an example of another approach to research centers. In 2000, there were eleven Conte centers (Hyman, 2000). Each of these centers is organized around a single hypothesis. The Centers are designed to optimize the use of resources to address a specific scientific problem. Center funding is not intended to provide full research support for investigators; they are expected also to have individual grant support. To coordinate the activities among these centers, the directors are expected to attend an annual meeting (NIMH, 1998). Funding varies with each center's needs. In 2001, Washington University was awarded $2 million over 3 years to establish a center for brain-mapping projects to enhance understanding of schizophrenia and other psychiatric disorders (Washington University, 2001). In 2000, Emory University received $13 million over 5 years to support their activities on clinical depression (Emory University, 2000).

The committee believes that suicide is best served by a similar mechanism that would allow a nationally coordinated effort that can be extended to global populations through international collaborations. As the discussion above points out, there are many options for organizing centers: core funding, hypothesis, theme, or flexible support. The committee did not find evidence that any one approach was preferable to another. Whatever structure is chosen, such centers would allow better estimates of incidence, improved evaluation of risk and protective factors, longitudinal studies that could assess intervention and prevention, and development of tissue repositories for genetic and other biological analyses. Ancillary benefits of such a center would be the wealth of data that would be collected on mental illness and substance abuse, major risk factors for suicide, and correlation with detailed social data. Because schizophrenia, mood disorders, substance abuse, and personality disorders are associated with increased incidence of suicide, studies of suicide will also address these important psychiatric conditions and lead to a better understanding of and possible interventions for the mental disorders. These are also the appropriate settings to conduct more rigorous evaluation of suicide prevention projects that link community- and individual-level evaluations.

Although suicide is less common than cancer, injury, Alzheimer's Disease, or tobacco use, suicide research has parallels to these other center-based research efforts. Like these other areas of investigation, suicide centers would focus an effort in an area of high significance for public health but where inroads toward solutions have been heretofore limited. While research in suicide has been stymied by inadequate populations for investigation, there is a wealth of understanding about many risk and protective factors including behavioral, psychological, and cultural aspects of the problem. As with other health areas, integration of multiple perspectives will generate new questions and hypotheses that can be expected to jump-start an understanding of mechanisms and possible interventions. Particularly because of the limits of our current knowledge about suicide, these centers are especially important for future progress. The same benefits that centers have provided to other disease initiatives can be expected for suicide.

Currently there are a small number of suicide research centers around the world. In the United States, for example, these include the Suicide Prevention Research Center at the University of Nevada School of Medicine funded by the CDC (NCIPC, 2002) and the University of Rochester's Center for the Study and Prevention of Suicide funded by NIMH (University of Rochester, 2001). Internationally there are centers in Oxford, England (University of Oxford, 2002); Gent, Belgium (Ghent University, 2001); Hamburg, Germany (University of Hamburg, 2000); Stockholm, Sweden (IPM, 2001); and others. The scale of these centers is relatively small; their interactions are limited. As proposed, the population research centers would enhance the population database for research among these investigators and provide an integrated network for coordination of effort and collaborative study.

Other alternatives might achieve some of these goals. Broad assessments of risk factors can be accomplished by including suicidal endpoints in all large epidemiological studies and this is an important approach to enhancing the research effort on suicide. Adding suicide cores to centers focussed on mental illness might also increase the collection of data regarding suicide. But these less expensive alternatives will not address the most serious obstacle to understanding suicide: the need for a large, a well-characterized population that would allow links to be made about causes, risks, protective factors, and successful interventions. Such a well-characterized and carefully studied population is essential for evaluating biological markers and genetic bases of suicide as well as the social and cultural influences. Currently the database is inadequate. Additionally, individual projects cannot access the large populations necessary to come to significant conclusions regarding this low base-rate event. As the statistical analysis above points out, at a suicide rate of 10 per 100,000 population, approximately 100,000 participants are needed to achieve statistical significance. In studying suicide among low-risk groups, the numbers needed are even greater.

While each center might be able to obtain a sufficiently large sample for studies in the general population, a consortium of centers will be necessary to fully explore differences based on region, economic environment, culture, urbanization, and other factors that vary across the country. In addition, one center might be responsible for coordinating international data to increase the understanding of suicide on a global scale. Furthermore, certain subpopulations may be sufficiently small or low risk to require broader recruitment than one center could access. The coordinated network of centers is an optimal way to achieve these goals. In addition, the centers will allow a comprehensive approach to understanding suicide from a truly interdisciplinary perspective with both cross sectional and longitudinal studies.

Suicide is responsible for over 30,000 deaths each year. Mental illness, the primary risk factor, afflicts over 80 million people in the United States; almost 15 million people have a serious mental illness (i.e, a mental disorder that leads to a functional impairment). For comparison, breast cancer claims the lives of about 40,000 women per year and between 10–15 million people are living with the diagnosis of breast cancer. In 1998 over $400 million from NCI and the Army programs was allocated to research into the prevention, treatment, and cure of breast cancer (IOM, 2001). From estimates of the portfolios of SAMHSA, CDC, and NIMH, the funding for suicide was less than $40 million in 2000. The committee finds that this is disproportionately low, given the magnitude of the problem of suicide. A substantial investment of funds is needed to make meaningful progress.

FINDINGS

• Suicidology has faced serious methodological limitations, including inconsistencies in definitions and misclassification of deaths by medical examiners or coroners. The quality of the data on suicide attempts is even less reliable than that for completed suicide. The low base-rate of suicide has necessitated the use of proximal endpoints in lieu of suicide itself and has created difficulties in computing the risk of suicide and statistically analyzing results.

The field should endorse common definitions and psychometrically sound measures. Better training of coroners and medical examiners in certification of suicide needs to be developed and provided. Registries of suicide attempts for clinical surveillance and research purposes that have the capacity to foster, among other things, international community-oriented studies that integrate clinical, biological, and social data should be created. Finally, novel applications of statistical analyses and research designs should be employed to advance research on suicide.

• Large sample sizes are required in order to provide statistical power for studies of events with a low base rate. For example, to determine the overall incidence rate of suicide in a general population within plus or minus 5 per 100,000 with 90 percent confidence, would require about 100,000 participants. Many statistical approaches exist that can be effectively applied to the field of suicide.

Researchers in suicide should seek out appropriate methodologies and statistical consultation to most effectively design protocols and analyze data.

- Suicidal individuals have been largely excluded from clinical trials. Evidence suggests, however, that high-risk participants can benefit from treatment trials and that certain research designs can increase the safety of participants. Evidence-based treatment protocols for suicidality are seriously lacking, making clinical trials critical.

Clinical trials of drug and psychotherapy treatment should include suicidal patients. Appropriate safeguards, including safe study designs, should be used with such populations.

- Treatment trials often exclude suicidal individuals because of liability concerns. Re-framing this mortality risk to include comparison with risks in other types of medical trials underscores that suicide is an unfortunately expectable outcome of mental illness for some percentage of afflicted individuals. Suicide is not a consequence of the research or therapeutic intervention.

Inform the public and Institutional Review Boards that mental illnesses are potentially fatal, and that for some percentage of individuals, suicide represents an unfortunately expectable outcome of mental illness.

- Lack of longitudinal and prospective studies remains a critical barrier to understanding and preventing suicide. Understanding the interactive risk and protective factors and their developmental course necessitates prospective, transactional research. Long-term assessment must occur for preventive interventions to be properly evaluated. Large, interconnected research centers have helped advance the science base regarding other societal problems, and are expected to do so for suicide, as well.

A national network of suicide research population laboratories devoted to interdisciplinary research on suicide and suicide prevention across the life cycle should be developed. Such an approach would redress many of the current methodological limitations and resultant lags in progress.

REFERENCES

AAST (American Association for the Surgery of Trauma). 2002. *National Violent Death Reporting System Receives Initial Funding*. [Online]. Available: http://www.aast.org/nvdrs.html [accessed April 15, 2002].

AdvanceMed. 2001. *Audit of the National Electronic Injury Surveillance System (NEISS) Hospitals. Final System-Wide Analysis Report to the U.S. Consumer Product Safety Commission.*

Agresti A, Lang JB. 1993. A proportional odds model with subject-specific effects for repeated ordered categorical responses. *Biometrika*, 80: 527-534.

Andreasen NC, Endicott J, Spitzer RL, Winokur G. 1977. The family history method using diagnostic criteria. Reliability and validity. *Archives of General Psychiatry*, 34(10): 1229-1235.

Andreasen NC, Rice J, Endicott J, Reich T, Coryell W. 1986. The family history approach to diagnosis. How useful is it? *Archives of General Psychiatry*, 43(5): 421-429.

Annest JL, Fingerhut LA, Conn JM, Pickett D, McLoughlin E, Gallagher S. 1998. *How States Are Collecting and Using Cause of Injury Data: A Survey on State-Based Injury Surveillance, External Cause of Injury Coding Practices, and Coding Guidelines in the 50 States, the District of Columbia, and Puerto Rico.* Washington, DC: American Public Health Association.

Annest JL, Mercy JA, Gibson DR, Ryan GW. 1995. National estimates of nonfatal firearm-related injuries. Beyond the tip of the iceberg. *Journal of the American Medical Association*, 273(22): 1749-1754.

Annest JL, Pogostin CL. 2000. *A Pilot Test of the Centers for Disease Control and Prevention Short Version of the International Classification of External Causes of Injury (ICECI). Report to the World Health Organization Collaborating Centers on the Classification of Disease.* Atlanta, GA: Office of Statistics and Programming, National Center for Injury Prevention and Control, Centers for Disease Control and Prevention.

Appelbaum PS, Grisso T. 1995. The MacArthur Treatment Competence Study. I: Mental illness and competence to consent to treatment. *Law and Human Behavior*, 19(2): 105-126.

Atkinson MW, Kessel N, Dalgaard JB. 1975. The comparability of suicide rates. *British Journal of Psychiatry*, 127: 247-256.

Azrael D, Barber C, Mercy J. 2001. Linking data to save lives: Recent progress in establishing a National Violent Death Reporting System. *Harvard Health Policy Review*, 2(2).

Baker JE, Channon S. 1995. Reasoning in depression: Impairment on a concept discrimination learning task. *Cognition and Emotion*, 9: 579-597.

Barber C, Hemenway D, Hargarten S, Kellermann A, Azrael D, Wilt S. 2000. A "call to arms" for a national reporting system on firearm injuries. *American Journal of Public Health*, 90(8): 1191-1193.

Beck AT, Davis JH, Frederick CJ, Perlin S, Pokorny AD, Schulman RE, Seiden RH, Wittlin BJ. 1973. Classification and nomenclature. In: Resnick HLP, Hathorne BC, Editors. *Suicide Prevention in the Seventies.* (pp. 7-12). Washington, DC: U.S. Government Printing Office.

Beck AT, Steer RA. 1987. *Beck Depression Inventory: Manual.* New York: Psychological Corporation.

Benowitz S. 1996. Gerontologist's provocative questions: Does NIA spend too much on Alzheimer's? *The Scientist*, 10(1): 5.

Berman AL. 2001. Assessing and recording violent injuries: The need for a national violent death reporting system. A panel discussion held at the 20th Annual American Medical Association Science Reporters Conference, October 28-29, 2001, San Francisco, CA. Summary available in: American Medical Association. *National Violent Death Reporting System Needed: Data From a National Reporting System Could Help Prevent Deaths* [Online]. Available: http://www.ama-assn.org/ama/pub/print/article/4197-5468.html [accessed April 15, 2002].

Beskow J, Runeson B, Asgard U. 1991. Ethical aspects of psychological autopsy. *Acta Psychiatrica Scandinavica*, 84(5): 482-487.

Böhning D. 1999. *Computer-Assisted Anaysis of Mixtures and Applications. Meta-Analysis, Disease Mapping and Others.* Boca Raton, FL: Chapman and Hall CRC.

Bostwick JM, Pankratz VS. 2000. Affective disorders and suicide risk: A reexamination. *American Journal of Psychiatry*, 157(12): 1925-1932.

Brent DA, Baugher M, Bridge J, Chen T, Chiappetta L. 1999. Age- and sex-related risk factors for adolescent suicide. *Journal of the American Academy of Child and Adolescent Psychiatry*, 38(12): 1497-1505.

Brent DA, Perper JA, Allman CJ. 1987. Alcohol, firearms, and suicide among youth: Temporal trends in Allegheny County, Pennsylvania, 1960 to 1983. *Journal of the American Medical Association*, 257(24): 3369-3372.

Brent DA, Perper JA, Kolko DJ, Zelenak JP. 1988. The psychological autopsy: Methodological considerations for the study of adolescent suicide. *Journal of the American Academy of Child and Adolescent Psychiatry*, 27(3): 362-366.

Brent DA, Perper JA, Moritz G, Allman CJ, Roth C, Schweers J, Balach L. 1993. The validity of diagnoses obtained through the psychological autopsy procedure in adolescent suicide victims: Use of family history. *Acta Psychiatrica Scandinavica*, 87(2): 118-122.

Bunk S. 1997. National HIV reporting approaches, but privacy remains paramount. *The Scientist*, 11(22): 1.

Cavanagh JT, Owens DG, Johnstone EC. 1999. Suicide and undetermined death in south east Scotland. A case-control study using the psychological autopsy method. *Psychological Medicine*, 29(5): 1141-1149.

CDC (Centers for Disease Control and Prevention). 1995. *Integrating Public Health Information and Surveillance Systems: A Report and Recommendations*. [Online]. Available: http://www.cdc.gov/od/hissb/docs/katz.htm [accessed April 24, 2002].

CDC (Centers for Disease Control and Prevention). 2001a. *National Electronic Disease Surveillance System: Frequently Asked Questions*. [Online]. Available: http://www.cdc.gov/nedss/About/faq.htm#injury _surveillance [accessed April 16, 2002].

CDC (Centers for Disease Control and Prevention). 2001b. *Supporting Public Health Surveillance Through the National Electronic Disease Surveillance System*. [Online]. Available: http://www.cdc.gov/od/hissb/docs. htm#nedss [accessed April 16, 2002].

CDC (Centers for Disease Control and Prevention). 1999. CDC guidelines for national human immunodeficiency virus case surveillance, including monitoring for human immunodeficiency virus infection and acquired immunodeficiency syndrome. *Morbidity and Mortality Weekly Report*, 48(RR-13): 1-29.

Chen T, Iyengar S, Brent D. unpublished. *A Hybrid Logistic Model for Case-Control Studies*. Unpublished manuscript, Bowling Green State University.

Cook PJ, Tauchen G. 1984. The effect of minimum drinking age legislation on youthful auto fatalities. *Journal of Legal Studies*, 13: 169-190.

Cooper J. 1999. Ethical issues and their practical application in a psychological autopsy study of suicide. *Journal of Clinical Nursing*, 8(4): 467-475.

CPSC (Consumer Product Safety Commission). 2001. *National Electronic Injury Surveillance System*. CPSC Document #3002. [Online]. Available: http://www.cpsc.gov/cpscpub/pubs/3002.html [accessed April 15, 2002].

Davies M, Connolly A, Horan J, Editors. 2001. *State Injury Indicators Report*. Atlanta, GA: Centers for Disease Control and Prevention, National Center for Injury Prevention and Control.

Davis Y, Annest JL, Powell KE, Mercy J.A. 1996. Evaluation of the National Electronic Injury Surveillance System for use in monitoring nonfatal firearm injuries and obtaining national estimates. *Journal of Safety Research*, 27: 83-91.

Ederer F, Meyers MH, Mantel N. 1964. A statistical problem in space and time: Do leukemia cases come in clusters? *Biometrics*, 20: 626-638.

Educational Development Center. 1999. *E Codes*. [Online]. Available: http://www.edc.org/HHD/csn/buildbridges/ bb2.2/ECODES.html [accessed April 15, 2002].

Elliot C. 1997. Caring about risks: Are severely depressed patients competent to consent to research? *Archives of General Psychiatry*, 54: 113-116.

Emanuel EJ, Wendler D, Grady C. 2000. What makes clinical research ethical? *Journal of the American Medical Association*, 283(20): 2701-2711.

Emory University. 2000. Does Abuse Breed Depression? *Emory Magazine*, 75(4): [Online]. Available: http://medicine.wustl.edu/~wumpa/news/2001/conte.html [accessed May 10, 2002].

Ethical considerations in suicide research debated. 2001. [Online]. Available: http://www.suicidology.org/ newslinksum42001.htm [accessed December 4, 2001].

Ezzet F, Whitehead J. 1991. A random effects model for ordinal responses from a crossover trial. *Statistics in Medicine*, 10: 901-907.

Feinstein AR. 1977. Clinical biostatistics. XLI. Hard science, soft data, and the challenges of choosing clinical variables in research. *Clinical Pharmacology and Therapeutics*, 22(4): 485-498.

Finkelstein MO, Levin B, Robbins H. 1996a. Clinical and prophylactic trials with assured new treatment for those at greater risk: II. Examples. *American Journal of Public Health*, 86(5): 696-705.

Finkelstein MO, Levin B, Robbins H. 1996b. Clinical and prophylactic trials with assured new treatment for those at greater risk: I. A design proposal. *American Journal of Public Health*, 86(5): 691-695.

Gallagher SS. 2001. *Critical Needs in Implementing a National Violent Death Reporting System—Results From a Process Evaluation.* Paper presented at the 129th annual meeting of the American Public Health Association in Atlanta, Georgia, October 21-25, 2001.

GAO (General Accounting Office). 1987. *Drinking-Age Laws: An Evaluation Synthesis of Their Impact on Highway Safety.* GAO/PEMD-87-10. Washington, DC: GAO.

GAO (General Accounting Office). 1997. *Consumer Product Safety Commission: Better Data Needed to Help Identify and Analyze Potential Hazards.* GAO/HEHS-97-147. Washington, DC: GAO.

Garenne M, Das Gupta M, Pison G, Aaby P. 1997. Introduction. In: Das Gupta M, Aaby P, Garenne M, Pison G, Editors. *Prospective Community Studies in Developing Countries.* (pp. 1-15). New York: Oxford University Press.

Garrison CZ, Lewinsohn PM, Marsteller F, Langhinrichsen J, Lann I. 1991. The assessment of suicidal behavior in adolescents. *Suicide and Life-Threatening Behavior*, 21(3): 217-230.

Georgetown University. 2001. *History of Demography Department.* [Online]. Available: http://www.georgetown. edu/departments/demography/main/AboutDept/history.htm [accessed May 10, 2002].

Ghent University. 2001. *Unit for Suicide Research.* [Online]. Available: http://allserv.rug.ac.be/~cvheerin/ [accessed May 10, 2002].

Gibbons RD. 1994. *Statistical Methods for Groundwater Monitoring.* New York: Wiley.

Gibbons RD, Clark DC, Fawcet J. 1990. A statistical method for evaluating suicide clusters and implementing cluster surveillance. *American Journal of Epidemiology*, 132 (Suppl 1): S183-S191.

Gist R, Welch QB. 1989. Certification change versus actual behavior change in teenage suicide rates, 1955-1979. *Suicide and Life-Threatening Behavior*, 19(3): 277-288.

Goodwin FK, Jamison KR. 1990. *Manic-Depressive Illness.* New York: Oxford University Press.

Gostin LO, Ward JW, Baker AC. 1997. National HIV case reporting for the United States. A defining moment in the history of the epidemic. *New England Journal of Medicine*, 337(16): 1162-1167.

Gould MS, Wallenstein S, Kleinman M. 1990. Time-space clustering of teenage suicide. *American Journal of Epidemiology*, 131(1): 71-78.

Grants for injury control research centers. Program announcement 01007. 2001. HIVDENT. [Online]. Available: http://www.hivdent.org/infctl/ic1679092000.htm [accessed December 19, 2001].

Guze SB, Robins E. 1970. Suicide and primary affective disorders. *British Journal of Psychiatry*, 117(539): 437-438.

Hahn GJ, Meeker WQ. 1991. *Statistical Intervals: A Guide for Practitioners*. New York: Wiley.

Hartlage S, Alloy LB, Vazquez C, Dykman B. 1993. Automatic and effortful processing in depression. *Psychological Bulletin*, 113(2): 247-278.

Harville DA, Mee RW. 1984. A mixed-model procedure for analyzing ordered categorical data. *Biometrics*, 40: 393-408.

Hawton K, Appleby L, Platt S, Foster T, Cooper J, Malmberg A, Simkin S. 1998. The psychological autopsy approach to studying suicide: A review of methodological issues. *Journal of Affective Disorders*, 50(2-3): 269-276.

Hawton K, Cole D, O'Grady J, Osborn M. 1982. Motivational aspects of deliberate self-poisoning in adolescents. *British Journal of Psychiatry*, 141: 286-291.

Hedeker D, Gibbons RD. 1994. A random effects ordinal regression model for multilevel analysis. *Biometrics*, 50: 933-944.

HICRC (Harvard Injury Control Research Center). 2001. *National Violent Injury Statistics System: Linking Data to Save Lives*. [Online]. Available: http://www.hsph.harvard.edu/hicrc/nviss/ [accessed April 15, 2002].

Holding TA, Barraclough BM. 1975. Psychiatric morbidity in a sample of a London coroner's open verdicts. *British Journal of Psychiatry*, 127: 133-143.

Holding TA, Barraclough BM. 1978. Undetermined deaths—suicide or accident? *British Journal of Psychiatry*, 133: 542-549.

Hopkins DD, Grant-Worley JA, Fleming DW. 1995. Fatal and nonfatal suicide attempts among adolescents—Oregon, 1988–1993. *Morbidity and Mortality Weekly Report*, 44(16): 312-315; 321-323.

Hosmer D, Lemeshow S. 1989. *Applied Logistic Regression*. New York: Wiley.

Hsieh FY. 1988. Sample size formulae for intervention studies with the cluster as unit of randomization. *Statistics in Medicine*, 7(11): 1195-1201.

Hyman SE. 2000. *Director's Column*. [Online]. Available: http://apu.sfn.org/NL/2000/May-June/articles/director.html [accessed May 10, 2002].

ICRIN (Injury Contol Research Information Network). 2001. *Status of Hospital Discharge E-Coding by State, U.S.* [Online]. Available: http://www.injurycontrol.com/icrin/Ecode%20tracking.htm [accessed April 22, 2002].

Injury prevention and control research and state and community based programs. 2001. Catalog of Federal Domestic Assistance. [Online]. Available: http://aspe.os.dhhs.gov/cfda/P93136.htm [accessed December 19, 2001].

Inskip HM, Harris EC, Barraclough B. 1998. Lifetime risk of suicide for affective disorder, alcoholism and schizophrenia. *British Journal of Psychiatry*, 172: 35-37.

IOM (Institute of Medicine). 1999. Bonnie RJ, Fulco CE, Liverman CT, Editors. *Reducing the Burden of Injury: Advancing Prevention and Treatment*. Washington, DC: National Academy Press.

IOM (Institute of Medicine). 2000. Pellmar TC, Eisenberg L, Editors. *Bridging Disciplines in the Brain, Behavioral, and Clinical Sciences*. Washington, DC: National Academy Press.

IOM (Institute of Medicine). 2001. Nass SJ, Henderson IC, Lashof JC, Editors. *Mammography and Beyond: Developing Technologies for the Early Detection of Breast Cancer*. Washington, DC: National Academy Press.

IPM (National Swedish Institute for Psychosocial Medicine)/Karolinska Institute. 2001. *National Centre for Suicide Research and Prevention of Mental Ill-Health*. [Online]. Available: http://www.ki.se/ipm/enheter/engSui.html [accessed May 10, 2002].

Ivarsson T, Gillberg C, Arvidsson T, Broberg AG. 2002. The Youth Self-Report (YSR) and the Depression Self-Rating Scale (DSRS) as measures of depression and suicidality among adolescents. *European Child and Adolescent Psychiatry*, 11(1): 31-37.

Jansen J. 1990. On the statistical analysis of ordinal data when extravariation is present. *Applied Statistics*, 39: 75-84.

Jenkins J, Sainsbury P. 1980. Single-car road deaths—disguised suicides? *British Medical Journal*, 281(6247): 1041.

Jobes DA, Berman AL, Josselson AR. 1987. Improving the validity and reliability of medical–legal certifications of suicide. *Suicide and Life-Threatening Behavior*, 17(4): 310-325.

Kann L, Kinchen SA, Williams BI, Ross JG, Lowry R, Hill CV, Grunbaum JA, Blumson PS, Collins JL, Kolbe LJ. 1998. Youth Risk Behavior Surveillance—United States, 1997. State and Local YRBSS Coordinators. *Journal of School Health*, 68(9): 355-369.

Kaufman J, Birmaher B, Perel J, Dahl RE, Stull S, Brent D, Trubnick L, al-Shabbout M, Ryan ND. 1998. Serotonergic functioning in depressed abused children: Clinical and familial correlates. *Biological Psychiatry*, 44(10): 973-981.

Keck PE Jr, McElroy SL, Strakowski SM, West SA, Sax KW, Hawkins JM, Bourne ML, Haggard P. 1998. 12-month outcome of patients with bipolar disorder following hospitalization for a manic or mixed episode. *American Journal of Psychiatry*, 155(5): 646-652.

Kelly TM, Mann JJ. 1996. Validity of DSM-III-R diagnosis by psychological autopsy: A comparison with clinician ante-mortem diagnosis. *Acta Psychiatrica Scandinavica*, 94(5): 337-343.

Kessler RC, Borges G, Walters EE. 1999. Prevalence of and risk factors for lifetime suicide attempts in the National Comorbidity Survey. *Archives of General Psychiatry*, 56(7): 617-626.

Knox G. 1964. The detection of space-time interactions. *Applied Statistics*, 3: 25-29.

Kraemer GW, Ebert MH, Schmidt DE, McKinney WT. 1989. A longitudinal study of the effect of different social rearing conditions on cerebrospinal fluid norepinephrine and biogenic amine metabolites in rhesus monkeys. *Neuropsychopharmacology*, 2(3): 175-189.

Lee MA, Ganzini L. 1992. Depression in the elderly: Effect on patient attitudes toward life-sustaining therapy. *Journal of the American Geriatrics Society*, 40: 983-988.

Liang KY, Zeger SL. 1986. Longitudinal data analysis using generalized linear models. *Biometrika*, 73: 13-22.

Linehan MM. 1986. Suicidal people. One population or two? *Annals of the New York Academy of Sciences*, 487: 16-33.

Linehan MM. 1997. Behavioral treatments of suicidal behaviors. Definitional obfuscation and treatment outcomes. *Annals of the New York Academy of Sciences*, 836: 302-328.

Longford NT. 1994. Logistic regression with random coefficients. *Computational Statistics and Data Analysis*, 17: 1-15.

Maudsley G, Williams EM. 1996. "Inaccuracy" in death certification—where are we now? *Journal of Public Health Medicine*, 18(1): 59-66.

McCarthy PD, Walsh D. 1975. Suicide in Dublin: I. The under-reporting of suicide and the consequences for national statistics. *British Journal of Psychiatry*, 126: 301-308.

Miller IW, Norman WH, Bishop SB, Dow MG. 1986. The Modified Scale for Suicidal Ideation: Reliability and validity. *Journal of Consulting and Clinical Psychology*, 54(5): 724-725.

Millon T. 1983. *Millon Clinical Multiaxial Inventory*. 2nd ed. Minneapolis, MN: National Computer Systems.

Mitchell RE. 1982. Social networks and psychiatric clients: The personal and environmental context. *American Journal Community Psychology*, 10(4): 387-401.

Mohandie K, Meloy JR. 2000. Clinical and forensic indicators of "suicide by cop". *Journal of Forensic Sciences*, 45(2): 384-389.

Moscicki EK, O'Carroll P, Rae DS, Locke BZ, Roy A, Regier DA. 1988. Suicide attempts in the Epidemiologic Catchment Area study. *The Yale Journal of Biology and Medicine*, 61: 259-268.

Murphy E, Lindesay J, Grundy E. 1986. 60 years of suicide in England and Wales. A cohort study. *Archives of General Psychiatry*, 43(10): 969-976.

Myers KA, Farquhar DR. 1998. Improving the accuracy of death certification. *Canadian Medical Association Journal*, 158(10): 1317-1323.

Nagelberg J. 1985. *Promoting Population Policy: The Activities of the Rockefeller Foundation, the Ford Foundation and the Population Council: 1959–1966*. Dissertation Abstract, Columbia University.

Nakashima AK, Horsley R, Frey RL, Sweeney PA, Weber JT, Fleming PL. 1998. Effect of HIV reporting by name on use of HIV testing in publicly funded counseling and testing programs. *Journal of the American Medical Association*, 280(16): 1421-1426.

National Bioethics Advisory Commission. 1998. *Research Involving Persons With Mental Disorders That May Affect Decisionmaking Capacity*. Rockville, MD. [Online]. Available: http://www.bioethics.gov/capacity/ TOC.htm [accessed December 19, 2001].

National Bioethics Advisory Commission. 2001. *Ethical and Policy Issues in Research Involving Human Participants*. Rockville, MD. [Online]. Available: http://bioethics.georgetown. edu/nbac/human/overvol1.html [accessed December 19, 2001].

NCHS (National Center for Health Statistics). 1988. *Vital Statistics of the United States, 1985. Volume II. Mortality, Part A*. DHHS publication number (PHS) 88-1101. Washington, DC: US Government Printing Office.

NCI (National Cancer Institute). 2000a. *The Cancer Center Branch of the National Cancer Institute. Policies and Guidelines Relating to the Cancer–Center Support Grant*. [Online]. Available: http://www3.cancer.gov/ cancercenters/download.html [accessed May 10, 2002].

NCI (National Cancer Institute). 2000b. *Fact Book: National Cancer Institute*. Bethesda, MD: U.S. Department of Health and Human Services, National Institutes of Health, Public Health Service. [Online]. Available: http://www.nci.nih.gov/admin/fmb/ Factbook2000.pdf [accessed December 19, 2001].

NCI (National Cancer Institute). 2001a. *Description of the Cancer Centers Program*. [Online]. Available: http://www.nci.nih.gov/cancercenters/description.html [accessed December 19, 2001].

NCI (National Cancer Institute). 2001b. *History of the NCI Cancer Centers*. [Online]. Available: http://www.nci.nih. gov/cancercenters/ccsg_comp_pt1_1to2.html#1history [accessed December 18, 2001].

NCI (National Cancer Institute). 2001c. *Major Policies on Budget*. [Online]. Available: http:// www.nci.nih.gov/ cancercenters/ccsg_comp_pt1_13to15.html#13major [accessed December 19, 2001].

NCIPC (National Center for Injury Prevention and Control). 2002. *Suicide Prevention Research Center. Announcement Number 98067*. [Online]. Available: http://www.cdc.gov/ ncipc/dvp/suinevada.htm [accessed May 9, 2001].

Nelson FL, Farberow NL, MacKinnon DR. 1978. The certification of suicide in eleven western states: An inquiry into the validity of reported suicide rates. *Suicide and Life-Threatening Behavior*, 8(2): 75-88.

NFFIRS (National Fatal Firearm Injury Reporting System) Workgroup. 2001. *Uniform Data Elements: National Fatal Firearm Injury Reporting System. Release 1.1*. [Online]. Available: http://www.hsph.harvard. edu/hicrc/nviss/about_parent_tech.htm [accessed May 14, 2002].

NHTSA (National Highway Traffic Safety Administration). 1996. *Traffic Safety Facts, 1996. Alcohol.* Washington, DC: NHTSA.

NHTSA (National Highway Traffic Safety Administration). 2001. *Fatality Analysis Reporting System.* [Online]. Available: http://www.nhtsa.dot.gov/people/ncsa/fars.html [accessed April 19, 2002].

NIA (National Institute on Aging). 1998. *NIH Guide: Amendment to Alzheimer's Disease Research Centers.* [Online]. Available: http://grants.nih.gov/grants/guide/notice-files/not98-025.html [accessed January 8, 2002].

NIA (National Institute on Aging). 2000. *NIH Guide: Alzheimer's Disease Core Centers.* [Online]. Available: http://grants.nih.gov/grants/guide/rfa-files/RFA-AG-00-002.html [accessed January 8, 2002].

NIDA (National Institute on Drug Abuse). 1999. *Federal Institutes and The Robert Wood Johnson Foundation Create Tobacco Use Research Centers.* [Online]. Available: http://www.nida.nih.gov/MedAdv/99/NR-1018.html [accessed May 10, 2002].

NIMH (National Institute of Mental Health). 1998. *Silvio O. Conte Centers for the Neuroscience of Mental Disorders.* [Online]. Available: http://grants1.nih.gov/grants/guide/pa-files/PAR-98-058.html [accessed May 10, 2002].

NVISS (National Violent Injury Statistics System) Workgroup. 2002. *Violent Death Reporting System Training Manual.* [Online]. Available: http://www.hsph.harvard.edu/hicrc/nviss/about_parent_tech.htm [accessed May 14, 2002].

O'Carroll PW. 1989. A consideration of the validity and reliability of suicide mortality data. *Suicide and Life-Threatening Behavior,* 19(1): 1-16.

O'Carroll PW, Berman AL, Maris RW, Moscicki EK, Tanney BL, Silverman MM. 1996. Beyond the tower of Babel: A nomenclature for suicidology. *Suicide and Life-Threatening Behavior,* 26(3): 237-252.

O'Donnell I, Farmer R. 1995. The limitations of official suicide statistics. *British Journal of Psychiatry,* 166(4): 458-461.

Ohberg A, Lönnqvist J. 1998. Suicides hidden among undetermined deaths. *Acta Psychiatrica Scandinavica,* 98(3): 214-218.

Ovenstone IM. 1973. A psychiatric approach to the diagnosis of suicide and its effect upon the Edinburgh statistics. *British Journal of Psychiatry,* 123(572): 15-21.

Pearson JL, King C, Stanley B, Fisher C. 2000. *Issues to Consider in Intervention Research With Persons at High Risk for Suicidality:* National Institute of Mental Health. [Online] Available: http://www.nimh.nih.gov/research/highrisksuicide.cfm [accessed December 19, 2001].

Pescosolido BA, Mendelsohn R. 1986. Social causation or social construction of suicide? An investigation into the social organization of official rates. *American Sociological Review,* 51(1): 80-100.

Phillips DP, Ruth TE. 1993. Adequacy of official suicide statistics for scientific research and public policy. *Suicide and Life-Threatening Behavior,* 23(4): 307-319.

PHS (Public Health Service). 2001. *National Strategy for Suicide Prevention: Goals and Objectives for Action.* Rockville, MD: U.S. Department of Health and Human Services.

Pine DS, Coplan JD, Wasserman GA, Miller LS, Fried JE, Davies M, Cooper TB, Greenhill L, Shaffer D, Parsons B. 1997. Neuroendocrine response to fenfluramine challenge in boys. Associations with aggressive behavior and adverse rearing. *Archives of General Psychiatry,* 54(9): 839-846.

Reynolds CF 3rd, Degenholtz H, Parker LS, Schulberg HC, Mulsant BH, Post E, Rollman B. 2001. Treatment as usual (TAU) control practices in the PROSPECT Study: Managing the interaction and tension between research design and ethics. *International Journal of Geriatric Psychiatry,* 16(6): 602-608.

Robbins H. 1993. Comparing two treatments under biased allocation. *La Gazette Des Sciences Mathematique De Quebec*, 15: 35-41.

Robbins H, Zhang CH. 1988. Estimating a treatment effect under biased sampling. *Proceedings of the National Academy of Sciences*, 85(11): 3670-3672.

Robbins H, Zhang CH. 1989. Estimating the superiority of a drug to a placebo when all and only those patients at risk are treated with the drug. *Proceedings of the National Academy of Sciences*, 86(9): 3003-3005.

Robbins H, Zhang CH. 1991. Estimating a multiplicative treatment effect under biased allocation. *Biometrika*, 78: 349-354.

Rudd MD, Rajab MH, Orman DT, Joiner T, Stulman DA, Dixon W. 1996. Effectiveness of an outpatient problem-solving intervention targeting suicidal young adults: Preliminary results. *Journal of Consulting and Clinical Psychology*, 64(1): 179-190.

Sainsbury P, Jenkins JS. 1982. The accuracy of officially reported suicide statistics for purposes of epidemiological research. *Journal of Epidemiology and Community Health*, 36(1): 43-48.

Schmidt CW Jr, Shaffer JW, Zlotowitz HI, Fisher RS. 1977. Suicide by vehicular crash. *American Journal of Psychiatry*, 134(2): 175-178.

Shaffer D, Gould MS, Fisher P, Trautman P, Moreau D, Kleinman M, Flory M. 1996. Psychiatric diagnosis in child and adolescent suicide. *Archives of General Psychiatry*, 53: 339-348.

Smith PG. 1982. Spatial and temporal clustering. In: Schottenfeld D, Fraumeni JF, Editors. *Cancer Epidemiology and Prevention*. (pp. 391-407). Philadelphia: WB Saunders.

STIPDA (State and Territorial Injury Prevention Directors Association). 1999. *STIPDA Resolutions: CSTE Position Statement #INJ-6*. [Online]. Available: http://www.stipda.org/resol/99nphss-intent.htm [accessed April 17, 2002].

Telcser SL. 1996. The psychological autopsy study of completed suicide: An experimental test of the impact of knowledge of the suicide upon informants' reports of psychopathology in the victim. Thesis (Ph.D.)—Loyola University of Chicago. *Dissertation Abstracts International*. Vol. 57-03. (pp. 2167).

Ten Have TR. 1996. A mixed effects model for multivariate ordinal response data including correlated failure times with ordinal responses. *Biometrics*, 52: 473-491.

Thomas N, Longford NT, Rolph J. 1992. *A Statistical Framework for Severity Adjustment of Hospital Mortality Rates*. Working paper. Santa Monica, CA: RAND.

University of Hamburg. 2000. *Center for Therapy and Studies of Suicidal Behavior*. [Online]. Available: http://www.uke.uni-hamburg.de/Clinics/Psych/TZS/TZS_e.html [accessed May 10, 2002].

University of Michigan. 2002. *Introduction to PSC (Population Studies Center)*. [Online]. Available: http://www.psc.isr.umich.edu/intro.html [accessed May 10, 2002].

University of North Carolina. 2001. *UNC Injury Prevention Research Center: Funding Description*. [Online]. Available: http://www.sph.unc.edu/iprc/aboutiprc/description.html [accessed December 19, 2001].

University of Oxford. 2002. *Centre for Suicide Research*. [Online]. Available: http://cebmh.warne.ox.ac.uk/csr/ [accessed May 10, 2002].

University of Rochester. 2001. Suicide study awarded $3.2 million. *Currents*, 29(21): [Online]. Available: http://www.rochester.edu/pr/Currents/V29/V29N21/story04.html [accessed May 10, 2002].

University of the Philippines. 2002. *Population Institute*. [Online]. Available: http://www.geocities.com/popinst/ [accessed May 10, 2002].

Velting DM, Shaffer D, Gould MS, Garfinkel R, Fisher P, Davies M. 1998. Parent-victim agreement in adolescent suicide research. *Journal of American Academy of Child and Adolescent Psychiatry*, 37(11): 1161-1166.

Wagenaar AC. 1993. Research affects public policy: The case of the legal drinking age in the United States. *Addiction*, 88(Supplement): S75-S81.

Wallenstein S, Gould M, Kleinman M. 1989. Use of the scan statistic to detect time-space clustering. *American Journal of Epidemiology*, 130: 1057-1064.

Washington Department of Health. 1997. New statewide system tracks firearm-related injuries to gather information for prevention strategies. *EpiTrends*, 2(3): 1-2.

Washington University. 2001. *Washington University Researchers Launch Silvio Conte Center.* [Online]. Available: http://medicine.wustl.edu/~wumpa/news/2001/conte.html [accessed May 10, 2002].

Wasserman D, Varnik A. 1998. Reliability of statistics on violent death and suicide in the former USSR, 1970-1990. *Acta Psychiatrica Scandinavica Supplement*, 394: 34-41.

Wolfgang ME. 1958. An analysis of homicide–suicide. *Journal of Clinical and Experimental Psychopathology*, 19: 208-218.

Zeger SL, Liang KY. 1986. Longitudinal data analysis for discrete and continuous outcomes. *Biometrics*, 42(1): 121-130.

To be, or not to be: that is the Question:
Whether 'tis Nobler in the Mind to suffer
The Slings and Arrows of outrageous Fortune,
Or to take Arms against a Sea of Troubles,
And by opposing end them; to die to sleep
No more, and by a Sleep to say we end
The Hart-ache, and the thousand Natural Shocks
That Flesh is heir to; 'tis a Consummation
Devoutly to be wish'd to die to sleep,
To Sleep, perchance to dream; ay there's the Rub,
For in that Sleep of Death what Dreams may Come . . .

—WILLIAM SHAKESPEARE
Hamlet, Act III, scene I.

11

Findings and Recommendations

ENHANCING THE INFRASTRUCTURE

Over 80 million people in the United States are at risk for suicide due to mental illness and substance use disorders; about 30,000 Americans each year die by suicide. It is estimated that the cost to society in lost productivity each year is approximately $11 billion. Yet, suicide has a low base-rate, approximately 11 individuals per 100,000 per year, which makes clinical investigation difficult. While this report discusses the wealth of knowledge about the risk and protective factors for suicide and promising treatments and prevention programs, important research gaps exist in the understanding of suicide and suicidal behavior. Most studies are cross-sectional or retrospective. Data are weakened by the constraint of using proximal endpoints instead of completed suicide and by inaccurate reporting of suicide and suicide attempts. The low base rate of suicide necessitates studies in large sub-populations to have adequate power to provide significant results. Most efforts to date have been disciplinary, single level approaches, limited by funding. To make fundamental advances requires a different scientific approach that will ensure a higher level of scientific rigor, integrate multiple levels of research, provide reliable national and international data on current rates of suicidal behavior and key risk and protective factors, and create the infrastructure for testing treatment and preventive interventions and implementing and institutionalizing the effective strategies. The following sections will briefly review the scientific gaps that are discussed throughout the report and will present a vision for a solution.

Magnitude of the Problem

Yearly, there are almost 30,000 reported suicides in the United States and a million worldwide. However, suicide rates are underestimates because of the lack of internationally accepted case definition and uniform ascertainment methods. Moreover, data are lacking on changing profiles of mental disorders and social factors associated with changes in suicide rates over time. Suicide attempt prevalence has been determined in some national epidemiological studies, but no data on changing rates are available in the United States. Suicide attempt rates estimated from cases presenting to emergency rooms or health care professionals are a significant underestimate of true rates. Because longitudinal studies are lacking, incidence cannot be estimated from existing data sets. Thus, accurate rates of suicide and particularly suicide attempts are not available at a national level. Data gathering must consider ethnic and social subgroups, including cross-cultural groups, in which rates may be strikingly different and where risk and protective factors may differ in relative importance.

Risk and Protective Factors

Biological, psychological, and cultural factors all have a significant impact on the risk of suicide in any individual. Risk factors associated with suicide include serious mental illness, alcohol and drug abuse, childhood abuse, loss of a loved one, joblessness and loss of economic security, and other cultural and societal influences. Resiliency and coping skills, on the other hand, can reduce the risk of suicide. Social support, including close relationships, is a protective factor.

However, knowledge regarding the relative importance of risk and protective factors is limited, and we are far from being able to integrate these factors in order to understand how they work in concert to evoke suicidal behavior or to prevent it. Where such knowledge is emerging, the results are difficult to generalize because of a lack of population level data. Without a combination of a population-based approach and studies at the level of the individual patient within higher risk sub-groups, macro-social trends cannot be related to biomedical measures. Most existing studies are retrospective or cross-sectional, involve a few correlates, and do not address prediction of risk. Without specific data from well-defined and characterized populations whose community level social descriptives are well-known, normative behavior and abnormality cannot be estimated.

Treatment and Prevention

Pharmacotherapy and psychotherapy can be effective in preventing suicide. Continued contact with a health care provider has been shown to be effective in reducing the risk of suicide, especially in the early weeks after discharge from a hospital. However, psychological autopsy studies and toxicological analyses indicate that many people who complete suicides are not under treatment for mental illness at the time of death. Accurate information on treatment utilization by persons at risk for suicidal behavior, efficacy or effectiveness of existing interventions and cost of treatment are not possible without accurate assessment of suicidal behaviors. Data on the reasons for under-treatment must be used to design corrective programs.

Several prevention programs have been developed that look promising. However, many prevention programs do not have the long-term funding that would allow them to assess reduction in the completion of suicide as an endpoint. The low base rate of suicide, combined with the short duration of assessment and the relatively small populations under study make it difficult to acquire sufficient power for such trials. As described in Chapter 10, to assess the incidence of suicide in a general population where the rates are between 5 and 15 per 100,000 with a 90 percent confidence requires almost 100,000 participants. These populations can only be recruited through large nationally coordinated efforts.

Population Perspectives

Extensive epidemiological data describe the suicide rates among various populations. The rates of suicide in the United States are exceptionally high in white males over 75 years of age, Native Americans, and certain professions, including dentists. Studies from across the world find higher rates of suicide in rural areas as compared to urban ones. Much is known about the general trends, but no data set provides a picture of evolving risk and protective factors at the national level. Globally, a million suicides are estimated to occur each year, but there is no coordinated effort to understand responsible factors or reduce the death toll. Major changes in rates of youth suicide remain unexplained. Population laboratories could provide data on a much larger population.

While each center might be able to obtain a sufficiently large sample for studies in the general population, a consortium of centers will be necessary to fully explore differences based on region, economic environment, culture, urbanization, and other factors that vary across the country. Furthermore, certain subpopulations may be sufficiently small or low risk to require broader recruitment than one center could access. For these reasons, multiple centers would be optimal to enhance the science of suicide. The integration of data across laboratories can provide an ongoing picture of the key factors influencing national suicide rates such that studies of risk and protective factors can be optimized, and permit rational prevention and treatment planning. The national impact of treatment and prevention interventions shown to be effective within a network can be estimated. This will permit translation into national implementation, and with systematic cross-cultural comparisons, global extension of United States studies would become more feasible.

Vision for a Solution: National Network of Population Laboratories

To obtain optimal data for the understanding, prevention, and treatment of suicide and suicidal behavior, a large population base is essential. The committee proposes a coordinated network of Population Laboratories that would allow stratified and repeated longitudinal surveys to provide more accurate data on rates of suicidal behavior, as well as long-term data on ethnographic, social, psychiatric, biological, and genetic measures necessary for increased success in prevention. Data on diagnoses associated with suicides would be obtained through the psychological autopsy method by the population laboratories for all suicides within their population, which would be enriched by highly focused ethnography. Similarly, data would be obtained on suicide attempts in the course of stratified population surveys that would be more complete than that obtained from reports generated from emergency rooms or health care providers. Thus, the population laboratory rates would correct underestimations of national rates through these registries of suicides and attempted suicides. The population laboratories would be the source of data on rates of suicidal ideation. Accurate ascertainment is essential for measurement of relative impact of risk and protective factors, and of preventive interventions.

Drawing smaller samples from these large population centers will allow the examination of risk and protective factors in far greater specificity. Multiple risk factors must be measured in the same high-risk group by multi-disciplinary groups of scientists to determine their interaction as well as their relative importance. This differs from the overwhelmingly typical approach of measuring only a few risk or protective factors in unrepresentative convenience samples. Sampling from within population laboratories allows measurement of generalizability. Deliberate sampling within ethnic and social subgroups as well as from groups with specific mental disorders can generate data applicable to at-risk groups all over the United States. In the course of obtaining data on completed suicides, the population laboratories can collect tissue samples from each individual that can be used for toxicological screens, biochemical analyses, and genetic research.

Finally, data on treatment utilization and barriers to treatment can be obtained at a population level and related to those considered to be at risk for suicidal behavior. A longitudinal data gathering strategy will be more powerful than a cross-sectional approach. A population-based approach is well suited for testing public health interventions. A sub-population high-risk group is best suited for randomized treatment studies that test efficacy at the level of the individual patient, and such studies can be feasibly extended to comparison studies in the developing world.

To address the problem of suicide effectively will require an integrated approach in which experts from many disciplines come together to tackle the problem. Only with such an interdisciplinary effort can a full understanding of the complex nature of suicide be obtained. And only through this full understanding can effective interventions be designed. A coordinated network of laboratories provides the infrastructure in which the many disciplines can be united. An interdisciplinary center also provides a) opportunities for training new scientists to think broadly about suicide and b) incentives to recruit established scientists to apply their expertise to this important area.

Because of the multidisciplinary nature of research on suicidal behavior, multiple federal agencies, foundations, and the pharmaceutical industry have a stake in enhancing the science and reducing the risk of suicide. The public health significance of suicidal behavior has been underscored by the World Health Organization and the United States Surgeon General and validates a substantial financial commitment to fostering biomedical research and improving the health of the public. The nation's experience and benefit from funding multiple Alzheimer Disease Research Centers, as well as centers of excellence in cancer, provides a useful precedent and analog for this initiative.

The committee believes that, to have a large public health impact, a network of Population Laboratories in the United States will be necessary. The longitudinal dimension of the proposed studies, necessary to provide a picture of the evolving rates of suicidal behaviors and of risk and protective factors, requires a 10-year funding period. The committee believes that population laboratories will eventually provide models of "reduced-suicide zones" that will have great benefit to public health.

Recommendation 1

The National Institute of Mental Health (in collaboration with other agencies) should develop and support a national network of suicide research Population Laboratories devoted to interdisciplinary research

on suicide and suicide prevention across the life cycle. The network of Population Laboratories should be administered by NIMH and funded through partnerships among federal agencies and private sources, including foundations. Very large study samples of at least 100,000 are necessary because of the relatively low frequency of suicide in the general public. A number of Population Laboratories (e.g., 5–10) are necessary to capture the data for numerous and complex interacting variables including the profound effects of demographics, region, culture, socioeconomic status, race, and ethnicity. Extending the efforts into the international arena where cultural differences are large may provide new information and can be fostered and guided by such global organizations as the World Health Organization and the World Bank and by the Fogarty International Center at NIH.

◆ **The network should be equipped to perform safe, high-quality, large-sample, multi-site studies on suicide and suicide prevention.**
   ❖ Each Laboratory would have a population base of approximately 100,000. At a base-rate of 10–12 suicides per 100,000 people, this population base of the network would significantly improve the available data for estimates of suicide incidence, capacity for longitudinal studies, development of brain repositories, access to representative samples for prevention and intervention studies, and studies of genetic risk for suicide. Several such laboratories would provide adequate data to assess the numerous and complex interacting variables including the profound effects of demographics, regions, culture, socioeconomic status, race, and ethnicity. Coordination and collaboration among centers should be encouraged to further enhance the breadth of the database.
   ❖ The laboratories would cover an ethnically and socially diverse and representative population and would recruit higher risk individuals and subgroups in communities within the population laboratories for longitudinal and more detailed studies.
   ❖ Treatment and prevention studies would be carried out in high-risk patients recruited from within the population laboratories.
   ❖ With these defined populations, the centers would conduct prospective studies—integrating biological, psychosocial, ethnographic, and ethical dimensions—that would be of great importance in advancing science and meeting public health needs. These studies would include such initiatives as identified in the committee report:

Intervention and Prevention Research

   Testing of promising programs at multiple sites with long term follow-up. It is critical to determine whether an intervention can be generalized to other sites. Long-term assessments are important for evaluation of the impact of interventions on suicide and suicide attempts rather than more proximal measures.

Intervention studies to evaluate means and effectiveness of promoting greater continuity of care, treatment adherence, and access to emergency services because patients recently discharged from inpatient care are among those at highest risk for suicide. Descriptive studies to identify markers for increased risk should aid in the design of intervention studies to decrease risk.

Psychological Risk and Protective Factors

Clinical trials on the specific effects of reducing hopelessness on suicide. Hopelessness is related to suicidality across age, diagnoses, and severity of disorder, yet the field lacks research on the pathways to hopelessness, interrelationships between hopelessness and other psychological aspects of suicide risk, and on the specific effects of reducing hopelessness on suicide.

Treatment Research

Carefully designed trials to understand the potential of pharmacotherapies to reduce suicidal behavior. Studies should include the antidepressants, anticonvulsants, lithium, and clozapine. The lack of long-term assessment of therapeutic strategies and the exclusion of high-risk patient from clinical trials represent critical gaps in the field.

Controlled clinical trials to determine the types and aspects of psychotherapy that are effective in reducing suicide for diverse individuals. Current evidence suggests that continued contact with a psychotherapist is critical. This needs to be rigorously evaluated.

Neurobiology

Longitudinal, prospective studies of the influence of HPA axis function on suicidality. The utility of assessing HPA axis function as a physiological screening tool for suicide risk should be explored. Medical and psychosocial treatments that attenuate HPA dysregulation should be further developed and tested for their efficacy in reducing suicide.

Biological predictors of suicidal behavior should be sought through brain mapping studies. Prospective, rather than cross-sectional studies, are crucial. Analyses *in vivo* would allow the examination of changes over time to elucidate response to treatment and remission from episodes of mental illness. Moreover, brain mapping studies may help to identify individuals at risk for suicidal behavior.

Molecular and Population Genetics

Genetic samples from psychiatric populations should be studied to examine the relationship between genetic markers and suicidal behavior. Genetic isolates (i.e., populations that have had few or no new genes added from outsiders for many generations) with a high rate of suicide and suicidal behavior should be identified for linkage studies. Studies searching for genes associated with suicidal behavior should be undertaken.

The relationship between suicide and aggression/impulsivity requires additional attention, particularly regarding its developmental etiology and genetic linkages. Genetic markers that have functional significance and correlate with impulsive aggression and suicidal behavior cross-sectionally may have the potential to identify individuals at risk and to suggest new molecular targets for treatment.

Clinical Epidemiology

Prospective studies of populations at high risk for the onset of suicidal behavior, such as the offspring of suicide completers or attempters, can allow for studies of neurobiologic, genetic, and non-genetic factors that predict the onset of suicidal behavior.

Interdisciplinary research that weaves together biological, cognitive, and social effects of trauma to elucidate the complex pathways from childhood trauma to mental illness and/or suicidality and thereby elucidate multiple possibilities for intervention.

Services Research

Research on the peri-hospital period to assess the risk and protective effects of hospitalization, the relationships between length of stay and outcomes, and the factors post-hospital that account for the increased risk for suicide would provide critical information for suicide reduction strategies. The efficacy of different approaches to follow-up care in reducing suicide across populations must also be established, and successful interventions should be replicated and widely disseminated.

Longitudinal research to assess outcomes of prophylactic/short-term versus maintenance/long-term treatment for suicidality. The course of suicidality across the life span suggests it may at times represent a lifelong condition requiring sustained treatment; further life-course research is required to verify this.

Economic and Cultural Studies

Interactions of genetics, psychosocial, socio-political, and socioeconomic context. The field requires interdisciplinary, multi-level research on the impact of individual and aggregate level variables on suicide. Contrasts among international suicide data also offer important insights into the influence of cultural/macro-social contexts on suicide. Ethnographic research and other qualitative methods to obtain greater detail about the setting, conditions, process, and outcome of suicide. These approaches should be developed to deepen and to increase the validity of psychological autopsy studies and prevention outcome studies.

◆ Funding should be provided for the necessary infrastructure for these centers. This should include support for dedicated full time staff at NIH to provide long-term (at least 10 years) continuity and consistency in these efforts. Furthermore, funding for centers should include support for the following:

❖ Population cores to coordinate the social science, ethnographic data and to maintain registries of deaths by suicide and suicide attempts.

❖ Pathology cores to maintain the repositories for tissue samples from suicide victims.

❖ Statistical cores to manage the databases on risk and protective factors including genetic markers and cultural contexts.

❖ Clinical cores to recruit patients and to ensure their safe and ethical treatment.

❖ Research efforts that encompass both program projects and individual projects. Centers should encourage collaborations across the centers and facilitate the sharing of data maintained by the cores.

◆ In an effort to recruit excellent scientists to research in suicide, supported sites should develop training programs, to provide local and distance mentoring, to attract new investigators from a wide variety of disciplines into the field, and to form research and research training partnerships with developed and developing countries.

ENHANCING THE DATABASE ON SUICIDE

Because suicide is a low base-rate event, special efforts are needed to ensure collection of sufficient data to allow meaningful analysis of risk factors and interventions. Long-term studies of suicidal behavior are potentially uniquely informative. Long-term studies such as the Framingham study offer populations that are studied over a long duration and from a variety of biological, behavioral, and sociological perspectives. Studies such as these provide an ideal opportunity to explore suicidal behavior prospectively if the correct measures and outcomes are incorporated. Managed care databases also offer unique opportunities to examine the development of suicidal behavior and the relationship between health behaviors, practice variation, and suicidal outcomes. Suicidal behaviors are likely much more common than generally thought, as found with child abuse and neglect (National Research Council report on Understanding Child Abuse and Neglect, 1993). Including measures of suicidality in ongoing long-term studies will broaden the understanding of the dimensions of the problem. Furthermore, addressing suicidality in these large studies would benefit the public by directing at-risk individuals to appropriate care.

As described in Chapter 10, exclusion of suicidal patients from clinical trials has serious repercussions. Analysis of the few trials that include suicidal participants reveals that only those studies that included high risk patients were able to demonstrate significant effects of an intervention. Currently, clinical trials exclude participants who exhibit suicidality. Suicidal participants can be included in clinical trials with appropriate safeguards consistent with the highest standards of human subjects' protection. Including suicidal participants in clinical trials is a critical step to improving the outcome of suicidal individuals by providing an evidence-base for treatment protocols. Such studies should be conducted with research designs and measures that touch on the etiopathogenesis of suicidal behaviors, as described throughout this report.

Surveillance is a cornerstone of public health, allowing realistic priority setting, the design of effective prevention initiatives, and the ability to evaluate such programs (Institute of Medicine report on Reducing the Burden of Injury, 1999). Non-uniformity in reporting suicide across jurisdictions introduces inaccuracies into data on prevalence and confounds the analysis of risk and protective factors. Ideally, coroners and medical examiners should receive uniform training to standardize diagnosis and information about suicide. However, given the limitations of funding, jurisdictional purview, and the influences of stigma and religion, the committee recognizes that this is unlikely to happen soon. The quality of data for suicide attempts is even less reliable than for completed suicides. The need for improved and expanded surveillance systems for suicide is highlighted as one of the central goals of the National Strategy for Suicide Prevention. National surveillance programs for HIV/AIDS and for motor vehicle deaths are currently in place and provide nationwide data that help form policies for prevention (see Chapter 10). Currently no such national program for suicide deaths or attempts exist. The National Violent Death Reporting System provides a promising framework that might be expanded into a national program that would provide the database for suicide deaths. The Oregon State Adolescent Suicide Attempt Data System is one of a few mechanisms that might inform the creation of a national system for reporting suicide attempts. Issues of confidentiality are a concern for surveillance of suicide as they are for HIV/AIDS. However, CDC found that reporting through a name-based system did not impact rates of testing for HIV/AIDS. As state and pilot programs have shown, there are options available that are sensitive to confidentiality yet allow the benefits of a reporting system (see Chapter 10). The committee is strongly committed to the principle of confidentiality and would urge that implementation of surveillance programs be done in a manner that respects the privacy of the individual and their families and communities. Yet examples exist of reporting systems that deal effectively with this issue. Consequently the committee sees no fundamental reason why these approaches cannot be applied to the reporting of suicide and suicide attempts.

Recommendation 2

National monitoring of suicide and suicidality should be improved. Steps toward improvement should include the following:

◆ **Funding agencies (including NIMH, NIA, NICHD, NIDA, NIAAA, CDC, SAMHSA and DVA) should encourage that measures of suicidality (e.g., attempts) be included in all large and/or long-term studies of health behaviors, mental health interventions, and genetic studies of mental disorder. Funding agencies should issue program announcements for supplements to ongoing longitudinal studies to include the collection and analysis of these additional measures.**

❖ **Suicidal patients should be included in clinical trials when appropriate safeguards are in place.**

❖ **A national suicide attempt surveillance system should be developed and coordinated through the CDC.** It might be developed as part of a broader injury reporting database. Modeled after Oregon's program for the reporting of adolescent suicide attempts and the HIV/AIDS registry, pilot programs should be developed, tested, and implemented as soon as feasible. State participation should be encouraged by requiring reporting as a prerequisite for receiving funding for related programs.

◆ **Federal funding should be provided to support a surveillance system such as the National Violent Death Reporting System that includes**

data on mortality from suicide. The system should have sufficient funding to support a national effort. CDC would be the most appropriate agency to coordinate this database given their experience with HIV/AIDS surveillance. Efforts to create such registries in other countries should be encouraged and, where feasible, assisted.

ENHANCING IDENTIFICATION OF
THOSE AT RISK FOR SUICIDE

In the United States, over 90 percent of completed suicides are associated with psychiatric diagnoses, yet single psychiatric diagnoses have low relative risk for suicide. Converging data indicate that *some portion* of risk for suicide is separable from these disorders. These data include: differential treatment effects for other symptoms associated with the disorder versus suicidality, differential heritability, ante- and post-mortem biological markers associated with suicide across psychiatric diagnoses, and psychological factors associated with suicidality across diagnoses.

Converging evidence across disciplines indicates that suicide is related to stress: developmental and adult trauma; cumulative stressors, including multiple morbidities; acute and chronic social and cultural stressors; and capacity to cope with stress. Suicide can be considered an expected outcome of a significant subgroup of mentally ill patients who experience accumulative life stresses, just as cardiac infarction is an expected outcome of untreated high blood cholesterol. The committee finds that mental illnesses are potentially fatal and that suicide is the most common cause of premature mortality in this group. This context for death from suicide conveys less blame for the physician and might be expected to lower the barriers to aggressive treatment, prevention, and reporting of suicide and its risk factors.

While much more needs to be learned about the processes leading to suicide detection and prevention, it is clear that existing knowledge and new findings are not adequately disseminated and practiced in the primary care and mental health professions. Case identification and treatment for those at risk of suicide is a serious problem. Although suicides in the United States are associated with a diagnosis of a mental illness, only about a third of those with mental illness receive services. The committee recognizes that several barriers exist to obtaining such treatment, including stigma, limited insurance coverage, and fragmentation of services. On the other hand, a significant proportion of those who do complete suicide visit a non-mental health clinician within the last month or even week of their lives. The committee finds that there is an important role for the primary care and mental health care providers as well as providers for special high-risk populations (e.g., aged, adolescents, and incarcerated individuals) in the identification and referral of patients with suicidal intent.

Many risk factors for suicide can be uncovered during a visit with a primary care physician. Depression is associated with a significant risk of suicide. Substance abuse, history of physical or sexual abuse, conduct disorder, and aggression/impulsivity also suggest greater risk of suicide, especially in combination. In addition, social and cultural contexts, such as family discord, economic hardship, and social isolation, deserve attention. Multiple concurrent risk factors increase the risk of suicide and should be heeded. Access to the means for suicide should also be noted.

Screening for suicidality would benefit from improved assessment tools. Currently available tools are inadequate to determine acute suicide risk or to predict when a person will attempt or complete suicide (see Chapter 7). Assessment tools may be specific only for the populations for which they were developed. Despite the limitations, tools for detection or risk assessment can be an important component of treatment when used appropriately.

Recommendation 3

Because primary care providers are often the first and only medical contact of suicidal patients, tools for recognition and screening of patients should be developed and disseminated. Furthermore, since over half of suicides occur in populations receiving treatment for mental disorders, it is critical to enhance the capacity of mental health professionals to recognize and address both chronic and acute suicide risk factors.

◆ **NIMH and other funding agencies should provide funds to clinical researchers to develop and evaluate screening tools that assess risk factors for suicide** such as substance use, history of abuse and/or trauma, involvement with the criminal justice system, mental illness, psychological and personality traits such as impulsivity and hopelessness, abnormal neurobiology or genetic markers, employment problems, bereavement and other relationship stresses, etc. Funding agencies should issue program announcements to encourage efforts in this area.

◆ **Physicians should refer patients with multiple risk factors to consultation with a mental health professional.** This should be standard in the same way finding high blood cholesterol levels dictates further medical and behavioral interventions. This will only be effective if the issue of parity is addressed and insurance benefits are expanded adequately to cover mental health care.

◆ **Professional medical organizations should provide training to health care providers for assessment of suicide risk and provide them with existing tools.** Mental health professional associations should encourage (or require, when appropriate) their memberships to increase their skills in suicide risk detection and intervention. National, state, county, and city public health organizations should build on their existing infrastructure to facilitate suicide screening especially in high-risk populations.

◆ **Medical and nursing schools should incorporate the study of suicidal behavior into their curricula or expand existing education.**

◆ **NIMH and Agency for Health Care Research and Quality (AHRQ) should work with physician associations including American College of Physicians, American College of Family Physicians, American Academy of Pediatricians, American Society of Internal Medicine to implement these recommendations.** In addition, through their health services research funds they should support efforts to improve approaches to identifying and treating those at risk.

ENHANCING PREVENTION AND INTERVENTIONS

As the Surgeon General's Call to Action states, prevention of suicide should be a national priority. The severity of the suicide problem nationally and globally demands that prevention programs be developed. Research is needed to rigorously test approaches at all levels of intervention. Successful experimental programs need to be expanded to larger populations. And effective approaches need to be implemented.

There are examples of promising universal, selective, and indicated interventions. Programs that integrate prevention at multiple levels are likely to be the most effective. Comprehensive, integrated state and national prevention strategies that target suicide risk and barriers to treatment across levels and domains appear to reduce suicide. Evaluation of such programs remains challenging given the multitude of variables on the individual and aggregate levels that interact to affect suicide rates. The value of intervention programs is frequently difficult to assess because of their short duration, inadequate control populations, and limited long-term follow up. Lack of adequate planning and funding for evaluation have seriously hampered prevention efforts.

Universal programs broadly blanketing a school or community have been shown to be effective in reducing suicide rates. For example, the Air Force's prevention program removed barriers; increased knowledge, attitudes, and competencies within that community; and increased access to help and support with a consequent decrease in suicide rates. Reducing the availability or the lethality of a method (such as using blister packs for pills or enacting stricter gun control laws) results in a decline in suicide by that method; method substitution does not invariably occur. Education of the media regarding appropriate reporting of suicides can change reporting practices. Such changes seem to reduce suicide in certain contexts but the data are limited.

Interventions that target groups with a greater likelihood of suicide (selective prevention measures) have also been shown to be effective. Screening programs, gatekeeper training programs, support/skills training groups, and school-based crisis response teams/plans can create a coordinated effort that identifies youth at suicide-risk and provides individual follow-up.

Indicated interventions directed toward individuals at high risk for suicide include medical and psychosocial approaches. Suicide is far more likely to occur in the first month after discharge from a psychiatric hospital than subsequently. Low treatment adherence poses a major risk factor for suicidal individuals. Long-term follow-up care of discharged suicidal individuals holds promise for reducing suicide. Controlling the underlying mental illness through pharmacology and psychotherapy is an important indicated prevention approach. Medication alone is not sufficient treatment for suicidality. Psychotherapy provides a necessary therapeutic relationship that reduces the risk of suicide. Cognitive-behavioral approaches that include problem-solving therapy appear to reduce suicidal ideation and attempts. However, major obstacles to utilizing these resources exist, including doctor–patient communication barriers, limitations on insurance or financing, and stigma of mental illness.

Providing skills and support for youth at risk through school programs appears to show promise. Optimism and coping skills, which enhance both mental and physical health, can be taught. Universal, selective, and indicated prevention programs that provide skills training reduce hopelessness. School-based programs employing a health promotion approach have been shown to effectively prevent and/or reduce suicide risk factors and correlates like adolescent pregnancy, delinquency, substance abuse, and depression. These programs also promote protective factors against suicide including self-efficacy, interpersonal problem solving, self-esteem, and social support. The data are limited, however, on the effectiveness of these programs to reduce completed suicides. Yet the known benefits and the links between these skills and suicide provide a logical rationale for recommending pilot studies in this area. Some international programs (see Chapter 8) have implemented similar efforts and it will be important to learn from their experiences.

Recommendation 4

Programs for suicide prevention should be developed, tested, expanded, and implemented through funding from appropriate agencies including NIMH, DVA, CDC, and SAMHSA.

◆ **Partnerships should be formed among federal, state, and local agencies to implement effective suicide prevention programs.** Collaboration should be sought with professional organizations (including the American Psychiatric Association, the American Psychological Association) and non-profit organizations dedicated to the prevention of suicide (such as the American Foundation for the Prevention of Suicide or the American Association of Suicidology). NIMH and SAMHSA should work with the Department of Education and the Administration on Aging to encourage national programs for youth and elderly populations.

◆ **Programs that have shown success within select populations should be expanded.** For example, the Air Force program should be adopted by hierarchical organizations that employ groups with increased suicide rates, including police and rescue workers. Gatekeeper training programs and screening programs for youth and elderly should be implemented more broadly within work and educational settings to identify and intervene with those at suicide-risk. There should be a systemic identification of high suicide risk groups for targeted intervention.

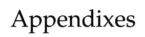

Appendixes

A

Statistical Details

One can naturally model the unobserved population heterogeneity or extra-population heterogeneity via mixture models. The simplest and most natural occurrence of the mixture model arises when one samples from a super population g which is a mixture of a finite number, say m, of populations $(g_1, ..., g_m)$, called the *components* of the population. Suppose a sample from a super population g is recorded as data (Y_i, J_i) for $i = 1, ...,$ n, where $Y_i = y_i$ is a measurement on the ith sampled unit and $J_i = j_i$ indicates the index number of the component to which the unit belongs. If sampling is done from the jth component, an appropriate probability model for the sampling distribution is given by

$$P(Y_i = y_i | J_i = j) = f_j(y_i; \theta_j)$$

The function $f_j(y_i; \theta_j)$ represents a density function, called the *component density* for the ith observation y_i and the parameter $\theta_j \in \Theta_j \subset \Re^{d_j}$ called the *component parameter*, that describes the specific attributes of the jth component population, g_j.

We treat the J_i as missing data and define the *latent random variable* $\Phi = (\Phi_1, ..., \Phi_n)$ to be the values of the parameter $\theta \in \{\theta_1, ..., \theta_m\}$ corresponding to the sampled components $J_1, ..., J_n$; i.e., if the ith observation came from the jth component, then define $\Phi_i = \theta_j$. Then the Φ_i are a random sample from the discrete probability measure Q that assigns a positive probability π_j to the support point θ_j for $j = 1, ..., m$. That is, the latent random variable Φ has a distribution Q, which is called the *mixing distribution*, defined by $P(\Phi = \theta_j) = Q(\{\theta_j\}) = \pi_j$. Thus the mixing distribution

$$Q = \begin{pmatrix} \theta_1 & \cdots & \theta_m \\ \pi_1 & \cdots & \pi_m \end{pmatrix}$$

puts a mass (or weight) of π_j on each parameter θ_j. We thus arrive at the *mixture distribution* $g(y_i; Q) = \sum_{j=1}^{m} Q(\{\theta_j\}) f_j(y_i; \theta_j)$, or equivalently

$$g(y_i; \theta, \pi) = \sum_{j=1}^{m} \pi_j f_j(y_i; \theta_j).$$

One can find the posterior probability that the ith observation comes from the jth component (i.e, $y_i \in G_j$) using

$$\tau_{ij} = \frac{\pi_j f_j(y_i; \theta_j)}{g(y_i; \theta, \pi)}.$$

In turn, one can assign each y_i to the population to which it has the highest estimated posterior probability of belonging; i.e., to G_j if $\tau_{ij} > \tau_{it}$ for $t = 1$, ..., m and $t \neq j$.

Estimation of the Parameters and the Mixture Components

One has to estimate the number of subpopulations or number of mixture components m as well as the parameters in the mixture distribution $g...$). This can be achieved via parametric or non-parametric maximum likelihood estimation (Laird, 1978; Böhning et al. 1992, Pilla and Lindsay, 2001). Laird (1978) considered nonparametric likelihood estimation of a mixing distribution and Lindsay (1983) linked its general theory, developed from a study of the geometry of the mixture likelihood, to the problem of estimating a discrete mixing distribution. One may also use an alternative approach to maximum likelihood for which menu driven software is provided by Böhning et al. (1998).

For a given m, one can estimate the parameters in the mixture distribution via the EM algorithm (Dempster et al. 1977) and several improvements of it which are discussed in McLachlan and Krishnan (1997). Let $\hat{\phi}$ = ($\hat{\pi}, \hat{\theta}$) be the vector of estimated parameters. Once $\hat{\phi}$ has been obtained, estimates of the posterior probability of population membership $\hat{\tau}_{ij}$ can be formed for each y_i to give a probabilistic clustering.

When m, the number of mixtures, is large, the EM algorithm can be excruciatingly slow. In that case, one can use alternative EM methods proposed by Pilla (1997) and Pilla and Lindsay (2001) in the nonparametric mixture setting. Their approach assumes that the θ's are known and the goal is to estimate the π's only. However, by setting up the problem in a nonparametric framework, one may find the maximum likelihood estimator (MLE) quite easily in a high-dimensional problem via Pilla and Lindsay's method. These methods are especially useful because $\theta_1 < \theta_2 < \dots$, i.e., the support points are ordered and hence the corresponding nearby densities can be paired to take advantage of the correlated densities.

Mixture Setting for Detecting Spatial Occurrence of Suicide

Suppose data are available on the spatial occurrence of suicide in N counties in a state or for the entire country over a five year period. Assume that the counties are a mixture of two groups $\mathcal{G}_1$ and $\mathcal{G}_2$, corresponding to normal and high risk with respect to suicide, in proportions of π_1 and π_2 respectively. The number of events y_i in the ith county is assumed to have a Poisson distribution with a rate of μ_j in $\mathcal{G}_j$ for $j = 1, 2; i = 1, \dots, n$. Let $\phi = (\mu_1, \mu_2, \pi_1, \pi_2)^T$ and $\theta_i = (\mu_1 N_i, \mu_2 N_i)^T$, where $N_i = M_i\, t_i$ is the mass of population at risk in the ith county assuming that there are M_i individuals at risk over time t_i. In this scenario, the log likelihood becomes

$$\log L(\phi; \boldsymbol{y}) = \sum_{i=1}^{n} \log \sum_{j=1}^{2} \pi_j f_j(y_i;\, \theta_i),$$

where $f_j(y_i;\, \theta_i) = exp(-\mu_j N_i)\, (\mu_j N_i)^{y_i}/y_i!$. One can use the EM algorithm to find the MLE of the parameters. The complete data log likelihood function becomes

$$\log L_{\text{com}}(\phi; \boldsymbol{y}, \boldsymbol{z}) = \sum_{i} \sum_{j} z_{ij} \{\log \pi_j + y_i\, \log(\theta_i \mu_i) - \theta_i \mu_i\} - \sum_{i} \log(y_i!),$$

where $z_{ij} = 1$ if $y_i \in \mathcal{G}_j$ and 0 otherwise. The MLE of the parameters are found iteratively via

$$\hat{\pi}_j = \frac{\Sigma_i \hat{\tau}_{ij}}{n}$$

and

$$\hat{\theta}_j = \frac{\Sigma_i x_i \hat{\tau}_{ij}}{\Sigma_i \hat{\tau}_{ij} \mu_i},$$

where $\hat{\tau}_{ij} = \hat{\pi}_j f_j(y_i;\, \theta_i) / \sum_{t=1}^{m} \hat{\pi}_t f_t(y_i;\, \theta_i)$ which is the estimated posterior probability that $y_i \in \mathcal{G}_j$.

Testing for the Number of Components in a Mixture

Testing for the number of components in a mixture is a very hard problem. Consider the problem of testing the hypothesis H_0: number of components = m against H_0: number of components = $m + 1$. The likelihood ratio test (LRT) statistic defined as $2 \log L_n = 2 [l(\hat{Q}_m) - l(\hat{Q}_{m+1})]$, where $l(\hat{Q}_m)$ is the log likelihood $\log L(Q_m) = \Sigma_{i=1}^n g(y_i \mid Q_m)$ evaluated at $\hat{Q}_m$, the nonparametric MLE under H_0 and similarly $l(\hat{Q}_{m+1})$ is the nonparametric MLE under H_1. The LRT statistic generally has an asymptotic X^2 distribution with d degrees of freedom, where d equals the difference between the number of parameters under the alternative and null hypothesis. However, this theory is known to fail for the mixture problem (Titterington et al., 1985:154). The reason for this is that the null hypothesis does not lie in the interior of the parameter space. The problem is not yet solved except for some special cases. However, the simulations or bootstrap can shed some light on the distributional properties of the LRT. See Lindsay (1995) and Böhning (1999) (including the references therein) for recent developments in theory and methods to test for the number of components in a mixture. There are other techniques for identifying the number of components of a mixing distribution including a variety of graphical techniques (Lindsay and Roeder, 1992).

The Choice of Initial Values and Multiple Mode Problem for the EM Algorithm

The continuous EM algorithm that finds the MLE of parameter estimators, for a given m, requires the specification of initial values for the number and location of the support points. Pilla and Lindsay (2001) show that if the number of support points is fixed in advance, then one could have multiple modes whereas the nonparametric ML approach corresponds to a unimodal likelihood. Böhning (1999) illustrates through an example where the choice of initial values is critical; for example, in testing for the number of components in the mixture. Through simulations, he demonstrates the effectiveness of several approaches that combat this problem. His recommendation is to choose the support points as values of certain order statistics of the data (see Böhning, 1999:68–70). In his simulation studies, the gold standard (the grid approach given below) seems to outperform the other methods. The optimization problem solved by the grid-based EM (where the support points are assumed known) proposed by Pilla and Lindsay (2001) has a unique optimum which in turn generates an estimated number of components. However, the continuous EM can converge to the suboptimal mode.

In light of the above characteristics, Pilla and Lindsay (2001) suggest the following: to obtain a continuous solution with a flexible number of support points, first start with one of the fast EM-based algorithms proposed by Pilla and Lindsay on a grid and next use the resulting solution as starting values for the continuous EM. This will protect against using an incorrect number of points or finding suboptimal solutions.

Convergence Criteria

Finding a natural stopping rule for iterative algorithms in the mixture problem when the final log likelihood is unknown is an important problem. In a potentially slow algorithm like EM, a far weaker convergence criterion based on the changes in the log likelihood value or on changes in the parameter estimates between iterations can be very misleading (Titterington et al. 1985:90). See Lindsay (1995:62–63) for further details. The following gradient-based stopping criterion proposed by Lindsay (1995:131–132) can be used to detect the convergence of the EM algorithm: we stop when $\sup_{j} D_Q(\theta) \leq \varepsilon$, with $\varepsilon = 0.005$, where the gradient function $D_Q(\theta)$ is defined as

$$D_Q(\theta) := \frac{1}{n} \sum_{i=1}^{n} \left\{ \frac{f(y_i; \theta)}{g(y_i \mid Q)} \right\} - 1 \text{ for all } j = 1, \ldots, m, \tag{1}$$

then we automatically satisfy the 'ideal stopping criterion': $|\log L_{\text{obs}}(\hat{\phi}; y) - \log L_{\text{obs}}(\phi^p; y)| \leq \varepsilon$, where ϕ^p is the estimate at the pth iteration. The gradient function therefore creates a natural stopping rule for iterative algorithms such as the EM when the final log likelihood is unknown, although it is more stringent than the ideal stopping rule.

Illustration of Poisson Mixture Model

To illustrate use of the Poisson mixture model we analyzed county-level suicide data for the US for the time period of 1996–1998. The three year period was used to obtain more stable estimates of the parameters. Application of the Poisson mixture model identified a mixture of four component distributions with proportions of .1125, .4523, .3119, and .1234, and means of 7.5, 10.9, 14.9, and 20.6 suicides per 100,000. Results of classifying counties into component distributions are displayed in Figure 1. Inspection of the map in Figure 1 reveals that those counties classified in the highest component distribution (20.6 suicides per 100,000), are predominantly in the western states with lowest population density, although there are exceptions throughout the country (see Figure A-1). Counties classified in the lowest component distribution (7.5 suicides per 100,000)

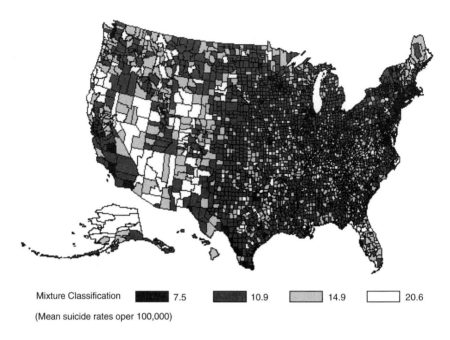

Mixture Classification   ▓▓▓ 7.5   ▓▓▓ 10.9   ▓▓▓ 14.9   ☐ 20.6
(Mean suicide rates oper 100,000)

FIGURE A-1 Annual Suicide Rates per 100,000 (1996–1998). The Poisson Mixture Model applied to county-level data.

appear to be clustered in the central United States. Finally, counties classified into the two intermediate groups are largely in the eastern portion of the United States. Unlike the earlier attempt at fitting a mixture distribution to temporal suicide data collected in Cook county (Gibbons et al., 1990) that was designed to identify "suicide epidemics" and failed to do so, the results of this analysis has focused on the spatial distribution of suicide and has identified qualitatively distinct geographic groupings of suicide rates across the United States. Note that this mixture distribution does not adjust for demographic disparity across the counties (e.g., age, sex, race, population density, etc.) that may have produced the mixture distribution in the first place.

POISSON REGRESSION MODELS

In the following sections, we present statistical details of both fixed-effects and mixed-effects Poisson regression models.

Fixed-Effects Poisson Regression Model

In Poisson regression modeling, the data are modeled as Poisson counts whose means are expressed as a function of covariates. Let y_i be a response variable and $x_i = (1, x_{i1}, ..., x_{ip})^T$ be a $[(p+1) \times 1]$ vector of co-variates for the ith individual. Then the Poisson regression model y_i is

$$f(y_i; \lambda_i) = \frac{\exp(-\lambda_i)(\lambda_i^{y_i})}{yi!} \text{ for } y_i = 0, ..., n, \tag{2}$$

where $\lambda_i = exp(\beta^T x_i)$ and $\beta = (\beta_0, \beta_1, ..., \beta_p)^T$ is a (p+1)-dimensional vector of unknown parameters corresponding to x_i. An important property of the Poisson distribution is the equality of the mean and variance:

$$E(y_i) = Var(y_i) = \lambda_i \tag{3}$$

From equation (2) one can write the likelihood and the log likelihood functions for the n independent observations as

$$L(\lambda; y) = \prod_{i=1}^{n} \frac{\exp(-\lambda_i)(\lambda_i^{y_i})}{y_i!}$$

and

$$\log L = -\sum_i [\lambda_i + y_i \log \lambda_i - \log(y_i!)]$$

respectively. The first and second partial derivatives with respect to the unknown parameters β are given by

$$\frac{\partial \log L}{\partial \beta} = \sum_i (y_i - \lambda_i) x_i$$

and

$$\frac{\partial^2 \log L}{\partial \beta \partial \beta^T} = -\sum_i \lambda_i x_i x_i^T$$

respectively. Since the above equations are not linear, iterative procedures such as the Newton-Raphson algorithm or Fisher's scoring algorithm are used to obtain the MLE of β, denoted by $\hat{\beta}$. A consistent estimator of the variance-covariance matrix of $\hat{\beta}$, $V(\hat{\beta})$ is the inverse of the information matrix, $I(\hat{\beta})$ — which is the negative of inverse of the matrix of second partial derivatives evaluated at the MLE. Inferences on the regression parameter β can be made using $V(\hat{\beta})$.

Mixed-Effects Poisson Regression Model

When we have a mixture of fixed and random effects, the more general mixed-effects Poisson regression model is used. Suppose that there are $n = \sum_i n_i$ nonnegative observations y_{ij} for $i = 1, ..., n_c$ clusters and $j = 1, ..., n_i$ observations and a $(p + 1)$ dimensional unknown parameter vector, β, associated with a covariate vector $x_{ij} = (1, x_{ij1}, ..., x_{ijp})^T$. Further, let the random effect v_i be normally-distributed with mean 0 and variance σ^2 and independent of the covariate vector x_{ij}. Then the conditional density function, $f(y_i; \theta_i)$, of the n_i suicide rates in cluster i is written as:

$$f(y_i; \theta_i) = \prod_{j=1}^{n_i} f(y_{ij}; \lambda_{ij})$$

$$= \prod_j \frac{\exp(-\lambda_{ij})\lambda_{ij}^{y_{ij}}}{y_{ij}!} \tag{4}$$

with

$$\lambda_{ij} = \exp(\beta^T x_{ij} + v_i)$$
$$= \exp(\beta^T x_{ij} + \sigma\theta_i),$$

where $\theta_i = v_i/\sigma$ such that $\theta_i \sim N(0,1)$. Thus the log-likelihood function corresponding to equation 4 becomes

$$\log L(y_i | \theta_i) = -\sum_{j=1}^{n_i} [\exp(\beta^T x_{ij} + \sigma\theta_i) + y_{ij}(\beta^T x_{ij} + \sigma\theta_i) - \log(y_{ij}!)].$$

The first and second derivatives of log L with respect to β and σ are

$$\begin{bmatrix} \dfrac{\partial \log L(y_i | \theta_i)}{\partial \beta} \\[3mm] \dfrac{\partial \log L(y_i | \theta_i)}{\partial \sigma} \end{bmatrix} = \begin{bmatrix} \sum_j (y_{ij} - \exp(\beta^T x_{ij} + \sigma\theta_i))x_{ij} \\[3mm] \sum_j (y_{ij} - \exp(\beta^T x_{ij} + \sigma\theta_i))\theta_i \end{bmatrix}$$

and

$$\begin{bmatrix} \dfrac{\partial^2 \log L(y_i | \theta_i)}{\partial \beta\, \partial \beta^T} \\[3mm] \dfrac{\partial^2 \log L(y_i | \theta_i)}{\partial \sigma\, \partial \sigma^T} \end{bmatrix} = \begin{bmatrix} -\sum_j \exp(\beta^T x_{ij} + \sigma\theta_i)x_{ij}x_{ij}^T \\[3mm] -\sum_j \exp(\beta^T x_{ij} + \sigma\theta_i)\theta_i^2 \end{bmatrix}.$$

The marginal density of y_i can be written as

$$h(\beta, \sigma, \theta_i; y_i) = h(y_i) = \int_\theta f(y_i \mid \theta_i) g(\theta) d\theta,$$

where $g(\theta)$ represents the multivariate standard normal density. One can approximate the above integral via the Gaussian quadrature as

$$\approx \sum_{q=1}^{Q} \left[\prod_{j=1}^{n_i} \frac{\exp(-\lambda_{ijq}) \lambda_{ijq}^{y_{ij}}}{y_{ij}!} \right] A(B_q), \tag{5}$$

where $\lambda_{ijq} = \exp(\beta^T x_{ij} + \sigma B_q)$, B_q is the quadrature node and $A(B_q)$ is the corresponding quadrature weight. From equation (5), one can obtain the first derivatives of the approximate log likelihood as

$$\frac{\partial \log L}{\partial \beta} = \sum_i \frac{1}{h(y_i)} \sum_q \sum_j (y_{ij} - \lambda_{ijq}) x_{ij} \frac{\exp(-\lambda_{ijq}) \lambda_{ijq}^{y_{ij}}}{y_{ij}} A(B_q)$$

and

$$\frac{\partial \log L}{\partial \sigma} = \sum_{i=1}^{n_c} \frac{1}{h(y_i)} \sum_q^{B_q} \sum_{j=1}^{n_i} (y_{ij} - \lambda_{ijq}) \theta_i \frac{\exp(-\lambda_{ijq}) \lambda_{ijq}^{y_{ij}}}{y_{ij}} A(B_q).$$

Solution of the above likelihood equations can be obtained iteratively using the Newton-Raphson algorithm. On the ith iteration, estimates for a parameter vector Θ are given by

$$\Theta_{i+1} = \Theta_i - \left[\frac{\partial^2 \log L}{\partial \Theta_i \partial \Theta_i^T} \right]^{-1} \frac{\partial \log L}{\partial \Theta_i} \tag{6}$$

where $\partial^2 \log L / \partial \Theta_i \partial \Theta_i^T$ is the matrix of second derivatives of the log-likelihood, evaluated at Θ_i. Alternatively, one can use the Fisher scoring method. This method replaces the matrix of second derivatives in (6) by their expected values:

$$E\left[\frac{\partial^2 \log L}{\partial \Theta \partial \Theta^T} \right]$$

which is equal to the negative of the information matrix. The scoring solution is often used in cases where the matrix of second derivatives is difficult to obtain. Note that when the expected value and the actual value of the Hessian matrix coincide, the Fisher scoring method and the Newton-Raphson method reduce to the same algorithm.

The convergence of the iterative procedure depends on the initial values of the parameters. Good starting values reduce the number of iterations needed to reach the final estimates. It is sometimes possible that a poor choice of starting values may reach some local maximum instead of the global maximum. For this reason, it is often desirable to re-estimate the parameters under a variety of starting values, or to use the EM algorithm to obtain starting values that are reasonably close to the final solution (Hedeker and Gibbons, 1994).

Estimation of Random Effects

Often, it is of interest to estimate values of the random effects θ_i within a sample. For this purpose the expected "a posteriori" (EAP) or empirical Bayes estimator $\bar{\theta}_i$ has been suggested by Bock and Aitkin (1981). The estimator $\bar{\theta}_i$ given y_i for cluster i can be obtained as:

$$\bar{\theta}_i = E(\theta_i \mid y_i) = \frac{1}{h(y_i)} \int_\theta \theta_i f(y_i \mid \theta_i) g(\theta) d\theta.$$

Similarly, the variance of the posterior distribution of $\bar{\theta}_i$, which may be used to make inferences regarding the EAP estimator (i.e., the posterior variance is an estimate of precision of the estimate of $\bar{\theta}_i$), is given by

$$Var(\bar{\theta}_i \mid y_i) = \frac{1}{h(y_i)} \int_\theta (\theta_i - \bar{\theta}_i)^2 f(y_i \mid \theta_i) g(\theta) d\theta.$$

Generalized Estimating Equations - GEE

An alternative approach to the analysis of clustered suicide rate data is based on Generalized estimating equations (GEEs) models, which were introduced by Liang and Zeger (1986) and Zeger and Liang (1986).

Let y_{ij} be the jth response for the ith unit (e.g., county) for $i = 1, ..., n_c$ and $j = 1, ..., n_i$ observations and $x_{ij} = (1, x_{ij1}, ..., x_{ijp})$ be a vector of covariates for the ith unit. Let y_i be the vector of the responses for the ith unit with corresponding mean vector μ_i and let V_i be an estimate of the covariance matrix of y_i. Then the GEE marginal model for estimating β is given by

$$\sum_{i=1}^{n_c} \frac{\partial \mu_i}{\partial \beta}' V_i^{-1} (y_i - \mu_i(\beta)) = 0 \tag{7}$$

and

$$g(\mu_{ij}) = g(E(y_i)) = \beta' x_{ij} \tag{8}$$

where g is the link function. Common choice for the link function might be the identity link for continuous data, log link for count data, and logit link for binary data. For example, the link functions for the Poisson and logistic regression models are $g(a) = \log(a)$ and $g(a) = \log(a/(1-a))$, respectively.

In addition to the marginal model, the covariance structure of the correlated observations for a given unit of y_i is modeled as

$$V_i = \psi A_i^{1/2} R(\alpha) A_i^{1/2},$$ (9)

where A_i is a diagonal matrix of variance functions and $R(\alpha)$ is the working correlation matrix of y_i specified by the vector of parameters α. Various types of working correlation structures such as exchangeable or autoregressive can be used in the model.

The maximum likelihood estimator $\hat{\beta}$ can be obtained by solving the above estimating equations iteratively:

$$\beta_{r+1} = \beta_r - \left[\sum_{i=1}^{n_c} \frac{\partial \mu_i'}{\partial \beta} V_i^{-1} \frac{\partial \mu_i}{\partial \beta} \right]^{-1} \left[\sum_{i=1}^{n_c} \frac{\partial \mu_i'}{\partial \beta} V_i^{-1} (y_i - \mu_i) \right]$$ (10)

Illustration of Poisson Regression Model

Returning to the national suicide data from the previous section, we now illustrate how Poisson regression models can be used to estimate the effects of age, race, and sex on clustered (i.e., within counties) suicide rate data. For the purpose of illustration, we considered the effects of age divided into five categories (5-14, 15-24, 25-44, 45-64, and 65 and older), sex, and race (African American versus Other) in the prediction of suicide rates across the U.S. for the period of 1996-1998. These categories were used so that there would be sufficient sample sizes available to compare observed and expected annual suicide rates for both GEE and mixed-effects (maximum marginal likelihood - MMLE) Poisson regression models. To this end, we fit a Poisson regression model with all main effects and two-way interactions using both GEE and a full likelihood mixed-effects model. Given the large sample sizes almost all terms in the model were statistically significant although of widely varying effect sizes. Table 2 displays a comparison of parameter estimates and standard errors for the GEE and mixed-effects models. In general, the GEE and MMLE parameter estimates were remarkably similar. The only nonsignificant terms were two terms in the race by age interaction. The comparison of rates for ages 5-14 versus 15-24 and 5-14 versus 25-44, did not depend on race.

Based on the parameter estimates in Table A-1, we estimated marginal suicide rates for both GEE and mixed-effects models. Table A-2

TABLE A-1 Comparison of Maximum Marginal Likeihood (MMLE) and Generalized Estimating Equations (GEE) for the Clustered Poisson Regression Model

	MMLE			GEE		
Effect	Estimate	SE	Prob	Estimate	SE	Prob
Intercept	−4.331	0.040	<0.0001	−4.408000	0.048000	<0.0001
Female	−1.009	0.076	<0.0001	−1.009000	0.073000	<0.0001
Black vs Other	−0.292	0.103	0.0046	−0.279000	0.112000	0.0127
15–24 vs 05–14	2.788	0.041	<0.0001	2.787000	0.043000	<0.0001
25–44 vs 05–14	3.030	0.040	<0.0001	3.021000	0.043000	<0.0001
45–64 vs 05–14	2.971	0.041	<0.0001	2.975000	0.046000	<0.0001
65+ vs 05–14	3.371	0.041	<0.0001	3.390000	0.047000	<0.0001
Female x Black	−0.345	0.036	<0.0001	−0.345000	0.041000	<0.0001
Female x 15–24	−0.664	0.080	<0.0001	−0.663000	0.077000	<0.0001
Female x 25–44	−0.355	0.077	<0.0001	−0.357000	0.074000	<0.0001
Female x 45–64	−0.223	0.077	0.0038	−0.223000	0.075000	0.0029
Female x 65+	−0.938	0.078	<0.0001	−0.945000	0.078000	<0.0001
Black x 15–24	0.065	0.106	0.5434	0.068000	0.107000	0.5297
Black x 25–44	−0.139	0.105	0.1829	−0.141000	0.107000	0.1877
Black x 45–64	−0.473	0.107	<0.0001	−0.486000	0.111000	<0.0001
Black x 65+	−0.740	0.112	<0.0001	−0.748000	0.117000	<0.0001
County Variance	0.280	0.003	<0.0001			

displays observed and expected annual suicide rates for both methods of estimation, broken down by age, sex, and race. Inspection of Table A-2 reveals several interesting results. In general, suicide increases with age, is higher in males, and is lower in African Americans. Black females have the lowest suicide rates across the age range. In white males, the suicide rate is increasing with age whereas in all other groups, the suicide rate either is constant or decreases after age 65. Comparison of the expected frequencies for the GEE and mixed-effects models reveal that they are quite similar and the GEE does a slightly better job of recovering the observed marginal rates.

A special feature of the mixed-effects model is the ability of estimating county-specific rates using empirical Bayes estimates of the random effects as described in the previous section. Using these estimates, we can accomplish two goals. First, we can estimate county-specific expected suicide rates, which directly incorporate the effects race, sex, and age of that county. Table A-3 provides a comparison of observed and expected numbers of suicides (1996-1998) for 100 randomly selected counties. In-

TABLE A-2 Observed and Expected Suicide Rates by Age, Race, and Sex. Data: CMF 1996–1998

Age Group	Race	Sex	Number of Suicides	Population	Observed Rate	Expected Rate(1)	Expected Rate(2)
05–14	Black	Male	79	9,256,227	0.000009	0.000010	0.000009
05–14	Black	Female	28	8,978,221	0.000003	0.000003	0.000002
05–14	Other	Male	620	50,356,003	0.000012	0.000014	0.000012
05–14	Other	Female	206	47,847,778	0.000004	0.000005	0.000004
15–24	Black	Male	1,333	8,389,386	0.000159	0.000177	0.000160
15–24	Black	Female	191	8,352,196	0.000023	0.000024	0.000021
15–24	Other	Male	9,482	47,906,710	0.000198	0.000222	0.000198
15–24	Other	Female	1,673	45,396,608	0.000037	0.000042	0.000037
25–44	Black	Male	2,546	15,274,935	0.000167	0.000184	0.000164
25–44	Black	Female	474	17,191,095	0.000028	0.000033	0.000030
25–44	Other	Male	27,209	109,106,670	0.000249	0.000283	0.000250
25–44	Other	Female	6,977	108,864,081	0.000064	0.000072	0.000064
45–64	Black	Male	861	7,741,680	0.000111	0.000124	0.000111
45–64	Black	Female	224	9,633,227	0.000023	0.000026	0.000023
45–64	Other	Male	17,358	72,740,945	0.000239	0.000267	0.000239
45–64	Other	Female	5,307	76,289,629	0.000070	0.000078	0.000070
65+	Black	Male	415	3,295,133	0.000126	0.000142	0.000131
65+	Black	Female	83	5,140,632	0.000016	0.000014	0.000013
65+	Other	Male	14,074	38,889,596	0.000362	0.000398	0.000361
65+	Other	Female	2,814	55,229,051	0.000051	0.000057	0.000051

Note: (1) Mixed-effect model
(2) GEE model

spection of Table A-3 reveals remarkably close agreement between observed and expected numbers of suicides.

Second, we can use the Bayes estimates directly to obtain county-level suicide rates adjusted for the effects of race, sex, and age. In the case of a Poisson model, the Bayes estimate for a given county is a multiple of the national suicide rate adjusted for the case mix in that county (i.e., race, sex and age). For example, a Bayes estimate of 1.0 represents an adjusted rate that is equal to the national rate. By contrast, a Bayes estimate of 2.0 represents a doubling of the national rate, and a Bayes estimate of 0.5 represents one-half of the national rate. Figure A-2 displays the Bayes estimates by county across the U.S. Inspection of Figure A-2 reveals that even after accounting for these important demographic variables, considerable spatial variability remains. Again, the highest adjusted rates are typically found in the less densely populated areas of the western U.S.

The map in Figure A-2 also provides a useful tool for qualitative research into the etiology of suicide. A natural approach is to examine the

TABLE A-3 Observed and Expected Number of Suicides for 100
Randomly Selected Counties

State	County	Observed # of Deaths	Expected # of Deaths	State	County	Observed # of Deaths	Expected # of Deaths
56	7	16	10.3	51	75	5	5.9
53	63	169	170.4	20	159	6	4.5
5	91	14	13.6	21	103	14	8.7
47	111	13	9.4	40	45	1	1.6
54	93	1	2.8	31	61	1	1.5
28	5	9	5.5	31	91	0	0.3
27	141	22	21.7	40	73	9	6.3
38	47	0	1.0	20	203	1	1.0
21	59	25	27.5	1	5	8	8.2
48	451	54	50.2	38	51	0	1.4
48	87	3	1.4	38	39	2	1.3
18	97	391	385.3	21	95	11	12.0
35	7	8	6.2	48	73	32	25.8
48	383	2	1.5	23	11	38	39.6
31	41	3	4.3	55	101	58	59.5
18	7	2	3.4	17	107	9	10.8
45	61	6	5.9	47	127	1	1.9
19	1	4	3.4	55	55	28	28.1
8	119	13	9.9	21	223	5	3.4
36	3	22	20.9	30	97	1	1.4
19	93	2	2.9	19	51	2	3.0
12	95	303	314.1	47	129	4	6.4
49	49	89	91.1	48	9	2	3.0
28	45	30	24.1	19	5	9	6.7
18	107	19	16.9	28	69	3	3.0
5	1	6	6.8	46	19	6	4.1
17	167	64	64.8	27	171	31	30.8
39	89	43	44.7	28	53	1	2.4
28	1	9	9.5	20	31	2	3.1
53	23	0	0.9	51	47	18	15.0
48	213	30	28.8	46	123	3	2.7
55	107	9	7.1	12	81	135	129.6
31	177	6	6.7	2	122	22	20.4
17	49	12	12.2	21	61	0	3.4
55	75	18	17.5	21	25	7	6.3
8	55	3	2.7	26	13	6	4.0
29	121	4	5.4	18	157	42	44.1
40	125	34	30.2	21	165	2	2.2
20	73	3	3.2	48	447	2	0.8
21	109	7	5.5	13	265	3	0.6
29	197	2	1.8	2	100	2	1.0
51	133	7	5.0	55	11	4	5.2
29	105	8	10.0	48	81	0	1.3
47	181	14	9.7	21	229	6	4.6
51	103	9	5.5	55	35	32	32.3
16	15	3	2.2	39	151	112	113.5
38	55	2	3.5	28	89	17	18.4
39	17	91	93.6	19	167	4	8.2
55	51	3	2.8	23	27	17	15.7
19	119	3	4.2	38	1	0	1.1

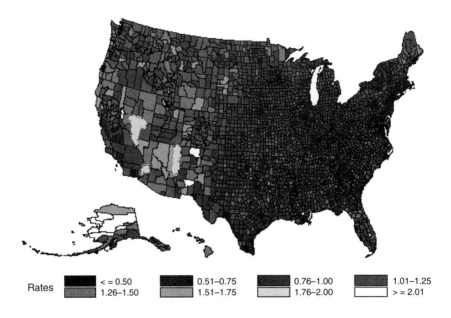

Rates
| | < = 0.50 | | 0.51–0.75 | | 0.76–1.00 | | 1.01–1.25 |
| | 1.26–1.50 | | 1.51–1.75 | | 1.76–2.00 | | > = 2.01 |

FIGURE A-2 Bayes Estimates of County-Level Deviations from the National Suicide Rates per 100,000 (1996–1998), Adjusted for Age, Sex, and Race.

spatial distribution of Bayes estimates in Figure A-2 for outliers. For example, in the western U.S. and Alaska where suicide rates are typically high there are a few counties that have Bayes estimates that are consistent with the national average. Similarly, in the central U.S. where there is a high concentration of counties with the lowest suicide rates, there are a few counties that exhibit the highest suicide rates. As an example, Table A-4 displays the Bayes estimates, observed and expected numbers of suicides and suicide rates for all counties in Alaska and New Mexico and the 8 counties with estimated adjusted suicide rates less than or equal to half of the national average (national average is 12.33 suicides per 100,000 during the period of 1996–1998). Table A-4 reveals that although there are generally elevated suicide rates in Alaska and New Mexico relative to the national average, there are several counties with low rates, similar to the national average. What are the protective factors that have produced these spatial anomalies? Are these spatial anomalies simply due to reporting bias or some other unmeasured characteristic that has produced the outlying Bayes estimate. Examining these spatial anomalies in greater detail is certainly a fruitful area for further research.

TABLE A-4 Observed and Expected rates per 100,000 for Alaska,
New Mexico, and Counties with BE <= 0.50

State	County Name	Observed # of Suicides	Expected # of Suicides
ALASKA	ALEUTIANS EAST	1	0.84
ALASKA	ALEUTIANS WEST	2	1.92
ALASKA	ANCHORAGE	118	115.66
ALASKA	BETHEL	22	10.17
ALASKA	BRISTOL BAY	1	0.58
ALASKA	DILLINGHAM	4	1.46
ALASKA	FAIRBANKS NORTH STAR	52	46.63
ALASKA	HAINES	2	0.96
ALASKA	JUNEAU	13	11.95
ALASKA	KENAI PENINSULA	22	20.38
ALASKA	KETCHIKAN GATEWAY	4	4.91
ALASKA	KODIAK ISLAND	5	5.17
ALASKA	LAKE AND PENINSULA	4	0.63
ALASKA	MATANUSKA-SUSITNA	29	25.80
ALASKA	NOME	14	5.02
ALASKA	NORTH SLOPE	10	3.35
ALASKA	NORTHWEST ARCTIC	15	3.87
ALASKA	PRINCE OF WALES-OUTER	3	2.64
ALASKA	SITKA	6	3.71
ALASKA	SKAGWAY-HOONAH-ANGOON	1	1.34
ALASKA	SOUTHEAST FAIRBANKS	6	2.69
ALASKA	VALDEZ-CORDOVA	1	3.31
ALASKA	WADE HAMPTON	18	4.37
ALASKA	WRANGELL-PETERSBURG	8	3.73
ALASKA	YAKUTAT	0	0.29
ALASKA	YUKON-KOYUKUK	16	5.91
ILLINOIS	MC LEAN	17	25.62
NEW JERSEY	HUNTERDON	13	22.23
NEW JERSEY	MORRIS	80	88.20
NEW JERSEY	UNION	80	88.66
NEW MEXICO	BERNALILLO	303	295.93
NEW MEXICO	CATRON	1	1.18
NEW MEXICO	CHAVES	24	23.46
NEW MEXICO	CIBOLA	12	9.84
NEW MEXICO	COLFAX	8	6.16
NEW MEXICO	CURRY	23	20.28
NEW MEXICO	DE BACA	2	1.05
NEW MEXICO	DONA ANA	63	62.45
NEW MEXICO	EDDY	30	26.30
NEW MEXICO	GRANT	23	17.83
NEW MEXICO	GUADALUPE	2	1.64
NEW MEXICO	HARDING	1	0.40
NEW MEXICO	HIDALGO	1	2.14
NEW MEXICO	LEA	15	16.90

Observed Rate/100,000	Expected Rate/100,000	Population	Bayes Estimate
15.66	13.08	2,128	1.01
16.27	15.61	4,098	1.00
16.90	16.56	232,752	1.24
52.75	24.37	13,902	2.58
26.75	15.50	1,246	1.03
34.00	12.44	3,921	1.22
22.51	20.19	76,998	1.50
32.20	15.52	2,070	1.08
15.56	14.30	27,850	1.07
16.65	15.43	44,035	1.11
10.28	12.62	12,967	0.92
12.42	12.85	13,415	0.97
87.45	13.69	1,524	1.31
19.23	17.10	50,276	1.26
58.89	21.11	7,924	2.05
53.11	17.80	6,276	1.70
87.41	22.54	5,720	2.45
15.29	13.45	6,541	1.02
25.55	15.80	7,827	1.19
9.36	12.58	3,561	0.97
38.23	17.13	5,232	1.30
3.47	11.51	9,597	0.82
105.40	25.59	5,692	3.00
41.81	19.47	6,377	1.40
0.00	12.45	764	0.97
73.37	27.08	7,269	2.24
4.31	6.49	131,572	0.48
3.86	6.59	112,392	0.46
6.27	6.91	425,476	0.49
5.73	6.35	465,455	0.49
20.70	20.22	487,809	1.48
12.76	15.02	2,613	0.98
13.88	13.57	57,623	1.02
16.81	13.78	23,799	1.17
20.83	16.03	12,799	1.15
17.94	15.82	42,733	1.22
29.93	15.64	2,227	1.08
13.81	13.69	152,009	1.02
20.25	17.76	49,371	1.31
26.42	20.48	29,022	1.49
17.59	14.42	3,790	1.02
38.83	15.70	858	1.05
5.77	12.35	5,775	0.90
9.68	10.91	51,633	0.84

continues

TABLE A-4 Continued

State	County Name	Observed # of Suicides	Expected # of Suicides
NEW MEXICO	LINCOLN	17	10.72
NEW MEXICO	LOS ALAMOS	8	7.68
NEW MEXICO	LUNA	22	15.23
NEW MEXICO	MC KINLEY	30	25.16
NEW MEXICO	MORA	3	2.05
NEW MEXICO	OTERO	16	17.58
NEW MEXICO	QUAY	3	3.72
NEW MEXICO	RIO ARRIBA	37	27.71
NEW MEXICO	ROOSEVELT	7	6.83
NEW MEXICO	SANDOVAL	30	29.60
NEW MEXICO	SAN JUAN	44	40.91
NEW MEXICO	SAN MIGUEL	19	14.81
NEW MEXICO	SANTA FE	81	75.18
NEW MEXICO	SIERRA	22	11.37
NEW MEXICO	SOCORRO	14	8.99
NEW MEXICO	TAOS	12	10.79
NEW MEXICO	TORRANCE	12	7.78
NEW MEXICO	UNION	1	1.53
NEW MEXICO	VALENCIA	29	26.99
NEW YORK	NASSAU	217	225.92
NEW YORK	ROCKLAND	30	40.87
NEW YORK	WESTCHESTER	163	167.11
TEXAS	HIDALGO	77	85.03

Observed and expected number of suicides : sum of 1996 - 1998
Population = Annual population

MIXED-EFFECTS ORDINAL REGRESSION MODELS

In motivating probit and logistic regression models, it is often assumed that there is an unobservable latent variable (y) which is related to the actual response through the "threshold concept." For a binary response, one threshold value is assumed, while for an ordinal response, a series of threshold values $\gamma_1, \gamma_2, ..., \gamma_{K-1}$, where K equals the number of ordered categories, $\gamma_0 = -\infty$, and $\gamma_K = \infty$. Here, a response occurs in category k ($Y = k$) if the latent response process y exceeds the threshold value γ_{k-1}, but does not exceed the threshold value γ_k.

The traditional ordinal regression model is parameterized such that regression coefficients α do not depend on k, i.e., the model asumes that the relationship between the explanatory variables and the cumulative logits does not depend on k. McCullagh (1980) calls this assumption of identical odds ratios across the $K - 1$ cut-offs, the *proportional odds assump-*

Observed Rate/100,000	Expected Rate/100,000	Population	Bayes Estimate
37.89	23.88	14,955	1.64
15.39	14.77	17,330	1.01
33.63	23.28	21,807	1.70
16.60	13.92	60,256	1.44
22.35	15.27	4,474	1.07
10.55	11.59	50,533	0.86
10.51	13.03	9,516	0.93
36.07	27.01	34,197	2.07
13.65	13.31	17,099	1.00
12.85	12.68	77,840	1.00
15.47	14.38	94,802	1.25
23.81	18.57	26,596	1.38
23.93	22.20	112,852	1.58
70.75	36.57	10,364	2.33
31.08	19.96	15,014	1.48
16.35	14.70	24,469	1.08
29.56	19.15	13,533	1.39
8.86	13.55	3,762	0.95
16.84	15.67	57,397	1.15
5.92	6.17	1,221,351	0.44
3.86	5.25	259,392	0.40
6.51	6.67	834,764	0.50
5.66	6.25	453,250	0.50

tion. This assumption implies that the effect of a regressor variable is the same across the cumulative logits of the model, or proportional across the cumulative odds. In the present context, this implies that the effect of an intervention is the same on the shift from no ideation to suicidal ideation, as it is from suicidal ideation to a suicidal attempt, an assumption that is questionable at best. As noted by Peterson and Harrell (1990), however, examples of non-proportional odds are not difficult to find. Recently Hedeker and Mermelstein (1998) have described an extension of the random effects proportional odds model to allow for non-proportional odds for a set of explanatory variables. For example, it sems reasonable to assume that the effects of the model covariates on suicidal ideation and suicidal attempts may not be the same. The resulting mixed-effects partial proportional odds model follows Peterson and Harrell's (1990) extension of the fixed-effects proportional odds model.

Proportional Odds Model

Assuming that there are $i = 1, ..., N$ level-2 units and $j = 1, ..., n_i$ level-1 units nested within the ith level-2 unit. The cumulative probabilities for the k ordered categories ($k = 1, ... K$) are defined for the ordinal outcomes Y as:

$$P_{ijk} = \Pr(Y \leq k \mid \beta_i, \gamma_k, \alpha),$$

where the mixed-effects logistic regression model for these cumulative probabilities is given as

$$\log \frac{P_{ijk}}{\left(1 - P_{ijk}\right)} = \gamma_k + x_{ij}^T \beta_i + w_{ij}^T \alpha,$$

with $K - 1$ strictly increasing model intercepts γ_k (i.e., $\gamma_1 > ... > \gamma_{K-1}$). As before, w_{ij} is the $p \times 1$ covariate vector and x_{ij} is the design vector for the r random effects, both vectors being for the jth level-1 unit nested within level-2 unit i. Also, α is the $p \times 1$ vector of unknown fixed regression parameters, and β_i is the $r \times 1$ vector of unknown random effects for the level-2 unit i. Since the regression coefficients, α do not depend on k, the model assumes that the relationship between the explanatory variables and the cumulative logits does not depend on k.

As in most mixed-effects models, it is convenient to orthogonally transform the response model. Letting $\beta = \Lambda t$, where $\Lambda \Lambda^T = \Sigma_\beta$ is the Cholesky decomposition of Σ_β, the reparameterized model is then written as

$$\log \frac{P_{ijk}}{(1 - P_{ijk})} = \gamma_k + x_{ij}^T \Lambda t_i + w_{ij}^T \alpha,$$

where t_i are distributed according to a multivariate standard normal distribution.

Partial-Proportional Odds Model

To allow for a partial proportional odds model the intercepts γ_k are denoted instead as γ_{0k}, and the following terms are added to the model:

$$\log \frac{P_{ijk}}{(1 - P_{ijk})} = \gamma_{0k} + (u_{ij}^*)^T \gamma_k^* + x_{ij}^T L t_i + w_{ij}^T a$$

or absorbing γ_{0k} and γ_k^* into γ_k,

$$\log \frac{P_{ijk}}{(1 - P_{ijk})} = u_{ij}^T \gamma_k + x_{ij}^T \Lambda t_i + w_{ij}^T \alpha$$

where, u_{ij} is a $[(h+1) \times 1]$ vector containing (in addition to a 1 for γ_{0k}) the values of observation ij on the subset of h covariates for which proportional odds are not assumed (i.e., u_{ij} is a subset of w_{ij}). In this model, γ_k is a $(h+1) \times 1$ vector of regression coefficients associated with the h variables (plus the intercept) in u_{ij}. Notice that the effects of these h covariates (u_{ij}^*) vary across the $(K - 1)$ cumulative logits. This extension of the model follows similar extensions of the ordinary fixed-effects ordinal logistic regression model discussed by Peterson and Harrell (1990) and Cox (1995). Terza (1985) discusses a similar extension for the ordinal probit regression model.

There is a caveat in this extension of the proportional odds model. For the explanatory variables without proportional odds, the effects on the cumulative log odds, namely $(u_{ij}^*)^T \gamma_k^*$, result in $(K - 1)$ non-parallel regression lines. These regression lines inevitably cross for some values of u^*, leading to negative fitted values for the response probabilities. For u^* variables contrasting two levels of an explanatory variable (e.g., gender coded as 0 or 1), this crossing of regression lines occurs outside the range of admissible values (i.e., < 0 or > 1). However, if the explanatory variable is continuous, this crossing can occur within the range of the data, and so, allowing for non-proportional odds is problematic. For continuous explanatory variables, other than requiring proportional odds, a solution to this dilemma is sometimes possible if the variable u has, say, m levels with a reasonable number of observations at each of these m levels. In this case $(m - 1)$ dummy-coded variables can be created and substituted into the model in place of the continuous variable u.

With the above mixed-effects regression model, the probability of a response in category k for the i-th level-2 unit, conditional on γ_k, α, and t is given by:

$$\log \frac{P_{ijk}}{\left(1 - P_{ijk}\right)} = \gamma_k + x_{ij}^T \beta_i + w_{ij}^T \alpha,$$

where, under the logistic response function,

$$P_{jk} = \frac{1}{1 + \exp(-z_{jk})},$$

with $z_{jk} = u_j^T \gamma_k + x_j^T \Lambda t + w_j^T \alpha$. Note that P_{j0} and $P_{jK} = 1$.

Estimation of the p covariate coefficients α, the population variance-covariance parameters Λ (with $r(r+1)/2$ elements), and the $(h + 1)(K - 1)$ parameters in γ_k ($k = 1, ..., K - 1$) is described in detail by Hedeker and Gibbons (1994).

Illustration

To illustrate application of the mixed-effects ordinal logistic regression model, we reanalyzed longitudinal data from Rudd et al. (1996) on suicidal ideation and attempts in a sample of 300 suicidal young adults (personal communication, M.D. Rudd, Baylor University, October 2001). 180 subjects were assigned to an outpatient intervention group therapy condition and 120 subjects received treatment as usual. In this analysis, we used an ordinal outcome measure of 0=low suicidal ideation, 1=clinically significant suicidal ideation, and 3=suicide attempt. Suicidal ideation was defined as a score of 11 or more on the Modified Scale for Suicide Ideation (MSSI; Miller et al., 1986). Model specification included main effects of month (0, 1, and 6) and treatment (0=control, 1=intervention), and the treatment by month interaction. Although data at 12, 18 and 24 months were also available, the drop-out rates at these later months were too large for a meaningful analysis. In addition, to illustrate the flexibility of the model, depression as measured by the Beck Depression Inventory (BDI; Beck and Steer, 1987) and anxiety as measured by the Millon Clinical Multiaxial Inventory (MCMI-A; Millon, 1983) were treated as time-varying covariates in the model, to relate fluctuations in depressed mood and anxiety to shifts in suicidality.

Table A-5 displays the observed proportions in each of the three ordinal suicide categories as a function of month and treatment. Table A-5 reveals that, if anything, the observed rate of attempts is as high or higher in the intervention group than the control group. Note that this is also true at baseline, therefore, these difference may be an artifact of randomization.

Table A-6 displays the model parameter estimates, standard errors, and associated probability estimates. A model with both random intercept and slope (i.e., month) effects failed to converge because the variance component for the intercept was close to zero. In light of this, the model was specified with a single random effect (i.e., a random slope model). Table A-6 reveals that both of the time-varying covariates, depression and anxiety, were significantly associated with suicidality. By contrast, the treatment by time interaction was not significant, indicating that the intervention did not significantly affect the rates suicide ideation or at-

TABLE A-5 Suicide as a Function of Treatment and Time, Observed
Frequencies

Month		None	Ideation	Suicide Attempt	Total	
0	Control	11	43	66		120
		9.2%	35.8%	55.0%		
	Active	11	56	113		180
		6.1%	31.1%	62.8%		
1	Control	70	18	2		90
		77.8%	20.0%	2.2%		
	Active	96	32	7		135
		71.1%	23.7%	5.2%		
6	Control	41	8	1		50
		82.0%	16.0%	2.0%		
	Active	61	11	3		75
		81.3%	14.7%	4.0%		

TABLE A-6 Mixed-effects Ordinal Regression Model, Suicide Data
(Rudd et. al., 1996)

Variable	Estimate	Stand. Error	Z	p-value
Month	−3.33237	0.44739	−7.44855	0.00000 (2)
Intercept	0.80413	0.39477	2.03695	0.04165 (2)
Treatment	0.34707	0.21230	1.63484	0.10208 (2)
Treatment × Time	−0.01756	0.32389	−0.05422	0.95676 (2)
Depression	0.02591	0.01047	2.47364	0.01337 (2)
Anxiety	0.00970	0.00462	2.09768	0.03593 (2)
Random effect variance term (standard deviation)				
Month	1.77373	0.25394	6.98491	0.00000 (1)
Thresholds (for identification: threshold 1 = 0)				
2	2.17069	0.17705	12.26010	0.00000 (1)

(1) = 1-tailed p-value
(2) = 2-tailed p-value

tempts over time. The random month effect was significant, indicating appreciable inter-individual variability in the rates of change over time.

It might be argued, that by including the effects of depression and anxiety in the model, the effect of treatment and the treatment by time interaction may be masked. For example, the intervention may work by modifying depression and anxiety which are in turn related to suicide ideation and attempts. In this case, including depression and anxiety in the model may mask the effect of the intervention. Reanalysis excluding depression and anxiety, however, also yielded nonsignificant treatment related effects, suggesting that this is not the case. Finally, a nonproportional odds model, in which the treatment by time interaction was allowed to be category-specific, also failed to identify any positive treatment related effects on suicide ideation or attempts.

INTERVAL ESTIMATION

Poisson Confidence Limits

A $(1 - \alpha)100\%$ confidence interval for the true suicide rate λ can be approximated as

$$\hat{\lambda} \pm z_{(1-\alpha/2)} \left(\frac{\hat{\lambda}}{n} \right)^{1/2} \tag{11}$$

where $\hat{\lambda} = y/n$, y is the total number of suicides over n time intervals (e.g., months) or geographic areas (e.g. counties), and z is an upper percentage point of the normal distribution. In general, the approximation will work extremely well for $y \geq 20$. When $y < 20$ tabled values are available in Hahn and Meeker (1991).

As an example, consider the case in which after 61 months of observation for a particular county, 123 suicides are recorded; therefore, $y = 123$ and $n = 61$. The 95% confidence limit for the population suicide rate λ is therefore

$$2.016 \pm 1.965 \left(\frac{2.016}{61} \right)^{1/2} = 1.659, \ 2.373. \tag{12}$$

In light of this, we can have 95% confidence that the true suicide rate is between 1.659 and 2.373 suicides per month.

Poisson Prediction Limits

Cox and Hinkley (1974) consider the case in which y has a Poisson distribution with mean μ. Having observed y their goal is to predict y^*, which has a Poisson distribution with mean $c\mu$, where c is a known constant. In the present context, y is the number of suicides observed in n previous time-periods, and y^* is the number of suicides observed in a single future time-period, therefore, $c = 1/n$. Alternatively, for a given time period, n may represent a number of counties, and our inference is to the predicted suicide rate in a single future county for the same length of time.

Following Cox and Hinkley (1974), Gibbons (1987) derived a prediction limit using as an approximation the fact that the left side of:

$$\left(y * - \frac{c(y+y^*)}{(1+c)}\right)^2 \Big/ \left(\frac{c(y+y^*)}{(1+c)^2}\right) < t^2_{[n-1,\alpha]} \tag{13}$$

is approximately a standard normal deviate, therefore, the $100\,(1-\alpha)\%$ prediction limit for y^* is formed from percentage points of the normal distribution. Upon solving for y^* the upper limit value is found as the positive root of the quadratic equation:

$$y^* = cy + \frac{z^2 c}{2} + zc\sqrt{y(1+1/c)+z^2/4}. \tag{14}$$

Returning to the previous example in which after 61 months of observation for a particular county, 123 suicides are recorded, we have $y = 123$ and $c = 1/61$. The 95% confidence Poisson prediction limit is given by

$$y^* = \frac{123}{61} + \frac{(1.645)^2}{2(61)} + \frac{1.645}{61}\sqrt{123(1+61)+(1.645)^2/4}$$
$$= 4.396 \text{ suicides in the next month.}$$

The prediction limit reveals that we can have 95% confidence that no more than four suicides will occur in the next month.

Poisson Tolerance Limits

The uniformly most accurate upper tolerance limit for the Poisson distribution is given by Zacks (1970). In terms of a future time interval, we can construct an upper tolerance limit for the Poisson distribution that will cover $P(100)\%$ of the population of future measurements with $(1-\alpha)100\%$ confidence. The derivation begins by obtaining the cumulative probability that a or more suicides will be observed in the next time period:

$$\Pr(a,\mu) = \sum_{x=a}^{\infty} f(x,\mu) \tag{15}$$

which can be approximated by:

$$\Pr(a,\mu) = \Pr(\chi^2[2a+2]) \geq 2\mu \tag{16}$$

where $\chi^2[f]$ designates a chi-square random variable with f degrees of freedom. This relationship between the Poisson and chi-square distribution was first described by Hartley and Pearson (1950). Given n independent and identically distributed Poisson random variables the sum

$$T_n = \sum_{i=1}^{n} x_i \tag{17}$$

also has a Poisson distribution. Substituting T_n for μ, we can find the value for which the cumulative probability is $1 - \alpha$, that is,

$$K_{1-\alpha}(T_n) = \frac{1}{2n} \chi^2_{1-\alpha}[2T_n + 2]. \tag{18}$$

The $P(100)\%$ upper tolerance limit is therefore $Pr^{-1}[P; K_{1-\alpha}(T_n)]$ = smallest j (≥ 0) such that

$$\chi^2_\gamma[2j+2] > 2K_{1-\alpha}(T_n). \tag{19}$$

The required probability points of the chi-square distribution can be most easily obtained using the Peizer and Pratt approximation described by Maindonald (1984:294).

Returning to the previous example, where after 61 months of observation for a particular county, 123 suicides are recorded, we have, $T_n = 123$ and $n = 61$. Furthermore, we require the resulting tolerance limit to have 99% coverage and 95% confidence. The cumulative 95% probability point is

$$K_{.95}(123) = \frac{1}{122} \chi^2_{.95}[2(123)+2] = 2.3421$$

The 99% upper tolerance limit is obtained by finding the smallest non-negative integer j such that:

$$\chi^2_{.01}[2j+2] > 2\,(2.3421) = 4.6842$$

Inspection of standard chi-square tables (extracted below for $j = 5$ to 7) reveals that the value of j that satisfies this equation is 7.

j	$\chi^2[2j+2]$
5	3.5706

6   4.6604
7   5.8122

Therefore, the P^{-1} [.99 ; $K_{.95}(123)$] upper tolerance limit is 7 suicides per month in the example posed.

REFERENCES

Beck AT, Steer RA. 1987. *Beck Depression Inventory: Manual*. San Antonio, TX: Psychological Corporation.

Bock RD, Aitkin M. 1981. Marginal maximum likelihood estimation of item parameters: an application of the EM algorithm. *Psychometrika*, 46: 443–459.

Böhning D, Schlattmann P, Lindsay BG. 1992. Computer-assisted analysis of mixtures (C.A.MAN): Statistical algorithms. *Biometrics*, 48: 283–303.

Böhning D, Dietz E, Schlattmann P. 1998. Recent developments in computer-assisted analysis of mixtures. *Biometrics*, 54: 525–536.

Böhning D. 1999. *Computer-Assisted Analysis of Mixtures and Applications. Meta-Analysis, Disease Mapping and others*. Chapman and Hall CRC: Boca Raton.

Cox C. 1995. Location-scale cumulative odds models for ordinal data: A generalized non-linear model approach. *Statistics in Medicine*, 14: 1191–1203.

Cox DR, Hinkley DV. 1974. *Theoretical Statistics*. Chapman and Hall: London.

Dempster AP, Laird NM, Rubin DB. 1977. Maximum likelihood from incomplete data via the EM algorithm (with discussion). *Journal of the Royal Statistical Society, Series B*, 39: 1–38.

Gibbons RD. 1987. Statistical models for the analysis of volatile organic compounds in waste disposal sites. *Ground Water*, 25: 572–580.

Gibbons RD, Clark DC, Fawcet J. 1990. A statistical method for evaluating suicide clusters and implementing cluster surveillance. *American Journal of Epidemiology*, 132 (Suppl 1): S183–S191.

Hahn GJ, Meeker WQ. 1991. *Statistical Intervals: A Guide for Practitioners*. Wiley: New York.

Hartley HO, Pearson ES. 1950. Tables of the chi-squared integral and of the cumulative Poisson distribution. *Biometrika*, 37: 313–325.

Hedeker D, Gibbons RD. 1994. A random effects ordinal regression model for multilevel analysis. *Biometrics*, 50: 933–944.

Hedeker D, Mermelstein RJ. 1998. A multilevel thresholds of change model for analysis of stages of change data. *Multivariate Behavioral Research*, 33: 427–455.

Laird N. 1978. Nonparametric maximum likelihood estimation of a mixing distribution. *Journal of the American Statistical Association*, 73: 805–811.

Liang KY, Zeger SL. 1986. Longitudinal data analysis using generalized linear models. *Biometrika*, 73: 13–22.

Lindsay BG. 1983. The geometry of mixture likelihoods, part I: A general approach. *Annals of Statistics*, 11: 783–792.

Lindsay BG. 1995. *Mixture Models: Theory, Geometry and Applications*. NSF-CBMS Regional Conference Series in Probability and Statistics, Vol. 5. Hayward, CA: Institute of Mathematical Statistics.

Lindsay BG, Roeder K. 1992. Residual diagnostics for mixture models. *Journal of the American Statistical Association*, 87: 785–794.

Maindonald JH. 1984. *Statistical Computation*. Wiley: New York.

McCullagh P. 1980. Regression models for ordinal data (with discussion). *Journal of the Royal Statistical Society, Series B*, 42: 109–142.

McLachlan GJ, Krishnan T. 1997. *The EM Algorithm and Extensions*. New York: Wiley.

Miller IW, Norman WH, Bishop SB, Dow MG. 1986. The Modified Scale for Suicidal Ideation: Reliablity and validity. *Journal of Consulting and Clinical Psychology*, 54(5):724–725.

Millon T. 1983. *Millon Clinical Multiaxial Inventory Manual*. 2nd ed. Minneapolis, MN: National Computer Systems.

Peterson B, Harrell FE. 1990. Partial proportional odds models for ordinal response variables. *Applied Statistics*, 39: 205–217.

Pilla RS. 1997. *Improving the Rate of Convergence of EM in High-Dimensional Finite Mixtures*. Ph.D. dissertation, The Pennsylvania State University.

Pilla RS, Lindsay BG. 2001. Alternative EM methods for nonparametric finite mixture models. *Biometrika*, 88: 535–550.

Rudd MD, Rajab MH, Orman DT, Joiner T, Stulman DA, Dixon W. 1996. Effectiveness of an outpatient problem-solving intervention targeting suicidal young adults: Preliminary results. *Journal of Consulting and Clinical Psychology*, 64(1):179–180.

Terza JV. 1985. Ordinal probit: A generalization. *Communications in Statistical Theory and Methods*, 14: 1–11.

Titterington DM, Smith AFM, Makov UE. 1985. *Statistical Analysis of Finite Mixture Distributions*. New York: Wiley.

Zacks S. 1970. Uniformly most accurate upper tolerance limits for monotone likelihood ratio families of discrete distributions. *Journal of the American Statistical Association*, 65: 307–316.

Zeger SL, Liang KY. 1986. Longitudinal data analysis for discrete and continuous outcomes. *Biometrics*, 42: 121–130.

B

Consultants

Robert Anderson, Ph.D.
National Center for Health
Statistics
Hyattsville, MD

Paul Appelbaum, M.D.
University of Massachusetts
Medical School
Worcester, MA

Bernard Arons, M.D.
National Center for Mental
Health Services
Rockville, MD

Aaron T. Beck, M.D.
Beck Institute for Cognitive
Therapy and Research;
University of Pennsylvania
School of Medicine
(emeritus)
Philadelphia, PA

Steven M. Berkowitz, Ph.D.
Department of Veterans Affairs
Washington, DC

Alan Berman, Ph.D.
American Association of
Suicidology
Washington, DC

C. Hendricks Brown, Ph.D.
University of South Florida
Tampa, FL

Gregory K. Brown, Ph.D.
University of Pennsylvania
Philadelphia, PA

William Byerley, M.D.
University of California, Irvine
Irvine, CA

Katherine Comtois, Ph.D.
University of Washington
Seattle, WA

Alexander Crosby, M.D., M.P.H.
Centers for Disease Control and
    Prevention
Atlanta, GA

Robert DeMartino, M.D.
Center for Mental Health
    Services
Rockville, MD

Lois Fingerhut, M.A.
National Center for Health
    Statistics
Hyattsville, MD

Robert Gebbia
American Foundation for Suicide
    Prevention
New York, NY

David Goldston, Ph.D.
Wake Forest University School of
    Medicine
Winston-Salem, NC

Madelyn Gould, Ph.D.
New York State Psychiatric
    Institute; Columbia
    University College of
    Physicians and Surgeons
New York, NY

David Hemenway, Ph.D.
Harvard School of Public Health
Boston, MA

Kwan Hur, Ph.D.
University of Illinois at Chicago
    Center for Health Statistics;
    Hines VA Hospital
Chicago, IL

David Jobes, Ph.D.
Catholic University of America
Washington, DC

Thomas Joiner, Ph.D.
Florida State University
Tallahassee, FL

John Kalafat, Ph.D.
Rutgers University
Piscataway, NJ

Scott Kim, M.D., Ph.D.
University of Rochester
Rochester, NY

David Litts, O.D.
Surgeon General's Office
Washington, DC

Ron Maris, Ph.D.
University of South Carolina
Columbia, SC

Eve Mościcski, Sc.D., M.P.H.
National Institute of Mental
    Health
Rockville, MD

Jacques Normand, Ph.D.
National Institute of Drug Abuse
Rockville, MD

Ghanshyam Pandey, Ph.D.
University of Illinois at Chicago
Chicago, IL

Jane Pearson, Ph.D.
National Institute of Mental
    Health
Rockville, MD

Bernice Pescosolido, Ph.D.
Indiana University
Bloomington, IN

Jeremy Pettit, M.A.
Florida State University
Tallahassee, FL

Ramani Pilla, Ph.D.
University of Illinois at Chicago
Chicago, IL

Robert Post, Ph.D.
National Institute of Mental
    Health
Rockville, MD

Deidra Roach, M.D.
National Institute of Alcohol
    Abuse and Alcoholism
Bethesda, MD

Edwin Shneidman, Ph.D.
UCLA (emeritus)
Los Angeles, CA

Herbert Schulberg, Ph.D.
Weill Medical College of Cornell
    University
Ithaca, NY

Morton Silverman, M.D.
University of Chicago
Chicago, IL

Martin Teicher, M.D., Ph.D.
Harvard Medical School; McLean
    Hospital
Boston, MA

Leonardo Tondo, M.D.
McLean Hospital; University of
    Cagliari
Boston, MA; Sardinia, Italy

Shirley Zimmerman, Ph.D.
University of Minnesota
    (emeritus)
St. Paul, MN

C
Workshop Agendas

WORKSHOP ON RISK FACTORS FOR SUICIDE

The Arnold and Mabel Beckman Center of
the National Academy of Sciences, Irvine, CA
March 14th, 2001

8:30–8:45   Remarks and introduction by chairs: *W. Bunney and A. Kleinman*

Topic 1: **Epidemiology & Measurement**

8:45–9:15   *Eve Mościcki*
"Epidemiology of suicide"

9:15–9:45   *David Goldston & Gregory Brown*
"Issues in measurement"

9:45–10:30   Discussion

Topic 2: **Socio-Cultural Factors**

10:45–11:15   *Ron Maris*
"Social and cultural factors in suicide risk"

11:15–11:45   Discussion

Topic 3: **Biologic Factors**

11:45–12:15   *Ghanshyam Pandey*
"Neurobiology of teenage and adult suicide: Possible
biological markers for identification of suicidal patients"

12:15–12:45   *William Byerley*
"Strategies to identify genes for complex diseases"

12:45–1:15   Discussion

Topic 4: **Developmental Factors & Trauma**

2:00–2:30   *Martin Teicher*
"Neurobiological consequences of childhood abuse and
neglect"

2:30–3:00   *Robert Post*
"Association of early physical or sexual abuse with suicide
attempts in bipolar illness"

3:00–3:30   Discussion

Topic 5: **Psychologic Factors**

3:45–4:15   *Ed Shneidman*
"Psychologic factors in suicide"

4:15–4:45   Discussion

4:45–5:15   Closing Comments

5:15   Adjourn

WORKSHOP ON SUICIDE PREVENTION

Green Building of the National Academy of Sciences, Room 104
2001 Wisconsin Avenue, NW, Washington, D.C.
May 14th, 2001

8:30-8:45   Remarks and introduction by the chair: *William Bunney*

8:45-9:15   *C. Hendricks Brown*
"Design choices and analytical strategies for population-
based prevention programs: Implications for suicide
prevention"

9:15-9:45   Discussion

9:45-10:15   *John Kalafat*
             "A systems approach to youth suicide prevention"

10:15-10:45 Discussion

10:45-11:15 *Madelyn Gould*
             "Suicide contagion"

11:15-11:45 Discussion

12:45-1:15   *Aaron T. Beck*
             "Cognitive approaches to suicide"

1:15-1:45   Discussion

1:45-2:15   *Kate Comtois*
             "Research and usual care prevention efforts across
             psychiatric diagnoses"

2:15-2:45   Discussion

3:00-3:30   *Herbert C. Schulberg*
             "Preventing suicide in ambulatory medicine patients: Does
             the primary care physician have a role?"

3:30-4:00   Discussion

4:00-4:30   *David Hemenway*
             "Firearm availability and suicide"

4:30-5:00   Discussion

5:00-5:30   Closing Comments

5:30   Adjourn

Index